PEDIATRIC SECRETS

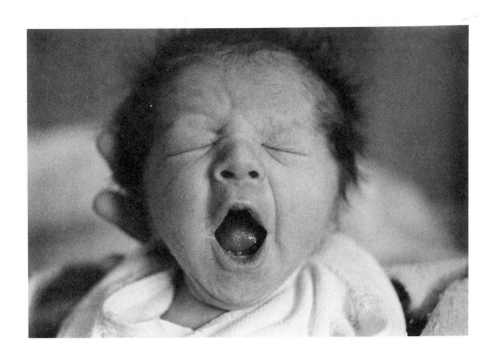

Photograph by Lionel J.M. Delevingne, Northampton, Massachusetts

PEDIATRIC SECRETS

Richard A. Polin, M.D.
Professor and Associate Chairman
Department of Pediatrics
University of Pennsylvania School of Medicine
Division of Neonatology, Department of Pediatrics
Children's Hospital of Philadelphia
Philadelphia, Pennsylvania

Mark F. Ditmar, M.D.
Clinical Director
Children's Seashore House
Atlantic City, New Jersey
Clinical Associate of Pediatrics
University of Pennsylvania School of Medicine
Children's Hospital of Philadelphia
Philadelphia, Pennsylvania

HANLEY & BELFUS, INC./Philadelphia
THE C.V. MOSBY COMPANY/St. Louis • Toronto • London

Publisher: HANLEY & BELFUS, INC.
210 S. 13th Street
Philadelphia, PA 19107

North American and worldwide sales and distribution:

THE C.V. MOSBY COMPANY
11830 Westline Industrial Drive
St. Louis, MO 63146

In Canada: THE C.V. MOSBY COMPANY
5240 Finch Avenue East
Unit 1
Scarborough, Ontario M1S 4P2
Canada

PEDIATRIC SECRETS   ISBN 0-932883-14-1

Library of Congress catalog card number   88-82169

Last digit is the print number: 9 8 7 6 5 4 3 2 1

CONTENTS

Cardiology 1
    Anthony Chang and Bernard J. Clark, III

Dermatology 29
    Paul J. Honig, Lawrence F. Eichenfield, and Linda G. Rabinowitz

Emergency Medicine 47
    Mark F. Ditmar

Endocrinology 65
    Daniel E. Hale

Gastroenterology and Nutrition 93
    David A. Piccoli

Genetics 121
    Alan E. Donnenfeld and Elaine H. Zackai

Growth, Development and Behavior 137
    Edward B. Charney and Mark F. Ditmar

Hematology 151
    Alan R. Cohen

Immunization 177
    Stephen D. Barbour and Adam Finn

Immunology 191
    Mary Ellen Conley

Inborn Errors of Metabolism 201
    Richard I. Kelley

Infectious Diseases 215
    David S. Hodes, Asher Barzilai, Alexander C. Hyatt, and Mark F. Ditmar

Neonatology 241
    Mary Catherine Harris and Philip Roth

Nephrology 315
    John W. Foreman

Neurology 335
    Robert R. Clancy

Oncology 361
    Beverly Lange

Orthopedics 377
    Douglas Boenning and Nancy R. Freedman

Pulmonology 389
    Robert W. Wilmott

Rheumatology 405
    Andrew H. Eichenfield

Toxicology 421
    Fred M. Henretig

Index 433

CONTRIBUTORS

Stephen D. Barbour, M.D., Ph.D.
Associate Professor of Pediatrics, Michigan State University School of Medicine, East Lansing, Michigan; Pediatric Infectious Diseases, Butterworth Hospital, Grand Rapids, Michigan

Asher Barzilai, M.D.
Assistant Professor of Pediatrics, Mt. Sinai School of Medicine, New York, New York

Douglas Boenning, M.D.
Associate Medical Director for Research, Emergency Medical Trauma Center, Children's Hospital National Medical Center, Washington, D.C.

Anthony Chang, M.D.
Instructor in Pediatrics, University of Pennsylvania School of Medicine; Fellow, Division of Cardiology, Department of Pediatrics, Children's Hospital of Philadelphia, Philadelphia, Pennsylvania

Edward B. Charney, M.D.
Associate Professor of Pediatrics, University of Pennsylvania School of Medicine; Division of Child Development, Department of Pediatrics, Children's Hospital of Philadelphia, Philadelphia, Pennsylvania

Robert R. Clancy, M.D.
Associate Professor of Neurology and Pediatrics, University of Pennsylvania School of Medicine; Director of Clinical Neurophysiology, Children's Hospital of Philadelphia, Philadelphia, Pennsylvania

Bernard J. Clark, III, M.D.
Assistant Professor of Pediatrics, University of Pennsylvania School of Medicine; Associate Cardiologist, Division of Cardiology, Department of Pediatrics, Children's Hospital of Philadelphia, Philadelphia, Pennsylvania

Alan R. Cohen, M.D.
Associate Professor of Pediatrics, University of Pennsylvania School of Medicine; Senior Physician, Division of Hematology, Department of Pediatrics, Children's Hospital of Philadelphia, Philadelphia, Pennsylvania

Mary Ellen Conley, M.D.
Professor of Pediatrics, University of Tennessee College of Medicine; St. Jude's Children's Research Hospital, Memphis, Tennessee

Mark F. Ditmar, M.D.
Clinical Director, Children's Seashore House, Atlantic City, New Jersey; Clinical Associate of Pediatrics, University of Pennsylvania School of Medicine and Children's Hospital of Philadelphia, Philadelphia, Pennsylvania

Alan E. Donnenfeld, M.D.
Director, Southern Maine Genetics Service, and Director, Prenatal Diagnostic Unit, Maine Medical Center, Portland, Maine

Andrew H. Eichenfield, M.D.
Assistant Professor of Pediatrics, University of Pennsylvania School of Medicine; Associate Physician, Children's Hospital of Philadelphia, Philadelphia, Pennsylvania; Attending Physician, Children's Seashore House, Philadelphia, Pennsylvania

Lawrence F. Eichenfield, M.D.
Chief Resident, Department of Pediatrics, University of Pennsylvania School of Medicine and Children's Hospital of Philadelphia, Philadelphia, Pennsylvania

Adam H.R. Finn, M.A., B.M., B.Ch., M.R.C.P. (UK)
Lecturer in Immunology, Institute of Child Health, London; Honorary Senior Registrar, Hospital for Sick Children, Great Ormond Street, London, England

John W. Foreman, M.D.
Associate Professor of Pediatrics, Medical College of Virginia, Virginia Commonwealth University, Richmond, Virginia

Nancy R. Freedman, M.S.N.
Formerly, Clinical Nurse Specialist in Orthopedics, Children's Hospital of Philadelphia, Philadelphia, Pennsylvania

Daniel E. Hale, M.D.
Assistant Professor of Pediatrics, University of Pennsylvania School of Medicine; Division of Endocrinology, Department of Pediatrics, Children's Hospital of Philadelphia, Philadelphia, Pennsylvania

Mary Catherine Harris, M.D.
Assistant Professor of Pediatrics, University of Pennsylvania School of Medicine; Division of Neonatology, Department of Pediatrics, Children's Hospital of Philadelphia, Philadelphia, Pennsylvania

Fred M. Henretig, M.D.
Assistant Professor of Pediatrics, University of Pennsylvania School of Medicine; Associate Director, Division of General Pediatrics, Department of Pediatrics, Children's Hospital of Philadelphia, Philadelphia, Pennsylvania

David S. Hodes, M.D.
Associate Professor of Pediatrics, Mt. Sinai School of Medicine, New York, New York

Paul J. Honig, M.D.
Associate Professor of Pediatrics and Dermatology, University of Pennsylvania School of Medicine; Division of Dermatology, Department of Pediatrics, Children's Hospital of Philadelphia, Philadelphia, Pennsylvania

Alexander C. Hyatt, M.D.
Associate Professor of Pediatrics, Mt. Sinai School of Medicine, New York, New York

Richard I. Kelley, M.D., Ph.D
Assistant Professor of Pediatrics, Johns Hopkins University School of Medicine; The Kennedy Institute, Baltimore, Maryland

Beverly Lange, M.D.
Associate Professor of Pediatrics, University of Pennsylvania School of Medicine; Division of Oncology, Department of Pediatrics, Children's Hospital of Philadelphia, Philadelphia, Pennsylvania

David A. Piccoli, M.D.
Assistant Professor of Pediatrics, University of Pennsylvania School of Medicine; Division of Gastroenterology, Department of Pediatrics, Children's Hospital of Philadelphia, Philadelphia, Pennsylvania

Richard A. Polin, M.D.
Professor and Associate Chairman, Department of Pediatrics, University of Pennsylvania School of Medicine; Division of Neonatology, Department of Pediatrics, Children's Hospital of Philadelphia, Philadelphia, Pennsylvania

Linda G. Rabinowitz, M.D.
Clinical Assistant Professor of Dermatology and Pediatrics, Jefferson Medical College of Thomas Jefferson University; Director of Pediatric Dermatology, Thomas Jefferson University Hospital, Philadelphia, Pennsylvania

Philip Roth, M.D., Ph.D.
Assistant Professor of Pediatrics, Division of Neonatology, Albert Einstein College of Medicine; Montefiore Medical Center and Bronx Municipal Hospital Center, Bronx, New York

Robert W. Wilmott, M.D.
Associate Professor, Department of Pediatrics, Wayne State University School of Medicine; Director, Division of Pulmonary Medicine; Children's Hospital of Michigan, Detroit, Michigan

Elaine H. Zackai, M.D.
Associate Professor of Pediatrics, Division of Genetics, Department of Pediatrics, Children's Hospital of Philadelphia, Philadelphia, Pennsylvania

ASSISTANT EDITORS

The editors gratefully acknowledge the following individuals for their time and assistance in helping to review and select questions for the book:

Jeffrey Avner, M.D.

Robert Baldassano, M.D.

Delma Broussard, M.D.

James Callahan, M.D.

Cindy Christian, M.D.

Richard Haupt, M.D.

Laurel Kruse, M.D.

Christopher Liacouras, M.D.

Andrew Mulberg, M.D.

Joseph W. St. Geme, III, M.D.

PREFACE

Medical school and residency are arduous and exhausting runs of discovery. It is through constant questioning and reappraisal that patient care is improved. Never should the spirit of inquiry be discouraged or curiosity be repressed, for according to a Chinese proverb: "He who asks a question may be a fool for five minutes, but he who does not ask a question remains a fool forever."

The transition from the beginnings of medical school to clerkships and residency is made more difficult because it is a transition from the written to the oral tradition. The relatively passive approach of lectures, notes, and textbooks is replaced in large part by vigorous give-and-take question and answer exchanges on rounds, in seminars, and even during exams. Depending on the point of view, the exchanges can be illuminating, intimidating, or constipating. Even in this age of computers, it is unlikely that the emphasis on the didactic oral tradition will lessen.

The purpose of this pediatric text is to address the questions that are commonly posed in the daily routine of a teaching hospital, in this case the Children's Hospital of Philadelphia. Most of the questions were submitted by housestaff and University of Pennsylvania medical students. The questions represent a wide spectrum of topics — from basic pathophysiology to general pediatric principles to practical management issues. Many of the questions have no right or wrong answer. However, we hope that points discussed in areas of controversy will stimulate efforts on the part of the reader to develop an ongoing appreciation of and interest in changing approaches to pediatric care.

We are indebted to the chapter authors for their diligent participation in the project; to Deborah H. Schaible, PharmD, for her editorial assistance; to Linda Belfus and Jack Hanley for their exceptional editorial expertise and tireless good nature in the conception and evolution of this book; to Carol Miller for her dedication and grace in preparation of the manuscript; to the Children's Hospital housestaff and medical students for their enthusiasm in times of fatigue; and to the hospital housekeeping department for not tearing down the illegal "Pediatric Secrets" question boxes posted on each floor.

Richard A. Polin, M.D.
Mark F. Ditmar, M.D.
Children's Hospital of Philadelphia

To David Cornfeld, M.D.

A constant questioner, teacher and friend

THE FAR SIDE

By GARY LARSON

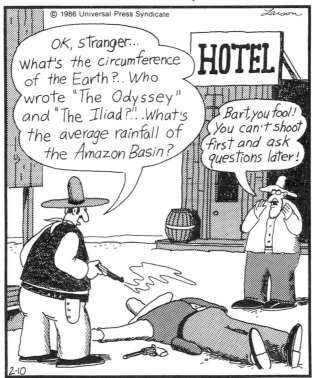

CARDIOLOGY

Anthony Chang, M.D.
Bernard J. Clark, M.D.

> When I first gave my mind to vivisection, as a means of discovering the
> motions and uses of the heart, and sought to discover these from actual
> inspection, and not from the writings of others, I found the task so truly
> arduous, so full of difficulties, that I was almost tempted to think with
> Fracastorius that the motion of the heart was only to be comprehended by
> God.
>
> William Harvey *(1578–1657)*
> *On the Motion of the Heart and*
> *Blood in Animals, Ch. 1*

1. What are the proven etiologies for congenital heart disease?
The vast majority of congenital heart disease is thought to be a result of genetic-environmental interaction, or multifactorial inheritance. Primary genetic factors include chromosomal aberrations and single mutant gene abnormalities (8% of total). The remainder involve primarily environmental factors such as drugs, infections, and maternal infections.

2. What is the recurrence risk for the common heart defects?
Recurrence risks of cardiovascular anomalies vary from 1–3% and are usually higher with the more common lesions (e.g., the recurrence risk for VSD is 3%—higher than the 1% recurrence risk for Ebstein's anomaly). The risk of congenital heart disease in pregnancies after the birth of one affected child is about 1–4%. With 2 first-degree relatives, the risk is tripled; with 3, the family may be considered "type C," in which recurrence risk may be even higher than mendelian inheritance.

3. Who first described a congenital heart defect in a human? (*Hint:* the defect was an ASD.)
Leonardo da Vinci in 1531.

4. When and where were the following landmark procedures in pediatric cardiology first reported? Mustard/TGA repair; Gibbon/heart-lung machine; Gross/PDA ligation; Blalock, Taussig/BT shunt; Rashkind/balloon atrial septostomy.
Mustard: Successful two-stage correction of transposition of the great vessels (Surgery 55:469–472, 1964)
Gibbon: Application of a mechanical heart and lung apparatus to cardiac surgery (Minnesota Med 37:171–177, 195, 1954)
Gross/Hubbard: Surgical ligation of a patent ductus arteriosus (Am Med Assoc J 112:729–731, 1939)
Blalock/Taussig: The surgical treatment of complete transposition of the aorta and pulmonary artery. (Surg Gynecol Obstet 90:1–15, 1950)
Rashkind/Miller: Creation of an atrial septal defect without thoracotomy: a palliative approach to complete transposition of the great arteries (Am Med Assoc J 196:991–992, 1966)

5. What are some hereditary diseases in which congenital heart disease is a frequent finding? (For example: Noonan's—dystrophic pulmonary valve)

Hereditary Disease in Which Congenital Heart Disease Is a Frequent Finding

HEREDITARY DISEASE	MODE OF INHERITANCE	COMMON CARDIAC DISEASE	IMPORTANT FEATURES
Apert's syndrome	AD	VSD	Irregular craniosynostosis with peculiar head and facial appearance Syndactyly of digits and toes
Crouzon's disease (craniofacial dysostosis)	AD	PDA, COA	Ptosis with shallow orbits Craniosynostosis, maxillary hypoplasia
Ehlers-Danlos syndrome	AD	Aneurysm of aorta and carotids	Hyperextensive joints, hyperelasticity, fragility and bruisability of skin
Ellis-van Creveld syndrome (chondroectodermal dysplasia)	AR	Single atrium	Neonatal teeth, short distal limbs. Polydactyly, nail hypoplasia
Friedreich's ataxia	AR	Cardiomyopathy	Late onset ataxia, skeletal deformities
Glycogen storage disease II (Pompe's)	AR	Cardiomyopathy	Large tongue and flabby muscles, cardiomegaly; ECG: LVH and short PR; normal FBS and GTT
Holt-Oram syndrome (cardiac-limb)	AD	ASD, VSD	Defects or absence of thumb or radius
Idiopathic hypertrophic subaortic stenosis (IHSS)	AD	Muscular subaortic stenosis	
Leopard syndrome	AD	PS, cardiomyopathy	Lentiginous skin lesion, ECG abnormalities, Ocular hypertelorism, Pulmonary stenosis, Abnormal genitalia, Retarded growth, Deafness
Long QT syndrome: Jervell and Lange-Nielsen, and Romano-Ward	AR / AD	Long QT interval, ventricular tachyarrhythmias	Congenital deafness (not in Romano-Ward), syncope due to ventricular arrhythmias. Family history of sudden death
Marfan's syndrome	AD	Aortic aneurysm, aortic regurgitation and/ or mitral regurgitation	Arachnodactyly, subluxation of lens
Mitral valve prolapse syndrome (primary)	AD	Mitral regurgitation, dysrhythmias	Thoracic skeletal anomalies (80%)
Mucopolysaccharidosis Hurler's (type I) Hunter's (type II) Morquio's (type IV)	AR / XR / AR	Aortic regurg./ mitral regurg., coronary artery disease	Coarse features, large tongue, depressed nasal bridge, kyphosis, retarded growth, hepatomegaly, corneal opacity (not in Hunter's), mental retardation
Muscular dystrophy (Duchenne's type)	XR	Cardiomyopathy	Waddling gait, "pseudohypertrophy" of calf muscle
Neurofibromatosis (von Recklinghausen's disease)	AD	PS, COA	Café-au-lait spots, acoustic neuroma, variety of bone lesions
Noonan's syndrome	AD	PS (dystrophic pulmonary valve)	Similar to Turner's syndrome but may occur in phenotypic male and without chromosomal abnormality
Rendu-Osler-Weber syndrome	AD	Pulmonary AV fistulas	Hepatic involvement; telangiectases, hemangiomas or fibrosis
Tuberous sclerosis	AD	Rhabdomyoma	Adenoma sebaceum (2–5 years of age), convulsion, mental defect
Williams's syndrome (supravalvular aortic stenosis)	AD	Supravalvular aortic stenosis, PA stenosis	Mental retardation, peculiar "elfin" facies, hypercalcemia of infancy?

AD = autosomal dominance, AR = autosomal recessive, XR = sex-linked recessive, FBS = fasting blood sugar, GTT = glucose tolerance test.

From Park MK: Pediatric Cardiology for Practitioners, 2nd ed. Chicago, Year Book Medical Publishers, 1988, pp 7–8, with permission.

Fetus and Newborn

6. When does the heart start to contract in a fetus?

Organized contractions of the heart begin by day 22 post conception and consist of peristalsis-like waves that begin in the sinus venosus and move through the atria and ventricles.

7. How does fetal circulation differ from neonatal circulation?

1. Intra- and extracardiac shunts are present: placenta, ductus venosus, foramen ovale, ductus arteriosus.

2. The two ventricles work in parallel rather than in a series.

3. The right ventricle pumps against a higher resistance than the left ventricle.

4. Blood flow to the lung is only a fraction of the right ventricular output.

5. The lung extracts oxygen from the blood instead of providing oxygen for it.

6. The lung continually secretes a fluid into the respiratory passages.

7. The liver is the first organ to receive maternal substances, such as oxygen, glucose, amino acids, etc.

8. The placenta is the major route of gas exchange, excretion, and acquisition of essential fetal chemicals.

9. The placenta provides a low resistance circuit.

Reference: Adams and Emmanouilides: Moss' Heart Disease in Infants, Children, and Adolescents. Baltimore, Williams and Wilkins, 1983, pp 11–17.

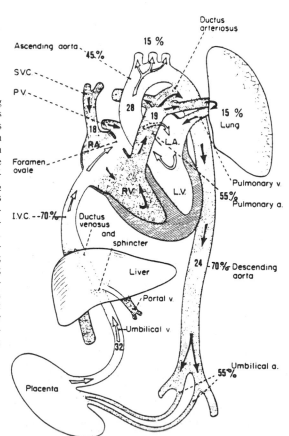

Diagram of fetal circulation showing four sites of shunt: placenta, ductus venosus, foramen ovale, and ductus arteriosus. Intravascular *shading* is in proportion to oxygen saturation, with the lightest shading representing the highest Po_2. The numerical value inside the chamber or vessel is the Po_2 for that site in mm Hg. The percentages outside the vascular structures represent the relative flows in major tributaries and outlets for the two ventricles. The combined output of the two ventricles represents 100%. A = artery; V = vein; IVC = inferior vena cava; PV = pulmonary vein; SVC = superior vena cava. (From Guntheroth WG, et al: Physiology of the Circulation: Fetus, Neonate and Child. In Kelley VC (ed): Practice of Pediatrics. Philadelphia, Harper and Row, 1982, vol. 8, ch. 23, p 70, with permission.)

8. What changes occur in stroke volume, cardiac output, and heart rate after birth?
Both stroke volume (SV) and cardiac output (CO) increase into adolescence, whereas heart rate falls.

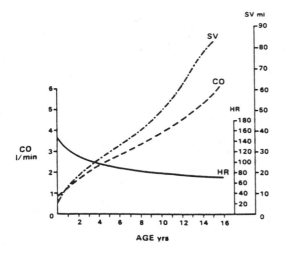

Changes in stroke volume *(SV)*, cardiac output *(CO)*, and heart rate *(HR)* after birth. (From Rudolph AM: Congenital Diseases of the Heart. Chicago, 1974, Year Book Medical Publishers, with permission).

9. What are the immediate postnatal changes in pH, pCO_2, and pO_2 in the term newborn infant?
During the first hours and days of life, pCO_2 and serum bicarbonate concentration *fall,* whereas paO_2 and pH *rise*. There are important changes in the cardiovascular system of the newborn immediately after birth: (1) pulmonary vascular resistance decreases, (2) pulmonary blood flow increases, (3) systemic vascular resistance increases, (4) blood flow through the ductus arteriosus becomes primarily left to right, and (5) foramen ovale closes. The premature infant differs from the full-term infant in two ways: (1) the ductus arteriosus is less responsive to oxygen for closure, and (2) pulmonary vascular resistance drops faster due to a less mature pulmonary arterial tree.

10. Are there any conditions during the newborn period in which prostaglandin use is contraindicated?
Prostaglandin maintains the patency of the ductus arteriosus, and is usually most effective in infants less than 96 hours of age. The use of prostaglandin may have *adverse* physiologic effects under certain situations: (1) transposition of the great arteries with a restrictive atrial septal defect, (2) tetralogy of Fallot without a patent ductus arteriosus, (3) total anomalous pulmonary venous return, and (4) persistent pulmonary hypertension of the newborn. Side effects of prostaglandins include: hypotension, tachycardia or bradycardia, vasodilatation, hyperpyrexia, seizure, hypoglycemia and hypocalcemia, apnea, and bleeding.

11. Which maternal medications increase the likelihood of premature closure of ductus arteriosus?
Aspirin, indomethacin, and other inhibitors of prostaglandin synthesis.

Cyanosis

12. A child with a chronic cyanotic heart disease develops polycythemia. At what level should phlebotomy or partial exchange be considered?

As a consequence of cyanosis, younger patients develop iron-deficiency anemia, whereas older patients develop polycythemia. Polycythemia secondary to cyanosis can lead to CNS complications such as cerebrovascular accident and brain abscess. Phlebotomy or partial exchange is usually performed when hematocrit is in excess of 60–65%.

13. What is the Blalock-Taussig shunt?

It is one of a number of operations used for cyanotic disease in the neonatal period when the congenital heart defect causes severe reduction in pulmonary blood flow. These systemic to pulmonary shunts are palliative procedures that increase pulmonary blood flow.

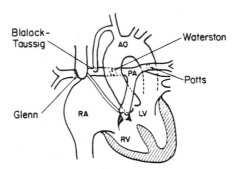

From Park MK: Pediatric Cardiology for Practitioners, 2nd ed. Chicago, Year Book Medical Publishers, 1988, p 173, with permission.

14. What is the Jatene operation?

First described in 1976, it is the "switch operation" done in cases of transposition of the great arteries. The operation involves reimplantation of the coronary arteries, bisection of the pulmonary artery and aorta, and resuturing of the two great vessels into their correct anatomic position. This operation contrasts with others whereby intra-atrial baffles are used to redirect blood along more proper anatomic paths (Senning and Mustard procedures).

15. What is a "tet" spell? What causes it?

It is an acute episode of increased cyanosis associated with hyperpnea in patients with tetralogy of Fallot, tetralogy of Fallot with pulmonary atresia, or complicated anatomy with tetralogy of Fallot "physiology" (such as double-outlet right ventricle with pulmonary stenosis). The specific cause is uncertain, but episodes are characterized by a *decrease* in systemic vascular resistance, an *increase* in pulmonary vascular resistance, and pulmonary outflow tract narrowing. These conditions result in a decrease in antegrade flow through the right ventricular outflow tract and an increase in right-to-left shunting.

16. What is the preferred method of treatment for a "tet" spell?

Knee-chest position	Morphine sulfate (0.1 mg/kg/dose)
Oxygen	Phenylephrine (bolus 50–100 µg/kg/dose IV)
Volume	Propranolol (0.1 mg/kg/IV)
Sodium bicarbonate	and importantly, a calm physician

17. What is the Fontan principle?

It is the establishment of a continuity between the systemic venous channels (RA/IVC/SVC) to the pulmonary arteries, thus bypassing a need for a ventricle to deliver blood to the pulmonary circulation (see figure). This surgery, initially introduced in 1971 for tricuspid atresia, has a more favorable outcome if: pulmonary artery pressure is normal, pulmonary vascular resistance is normal, pulmonary arteries are of adequate size, and end-diastolic pressure is low. Complications include superior vena cava syndrome, right ventricular failure, pleural and pericardial effusions, and arrhythmias.

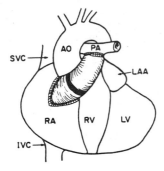

The Fontan procedure in which a conduit, valved or not, is placed between the dilated RA and the PA. The Glenn operation prior to the Fontan procedure is recommended by some. (From Park MK: Pediatric Cardiology for Practitioners. Chicago, Year Book Medical Publishers, 1984, p 161, with permission.)

18. What is the differential diagnosis of pulmonary hypertension in children?
Main categories include (1) large left-to-right shunt lesions, (2) alveolar hypoxia, (3) pulmonary venous hypertension, and (4) pulmonary vascular disease.

Causes of Pulmonary Hypertension

Large left-to-right shunt lesions ("hyperkinetic" pulmonary hypertension, VSD, PDA, etc.
Alveolar hypoxia
  Pulmonary parenchymal disease
    Bronchopulmonary dysplasia (BPD)
    Interstitial lung disease (Hamman-Rich syndrome)
    Wilson-Mikity syndrome
  Airway obstruction
    Upper airway obstruction (large tonsils)
    Lower airway obstruction (bronchial asthma, cystic fibrosis)
  Inadequate ventilatory drive (CNS diseases)
  Disorders of chest wall or respiratory muscles
    Kyphoscoliosis
    Weakness or paralysis of skeletal muscle
  High altitude (in certain hyperreactors)
Pulmonary venous hypertension
  Mitral stenosis, cor triatriatum, TAPVR with obstruction, chronic left heart failure
Pulmonary vascular disease
  Persistent pulmonary hypertension of the newborn
  Primary pulmonary hypertension—a rare, fatal form of pulmonary hypertension with obscure
    etiology
  Eisenmenger's physiology, secondary to long-standing "hyperkinetic" pulmonary hypertension
  Thromboembolism
    Ventriculovenous shunt for hydrocephalus, sickle cell anemia, etc.
  Collagen disease
    Rheumatoid arthritis, scleroderma, mixed connective tissue disease

From Park MK: Pediatric Cardiology for Practitioners, 2nd ed. Chicago, Year Book Medical Publishers, 1988, p 326, with permission.

19. In children with congenital heart disease and RSV pneumonitis, which preexisting abnormalities are associated with a poor outcome?
Cyanosis, pulmonary hypertension, and certain surgeries (such as the Fontan procedure).

Congestive Heart Failure

20. What are the clinical signs and symptoms associated with congestive heart failure (CHF)?

They may be grouped into three categories (* = often seen in infants):

1. *Signs of impaired myocardial performance:* cardiomegaly*, tachycardia*, gallop rhythm, cold extremities or mottling, pulsus paradoxus and pulsus alternans, growth failure*, and sweating*.

2. *Signs of pulmonary congestion:* tachypnea*, wheezing, rales, cyanosis, dyspnea, and cough.

3. *Signs of systemic venous congestion:* hepatomegaly*, neck vein distention, and peripheral edema.

21. What are the causes of heart failure due to congenital heart disease that appear at birth, at one week of age, and at one month of age?

Causes of CHF Due to Congenital Heart Disease According to Age

At birth	Hypoplastic left heart syndrome (HLHS)
	Severe birth asphyxia (hypoxia + acidosis)
	Volume overload lesions:
	Severe tricuspid or pulmonary insufficiency
	Large systemic AV fistula
First week	PDA in small premature infants
	HLHS (with more favorable anatomy)
	TAPVR, particularly those with pulmonary venous obstruction
	Others:
	Systemic AV fistula
	Critical AS or PS
1–4 wk	Coarctation of the aorta (preductal, with associated anomalies)
	Critical aortic stenosis
	Large left-to-right shunt lesions (VSD, PDA) in premature infants
	All other lesions listed above
4–6 wk	Some left-to-right shunt lesions such as complete A-V canal defect
6 wk–4 mo.	Large VSD
	Large PDA
	Others such as anomalous left coronary artery from the pulmonary artery

From Park MK: Pediatric Cardiology for Practitioners, 2nd ed. Chicago, Year Book Medical Publishers, 1988, p 310, with permission.

22. What is the differential diagnosis of cardiomegaly without heart murmur?
The differential diagnosis includes three main categories: myocardial disease, coronary artery diseases, and congenital heart disease.

Differential Diagnosis of Cardiomegaly Without Heart Murmur in Pediatric Patients

Myocardial diseases
   Endocardial fibroelastosis
   Myocarditis (viral or idiopathic)
   Glycogen storage disease (Pompe's disease)
Coronary artery diseases resulting in myocardial insufficiency
   Anomalous origin of the left coronary artery from the pulmonary artery
   Collagen disease (periarteritis nodosa)
   Kawasaki's disease (mucocutaneous lymph node syndrome)
   Calcification of coronary artery
   Medial necrosis of coronary artery
Congenital heart disease with severe heart failure
   Coarctation of the aorta in infants
   Ebstein's anomaly

Table continued on next page.

Differential Diagnosis of Cardiomegaly Without Heart Murmur *(Continued)*

Miscellaneous conditions
    CHF secondary to respiratory disease (upper airway obstruction, chronic alveolar hypoxia such as
        seen with bronchopulmonary dysplasia, extensive pneumonia)
    Paroxysmal atrial tachycardia with CHF
    Pericardial effusion
    Severe anemia
    Tumors of the heart
    Neonatal thyrotoxicosis
    Malnutrition (infantile beriberi, protein calorie malnutrition)
    Toxicity (drugs, such as adriamycin, or radiation)

From Park MK: Pediatric Cardiology for Practitioners, 2nd ed. Chicago, Year Book Medical Publishers,
1988, p 219, with permission.

23. What are the acid-base changes associated with CHF?

1. Mild CHF: respiratory alkalosis—as a result of tachypnea (stimulation of J receptors
by increasing pulmonary edema).

2. Moderate or severe CHF: respiratory acidosis—as a consequence of pulmonary
edema and reduced compliance; and metabolic acidosis—as a result of decreased tissue
perfusion.

24. How is CHF managed in children?

Treatment of Congestive Heart Failure

  I. General interventions
        Rest (occasional sedation)
        Temperature and humidity control
        Oxygen
        Decrease sodium load
        Avoid aspiration
        Treat infection, if present
 II. Specific interventions
        Preload
            Move ventricular function curve up by volume infusion to increase venous return
            Move ventricular function curve down with diuretics, venodilators
        Afterload reduction
            Facilitate ventricular emptying by reducing wall tension
            Reduce blood viscosity
            Drugs, arteriolar dilators, mechanical counterpulsation
        Inotropic stimulation
            Improve physical and metabolic milieu: pH, Pao_2 glucose, calcium, hemoglobin
            Common drugs: digitalis, catecholamines
            Newer drugs: amrinone, milrinone, prenalterol, TA-064
        Heart Rate
            Control rhythm disturbances with pacing, drugs
        Other
            Mechanical ventilation
            Prostaglandin manipulation
            Peritoneal dialysis
III. Surgery

From Friedman WF, George BL: Treatment of congestive heart failure by altering loading conditions of
the heart. J Pediatr 1985, p 698, with permission.

25. What are some laboratory findings in CHF?

1. Electrolyte imbalance: hyponatremia, hypochloremia, and hypocalcemia.
2. Hematologic: anemia and leukocytosis.
3. Urinalysis: albuminuria and microscopic hematuria.
4. Hypoglycemia.

Anatomy

26. What is the "segmental approach" to congenital heart disease?
This approach, developed by Dr. van Praagh, views the heart and the great arteries as three separate segments.

1. The *atria*—normally, the right atrium is on the same side as the liver: *S* (solitus). Other possibilities: I (inversus) and A (ambiguous).

2. The *ventricles*—normally, the ventricles are related in a D-loop as a result of right-sided "bending" of the heart tube in embryogenesis: *D* (D-loop). Other possibilities: L (L-loop) and X (indeterminate).

3. The *great arteries*—normally, the aorta is posterior and to the right of the pulmonary artery: *S* (solitus). Other possibilities: I (inversus), D (D-transposition), and L (L-transposition).

Therefore, a normal heart has segments *S, D, S*.

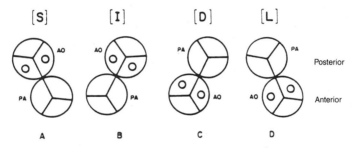

Relationship between the great arteries. A, solitus. B, inversus. C, D-transposition. D, L-transposition. (From Park MK: Pediatric Cardiology for Practitioners, 2nd ed. Chicago, Year Book Medical Publishers, 1988, p 204, with permission.)

27. What are the most common vascular rings and slings? How do they present and how are they diagnosed and treated?

	Frequency	Symptoms	Treatment
"Complete" rings Double aortic arch	40%	Respiratory difficulty (onset <3 mos.) Swallowing dysfunction	Surgical division of a smaller arch
Right aortic arch with left ligamentum arteriosum	30%	Mild respiratory difficulty (onset >1 year) Swallowing dysfunction	Surgical division of the lig. arteriosum
"Incomplete" rings Anomalous innominate artery	10%	Stridor and/or cough in infancy	Conservative management, or surgical suturing of the artery to the sternum
Aberrant right subclavian artery	20%	Occasional swallowing dysfunction	Usually no treatment is necessary
Vascular sling or anomalous left pulmonary artery	rare	Wheezing and cyanotic episodes since birth	Surgical division of the anomalous LPA (from the RPA) and anastomosis to the MPA

In addition to barium swallow, other diagnostic evaluations such as arteriogram, echocardiogram, or MRI are helpful in diagnosis. (Modified from Park MK: Pediatric Cardiology for Practitioners. Chicago, Year Book Medical Publishers, 1984, p 175).

Physical Examination

28. What are abnormal findings of the second heart sound (S2) and their significance?
1. Widely split S2
   (a) prolonged right ventricular (RV) ejection time:
      (i) RV volume overload—atrial septal defect (ASD), partial anomalous pulmonary venous return (PAPVR)
      (ii) RV pressure overload—mild pulmonary stenosis (PS)
      (iii) RV conduction delay—right bundle branch block
   (b) shortened left ventricular (LV) ejection time:
      early aortic closure—mitral regurgitation (MR)
2. Single S2
   (a) presence of only one semilunar valve—aortic or pulmonary atresisa, truncus arteriosus
   (b) P2 not audible—tetralogy of Fallot (TOF), transposition of the great arteries (TGA), pulmonary stenosis (PS), and pulmonary hypertension
   (c) A2 delayed—severe aortic stenosis (AS)
   (d) May be normal in a newborn
3. Paradoxically split S2 (A2 follows P2): present in severe AS, left bundle branch block (LBBB), and pulmonary hypertension.
4. Loud P2: present in pulmonary hypertension.

29. When can S3 and S4 be considered a normal finding during a pediatric cardiac examination?
An S3, or "ventricular" gallop, occurs early in diastole. It is usually benign but can be abnormal in children with dilated ventricles and decreased compliance (as in congestive heart failure). An S4, or "atrial" gallop, occurs late in diastole. It is usually abnormal in children (although it can be normal in an older adult).

30. What is the difference between a heave and a tap?
A *heave* is a slow-rising, diffuse impulse associated with a volume-overloaded ventricle (as in a ventricular septal defect). A *tap* is a rapid-rising, localized impulse associated with a pressure-overloaded ventricle (as in pulmonary stenosis). Some authorities also differentiate between a thrust and a heave. A thrust is substernal and thus associated with right ventricular hypertrophy, whereas a heave is apical and therefore associated with left ventricular hypertrophy.

31. What is an ejection click and what are the possible etiologies?
An ejection click occurs at the onset of ventricular ejection, follows S1, and is best heard at the base of the heart. Possible etiologies include (1) stenosis of semilunar valves: aortic stenosis or pulmonary stenosis (not infundibular or supravalvular PS); (2) dilatation of great arteries: tetralogy of Fallot (dilated aorta), truncus arteriosus, hypertension, or coarctation of the aorta; (3) mitral valve prolapse (produces a midsystolic click); and (4) other (rare): cardiac tumors, atrial septal aneurysms, and dissecting aortic aneurysms.
   Reference: Park MK: Pediatric Cardiology for Practitioners. Chicago, Year Book Medical Publishers, 1984, p 18.

32. Name the common innocent murmurs. Which murmurs are usually *not* innocent?
Usually not innocent: diastolic murmurs, pan-systolic or late-systolic murmurs, and loud (grade 4 or louder) murmurs.

Common Innocent Heart Murmurs

TYPE (TIMING)	DESCRIPTION OF MURMUR	AGE GROUP
Classic vibratory murmur (Still's murmur) (systolic)	Maximal at MLSB or between LLSB and apex Grade 2–3/6 Low-frequency vibratory, "twanging string," groaning, squeaking, or musical	3–6 yr Occasionally in infancy
Pulmonary ejection murmur (systolic)	Maximal at ULSB Early to midsystolic Grade 1–3/6 in intensity Blowing in quality	8–14 yr
Pulmonary flow murmur of newborn (systolic)	Maximal at ULSB Transmit well to the left and right chest, axillae, and back Grade 1–2/6 intensity	Prematures and fullterm newborns Usually disappears by 3–6 months of age
Venous hum (continuous)	Maximal at right (or left) supra- and infra-clavicular areas Grade 1–3/6 intensity Inaudible in the supine position Intensity changes with rotation of the head and compression of the jugular vein	3–6 yr
Carotid bruit (systolic)	Right supraclavicular area and over the carotids Grade 2–3/6 in intensity Occasional thrill over a carotid	Any age

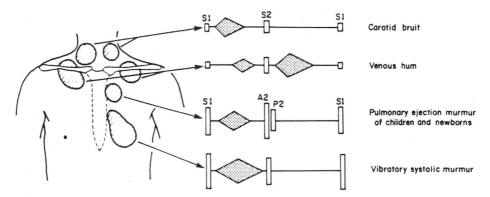

Table and figure from Park MK: Pediatric Cardiology for Practitioners, 2nd ed. Chicago, Year Book Medical Publishers, 1988, p 31, with permission.

33. What is the differential diagnosis for a systolic murmur in each auscultatory area?

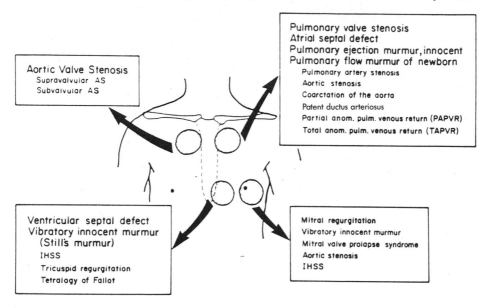

Pulmonary valve stenosis
Atrial septal defect
Pulmonary ejection murmur, innocent
Pulmonary flow murmur of newborn
Pulmonary artery stenosis
Aortic stenosis
Coarctation of the aorta
Patent ductus arteriosus
Partial anom. pulm. venous return (PAPVR)
Total anom. pulm. venous return (TAPVR)

Aortic Valve Stenosis
Supravalvular AS
Subvalvular AS

Ventricular septal defect
Vibratory innocent murmur
(Still's murmur)
IHSS
Tricuspid regurgitation
Tetralogy of Fallot

Mitral regurgitation
Vibratory innocent murmur
Mitral valve prolapse syndrome
Aortic stenosis
IHSS

Systolic murmurs audible at various locations. Less common conditions are shown in smaller type. (From Park MK: Pediatric Cardiology for Practitioners, 2nd ed. Chicago, Year Book Medical Publishers, 1988, p 28, with permission.)

34. Which diastolic murmurs are considered benign?
There are very few innocent diastolic murmurs. A benign transient diastolic murmur can sometimes be heard in the neonatal period due to the ductus arteriosus. In addition, diastolic murmurs due to pulmonary insufficiency as a result of surgery (any RV-PA nonvalved conduit or full corrective TOF repair) are often well-tolerated.

35. What is the differential diagnosis of a continuous murmur?
A continuous murmur begins in systole and continues beyond S2. It may be caused by:
    1. Aortopulmonary or arteriovenous connections: aortopulmonary window, patent ductus arteriosus, truncus arteriosus, AV fistula (systemic, pulmonary or coronary), and systemic-pulmonary shunts.
    2. Disturbances of flow patterns in veins: venous hum.
    3. Disturbances of flow patterns in arteries: pulmonary artery stenosis, collaterals (tetralogy of Fallot or coarctation of the aorta), or ruptured sinus of Valsalva aneurysm.
    Reference: Park MK: Pediatric Cardiology for Practitioners. Chicago, Year Book Medical Publishers, 1984, pp 27–28.

36. What is the differential diagnosis of an intracranial bruit?
An intracranial bruit can be found in 50% of normal children. The following conditions, however, may also be associated with an intracranial bruit:

fever	cerebral aneurysm
thyrotoxicosis	cerebral AVM
anemia	intracerebral tumors
cardiac murmurs	any cause of increased intracranial pressure
cerebral angioma	

In addition, up to 80% of children with meningitis may have an associated intracranial bruit.
    Reference: Mace JW, Peters ER, Mathies AW: N Engl J Med 278:1420, 1968.

37. What is the difference between pulsus alternans and pulsus paradoxus?

1. Pulsus alternans is a pulse pattern in which there is alternating (beat-to-beat) variability of pulse strength due to decreased ventricular performance (sometimes seen in congestive heart failure.)

2. Pulsus paradoxus indicates an exaggeration of normal reduction of systolic blood pressure during inspiration. Associated conditions include cardiac tamponade (effusion or constrictive pericarditis), respiratory illness (asthma or pneumonia), and myocardial disease affecting wall compliance (endocardial fibroelastosis or amyloidosis).

38. After what age does a presumed peripheral pulmonic stenosis murmur deserve more detailed study?

The murmur of peripheral pulmonic stenosis (PPS), a low-intensity systolic ejection murmur heard frequently in newborns, is due to the relative hypoplasia as well as the acute angle of the branch pulmonary arteries in the early newborn period. This murmur usually persists until 3–6 months of age.

39. Name four conditions associated with dextrocardia.

1. Mirror image dextrocardia
2. Displacement of a normal heart (dextroversion)
3. L-TGA
4. Heterotaxy syndromes (asplenia and polysplenia)

40. What EKG and chest x-ray findings are considered characteristic for certain congenital heart malformations?

EKG:

1. LAD (left axis deviation)—ASD (primum), endocardial cushion defect, tricuspid atresia
2. WPW (Wolff-Parkinson-White)—Ebstein's anomaly, L-TGA
3. CHB (complete heart block)—L-TGA, polysplenia

CXR:

1. Boot-shaped heart—tetralogy of Fallot or tricuspid atresia
2. Egg-shaped heart—transposition of the great arteries
3. Snowman—total anomalous pulmonary venous return

41. What are the EKG criteria for chamber enlargement or hypertrophy?

Chamber Enlargement (Hypertrophy)

Right Ventricular
QR pattern V_4R, V_3R, or V_1 (may be ventricular inversion)
Upright T wave V_4R, V_3R, or V_1—5 days to adolescence (if R/S > 1) (may be reciprocal from left chest)
Abnormal R/S ratio V_1 or V_6 (see above values)
Abnormal Amplitude R V_1 or S V_6

Left ventricular
R V_6 + S V_1 ≥ 60 (do not use transition leads; use V_5 if R V_5 > R V_5)
S V_1 > twice R V_5
Abnormal R/S ratio
Abnormal amplitude S V_1 or R V_6

Combined ventricular
Meets criteria for RVH and in addition S V_1 or R V_5 exceeds *mean* for age
Meets criteria for LVH and in addition R V_1 or S V_6 exceeds *mean* for age
Equiphasic large midprecordial voltage—weak criterion ("Katz-Wachtel") 65 mm in one lead, 45 mm in four leads

Table continued on next page.

Chamber Enlargement (Hypertrophy) *(Continued)*

Right atrial
  Peaked P wave > 3.0 mm if < 6 months or > 2.5 mm if > 6 months

Left atrial
  Lead II: > 0.09 sec duration
  Lead V_1: late negative deflection > 0.04 sec duration *and* > 1 mm deflection

Combined atrial
  Early portion of P wave peaked and > 2.5 mm *and* duration of P wave > 0.09 sec

  *If QRS duration is normal, add R + R' and compare total (R + R') with standards. In the presence of complete bundle branch block criteria for ventricular hypertrophy are invalid.
  †R/S undefined because S can be equal to 0.
  ‡Minimum-maximum (mean).
  From combined sources. Revised July 1978 by Garson, Gillette, and McNamara. (From Gillette PC, Garson A: Pediatric Cardiac Dysrhythmias. New York, Grune and Stratton, 1981, p 453, with permission.)

42. What are the most helpful clues for diagnosing right ventricular hypertrophy (RVH) by EKG in a newborn?
  1. Pure R wave (with no S wave) in V1 greater than 10 mm.
  2. R in V1 greater than 25 mm or R in AVR greater than 8 mm.
  3. A qR pattern in V1 (also present in 10% of normal newborns).
  4. Upright T in V1 after 3 days of age.
  5. RAD greater than + 180 degrees.

43. What are the developmental changes in the pediatric EKG during childhood?
  1. Lengthening of most, not all, intervals: p wave duration, PR interval, and QRS duration. (An exception is QTc interval.)
  2. Decrease in RV forces with increasing age: R in V1 and S in V6 decrease in magnitude. (Axis shifts as well from + 75 to + 180 in a newborn to − 15 to + 110 in an adolescent.)

44. What are the EKG abnormalities associated with potassium imbalance? calcium imbalance? magnesium imbalance?
  1. Potassium imbalance (see figure 1)
  2. Calcium imbalance (see figure 2)
  3. Magnesium imbalance:
Hypermagnesemia—simulates hypercalcemia. The few EKG changes include PR prolongation and intraventricular conduction delay.
Hypomagnesemia—simulates hypokalemia. The EKG changes include large U waves and flattened T waves.

SERUM K

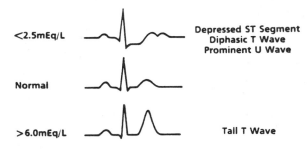

<2.5mEq/L	Depressed ST Segment / Diphasic T Wave / Prominent U Wave
Normal	
>6.0mEq/L	Tall T Wave

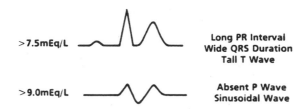

ECG findings of hypokalemia and hyperkalemia. (From Park MK, Guntheroth WG: How to Read Pediatric ECGs, 2nd ed. Chicago, Year Book Medical Publishers, 1987, p 96, with permission.)

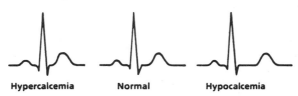

ECG findings of hypercalcemia and hypocalcemia. Hypercalcemia shortens and hypocalcemia lengthens the ST segment. (From Park MK, Guntheroth WG: How to Read Pediatric ECGs, 2nd ed. Chicago, Year Book Medical Publishers, 1987, p 96, with permission.)

45. How is the Qo-Tc measured, and what is its clinical significance? How is it different from QTc?

Qo-Tc is the interval from the onset of the QRS complex to the onset of the T wave, corrected for heart rate:

$$Qo\text{-}Tc = Q - oT/\sqrt{R - R'}$$

Qo-Tc is increased in hypocalcemia since the ST segment is prolonged. An estimation of calcium (total and ionized) could be made using the calculated Qo-Tc and reference tables. QTc is the interval from the onset of the QRS complex to the end of the T wave, corrected for heart rate.

$$QTc = QT/\sqrt{R - R'}$$

46. What causes prolongation of the QT interval?

1. Congenital long QT syndrome
   Hereditary form
      Jervell-Lange-Nielsen syndrome (associated with deafness)
      Romano-Ward syndrome
   Sporadic type
2. Acquired long QT syndrome

Drug induced	Metabolic/electrolyte abnormalities
Antiarrhythmic agents	Very-low-energy diets
Phenothiazines	Central and autonomic nervous system disorders
Tricyclic antidepressants	Miscellaneous
Lithium carbonate	Coronary heart disease, mitral valve prolapse

Reference: Moss AJ: Prolonged QT-interval syndromes. JAMA 21:2986, 1986.

47. How abnormal are premature atrial contractions (PACs)?

Premature atrial beats are usually benign, with two exceptions:

1. Infants under 1 year of age have a small risk of developing supraventricular tachycardia or atrial flutter if PACs occur frequently.
2. Children on digoxin—PACs may be an early sign of digoxin toxicity.

48. What are the common causes of supraventricular tachycardia?

1. Idiopathic (with a structurally normal heart),
2. Congenital heart disease (preoperative): such as Ebstein's anomaly, L-transposition of the great arteries, or single ventricle.
3. Congenital heart disease (postoperative): atrial surgery
4. Drugs: sympathomimetics (cold medications, theophylline, beta agonists)
5. Infections: myocarditis or fever
6. Others: Wolff-Parkinson-White syndrome, hyperthyroidism

49. How does one differentiate aberrancy from ventricular tachycardia?

Aberrancy occurs when a supraventricular impulse reaches the AV node or the His bundle prematurely and finds only one bundle branch excitable and the other refractory. This results in a QRS complex resembling a bundle branch block. Premature wide QRS complexes due to aberrancy (vs. one due to a premature ventricular contraction) may be identified by these characteristics: (1) the mean ventricular rate is relatively fast, (2) there is QRS variability (in morphology), (3) there is variation of the coupling interval, (4) there is no attempt at a compensatory pause, and (5) it is not associated with A-V dissociation. A widened QRS complex could also be due to: bundle branch blocks, pre-excitation syndrome (WPW), intraventricular blocks (such as metabolic disturbances), or pacemakers.

50. What are the common causes of atrial flutter and fibrillation in childhood?

Intra-atrial surgery (Mustard, atrial septal defect repair)	Idiopathic with an otherwise normal heart
	Cardiomyopathy
Congenital heart disease (Ebstein's anomaly)	Wolff-Parkinson-White syndrome
	Sick sinus syndrome
Heart disease with dilated atria (atrioventricular valve regurgitation)	Myocarditis

51. When are isolated premature ventricular contractions (PVCs) acceptable in the otherwise healthy school-aged child?

1. EKG intervals, especially QTc, are normal.
2. There are no paired or multiform PVCs or "R-on-T" phenomena.
3. There is no evidence of myocarditis, cardiomegaly, or ventricular tumor.
4. There is no history of drug use.
5. The electrolytes and glucose are normal.
and *especially* if
6. The PVCs decrease with exercise.

52. What is sick sinus syndrome (SSS)? What is the etiology? Clinical presentation?

SSS is a disorder of the atria, the sinus node, and the AV junctional tissue resulting in depression of automaticity leading to a brady (sinus bradycardia, sinoatrial block or sinus arrest)—tachy (atrial flutter, atrial fibrillation or SVT) arrhythmia. The most common etiologies are intra-atrial repairs for transposition of the great arteries, atrial septal defect repair, Blalock-Hanlon septectomy, myocarditis, or idiopathic. Clinical presentations include dizziness, syncope, palpitations, and exercise intolerance.

53. What is a vectorcardiogram and in what clinical settings is it useful?

It is a recording of cardiac electrical activity in an orthogonal system (i.e., in three planes), thus indicating the magnitude and direction of the maximum QRS vector. It is seldom used now, but can be useful in the evaluation of patients with complex ventricular anatomy.

54. What are indications for Holter monitors in children?

General indications: evaluation of rate or rhythm disturbances that cannot be accurately diagnosed and properly managed by routine EKG.

Specific indications: examples:

1. Following corrective surgery for defects such as TGA (especially corrected by atrial baffle procedure), tetralogy of Fallot, and complete atrioventricular canal
2. Mitral valve prolapse with associated chest pain, palpitations, or syncope
3. Unexplained fainting
4. Near-miss sudden infant death syndrome
5. Unexplained sudden death in a close family member, particularly one of young age
6. Evaluation of drug therapy for rhythm disturbances
7. Patient complaints suggestive of episodic tachycardia.

Reference: Graham TP, et al: Recommendations for use of laboratory studies for pediatric patients with suspected or proven heart disease. Circulation 72:443A–450A, 1987.

55. What are the indications for, and the most common type of pacemaker used in children?

The most frequent indication for pacemakers in children is symptomatic bradycardia. Other indications include sick sinus syndrome, supraventricular tachycardia refractory to medical management, and ventricular tachycardia refractory to medical management. The most commonly used pacemaker is the VVI. A quick review of the three-letter system:

- first letter: chamber paced
  V = ventricular
  A = atrial
  D = dual
- second letter: chamber sensed
  V = ventricular
  A = atrial
  D = dual

- third letter: mode
  I = inhibited
  T = trigger
  O = not applicable
- The VVI unit is also called:
  V demand
  R wave inhibited
  V inhibited
  pacemaker

Catheterization

56. What are normal pressures and saturations in the heart and great vessels?

NORMAL CARDIAC CATHETERIZATION DATA

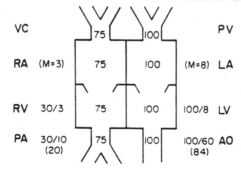

Pressure and oxygen saturation values in normal children. (From Park MK: Pediatric Cardiology for Practitioners. Chicago, Year Book Medical Publishers, 1984, p 299, with permission.)

57. What is meant by Qp/Qs and how is it calculated?

Qp/Qs is the ratio of pulmonary blood flow (Qp) to systemic blood flow (Qs), thus quantifying the amount of left to right shunt. (It is 1:1 in a normal heart.) A quick way of estimating Qp/Qs is to take the difference of O_2 saturations of aorta and SVC, and divide this by the difference of O_2 saturations in the pulmonary vein and artery (assuming pulmonary vein to be 99% saturated):

$$Qp/Qs = (Ao\ sat\ -\ SVC\ sat)/(PV\ sat\ -\ PA\ sat)$$

58. What are present interventional cardiac catheterization procedures?

1. Balloon atrial septostomy/blade atrial septectomy for transposition of the great arteries

2. Balloon valvuloplasty/angioplasty for aortic stenosis/pulmonary stenosis/coarctation of the aorta

3. Umbrella plugging for patent ductus arteriosus, and coil embolization for collateral and arteriovenous fistulae

Other interventional procedures that may be developed in the future are umbrella plugging for atrial septal defect, ventricular septal defect, and aorto-pulmonary window; stents (short tubes) for coarctation, pulmonary arteries, vena cavae; and contracting ring for mitral regurgitation or Ebstein's anomaly.

Reference: Garson A: The science and practice of pediatric cardiology in the next decade. Am Heart J 114:462–468, 1988.

59. What are the complications of cardiac catheterization?

Arrhythmias: ventricular tachycardia, paroxysmal atrial or junctional tachycardia, atrioventricular block, and bradycardia.

Arterial Complications: weak or absent pulse.

Rare complications include superficial wound infections, allergic reactions to contrast, air embolus, and perforation of chambers of the heart.

Noninvasive Modalities

60. What are the indications for echocardiography?

1. Unexplained cyanosis
2. Congestive heart failure
3. Clinical findings suggestive of a significant cardiac lesion
4. Evaluation of a patient undergoing cardiac catheterization or cardiac surgery
5. Presence of clinically important arrhythmias
6. Clinical suspicion of inflammatory disease of the heart (such as endocarditis, myocarditis, pericardial effusion, or Kawasaki disease)
7. Assessing chamber size and function
8. Exposure to cardiotoxic agents (such as anthracyclines)
9. Strong family history of cardiomyopathy
10. Evaluation of anticongestive therapy or pharmacologic closure of patent ductus
11. Postoperative evaluation
12. Fetal indications

Reference: Graham TP et al: Recommendations for use of laboratory studies for pediatric patients with suspected or proven heart disease. Circulation 72-207:443A–450A, 1987.

61. What are the indications for fetal echocardiography?

1. Polyhydramnios or oligohydramnios
2. Suspected cardiac malformation on obstetrical ultrasound
3. Sustained fetal tachy- or bradycardia
4. Irregular fetal rhythm
5. Family history of congenital heart disease
6. Family history of chromosomal disorders
7. Known fetal chromosomal disorders
8. Maternal drug ingestion: lithium, amphetamines, alcohol, anticonvulsants, chemotherapy, or hormones
9. Maternal diabetes
10. Maternal collagen vascular disorders
11. Intrauterine growth retardation
12. Rh sensitization
13. Ultrasonic evidence of pleural, pericardial or peritoneal fluid
14. Rubella exposure

62. What is Doppler echocardiography and what are indications for its use?

The Doppler principle, described initially by Christian Doppler in 1842, states that motion causes a frequency shift under certain situations. Application of noninvasive cardiac Doppler technology began in 1967 after the Fast Fourier transform (FFT) circuitry was developed for the Doppler echocardiographic system. Clinical applications include detection of turbulent flow, measurement of valvular gradients across stenotic valves, and quantitative measurement of flow by multiplying velocity by area.

63. How is shortening fraction calculated by echocardiography?

$$(LVED - LVES / LVED) \times 100$$

LVED = left ventricular end-diastolic dimension
LVES = left ventricular end-systolic dimension
Normal range = 28–38%

64. When is exercise testing indicated in a child?

Exercise testing is generally performed on children 4 years of age and over since certain coordination and cooperation are needed for the treadmill or the bicycle ergometer.

Indications include (1) diagnosis of exercise-induced symptoms: such as syncope, chest pain, or palpitations; (2) evaluation of patients with known or suspected arrhythmias: usually tachyarrhythmias or ectopy; (3) evaluation of exercise tolerance: especially postoperatively; (4) assessment of potential myocardial ischemia: useful in left ventricular outflow tract obstruction, cardiomyopathies, or coronary artery diseases; and (5) assessment of blood pressure responses: especially in coarctation of the aorta.

Important *contraindications* include active inflammatory cardiac disease, acute heart failure, critical cardiac outflow obstruction, known ischemic disease with angina, severe pulmonary vascular disease, severe hypertension, and serious rhythm disturbance.

Reference: Graham TP, et al: Recommendations for use of laboratory studies for pediatric patients with suspected or proven heart disease. Circulation 72:207 443A–450A, 1987.

65. What are the best noninvasive methods of measuring cardiac output?

Physical exam—mental status, perfusion, urine output, etc.; exercise testing; and echocardiography. Calculation of cardiac output can be done by using Doppler flow velocities measured in the ascending aorta:

$$SV = CSA \times FVI$$

where SV = stroke volume, CSA = calculated surface area (of the valve), and FVI = flow velocity integral (derived by integrating areas under the velocity curves).

$$CO = HR \times SV$$

where CO = cardiac output, HR = heart rate, and SV = stroke volume.

It is important to remember that there are limitations to this non-invasive method of calculating cardiac output. For instance, the elasticity of the aorta and the error of measurement of the valve area both contribute to error in the calculation.

Subacute Bacterial Endocarditis

66. Which cardiac lesions do not require prophylactic antibiotics?

There are four conditions in which endocarditis prophylaxis is *not* recommended:
   1. Isolated secundum atrial septal defect
   2. Secundum atrial septal defect repaired without a patch six or more months earlier
   3. Patent ductus arteriosus ligated and divided six or more months earlier
   4. Postoperative coronary artery bypass graft (CABG) surgery

Ventriculoatrial shunts for hydrocephalus, dialysis fistulae and shunts, and transvenous pacemakers are probable indications for SBE prophylaxis.

67. How reliable is the echocardiogram for diagnosing subacute bacterial endocarditis (SBE)?

Although the yield for diagnosing SBE by echocardiogram is low, the likelihood of a positive finding is increased under certain conditions: indwelling catheters, prematurity, immunosuppressed patients on antibiotics, and evidence of peripheral embolization. SBE is still a clinical and laboratory diagnosis (physical examination and blood cultures, respectively) and *not* an "echocardiographic" diagnosis. A negative study does not "rule out" SBE.

68. Which cardiac lesions are most at risk for bacterial endocarditis?

Tetralogy of Fallot (TOF)	Ventricular septal defect (VSD)
Patent ductus arteriosus (PDA)	D-Transposition of the great arteries (D-TGA)
Aortic stenosis (AS)	AV canal
Pulmonary stenosis (PS)	

Reference: Johnson DH, Rosenthal A, Nadas AS: A forty-year review of bacterial endocarditis in infancy and childhood. Circulation 51:581–588, 1975.

69. How many blood cultures should be obtained to rule out SBE?

Three separate blood cultures should be obtained. In 10–30% of children, the first two blood cultures may be negative. The timing of blood cultures in relation to fever has been found to be unimportant; however, the use of multiple sites may decrease the likelihood of mistaking a contaminant for the true etiologic agent.

70. What is the single drug regimen of SBE prophylaxis for a penicillin-allergic patient?

Vancomycin or erythromycin.

Antibiotic Prophylaxis to Prevent Endocarditis

I. For Dental, Otolaryngologic, and Bronchoscopic Procedures
  A. Single drug
    1. Parenteral and oral penicillin
      Aqueous penicillin G (30,000 units/kg) mixed with procaine penicillin G (600,000 units) intramuscularly 30–60 min before procedure followed by penicillin V orally 500 mg (250 mg for <60 lbs) every 6 hr for 8 doses.
    2. Oral penicillin
      Penicillin V (2.0 gm) orally 30–60 min before procedure and then 500 mg orally every 6 hr for 8 doses (half-doses for children <60 lbs)
    3. For penicillin-allergic patients
      a. Vancomycin (20 mg/kg) intravenously over 60 min beginning 30–60 min before procedure, followed by erythromycin (10 mg/kg) orally every 6 hr for 8 doses. Or
      b. Erythromycin (20 mg/kg) orally 1½ to 2 hr prior to procedure, followed by 10 mg/kg every 6 hr for 8 doses.
  B. Two drugs
    1. Aqueous penicillin G (30,000/kg) mixed with procaine penicillin (600,000 units) intramuscularly plus steptomycin (20 mg/kg) intramuscularly, both given 30–60 min before procedure, followed by penicillin V 500 mg orally (250 mg for 60 lbs) every 6 hr for 8 doses.
    2. For penicillin-allergic patients
      Vancomycin (20 mg/kg) intravenously over 60 min, beginning 30–60 min before procedure followed by erythromycin (10 mg/kg) orally every 6 hr for 8 doses.
II. For Genitourinary or Gastrointestinal Tract Procedures
  A. For nonpenicillin-allergic patient
    1. Aqueous penicillin G (30,000 units/kg) IM or IV
    2. Ampicillin (50 mg/kg) IM or IV
          plus
    3. Gentamicin (2.0 mg/kg) IM or IV or

Table continued on next page.

Antibiotic Prophylaxis to Prevent Endocarditis *(Continued)*

4. Streptomycin (20 mg/kg) IM. Doses should be given 30–60 min prior to procedure and should be repeated every 8 hr times 2 if gentamicin is used, or every 12 hr times 2 if streptomycin is used.
B. For Penicillin-Allergic Patients
   Vancomycin (20 mg/kg) given IV over 60 min beginning 30–60 min before procedure plus streptomycin (20 mg/kg) IM 30–60 min before the procedure and repeated once in 12 hr.

From Adams FH, Emmanouilides GC: Moss' Heart Disease in Infants, Children, and Adolescents. Baltimore, Williams and Wilkins, 1983. Modified from: The Committee on Prevention of Rheumatic Fever and Bacterial Endocarditis of the American Heart Association.

In no instance should the dose of drugs exceed the adult dosage (aqueous penicillin G, 1,000,000; streptomycin, 1 gm; vancomycin, 1 gm; erythromycin, 1 gm; ampicillin, 1 gm; gentamicin, 80 mg). Doses may need modification for patients with compromised renal function.

Older Children and Adolescents

71. Which congenital heart defects present in later childhood?
In order of frequency:
   Ventricular septal defect
   Patent ductus arteriosus
   Atrial septal defect
   Tetralogy of Fallot
   Pulmonary stenosis
   Coarctation of the aorta
   Aortic stenosis

72. What methods have a high accuracy in the diagnosis of mitral valve prolapse (MVP)?
1. Auscultation—especially with midsystolic click and late systolic murmur.
2. Echocardiography—most accurate in parasternal long-axis view.
3. Angiography—usually not indicated.

Major Criteria that Establish the Diagnosis of MVP

Auscultation
   Mid to late systolic clicks and a late systolic murmur at the cardiac apex
   Mobile mid to late systolic clicks at the cardiac apex
   Late systolic murmur at the cardiac apex in the young patient
Auscultation plus echocardiography
   Apical holosystolic murmur of mitral regurgitation plus echocardiographic criteria
Two-dimensional/Doppler echocardiography

Minor Criteria that Arouse Suspicion but Do Not Establish the Diagnosis of MVP

History
   Focal neurologic attacks or amaurosis fugax in the young patient
First-degree relatives with major criteria
   Recurrent supraventricular tachycardia (documented)
Auscultation
   Soft, inconstant, or equivocal mid to late systolic sounds at the cardiac apex
Other physical signs
   Low body weight, asthenic habitus
   Low blood pressure
   Thoracic bony abnormalities
Two-dimensional/Doppler/color flow echocardiography

Tables modified from MacMahon SW, Devereau RB, Schron E: Clinical and epidemiological issues in mitral valve prolapse. Proceedings of a National Heart, Lung and Blood Institute Symposium. Am Heart J 113:1330-1331, 1987.

73. What are the possible (and usual) presentations of MVP?

Most are asymptomatic with click or murmur heard on physical examination. Other possible presentations include palpitations, shortness of breath, dyspnea on exertion, chest pain, congestive heart failure, subacute bacterial endocarditis, and cerebrovascular accident.

Mitral valve prolapse is classified as below:

Primary

Secondary

1. An associated systemic disease of connective tissue (Marfan's syndrome, Ehlers-Danlos syndrome, pseudoxanthoma elasticum, osteogenesis imperfecta, Hurler's syndrome).

2. A reduction in left ventricular cavity size (ostium secundum, atrial septal defect, anorexia nervosa, Ebstein's anomaly).

Reference: MacMahon SW, Devereux RB, Schron E: Clinical and epidemiological issues in mitral valve prolapse. Proceedings of a National Heart, Lung, and Blood Institute Symposium. Am Heart J 113:1265–1332, 1987.

74. What is the significance of MVP and does this condition require subacute bacterial endocarditis prophylaxis?

The incidence of endocarditis in patients with MVP and systolic murmur is 1/2000 per annum. Three factors, the *male* gender, the *elderly* population, and the presence of *systolic murmur,* seem to be associated with an increased risk of endocarditis in patients with MVP. Thus, there is some agreement that only patients with MVP and systolic murmur (mitral regurgitation) should have SBE prophylaxis.

75. How common is chest pain in children and what are the common causes of chest pain?

In one study, the occurrence (per patient visits) was 0.3%. In order of decreasing frequency, the diagnostic categories were: idiopathic (45%), costochondritis (22.5%), bronchitis (12.5%), miscellaneous (10%), muscle strain (5%), and trauma (5%).

Reference: Driscoll DJ, Glicklich LB, Gallen WJ: Chest pain in children: a prospective study. Pediatrics 57:648–651, 1976.

76. When should lipid screening be done in children to evaluate their risk for premature atherosclerosis?

Lipid screening should be done when there is a family history of: diabetes mellitus, hypertension, coronary artery disease (especially at an early age), sudden death, xanthomata, or elevated cholesterol.

77. Which types of hyperlipidemias have their onset in childhood?

1. Type I—elevated triglycerides due to lipoprotein lipase deficiency.

2. Type IIA—elevated cholesterol and increased low-density lipoproteins (LDL).

3. Type IIB—elevated cholesterol and triglyceride and increased low-density lipoproteins (LDL) and very low-density lipoproteins (VLDL).

78. At what age are patients with Marfan's syndrome at risk for serious vascular complications?

In Marfan's syndrome, mitral valve abnormalities (such as dilatation of the annulus, distortion of leaflets, or abnormalities of the chordae tendineae) are more evident in children, whereas aortic valve pathology (such as dilatation of ascending aorta, aortic insufficiency, or aneurysms of sinuses of Valsalva) is predominantly found in adults. Clinically evident cardiovascular disease is present in 50% of patients with Marfan's syndrome by age 21 years.

79. What causes sudden death in anorectics?

The chronic emaciation takes its toll on the myocardium. Anorectics develop depressed cardiovascular functions and an altered conduction system. EKG changes are common, including bradycardia, QRS amplitude decreases, prolonged Q-T intervals, and nonspecific ST segment changes. These EKG changes often occur without underlying electrolyte abnormalities. The arrhythmogenic potential is heightened if electrolytes (specifically potassium) are distorted by excessive vomiting or laxative abuse. Sudden death is likely due to the culmination of chronic myocardial injury in emaciated patients (less than 35–40% below ideal weight) with resultant failure and arrhythmia.

80. What percentage of hypertensive adolescents become hypertensive adults?
Of adolescents with primary or essential hypertension, two-thirds become hypertensive adults.

Inflammatory Heart Disease

81. What are the common clinical symptoms and signs of pericarditis?
Symptoms: chest pain, fever, cough, palpitations, irritability, abdominal pain, and decreased feeding.
Signs: friction rub, pallor, pulsus paradoxus, muffled heart sounds, and neck vein distention.

82. What is the diagnostic test of choice in pericarditis?
Although these signs and symptoms are frequently associated with electrocardiographic changes (ST elevation, T wave inversion, and decreased QRS voltage) and chest x-ray abnormalities (cardiomegaly), the diagnostic test of choice is an echocardiogram.

83. What are the common causes of infectious and noninfectious pericarditis?
Infectious:
bacterial:	*Staphylococcus aureus*
	Streptococcus pneumoniae
	Hemophilus influenzae
	Neisseria meningitidis
viral:	coxsackie virus
	ECHO virus
	adenovirus
	influenza virus
	mumps virus
	tuberculosis
	mycotic

Noninfectious:
collagen vascular disease:	systemic lupus erythematosus
	rheumatoid arthritis
rheumatic:	acute rheumatic fever
renal:	uremic pericarditis
malignancy:	radiation-induced Hodgkin's disease
	post-pericardiotomy syndrome

84. When should steroids be given to a child with myocarditis?
The use of steroids in myocarditis is controversial at present. Some authorities feel that the use of steroids may inhibit interferon synthesis and thus increase virus replication. If the inflammatory process is secondary to rheumatic disease, however, steroids may be indicated.

85. What is the differential diagnosis for myocarditis?
1. Active myocardial disease
    Infections:
        Bacterial: diphtheria
        Viral: coxsackie, human immunodeficiency virus
        Mycoplasma
        Rickettsial: typhus
        Fungal and protozoal: histoplasmosis, toxoplasmosis
        Others: Kawasaki disease, systemic lupus erythematosus,
        rheumatoid arthritis
    Chemical/Physical Agents:
        Radiation injury
        Drugs: adriamycin
        Toxins: lead
        Animal bites: snakes, scorpion
2. Chronic muscle disease
    Systemic/Metabolic Diseases:
        Cardiac glycogenesis: Pompe's
        Neuromuscular: Friedreich ataxia
        Nutritional: beri-beri
        Others: Hurler's, muscular dystrophy
    Congenital Defects:
        Outflow obstruction: aortic and pulmonary stenosis
        Coronary anomalies: anomalous coronary from pulmonary artery
        Neoplasia: rhabdomyoma
Note: tachyarrhythmias, especially supraventricular tachycardia, should also be considered.
Reference: Hohn AR, Stanton RE: Myocarditis in children. Pediatr Rev 9:83–88, 1987.

86. What is the recommended guide for medical therapy and for rest and ambulation in a child with minimal rheumatic carditis?
Medical therapy: aspirin for 2–4 weeks at 100 mg/kg/day, tapering to 60 mg/kg/day after 2 weeks if clinically improved.
Rest and ambulation: 3 weeks of bedrest followed by 3 weeks of indoor ambulation.

Intensive Care

87. Is there a clever way to remember how to order emergency drips for cardiac resuscitation?
    Example:
        0.1 µg/kg/min Isuprel for a 10 kg child:
        0.6 mg × weight (10 kg) in 100 cc =
        6 mg in 100 cc at 1 cc/hr

Preparation of Catecholamine Infusions in Children

CATECHOLAMINE	PREPARATION	DOSE
Isoproterenol Epinephrine Norepinephrine	0.6 mg × body weight (in kg), added to diluent to make 100 ml	Then 1 ml/hr delivers 0.1 µg/kg/min
Dopamine Dobutamine	6 mg × body weight (in kg), added to diluent to make 100 ml	Then 1 ml/hr delivers 1 µg/kg/min

Adapted from Zaritsky A, Chernow B: Catecholamines, sympathomimetics. In Chernow B, Lake CR (eds): The Pharmacologic Approach to the Critically Ill Patient. Baltimore, Williams & Wilkins, 1983.

Surgical Procedures

88. What are approximate costs for common cardiology procedures?

EKG—$75.00, Holter—$300.00, 2D Echo—$700.00–$1,000.00, cardiac catheterization—$1,500.00, exercise test—$500.00–$1,000.00.

89. What are the indications for endomyocardial biopsy (EMB)?

1. Cardiac transplant rejection—EMB is still the most reliable technique for diagnosing rejection, even though cyclosporine has altered biopsy findings.

2. Doxorubicin cardiotoxicity—EMB is the most sensitive method for determination of extent of myocardial injury. This has lead to a decrease in deaths due to cardiomyopathy-related CHF.

Other potential uses for EMB include: myocarditis, glycogen storage disease, cardiac tumors, and rheumatic carditis.

90. What are the most common cardiothoracic postoperative syndromes?

1. Postcoarctectomy syndrome—arteritis in the mesenteric circulation, causing abdominal pain (2–8 days following surgery).

2. Postpericardiotomy syndrome—immunologic phenomenon leading to pericardial effusion, causing chest pain and vomiting (2–3 weeks following surgery).

3. Postperfusion syndrome—CMV infection causing fever and splenomegaly (3–6 weeks following surgery).

4. Hemolytic anemia syndrome—trauma to red cells leading to fever, jaundice, and hepatomegaly (1–2 weeks following surgery).

91. What is the current survival rate in heart transplantation in children?

In recent review of cardiac transplantation in children with heart disease (underlying diseases were cardiomyopathy, congenital heart disease, and endocardial fibroelastosis), 1-year survival was reported to have increased from 22% in 1968 to 83% in 1986. Increased survival has been mainly attributed to introduction of the new immunosuppressive agents, especially cyclosporine.

Reference: Starnes V, et al: Cardiac transplantation in children and adolescents. Circulation 76:43–51, 1987.

Pharmacologic Agents

92. What are the recommended enteral and parenteral digitalizing doses for an infant, toddler, and older child?

Dosage Regimens for Inotropic Agents—Digoxin

AGE AND WEIGHT	DOSE AND ROUTE*	
	Acute Digitalization	*Maintenance*
Prematures	10-20 μg/kg IV	4 μg/kg/day IV
<1.5 kg	Total Digitalizing Dose (TDD): ½, ¼, ¼ of dose q 8h	(may increase to 4 μg/kg q 12h at age 1 month)
1.5–2.5 kg	Same as above	4 μg/kg q 12h IV
Full-term newborns	30 μg/kg IV, TDD	4–5 μg/kg q 12h IV
Infants (1–12 months)	35 μg/kg IV, TDD	5–10 μg/kg q 12h IV

Table continued on next page.

Dosage Regimens for Inotropic Agents—Digoxin *(Continued)*

	DOSE AND ROUTE*	
AGE AND WEIGHT	*Acute Digitalization*	*Maintenance*
>12 months	40 µg/kg IV, TDD (maximum 1.0 mg)	5–10 µg/kg q 12h IV
Older children (over 20 kg)	1.0–2.0 mg IV, TDD over 48 hours	0.125–0.250 mg IV q day

*P.O. dose approximately 20% greater than IV dose except in "older children." In older children, IV = P.O.

From Friedman WF, George BL: New concepts and drugs in the treatment of congestive heart failure. Pediatr Clin North Am 31:1200, 1984, with permission.

93. How valuable are digoxin levels?

Digoxin levels may not be helpful in children because: the presence of endogenous DLIS (digoxin-like immunoreactive substances), which cross-react with immunoassay antibodies to digoxin; and in children, the concentration of digoxin is much higher in the myocardium than in the plasma. Digoxin levels may be helpful, however, in older children (especially in presence of dysrhythmias).

94. How long before oral digoxin begins to work?

Oral digoxin reaches peak plasma levels 1 to 2 hours after administration. However, peak "hemodynamic" effect is not evident until 6 hours after administration (versus 3 hours for intravenous digoxin).

95. What factors may predispose a patient to digitalis toxicity?

1. High serum digoxin level
     high-dose requirement as in treatment of certain
          arrhythmias
     decreased renal excretion:
          premature infants
          renal disease
     hypothyroidism
2. Increased sensitivity of myocardium
     status of myocardium
          myocardial ischemia
          myocarditis (rheumatic, viral)
     systemic changes
          electrolyte imbalance (hypokalemia, hypercalcemia)
          hypoxia
          alkalosis
          adrenergic stimuli or catecholamines

Finally, certain drugs may raise plasma level of digoxin: quinidine, verapamil, amiodarone, indomethacin, and penicillins.

96. Which drugs are most effective in treating digoxin-induced atrial and ventricular dysrhythmias?

Lidocaine and diphenylhydantoin.

97. What are the ECG signs of digitalis toxicity?

ECG Changes Associated with Digitalis

Effects
    Shortening of QTc, the earliest sign of digitalis effect
    Sagging ST segment and diminished amplitude of T wave (the T vector does not change)
    Slowing of heart rate
Toxicity
    Prolongation of PR interval
        Some normal children have prolonged PR interval making it mandatory to obtain a baseline
        ECG.
        The prolongation may progress to second-degree AV block.
    Profound sinus bradycardia or SA block
    Supraventricular arrhythmias, such as atrial or nodal ectopic beats and tachycardias (particularly if
        accompanied by AV block), are more common than ventricular arrhythmias in children.
    Ventricular arrhythmias such as ventricular bigeminy or trigeminy are extremely rare in children,
        although they are common in adults with digitalis toxicity. Ventricular premature beats are not
        uncommon in children as a sign of toxicity.

From Park MK: Pediatric Cardiology for Practitioners, 2nd ed. Chicago, Year Book Medical Publishers, 1988, p 314, with permission.

98. When is afterload reduction indicated in the treatment of congestive heart failure?
Impaired ventricular function in the immediate postoperative period, chronic ventricular dysfunction, mitral and/or aortic regurgitation, and systemic-to-pulmonic shunts.

99. What are the indications for the following inotropic agents: isoproterenol, dobutamine, dopamine? How do the physiologic effects of these agents differ?
    1. Isoproterenol: mainly beta-1 and beta-2 effects
        Indications
            bradycardia (unresponsive to atropine)
            status asthmaticus
            pulmonary hypertension (controversial)
    2. Dobutamine: mainly beta-1 effects
        Indications
            cardiogenic shock
            septic shock
    3. Dopamine: mainly beta-1, beta-2, and dopaminergic (renal) effects, but has also alpha effects depending on dose
        Indications
            hypotension
            low cardiac output (especially post-operative)

Bibliography

1. Adams FH, Emmanouilides GC: Moss' Heart Disease in Infants, Children, and Adolescents. Baltimore, Williams and Wilkins, 1983.
2. Behrman RE, Vaughan VC: Nelson Textbook of Pediatrics, 13th ed. Philadelphia, W.B. Saunders Co., 1987.
3. Degowin EL, Degowin RL: Bedside Diagnostic Examination. New York, Macmillan Publishing Co., 1981.
4. Garson A: The Electrocardiogram in Infants and Children. Philadelphia, Lea and Febiger, 1983.
5. Gillette PC, Garson A: Pediatric Cardiac Dysrhythmias. New York, Grune and Stratton, 1981.
6. Hurst JW: The Heart, 6th ed. New York, McGraw-Hill Book Co., 1986.
7. Keith JD, Rowe RD, Vlad P: Heart Disease in Infancy and Childhood, 3rd ed. New York, Macmillan Publishing Co., 1978.

8. Park MK: Pediatric Cardiology for Practitioners. Chicago, Year Book Medical Publishers, 1984; 2nd edition 1988.
9. Park MK, Guntheroth WG: How to Read Pediatric EKGs. Chicago, Year Book Medical Publishers, 1987.
10. Perloff JK: The Clinical Recognition of Congenital Heart Disease. Philadelphia, W.B. Saunders Co., 1987.
11. Rudolph AM, Hoffman J: Pediatrics, 18th ed. Norwalk, CT, Appleton-Century-Crofts, 1987.
12. Schneeweiss A: Drug Therapy in Infants and Children with Cardiovascular Diseases. Philadelphia, Lea and Febiger, 1986.

DERMATOLOGY

Paul J. Honig, M.D.
Lawrence F. Eichenfield, M.D.
Linda G. Rabinowitz, M.D.

1. How is tinea versicolor diagnosed?

A very common superficial disorder of the skin, tinea versicolor is caused by the fungus *Pityrosporum orbiculare* (also known as *Malassezia furfur*). It presents as multiple macules and patches, with fine scales, over the upper trunk, arms, and occasionally the face and other areas. Lesions may be hypo- or hyperpigmented, appearing lighter than tanned skin in the summer and relatively darker in winter—thus "versatile" in color, "versicolor." Diagnosis can be confirmed by KOH preparation of a scraping from involved skin, which has characteristic fungal hyphae and a grape-like spore pattern referred to as the "spaghetti and meatball" appearance. Wood's light will also display fluorescence (yellow-brown).

2. What is the treatment for tinea versicolor?

(1) Selenium sulfide suspension (2.5% concentration) applied over the affected area overnight multiple times during the first week, with decreasing frequency over the ensuing weeks; (2) topical antifungal creams (these can be quite expensive); and (3) oral ketoconazole. The latter has been shown to be effective in adults in a single one-time dose, and may be considered for use in older adolescents, although side effects may occur. There are reports that this fungus causes central line sepsis in neonates on hyperalimentation. So interest in this fungus isn't only skin deep.

3. How do the commonly used topical steroids vary in potency?

There is a myriad of topical corticosteroids for inflammatory lesions of the skin. Here is a list of the relative potency of some of the commonly used preparations (group 1, very potent; group 6, mild):

1. Betamethasone dipropionate (Diprolene) 0.05%
   Clobetasol propionate (Temovate) 0.05%
2. Amcinonide (Cyclocort) 0.1%
   Desoximetasone (Topicort) 0.25%
   Diflorasone diacetate (Florone, Maxiflor) 0.05%
   Fluocinonide (Lidex) 0.05%
   Halcinonide (Halog) 0.1%
3. Amcinonide cream (Cyclocort) 0.1%
   Betamethasone valerate (Valisone) 0.1%
   Fluocinolone acetonide (Synalar, Fluonid) 0.2%
   Flurandrenolide (Cordran) 0.05%
   Triamcinolone acetonide (Aristocort, Kenalog) 0.5%
4. Fluocinolone acetonide 0.025%
   Hydrocortisone valerate (Westcort) 0.2%
   Triamcinolone acetonide 0.1%
5. Desonide (Tridesilon) 0.05%
   Flumethasone pivalate (Locorten) 0.03%
   Hydrocortisone 1% (with urea)
6. Dexamethasone 0.1%
   Hydrocortisone 1% (alcohol or acetate)

Reference: Int J Dermatol 24:436, 1985, with permission.

4. What is the medical significance of cutis marmorata?
Cutis marmorata is the bluish mottling of the skin often seen in infants and young children exposed to low temperatures or chilling. The reticulated marbling effect is due to dilated capillaries and venules causing darkened areas on the skin. This disappears with warming. This disorder is of no medical significance and no treatment is indicated; however, persistent cutis marmorata is associated with trisomy 21, trisomy 18, and Cornelia de Lange syndromes.

5. What is the "harlequin color change"?
Seen in newborns and more commonly in premature infants, this entity consists of reddening of one side of the body with a sharp line of demarcation along the midline. It is not uncommon, occurring in up to 10% of infants. The change occurs only when the child is lying on one side—the superior half is light, whereas the dependent half is dark and subfused. The cause is thought to be an imbalance in autonomic regulation of peripheral blood vessels. Don't flip out over this problem—rather flip the child, and the color pattern will reverse; place the child prone or supine and the color change will disappear.

6. What is the appearance and clinical significance of subcutaneous fat necrosis?
Subcutaneous fat necrosis consists of sharply circumscribed, indurated nodular lesions usually seen in healthy term newborns and infants in the first few days to weeks of life. The stony hard areas of panniculitis are generally movable and slightly elevated, and the overlying skin is a reddish, violaceous color. While the cause is unknown, it is thought that obstetric trauma and pressure on bony prominences may contribute to the problem. The usual sites (cheeks, back, buttocks, arms, and thighs) are consistent with this. Histologically the lesions display extensive inflammation in the subcutaneous tissue with large fat lobules. Most lesions are self-limiting and require no therapy; however, occasionally they may extensively calcify and spontaneously drain with subsequent scarring. Remember that significant hypercalcemia may be present in a small number of patients. Therefore, a serum calcium should be ordered.

7. How does sclerema differ from scleredema?
Sclerema neonatorum, a wax-like hardening of the skin and subcutaneous tissue, occurs in premature and debilitated infants in the first few weeks of life. It is usually associated with serious underlying disease (sepsis, congenital heart disease, respiratory distress, diarrhea, dehydration). It frequently starts on the legs and buttocks, and as it spreads the skin takes on a stony hard, whitish, cadaver-like appearance. The prognosis is poor, with mortality occurring in greater than 50% of infants. Scleredema is a rare disorder characterized by diffuse woody induration of large areas of the skin. Often of sudden onset following a febrile illness, it is twice as common in females as in males. It usually affects the posterior and lateral aspects of the neck and shoulders, with extension to the face, shoulders, arms, and thorax. In adults it has been associated with diabetes mellitus and following streptococcal infection. While the pathogenesis is unknown, the prognosis is good and spontaneous resolution usually occurs.

8. What is the appearance of erythema toxicum neonatorum?
Erythema toxicum is a common eruption composed of erythematous macules, papules, and pustules occurring in newborns usually in the first few days of life. The lesions may start as irregular, blotchy, red macules, varying in size from millimeters to several centimeters. They often develop into 1–3 mm yellow-white papules and pustules on an erythematous base, giving a "flea-bitten" appearance. They occur all over the body except on the palms and soles, which are spared because the lesions occur in pilosebaceous follicles, which are absent on the palmar and plantar surfaces. The rash is less common in premature infants, with incidence proportional to gestational age and peaking at 41–42 weeks. While it may be seen at birth, it is most common in the first 3–4 days of life and is occasionally noted as late as 10 days of life. Erythema toxicum usually lasts 5–7 days and heals without pigmentation.

9. How is the diagnosis of erythema toxicum confirmed?

There seems to be nothing "toxic" about this eruption, but it should be differentiated from impetigo neonatorum, herpes simplex, transient neonatal pustular melanosis, milia, or miliaria. The diagnosis can be confirmed by staining the contents of a pustule with Wright or Giemsa stain. Clusters of eosinophils confirm the presence of erythema toxicum.

10. What is the appearance and distribution of transient neonatal pustular melanosis?

Consisting of small vesicopustular lesions, 3–4 mm in size, transient pustular melanosis occurs in almost 5% of black and less than 1% of white newborns. It may be present at birth or appear shortly after birth. The lesions most often cluster on the neck, chin, palms, and soles, although they may occur on the face and trunk. They are easily ruptured, and progress to brown pigmented macules with a fine collarette of scale. Transient neonatal pustular melanosis is a benign disorder without associated systemic manifestations.

11. What are the causes of alopecia in children?

Some hair loss is due to disorders of the hair itself—follicles, sebaceous glands, growing phase, etc. Others are secondary to diseases of the scalp. A useful approach is to classify loss by pattern (diffuse vs. localized) and time of presentation (congenital vs. acquired):

Classification of Hair Loss

Congenital localized	Congenital diffuse
Sebaceous epidermal nevi	Hair shaft abnormalities
Melanocytic nevi	Trichorrhexis nodosa
Hemangiomas	Proximal
Lymphangiomas	Distal
Aplasia cutis	Familial
Incontinentia pigmenti	Arginosuccinicaciduria
Focal dermal hypoplasia	Pili torti
Chondrodysplasia punctata	Trichorrhexis invaginata
Sutural alopecia of the Hallermann-Streiff	(Netherton syndrome)
syndrome	Menkes' syndrome
Intrauterine trauma (e.g., scalp electrodes)	Monilethrix
Infection (e.g., gonococcal, herpes)	Trichoschisis
	Genetic syndromes:
	Ectodermal dysplasias
	Congenital hypothyroidism
	Marinesco-Sjögren syndrome
	Atrichia congenita
	Cartilage-hair hypoplasia
	(McKusick syndrome)
	Cockayne syndrome
	Amino acid disorders
Acquired localized	**Acquired diffuse**
Alopecia areata	Telogen effluvium
Tinea capitis	Anagen effluvium
Traumatic scarring	(may be drug, diet, or endocrine induced)
trichotillomania	Proximal trichorrhexis nodosa
friction	Lamellar ichthyosis
traction	Acrodermatitis enteropathica
burns	Endocrinopathies (e.g., hypothyroidism,
Seborrheic dermatitis	hypopituitarism)
Androgenic alopecia (male pattern baldness)	
Neonatal lupus	
Acne keloidalis	
Histiocytosis	
Linear scleroderma	

Adapted from Datloff and Esterly, Contemp Pediatr Oct 1986, pp 53–72.

12. Cutis aplasia of the scalp is commonly associated with which chromosomal abnormality?

Aplasia cutis congenita (more simply congenital absence of the skin) presents on the scalp as solitary or multiple well-demarcated ulcerations or atrophic scars. Of variable depth, the lesions may be limited to epidermis and upper dermis or occasionally extend to the skull and dura. While most children with this lesion are normal, scalp cutis aplasia has been classically associated with trisomy 13 syndrome.

13. How do strawberry hemangiomas differ from port-wine stains?

Strawberry hemangiomas are superficial, palpable, vascular nevi that usually involute with time. Port-wine stains, sometimes called nevus flammeus or salmon patches, are flat vascular malformations that do not involute.

Strawberry Hemangiomas	Port-Wine Stains
Palpable	Flat, macular
Common (approx. 10% of children < 1 yr)	Less common (0.1–0.3%)
Often inapparent at birth (most apparent at 2 weeks up to 1 yr)	Present at birth
Bright red	Pale pink to blue-red (darkens with age)
Well-defined borders	Borders variable
Blanch and compress with palpation	Incomplete blanching with pressure
Predilection for head and neck (40–60%)	May be anywhere, increased percentage on head and face
Pathology: proliferating angioblastic endothelial cells with variable blood-filled capillaries	Pathology: no abnormality until adolescence; then capillary dilatation is seen in the dermis
At 5 years, 50% involute; 7 years: 75–90% involute	No involution—may in fact worsen (elevate and darken)
May have rapid growth phase	Grows in proportion to child
Suggested Rx: allow for spontaneous involution	Laser (tunable dye laser seems promising)

14. When are systemic corticosteroids indicated in the treatment of cavernous or capillary hemangiomas?

While the approach to palpable hemangiomas generally involves observation over time (and perhaps compression therapy), indications for systemic corticosteroids include (1) Kasabach-Merritt syndrome with severe persistent thrombocytopenia (e.g., less than 40,000 platelets), (2) rapidly growing hemangiomas that involve vital structures, and (3) periocular hemangiomas that obstruct vision (to prevent amblyopia).

15. What is Kasabach-Merritt syndrome?

Kasabach-Merritt syndrome is thrombocytopenia associated with cavernous hemangiomas. The platelets are sequestered within the lesions. Usually presenting in the first few months of life, there is significant risk of ecchymosis and precipitous hemorrhage. While most of the lesions are cutaneous, the syndrome may be seen with hidden visceral hemangiomas as well.

16. What are the common varieties of diaper dermatitis?

Common Varieties of Diaper Dermatitis

	LOCALIZATION	SYMPTOMS	CHARACTERISTICS
Generic	Abdomen, thighs, buttocks, spares deep folds	Minimal	Moderate erythema, poorly marginated, dry, wrinkled skin
Candidal	Involves deep folds—may spread to entire diaper area	Moderate–substantial	Satellites, bright red *erosions*
Noduloulcerative	Prominent anterior parts, thigh, penis, scrotum, labia	Minimal	2- to 4-cm *firm* nodules with central ulcer; no cellulitis or adenopathy
Impetigo	Any site, but not usually the deep folds	Minimal	Usually blisters rupture rapidly leaving thin scale/crust; spreads rapidly to sites not covered by diaper
Infantile seborrheic dermatitis	Large confluent anterior surface of groin—usually spares posterior diaper area	None	Sharply marginated bright red plaques and satellites; no erosions–rapidly spreads to face, scalp, extremities, and other flexures
Intertrigo	Deep folds; slight white or yellow exudate	None moderate	Diffuse margins; no satellites; mild erythema

From Rasmussen J: Diaper dermatitis. Pediatr Rev 6:77–82, 1984, with permission.

17. What causes diaper dermatitis?

Generic irritant diaper rash has an unclear etiology, although it has been ascribed to ammonia, fecal material, pH, *Candida albicans,* and bacterial overgrowth, among others. The full story has yet to be uncovered, though uncovering is not a bad treatment for the condition. Uncommon causes include histiocytosis X, psoriasis, atopic dermatitis, granuloma gluteale infantum, tinea cruris, scabies, cutaneous larvae migrans, acrodermatitis enteropathica, congenital syphilis, and allergic contact dermatitis.

18. Are cloth diapers "better" than disposables?

There is no clear answer here, though there are parties who would swear by one or the other. Some studies have shown a decreased incidence of diaper rash with disposable diapers, and a further documented decrease in skin moisture and incidence of rash with superabsorbent diapers. The adjective "better" implies a value judgment, and other factors such as cost and convenience must be considered.

19. What are the cutaneous manifestations of histiocytosis X?

Clinical Feature	Examples
1. Rash in "seborrheic" distribution	Scalp, posterior auricular folds, diaper area, trunk
2. Biologically aggressive process	Petechiae, purpura, vesicles or bullae, erosions with crusting, ulceration, nodules, atrophy
3. Failure to respond to mild topical therapies for seborrheic dermatitis	Frequent shampooing, 1% hydrocortisone
4. Characteristic histopathology	Infiltrate with atypical histiocytes, electron microscopic identification of Birbeck granule, cytochemical markers for Langerhans cell histiocytes

From Williams M: Pediatr Rev 7:207, 1986, with permission.

20. What is the appearance of condyloma acuminatum and how is it acquired?

Condylomata acuminatum (anogenital warts) are soft, fleshy, wet, polypoid or pedunculated papules that appear in the genital and perianal area. They may coalesce and take on a cauliflower appearance. Of viral etiology, they may be transmitted by sexual contact (so-called venereal warts), and their presence in children should alert the examining physician to the possibility of sexual abuse.

21. What is the therapy for condyloma acuminatum?
A reasonable approach is 25% podophyllin resin in benzoin carefully applied and washed off well in 4–6 hours. Other approaches include trichloracetic acid, excision, and laser.

22. What is the triad of findings in acrodermatitis enteropathica?
Diarrhea, hair loss, and dermatitis are the presenting signs of this rare autosomal recessive disorder. The name nicely describes the disorder: (1) there is a classic acral distribution of the rash; it is usually eczematous, often with a vesiculobullous or pustular component, and involves skin around body orifices as well. (2) Enteropathica: serum zinc levels are extremely low, secondary to impaired gastrointestinal absorption. Dietary insufficiency of zinc may give an identical clinical picture. This has been found in children on long-term total parenteral nutrition without sufficient zinc, and in very premature infants due to decreased stores and increased requirement.

23. What is the differential diagnosis of seborrheic dermatitis in infancy and childhood?

Common Disorders	Rare Disorders
Seborrheic dermatitis	Histiocytosis X
Atopic dermatitis	Graft vs. host disease
Irritant contact dermatitis	Leiner disease
Candidal diaper dermatitis	Multiple carboxylase deficiency
Uncommon Disorders	Biotin deficiency
Psoriasis	Essential fatty acid deficiency
Dermatophytic (tinea) infections	Acrodermatitis enteropathica
Psoriasiform-id reaction	Zinc deficiency
Allergic contact dermatitis	

From Williams M: Pediatr Rev 7:205, 1986, with permission.

24. What is the difference between eczema and atopic dermatitis?
The term "eczema" derives from the Greek word "exzein," to erupt—ex (out) plus zein (to boil). To most physicians, eczema is synonymous with atopic dermatitis, a chronic skin disease manifested by intermittent skin eruption. Eczema is primarily a morphologic term used to describe an erythematous, scaling, inflammatory eruption with itching, edema, papules, vesicles, and crusts. There are other "eczematous eruptions" (nummular eczema, Wiskott-Aldrich syndrome) but "garden variety" eczema is certainly the most common. Atopic dermatitis is a broader allergic tendency with multiple dermal manifestations mostly secondary to pruritus. Jacquet stated that atopic dermatitis is an "itch that rashes, not a rash that itches." Its manifestations are dry skin, low threshold to pruritus, hyperlinear palms, eyelid pleats (Dennie's lines), pityriasis alba, and keratosis pilaris, among others.

25. What is cradle cap and how is it treated?
Seborrheic dermatitis of the scalp in infancy. It presents as a scaly rash on the scalp and may spread to the forehead, eyes, ears, eyebrows, nose, and back of head. It appears in the first few months of life and generally resolves in several weeks to a few months. Treatment consists of frequent shampooing with baby shampoo, use of an antiseborrheic shampoo, and removal of thick scales with mineral oil or petrolatum with gentle scrubbing. Occasional refractory cases respond to topical corticosteroid lotion. Seborrheic dermatitis is rare after 6 months of age and before adolescence.

26. Which dietary deficiencies are associated with an eczematous dermatitis?
Zinc, biotin, essential fatty acids, histidine, and protein (kwashiorkor).

27. Are there consistent immunologic alterations in children with atopic dermatitis?
Humoral changes include elevated IgE levels and a higher than normal number of positive skin tests (type 1 cutaneous reactions) to common environmental allergens. Cell-mediated abnormalities have been found only during acute flares of the dermatitis. These include: mild to moderate depression of cell-mediated immunity, a 30–50% decrease in lymphocyte-forming E-rosettes, decreased phagocytosis of yeast cells by neutrophils, and chemotactic defects of polymorphonuclear and mononuclear cells.

28. How is atopic dermatitis treated?
Atopic dermatitis is a chronic disorder for which there is no cure. (This needs to be explained to parents who often expect that once their child is clear, he or she will remain clear). Despite the chronicity of this skin condition, measures can be taken to reduce pruritus, hydrate the skin, reduce inflammation, control infection, and protect the skin from irritants and "triggers." (Note that treatment plans may vary from physician to physician).
    1. *Reduce pruritus.* This is crucial! It is important to break the itch-scratch cycle and to prevent new lesions from forming. Oral antihistamines should be used and titrated as needed to control itching. Some children may need higher than the recommended doses of Atarax and Benadryl.
    2. *Hydrate the skin.* Emollients (Vaseline, Eucerin, Nivea cream) prevent evaporation of moisture via occlusion and are best applied right after bathing, when the skin is maximally hydrated. Frequent bathing can actually dry out the skin; thus bathing should be limited to 2-3 times per week. Room humidifiers may also be beneficial.
    3. *Reduce inflammation.* Topical steroids are invaluable as anti-inflammatory agents and can hasten clearing of eruptions that are erythematous (inflamed). Medium-strength corticosteriods can be used on areas other than the face and perineum; low-strength steroids (such as 1% hydrocortisone) may be used in these thin-skinned areas.
    4. *Control infection.* Superinfection with *Staphylococcus aureus* is extremely common. Skin can be cultured and sensitivities obtained. Erythromycin and cephalosporins are the usual antibiotics of choice for infected atopic dermatitis. Resistance to erythromycin occurs frequently.
    5. *Avoid irritants.* Gentle soaps and shampoos should be used; wool should be avoided; tight garments may help minimize the "itchy" feeling; consider furniture, carpeting, pets and dust mites as possible irritants and/or trigger factors.

29. Do soaps or clothes make any difference in atopic dermatitis?
    Soaps: less drying, non-detergent soaps such as Dove, Tone, and Caress are better than more drying soaps such as Ivory. Other mild soaps include Purpose, Aveeno bar, and Basis; the latter is a superfatted soap.
    Clothing: avoid woolen clothes—the fibers can irritate the skin and trigger the itch-scratch cycle. If woolens must be used, they should be lined. Soft fibers are the least irritating and itchy (cotton jerseys).

30. Which bacteria commonly infects children with atopic dermatitis?
Children with atopic dermatitis frequently have a secondary infection with *Staphylococcus aureus* or possibly group A β-hemolytic streptococcus. The disruption of the epidermis allows bacteria to "set up shop" on the skin. Infected atopic dermatitis commonly resists therapy with topical steroids and emollients unless a systemic antibiotic is added to the regimen.

31. What is the usual distribution of the rash in eczema?

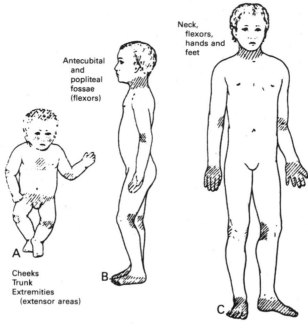

From Fleisher G, Ludwig S (eds): Textbook of Pediatric Emergency Medicine. Baltimore, Williams and Wilkins, 1983, p 654, with permission.

32. What features help to differentiate seborrheic from atopic dermatitis in infancy?

	Seborrheic dermatitis	Atopic dermatitis
Color	salmon	pink, red (if inflamed)
Scale	yellowish, greasy	whiter, non-greasy
Age	infants less than 6 months or adolescents	may begin 2–12 months and continue through childhood
Itching	not present	may be severe
Distribution	face; postauricular, scalp axillae and groin	(see previous diagram)
Associated features	none	Dennie's pleats, allergic shiners, palmar creases
Lichenification (thickening of skin with exaggerated skin markings)	none	may be prominent
Response to topical steroids	rapid	slower

33. What is dermographism and what is its clinical significance?

Dermographism occurs when the skin is stroked firmly with a pointed object. The result is a *red line*, followed by an *erythematous flare*, which is eventually followed by a *wheal*. This "triple response of Lewis" usually occurs within 1-3 minutes. Dermographism (or "skin writing") is an exaggerated triple response of Lewis and is seen in patients with urticaria. The tendency to be "dermographic" can appear at any age and may last for months to years. The cause is often unknown. "White" dermographism is seen in patients with an atopic diathesis. The red line is replaced by a white line without a subsequent flare and wheal.

34. What clinical features are useful for differentiating staphylococcal from streptococcal impetigo?

	Staphylococcal	Streptococcal
Etiology	*Staphylococcus aureus* (phage group II)	group A beta-hemolytic streptococcus (culture may grow *S. aureus* also)
Clinical lesions	flaccid blisters with erythematous areola	golden, honey-colored crusts develop after vesicles ooze serous fluid; lesions also consist of erythematous papules
Contagious?	yes	yes
Age affected	infants and children	infants and children
Seasonal?	no	summer more common
Distribution	face, trunk and extremities	legs, face
Fever, lymphadenopathy	late	early
Treatment	need antistaphylococcal antibiotic—dicloxacillin, erythromycin, or Keflex. Cultures should be done if lesions do not respond to treatment. Resistance to various antibiotics is common.	penicillin

35. What is Nikolsky's sign?

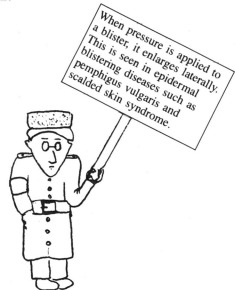

When pressure is applied to a blister, it enlarges laterally. This is seen in epidermal blistering diseases such as pemphigus vulgaris and scalded skin syndrome.

36. Which diseases should be considered in the differential diagnosis of impetigo?
Insect bites, nummular eczema, staphylococcal scalded skin syndrome, and staphylococcal folliculitis.

37. When should systemic antibiotics be used in infants with impetigo?
Impetigo should be treated with systemic antibiotics when it is extensive, and when localized areas are not clearing with conservative measures. Systemic antibiotics result in a higher and more predictable cure rate. The M. serotypes associated with nephritis are 2.49, 55, 57 and 60.

Note: A new topical antibiotic mupirocin (Bactroban, Beecham Labs., Bristol, TN) is now on the market and thus far has been shown to be more effective in treating impetigo than oral erythromycin.

38. What is the characteristic rash of hepatitis B infection?
Circulating immune complexes contribute to the pathogenesis of cutaneous manifestations of hepatitis B. The most common cutaneous associations of hepatitis B are urticaria and Gianotti-Crosti syndrome (papular acrodermatitis of childhood).
    1. *Urticaria.* "Hives" may be the major feature of the prodrome of hepatitis B infection. The rash may precede the arthralgias and the icterus and may last several days; it may also be maculopapular or petechial.
    2. *Gianotti-Crosti.* This syndrome consists of nonpruritic, erythematous, 1–5 mm papules arranged symmetrically on the face, buttocks, and extremities. The lesions erupt over a few days and do not become confluent. They may last for 3 weeks; lymphadenopathy may persist for months. This rash is classically associated with anicteric hepatitis, which develops at the same time as the rash or weeks later. Other viruses such as EBV may also be associated with these cutaneous findings.

39. When does the rash in poison ivy appear relative to exposure?
Poison ivy, or rhus dermatitis, is a typical delayed hypersensitivity reaction. The time between exposure and cutaneous lesions is usually 2–4 days. However, the eruption may appear as late as a week or more after contact (this explains why lesions continue to erupt after the initial "outbreak" of rash).

40. Can the allergen in poison ivy be transmitted from body part to body part?
The allergen in poison ivy can be transmitted only by that which has the plant's oleoresin on it. Direct contact with the plant, hands, clothing, or pets that have the oleoresin on them may produce transmission to any body part.

41. Are the vesicles in poison ivy contagious?
The contents of blisters do not contain the allergen. Washing the skin removes all surface oleoresin and prevents further contamination. The potent sensitizing oleoresin is called urushiol and is contained in all parts of the plants belonging to the anacardiaceae family (genus Rhus).

42. What is the Koebner reaction and in which diseases is it noted?
Koebnerization is an isomorphic response in which skin lesions occur at sites of local injury. The mechanism is unknown. The Koebner phenomenon is seen in psoriasis, warts, and lichen planus—to name a few.

43. What is the differential diagnosis of dermatoses of the feet in children?
The seven wonders of the foot: (1) juvenile plantar dermatosis, (2) allergic contact dermatitis, (3) tinea pedis, (4) scabies, (5) psoriasis, (6) granuloma annulare, and (7) plantar warts.

44. What is the classic appearance of "shoe dermatitis" and how can it be differentiated from tinea pedis?
Allergic contact dermatitis ("shoe dermatitis") involves the dorsa of the toes and distal third of the foot. The rash is red, scaly, and vesicular. KOH preparations of scrapings are negative. In tinea pedis ("athlete's foot") redness and scaling occur primarily on the instep or entire weightbearing surface, with maceration between the toes. The nails may be yellowed and thickened. The KOH preparation is positive for hyphae. Tinea pedis is very uncommon in prepubertal children.

45. What are the long-term adverse effects of ultraviolet radiation on the skin?

Wrinkling	Actinic keratoses ("pre" skin cancers)
Hyperpigmentation	Skin cancers

Hypopigmentation	"Leathery" changes of skin
Telangiectasias	Solar elastosis (degeneration of elastic
Atrophy	tissue)
	Increased suppressor T cells and
	decreased helper T cells.

It is important to remember that children need sunscreens too. Ultraviolet radiation can damage the skin whether or not a sunburn results.

46. What are the common photosensitivity disorders?
Polymorphous light eruption, solar urticaria, photoallergic and phototoxic reactions, phyto-photodermatitis (seen after contact with peels of lime/citrus fruits), and drug-induced photosensitivity.

47. What is the appearance of polymorphous light eruption and how is it diagnosed?
It is characterized by itchy red papules; plaques or papulovesicles appear several hours to days after ultraviolet light exposure. It can be diagnosed by phototesting (induction of lesions by intentional UV light exposure) and by skin biopsy. It is usually diagnosed by the classic history and exclusion of other photosensitivity disease.

48. Photosensitivity disorders are associated with which systemic diseases in children?
Lupus, the porphyrias, Bloom syndrome, xeroderma pigmentosum, Rothmund-Thomson syndrome, Cockayne syndrome, and Hartnup disease.

49. What drugs cause phototoxic and photoallergic reactions? Which type of reaction is more common?
Phototoxic: psoralens, tetracyclines, phenothiazines, sulfonamides, thiazides, and retinoic acids. *Photoallergic:* phenothiazines, sulfonamides, para-aminobenzoic acid esters (glyceryl p-aminobenzoate, Escalol 106), halogenated salicylanilides (tetrachlorosalicylanilide and tribromosalicylanilide). Phototoxic reactions are more common (e.g., sunburn) than pho-toallergic, which depend on circulating antibodies and occur either with or without a photosensitizer. Photopatch tests help to confirm the allergen.
Reference: Pediatr Rev 5:July 1983.

50. What are the wavelengths of light responsible for tanning and sunburns?
290–400 nm = tanning; 290–320 nm = burning

51. How do sunscreens work?
Sunscreens either form a physical barrier (zinc oxide) or absorb UVB (PABA) or block UVA (benzophenones). The SPF (sun protection factor) is the ratio of time it takes to develop erythema with sunscreen on the skin to the time it takes to develop erythema without a sunscreen applied. An SPF of 15 means a person can spend 15 times longer in the sun without burning. The lifetime incidence of squamous and basal cell carcinomas could be reduced by almost 80% if sunscreens (SPF 15 or higher) were used regularly during the first 18 years of life!

52. Are steroids effective in the treatment of severe sunburn?
Steroids may be useful in treating severe sunburn. A short course of prednisone (1–2 mg/kg/day) with tapering after 4–8 days may abort severe sunburn reactions and provide relief.

53. What is "berloque dermatitis" and how did it get its name?
Berloque dermatitis (French "berloque" = pendant) is an irregularly patterned hyperpigmen-tation of the neck due to photosensitization by 8-methoxypsoralen and other furocoumarins in perfumes. It is caused by fragrances that contain oil of bergamot, an extract from the peel of an orange grown in southern France and Italy. Oil of bergamot contains 5-methoxypsoralen, which enhances the erythematous and pigmentary response of UVA.

54. What is the "Auspitz sign" and in which disorder is it noted?

The appearance of punctate bleeding points after removal of a scale. It is seen in psoriasis and is related to the rupture of capillaries high in the papillary dermis of lesions (near the skin surface).

55. What is the usual distribution and appearance of the lesions of childhood psoriasis?

A bilaterally symmetrical pattern with a distinct predilection for scalp, knees, elbows, presacral and genital regions. The classic lesions are either guttate (tear-drop) or round, erythematous, well-demarcated plaques covered with a silvery white micaceous scale.

56. What percentage of children with psoriasis have nail involvement?

Although pitting is said to be seen less often in childhood psoriasis than in the adult form, it is more common than is realized. Approximately 80% of children with psoriasis demonstrate pitting of the nails. Other nail changes include onycholysis (separation of nail plate from nail bed at distal margin) and thickening of the nail plate, often with white-yellow discoloration.

57. Which joints are classically involved in psoriatic arthritis?

The distal interphalangeal joints of the hands and feet. Juvenile psoriatic arthritis (<16 years old) often presents as an acute monoarthritis. Joint changes often precede the skin changes. Psoriatic arthritis is more common in patients who have severe psoriasis. Flares are unrelated to the skin condition.

58. What is Mucha-Habermann disease?

Another name for this disorder, often confused with chickenpox, is PLEVA (pityriasis lichenoides et varioliformis acuta). Generally speaking, the longer the name assigned to a particular dermatologic entity, the less likely a clear etiology has been established. Successive crops of papules appear which progress to form vesicles or necrotic centers. Frequently, the skin changes last a few weeks or months. At times, recurrences continue for several years. Other than chickenpox, this entity is often misdiagnosed as impetigo, vasculitis, or scabies. Rickettsialpox may even be considered. A skin biopsy clearly establishes the diagnosis (i.e., perivascular lymphocytic infiltrate with red blood cells migrating from the dermis to the epidermis). Sunlight, natural or artificial, ameliorates the pruritus and the skin changes. Oral erythromycin may help to clear the eruption.

59. What are the histopathologic differences between a "blackhead" and a "whitehead"?

Both lesions are produced by obstruction and distention of the sebaceous follicle with sebum and cellular debris. When the follicular contents tent the overlying skin but are not exposed to the atmosphere, a whitehead occurs. If the contents project out of the follicular opening, oxidation of the exposed mass of debris produces a color change, "black" head.

60. What is a current accepted treatment of acne and when should a child with acne be referred to a dermatologist?

Therapy of acne is two-pronged and directed at several hypothesized abnormalities that acne patients exhibit. The lining cells of the follicular channel do not desquamate, which leads to obstruction of the sebaceous follicule. Debris and sebum are trapped and the bacterium responsible for acne (*Propionibacterium acnes*) replicates. Low molecular weight particles produced by this organism attract white blood cells, which insinuate through the follicular wall. Following ingestion of *P. acnes* the white blood cell releases enzymes, which rupture the follicular wall. Once the contents of the follicle are emptied into the dermis, an inflammatory response is triggered (including the complement cascade). This results in inflammatory lesions (papules, pustules, and cysts). Retinoic acid cream is used to unstick the follicular cells that form the lining of the follicle. Obstruction is therefore prevented. Topical and systemic antibiotics reduce the concentration of bacteria responsible for the acne process. Acne that is difficult to control (progressing rapidly, producing scarring, or is cystic), should be treated by a dermatologist. Many times alterations in the use of current medications is all that is necessary. In other instances, Accutane will be required.

61. Does chocolate make a difference in outbreaks of acne?
According to "controlled" studies, no! However, never let it be said that I forced an acne patient to eat chocolate just to prove a point. If a patient says that chocolate makes the acne worse, I say don't eat it!

62. Should systemic antibiotics be given to children with severe acne?
Absolutely! Acne can leave permanent scars (cosmetic and psychological), and prolonged courses of tetracycline or erythromycin may be required to try to prevent a negative outcome. Patients have been on these antibiotics for more than five straight years without ill effects.

63. What is the importance of facial cleansing in acne control?
It certainly is a good idea to wash the face to remove previously applied medications. However, vigorous scrubbing can actually worsen acne by causing the clogged distended follicles to rupture. This then sets off the inflammatory cycle. One must also caution acne patients to pat the skin dry with a towel rather than rub it dry. Same reason!

64. What are the principles of topical acne therapy?
1. Never apply a topical medication to wet skin! (wait ½ hour after washing)
2. Dispense no more than a "pea-sized" amount of medication onto the finger.
3. Touch affected areas of skin with a dab of medication (not each comedone or pimple)
4. Gently spread medication over acne-prone region of skin.
5. Wash finger that was in contact with medication.
6. Warn patients of possible side effects:
   Benzoyl peroxide (1 in 10 have allergic reaction and get fiery red skin).
   Retin A cream (erythema and peeling are normal initially; marked redness and severe stinging are not!)
7. Don't apply lotions, creams, makeups, or other potions that are comedogenic.

65. What are the side effects and toxicity of oral cis-retinoic acid?

Side Effects		Toxicity
Common	*Uncommon*	
Dry skin	Musculoskeletal pain	Dysmorphogenesis
Dry mucous membrane	Corneal opacities	Liver (increase SGOT, SGPT)
Epistaxis	Edema	Pseudotumor cerebri
Pruritus	GI complaints	
Alopecia	Headaches	
Curly hair	Tiredness	
Paronychia	Permanently dry eyes	
Dry eyes	Increased triglycerides	
Conjunctivitis	Increased cholesterol	
	Skeletal hyperostosis	
	Premature epiphysial closure	
	Exuberant granulation tissue	

66. What is acne fulminans?
The acute onset of numerous inflamed, painful, ulcerated, and crusted acne lesions in association with fever, chills, malaise, weight loss, and musculoskeletal pain (polyarthralgia) indicates the presence of acne fulminans. These individuals may have leukocytosis, an increased sedimentation rate, anemia, hematuria, and osteolytic lesions. Unlike acne conglobata, which occurs more frequently in females, most patients with acne fulminans are males. Comedones are absent in contrast to acne conglobata. Although no known etiology has been determined, immune complexes are thought to be involved. Prednisone is the drug of choice.

67. How is neonatal acne differentiated from milia and erythema toxicum?

	Neonatal acne	Milia	Erythema toxicum
Distribution	face	face +	face +
Appearance	papule or pustule	yellow or white papule	yellow or white papule
Erythematous	+	−	+
Contents on smear	PMNs	keratin + sebaceous material	eosinophils
Incidence	occasional	40–50% of infants	30–70% of infants (premie to fullterm), 0%–59% of infants 30–42 wks
Course	last several months	disappear in 3–4 weeks	disappear in 2 weeks

68. What is "prickly heat"?

The scientific name for this condition is miliaria. It is due to sweat retention. Its clinical morphology is determined by the level at which sweat is trapped. Sweat trapped at a superficial level produces clear vesicles without surrounding erythema (sudamina); miliaria rubra (prickly heat, erythematous papules, vesicles, papulovesicles) is produced by sweat trapped at a deeper level; pustular lesions are produced with sweat retention at the deepest of levels (infants rarely develop this type). With the advent of air conditioning, this problem now rarely occurs in newborn nurseries.

69. What is the malignant risk of congenital pigmented nevi?

Unfortunately the answer is as clear as melanin. No prospective studies have been done as yet to clarify this issue. Although one author suggested malignant conversion in 10% of cases, the actual incidence is probably far below that level. Melanoma is rare during the preadolescent period! Prospective studies are currently under way. It is, therefore, very difficult to counsel families as to what action should be taken. Some feel it is better to be safe than sorry. Others feel if all congenital nevi were removed many unnecessary procedures would have to be carried out. Remember the greatest risk from general anesthesia occurs in the first year of life. Psychologically, any procedure is tolerated better when the child is 4 to 5 years of age or older.

70. What are the causative organisms of tinea capitis?

Until 1950 Microsporum was the agent most frequently responsible for tinea capitis. However, since that time the "tide has turned." Currently, Trichophyton is the predominant organism:

> *Trichophyton tonsurans*   *Trichophyton verrucosum*
> *Microsporum audouini*   *Trichophyton violaceum*
> *Microsporum canis*   *Trichophyton schonleinii*

71. What is the treatment for tinea capitis?

Griseofulvin: 15 mg/kg/day of the microsize preparation is given in two divided doses with a glass of milk. The child is shampooed biweekly with 2.5% selenium sulfide to decrease the risk of spread of spores.

72. How is scabies treated?

The best therapeutic agent currently is lindane (5% permethrin cream, a safer preparation, is currently awaiting FDA approval). Simultaneous treatment of all contacts is most effective. Lindane applied for 6 hours is almost as effective in clearing a mite infestation as when it is kept on for 24 hours (i.e., 96% effective vs 98% cure rate). Unfortunately, reports of adverse effects (CNS toxicity due to preferential deposition in the fatty tissue of the brain) have led some to question the safety of this preparation. It certainly should not be used in pregnant females and malnourished individuals (whose only fatty tissue is brain substance). Whether it should be used in children in a stage of rapid brain development (i.e., under 1 year of age) is debatable. The alternative therapies are not as effective. Studies show crotamiton to be much less likely to eradicate the mite. Some suggest that a greater number of consecutive days of therapy (i.e., more than the two recommended above) may produce better results. An added benefit of this preparation is its antipruritic effects. The sulfur ointment is not only less effective, it causes a dermatitis that develops in the flexors and on the nipples. It must be stressed that all family members and all close contacts should be treated simultaneously. Treatment failures are frequently related to this omission or to poor compliance. Thick crusting in debilitated and immunosuppressed individuals may protect the mites and prevent adequate therapy (removal of these crusts is essential). A subungual reservoir of mites has also been reported to be a cause of treatment failures. Although the issue of resistance to scabicides has been raised when treatment failures occur, no such instances have been proved in the United States. Physicians must make their patients aware of the fact that lesions and pruritus may linger for one or two weeks after effective threapy. One must be supportive during this time to prevent unnecessary retreatment by parents. Antihistamines and topical steroids can be helpful for the symptoms. Intralesional steroids may be necessary for persistent nodular lesions.

73. What causes "swimmer's itch"?

Penetration of the skin by the cercariae of schistosomes. Schistosomes are parasitic flatworms that are microscopic in size.

74. What are the varieties of epidermolysis bullosa and how are they inherited?

Classification of Epidermolysis Bullosa (EB)

Disease	Inheritance	Other designation
Nonscarring		
Generalized EB simplex	Autosomal dominant	EB simplex
Localized EB simplex	Autosomal dominant	Recurrent bullous eruption of the hands and feet (Weber-Cockayne)
Junctional EB	Autosomal recessive	EB letalis Herlitz disease
Scarring		
Dystrophic EB	Autosomal dominant	
Dystrophic EB	Autosomal recessive	
Acquired EB		EB acquisita

From Honig PJ: Epidermolysis bullosa. Ostomy/Wound Management 10:18–20, 1986, with permission.

75. What are some of the associated findings of acquired epidermolysis bullosa?

This disorder is very similar to the inherited form of EB. It is acquired rather than genetic and seen first during adolescence or adulthood. Immunoelectron-microscopy localizes the immune deposits below the basement membrane. Therefore, the split is in a location similar to the dominantly inherited *dystrophic* form of EB. These patients blister following trauma. Scarring, milia formation, and nail dystrophy occur. Only the oral mucous membranes are involved. Other diseases associated with acquired EB and thought to be possible precipitants include amyloidosis, dermatitis herpetiformis, Ehlers-Danlos syndrome, impetigo, ingestions (arsenic, penicillamine, sulfonamides), inflammatory bowel disease, poison oak, porphyria, scarlet fever, and tuberculosis.

76. What are the metabolic causes of hyperpigmentation?

Hepatobiliary disorders
Hemochromatosis
Addison's disease
Hyperthyroidism
Hypothyroidism
Acromegaly
Cushing's syndrome
Heavy metals (silver, gold, mercury)
Drugs (thorazine, antimalarials)

Fixed drug eruptions (phenolphthalein,
barbiturates, bisulfan, Cytoxan, ASA,
phenacetin, Dilantin, gold, arsenic,
sulfur, tetracycline)
Porphyria cutanea tarda, variegate
porphyria
Gaucher's disease
Niemann-Pick disease
B_{12} deficiency
Wilson's disease
Hyperparathyroidism

77. Which trace element deficiency is associated with Menkes' kinky hair syndrome? What are the features of this syndrome?

This syndrome is thought to be secondary to inappropriate systemic copper distribution and storage. Plasma copper and ceruloplasmin levels are low. Features include:

X-linked recessive
Coarse facies
Pili torti, monilethrix, trichorrhexis
nodosa
Hypothermia
Seizures

Psychomotor retardation
Growth failure
Arterial abnormalities
Poorly pigmented hair
Scorbutic bone changes (similar to child
battering)

78. What are the characteristic findings of urticaria pigmentosa?

The characteristic lesions of urticaria pigmentosa are red-brown, brown, yellow-brown, or yellow macules, papules, plaques, or nodules that have a rippled surface (peau de orange). The lesions are oval or round and frequently are mistaken for pigmented nevi or xanthoma. They vary in size from several millimeters to many centimeters. They occur on any portion of the skin surface but tend to concentrate on the trunk. The diagnosis is clinched by stroking the lesion. This maneuver causes degranulation of the collection of mast cells, release of histamine, and urtication (Darier's sign).

79. What is the characteristic clinical picture of erythema nodosum?

A prodrome of fever, chills, malaise, and arthralgia may precede the typical skin findings. Crops of red to blue tender nodules appear over the anterior shins. Lesions may be seen on the knees, ankles, thighs, and occasionally, lower extensor forearms and face. They may evolve through a spectrum of colors that resemble a bruise. Often the changes are misdiagnosed as cellulitis or secondary to a traumatic event.

80. What infectious and noninfectious conditions are associated with erythema nodosum?

Infectious
Group A beta-hemolytic strep.
Tuberculosis
Yersinia
Coccidioidomycosis
Histoplasmosis
North American blastomycosis
Psittacosis
Lymphogranuloma venereum
Ornithosis
Cat-scratch fever
Measles

Noninfectious
Sarcoidosis
Ulcerative colitis
Regional ileitis
Hodgkin's disease
Lymphosarcoma
Leukemia
Bençet's syndrome
Sulfonamides
Halogens
Contraceptives

81. What are Gottron's papules?

These skin changes are pathognomonic for dermatomyositis. They begin as inflammatory papules over the dorsal interphalangeal joints. The papules become violaceous in color and flat-topped. Finally, atrophy, telangiectasia, and hypopigmentation are left behind.

82. What are skin findings in tuberous sclerosis?

Age at Onset	Skin findings	Incidence
Birth or later	Hypopigmented macules	80%
2–5 years	Angiofibromas	70%
2–5 years	Shagreen patches	35%
Puberty	Periungual and gingival fibromas	20–50%
Birth or later	Café au lait spots	26%

83. What syndromes are associated with café-au-lait spots?

Neurofibromatosis
Bloom syndrome
Tuberous sclerosis
Ataxia telangiectasia
Multiple lentigenes syndrome
Russell-Silver syndrome
Epidermal nevus syndrome
Pulmonary stenosis
Temporal lobe dysrhythmias
Basal cell nevus syndrome

84. What are "mongolian spots"?

Deep collections of spindle-shaped melanocytes. Because of their depth they appear blue-black or slate-gray. Seen mainly in dark-skinned individuals [Black (90%), American Indian (90%), Oriental (80%), Latin (70%), Caucasian (10%)] they usually fade by 2 years of age and disappear by 10 years of age. They are typically found on the buttocks, lumbosacral areas, extremities, back, and shoulders. On rare occasions they may be diffuse.

85. What are "salmon patches" and what is their usual distribution?

Salmon patches are distended dermal capillaries. When seen at the nape of the neck (20%), they have been termed "stork bites." They are one of the most common vascular lesions seen at birth. They also occur on the glabella (5%), upper eyelids (5%), or on both sites (20%). The nasolabial skin may also be involved. They tend to become less prominent over time.

Bibliography

1. Hurwitz S: Clinical Pediatric Dermatology. Philadelphia, W.B. Saunders Co., 1981.
2. Rasmussen J: Diaper dermatitis. Pediatr Rev 6:77–82, 1984.
3. Schachner LA, Hansen RC: Pediatric Dermatology. New York, Churchill Livingstone, 1988.
4. Weinberg S, Leider M, Shapiro L: Color Atlas of Pediatric Dermatology. New York, McGraw Hill, 1975.
5. Weston W: Practical Pediatric Dermatology. Boston, Little, Brown and Co., 1985.

EMERGENCY MEDICINE

Mark F. Ditmar, M.D.

1. Why is the airway of an infant or child prone to obstruction?

1. Simple physics. Because airflow is inversely proportional to the airway radius raised to the fourth power (the oft-cited Poiseuille's law), small changes in the diameter of the trachea can result in very large drops in airflow. An infant has less margin of safety.

2. An infant has relatively looser mucosal tissue than an adult and this tissue can readily swell with infection or inflammation.

3. The relative lack of cartilage in an infant's trachea can result in collapse with hyperextension. This is particularly important if CPR is performed with vigorous extension of the neck. Air exchange may then be obstructed.

4. Children have a normal narrowing of the trachea at the level of the cricoid ring.

5. The typical peanut and an infant's mainstem bronchus always seem to fit hand-in-glove.

2. How is the jaw-thrust maneuver performed?

With the neck in slight extension, lift the jaw by the bases (rami) of the mandible. This lifts the tongue as well, often clearing an obstructed airway.

3. Is there any use for the "precordial thump" in pediatric CPR?

Even in witnessed and documented ventricular fibrillation, the thump is felt not to be more effective than routine external compressions in terms of converting the abnormal rhythm, and there is increased risk of internal organ damage.

4. What emergency drugs can be given down an endotracheal tube?

E–LAINE (Endotracheally–Lidocaine, Atropine, Isuprel, Narcan, and Epinephrine).

5. Is there ever an indication for intracardiac epinephrine?

Epinephrine is rarely administered via the intracardiac route: it interrupts CPR and can cause tamponade, coronary artery laceration, or pneumothorax. If epinephine is accidently given into the cardiac muscle rather than the ventricular chamber, intractable ventricular fibrillation or cardiac standstill may result.[25] Intracardiac epinephine may be tried as a last resort if all other treatments have failed. It may be used as an initial treatment if other vascular access (peripheral or central IV, intraosseous or endotracheal tube) is not available.

6. When is atropine indicated during resuscitation?

For bradycardia, particularly when the etiology of the slow heart rate is excessive parasympathetic stimulation of the heart (e.g., digoxin or hyperactive carotid sinus reflex) and other resuscitative measures (such as ventilation) have already been initiated. The deleterious effects of a slow heart rate are more likely to occur in a younger child, whose cardiac output is more dependent on rate changes than volume or contractility changes. Atropine may also be of transient help in overcoming second and third degree block and slow idioventricular rates.

7. What risks are associated with administration of atropine?

If the dose of atropine is too small, paradoxically worsening bradycardia may result. This is due to atropine's central stimulating effect at lower doses on the medullary vagal nerve, which in turn slows AV conduction and heart rate. Standard dosing of atropine in a setting of bradycardia is 0.01 mg/kg IV. However, at least 0.2 mg should be used even in the youngest patient.

8. When is calcium useful during a resuscitation?
Calcium is used much less than in the past and is no longer felt to have a role in the treatment of ventricular fibrillation or asystole. There is evidence that calcium may increase post-ischemic injury in the intracranial reperfusion phase following resuscitation. Calcium may be justified in four settings of resuscitation: (1) an overdose of a calcium channel blocker, (2) hyperkalemia resulting in cardiac dysrhythmia, (3) electromechanical dissociation of the heart if there is no mechanical cause (e.g., pneumopericardium) and no response to bicarbonate or epinephrine therapy, and (4) infants and children with a low serum calcium. For an excellent review of calcium's role in resuscitation and its historical decline, see Hughes and Ruedy.[13]

9. How do pediatric and adult defibrillation differ?
Smaller dosing: 2 watt-sec/kg and then doubled as needed; smaller paddles: standard pediatric paddles are 4.5 cm in diameter (vs. 8 cm in adults); and rarer use in pediatrics: ventricular fibrillation is quite uncommon in children.

10. What is an intraosseous line?
An intraosseous line is a rapid means of vascular access utilizing the readily reachable marrow cavity of bone which drains into the central venous system. Fluid and drug distribution and rates appear to be comparable to intravenous infusions, including circumstances of closed chest massage. The technique is straightforward and involves placing a needle with stylet into the proximal or distal tibia or distal femur. Intraosseous lines are becoming an accepted second line of emergency access if rapid venous access is not obtained.[31]

11. What size endotracheal tube should be used for resuscitation?
A good rule of thumb:
$$\text{internal diameter (mm): } \frac{16 + \text{ age in years}}{4}$$
For example, a 2-year-old would warrant a 4.5 mm tube by this formula. Since this is an approximation, the next smaller or larger size tubes should be available. To convert internal diameter size to French catheter size, multiply x 4. A 5.0 tube is 20 French.

12. If a child suddenly becomes asystolic and resuscitation is not initiated, what is the time course of pupillary changes?
15 seconds after the arrest, pupillary dilatation begins and is complete at 1 minute and 45 seconds.

13. What is the average amount of time needed to establish intravenous access in a pediatric emergency room resuscitation?
In one study by Rossetti,[28] 7.8 minutes. In nearly 25%, at least 10 minutes was required. In 6% of the arrests, IV access was not obtained. An IV cutdown took an average of 24 minutes. A strong case can be made for intraosseous infusions.

14. How successful is pediatric emergency room resuscitation?
Unobserved cardiorespiratory arrest in children carries a grim prognosis, much worse than in adults. More than 90% do not survive. Of the survivors, nearly 100% are vegetative or have severe neurological sequelae.

15. Why is resuscitation less successful in children than in adults?
A large percentage of adults collapse and arrest from primary cardiac disease and associated arrhythmias—ventricular tachycardia and fibrillation. These are more readily reversible and carry a better prognosis. Children, however, have cardiac arrest as a secondary phenomenon

from other processes such as respiratory obstruction or apnea often associated with infection, hypoxia, acidosis, or hypovolemia. Primary cardiac arrest is rare. By the time a child has cardiac arrest, severe neurological damage is usually present and other disease processes make resuscitation more difficult.

16. What factors in non-hospital arrests have a better prognosis for survival?
Witnessed arrest, ventricular fibrillation, non-SIDS patients, non-trauma patients, and intubation done on-site by EMT personnel.[19]

17. What are the criteria for stopping a resuscitation?
There is no precise answer. A review of resuscitation at Children's Hospital of Philadelphia following cardiopulmonary arrest found that long-term survival improved when the duration of CPR was less than 15 minutes. There were no survivors when two rounds of medication (epinephine and bicarbonate) were given without improvement.[23] Unwitnessed out-of-hospital arrests in children are nearly always associated with death or neurologic devastation.[32] In hypothermia, asystolic patients should be rewarmed to 36°C before resuscitation is discontinued.

18. What is the difference between livor mortis and rigor mortis?
Livor mortis or dependent lividity is the gravitational pooling of the blood that results in a line of mauve staining in the dependent half of a recently deceased body. It usually is noticeable 30 minutes after death and is very marked at 6 hours. Rigor mortis is the muscular stiffening and shortening that results from ongoing cellular activity and depletion of ATP after death with increasing lactate and phosphate and salt precipitation. Neck and facial changes begin at 6 hours, shoulders and upper extremities at 9 hours, and trunk and lower extremities at 12 hours. Livor mortis and rigor mortis are absolute indications not to initiate a resuscitation. They should be looked for during the initial rapid assessment. In the confusion of the moment, they may be easily overlooked.

19. What are the top ten errors in running a resuscitation?
One subjective list in order of increasing frequency is as follows:
    Leader of code not clearly designated
    Failure to place nasogastric tube
    Failure to give proper meds in response to situation
    Failure to periodically assess breath sounds, pupils, pulses
    Delay in access before attempting intraosseous line or other
    Leader of code too involved with individual procedure
    Failure to assign roles
    Failure to assess patient initially
    Failure to observe adequate cardiac compressions
    Excessively lengthy resuscitations for out-of-hospital arrests

20. What is the Glasgow coma scale and what is its prognostic significance?
Developed in 1974 by the neurosurgical department at the University of Glasgow, the scale was an attempt to standardize the assessment of the depth and duration of impaired consciousness and coma, particularly in the setting of trauma. The scale is based upon eye opening, verbal responses, and motor responses, with a total score ranging from 3 to 15.

Glasgow Coma Scale

Best verbal response	5	oriented, appropriate conversation
	4	confused conversation
	3	inappropriate words
	2	incomprehensible sounds
	1	no response

Table continued on next page.

Glasgow Coma Scale *(Continued)*

Best motor response	6	obeys a verbal command
(to command or pain,	5	localizes
such as rubbing	4	withdraws
knuckles	3	abnormal flexion (decorticate posturing)
on sternum)	2	abnormal extension (decerebrate posturing)
	1	no response
Eye opening	4	spontaneous
	3	in response to verbal command
	2	in response to pain
	1	no response

A Glasgow score greater than 5 generally indicates a good prognosis for full recovery. A score of 5 or less has a poorer prognosis, but not grim. For a look at the remarkable recuperative powers of pediatric patients in coma, see Mahoney et al.[20] In this study, nearly two-thirds of patients in coma with initial Glasgow scores less than 5 survived, and of those, nearly two-thirds returned to their pretraumatic state.

21. How should a child with suspected epiglottitis be evaluated in the emergency room?
Rapid, calm evaluation is needed. Because of the risk of airway obstruction with agitation, the patient should be: allowed to remain with parents, free from restraint, and examined as delicately as possible. If necessary, this may be done from a distance, and always without inspection of the oropharyanx because of the risk of provoking obstruction. No blood studies should be drawn. In children with typical signs of epiglottitis—ill-appearing, anxious or limp, drooling, protruding jaw, febrile—there must be rapid mobilization of equipment and personnel for the placement of an artificial airway. This is most properly done in an operating room. If the diagnosis is uncertain (e.g., croup or retropharyngeal abscess or other possibilities), a lateral x-ray should be obtained, but always with a physician and intubation equipment.

22. What are the criteria for admission of a child with viral croup?
    1. Clinical signs of impending respiratory failure: marked retractions, depressed level of consciousness, cyanosis, hypotonicity, and diminished or absent inspiratory breath sounds.
    2. Laboratory signs of impending respiratory failure: PCO_2 >45 mm Hg, PAO_2 <70 mm Hg in room air.
    3. Clinical signs of dehydration.
    4. Social considerations: unreliable parents, excessive distance from hospital.
    5. Historical considerations: high-risk infant with history of subglottic stenosis, prior intubations.
    6. Previous administration of racemic epinephine to decrease stridor. Hospitalization is warranted in this situation due to the risk of "rebound" obstruction.

23. Is a chest x-ray (CXR) necessary for all children who wheeze for the first time?
Statistically, children over 1 year of age who wheeze for the first time are having their initial presentation of asthma. In infants less than 1 year of age, asthma and bronchiolitis are the two most common diagnoses. An oft-heard slogan is "all that wheezes is not asthma" and CXRs are often recommended for children on their initial wheezing to rule out other diagnostic possibilities such as heart failure, pneumonia, or foreign body aspiration. If the history or physical exam is suspicious for a non-asthmatic diagnosis, such as weight loss and adenopathy suggesting a mediastinal mass, then clearly a CXR is indicated. For wheezing alone, the vast majority of CXRs will not add any new information for diagnosis or treatment. A CXR might be considered in the following situations:
    1. A first-time wheezing patient, especially an older child, with no family history of asthma or atopy.
    2. Suspected pneumonia (high fever, localized rales or locally diminished breath sounds).

3. Suspected foreign body aspiration.

Even though the proper evaluation is far from clear, if you don't order a CXR on a first-time wheezer, be prepared for stern questioning on rounds. The heartland of pediatrics is filled with anecdotes of the simple wheeze that turned out to be a multiloculated fascinoma.

24. When should hydrocortisone be given during the initial management of an asthmatic attack?

Corticosteroids arguably are beneficial in the treatment of asthma. They increase sensitivity to bronchodilators, diminish production of tenacious sputum, and lessen mucosal edema. With short-term therapy (less than 2 weeks), there is almost no risk of serious toxicity.[34] Mild attacks usually can be managed without steroids. Moderate to severe asthmatic attacks warrant the use of steroids if: (1) an attack is incompletely relieved by bronchodilator therapy in an outpatient setting, but the patient is not sick enough to be hospitalized; or (2) an attack is severe enough to warrant hospitalization, in which case intravenous hydrocortisone is appropriate.

The use of steroids prophylactically at the first sign of an upper respiratory infection to prevent a virally induced exacerbation is generating interest. Brunette et al.[5] found a 90% decrease in hospitalization and a 56% decrease in attacks in known asthmatic children younger than 6 years given 1 mg/kg/day of prednisone along with their usual medications at the onset of coryza, cough, or sore throat.

25. Which asthmatics should be admitted to the hospital?

Admission is warranted if after therapy a patient has depressed level of consciousness, severe retractions, cyanosis, severe wheezing, or markedly diminished breath sounds. Other considerations that usually require admission include dehydration, arrhythmias (usually due to inhaled bronchodilators), pneumothorax, history of severe attacks involving prolonged hospitalization and/or intubation, or parental unreliability. A more difficult (but unanswerable) question relates to which patients will relapse after responding to therapy and subsequently require hospitalization. This is a major problem, as rates of relapse can approach 20–30%.

26. What laboratory studies are needed in suspected carbon monoxide poisoning?

The main physiologic problem in carbon monoxide poisoning is tissue hypoxia due to hemoglobin's much stronger binding of carbon monoxide at the expense of oxygen carriage and release. Primary laboratory studies should include:

1. Blood carboxyhemoglobin concentration: 20%—mild intoxication; 60%—coma and possible death

2. Hemoglobin concentration to evaluate a correctable anemia

3. Arterial pH to evaluate acidosis

4. Urinalysis for myoglobin

Patients with carbon monoxide poisoning are susceptible to tissue and muscle breakdown with possible acute renal failure resulting from renal myoglobin deposition.

Reference: Thompson AE: Environmental emergencies. In Fleisher G, and Ludwig S (eds): Textbook of Emergency Medicine. Baltimore, Williams and Wilkins, 1983, pp 591–592

27. What is the treatment of carbon monoxide poisoning?

1. Very close monitoring

2. 100% oxygen until carboxyhemoglobin levels fall to 5%: the half-life of carboxyhemoglobin is 4 hours if the subject is breathing room air (at sea level), 1 hour in 100% oxygen (at sea level) and <1 hour in a hyperbaric oxygen chamber with 100% oxygen.

3. Correct metabolic acidosis if pH < 7.3.

4. Transfuse with packed red blood cells for a hemoglobin concentration < 10 gm/dl.

5. If myoglobinuria is present, consider vigorous hydration and furosemide and/or mannitol therapy to maintain a urine output of at least 1 ml/kg/hr.

28. What is the differential diagnosis of hyperglycemic coma?
Diabetes mellitus
Hypernatremic dehydration
Salicylate overdose (although hypoglycemia is more common)
Iron overdose
Acute pancreatitis
Central nervous system hemorrhage or asphyxia
Coma with chronic liver or chronic renal disease

29. Up to what age should patients with fever be admitted?
This is controversial. A 1981 survey demonstrated the enormous variance in management styles for neonatal fever. In this study, neonatal fever was defined as temperature greater than 37.8°C in infants during the first 2 months of life. Of pediatric chief residents, about 95% recommended hospitalization, whereas only 9% of general pediatricians felt hospitalization was warranted.[18] Generally, larger teaching hospitals empirically admit infants less than 2 months of age with fever, while general pediatricians do not, owing in large part to the latter's certainty of careful follow-up. It is an area of pediatric care in vigorous search of more precision.

30. What is occult bacteremia?
The clinically unsuspected finding of bacteria in the blood of patients, usually between 3 months and 24 months of age, who are febrile without an apparent focus of infection. This term should be distinguished from "septicemia"—the growth of bacteria in the blood from a child with the clinical picture of toxicity and shock.

31. How should children with "occult bacteremia" be managed?
The typical scenario addressed here is the telephone call at 48 hours into an illness when the microbiology lab announces a positive blood culture result. The child should then be reexamined.
    1. If the examination is normal and the organism recovered is *S. pneumoniae*, it is generally safe to reculture the child and observe. If the blood culture is positive for *Hemophilus influenzae, N. meningitidis* or salmonella, the child should be admitted and treated.[22]
    2. If the examination is abnormal, the child should be admitted and begun on antibiotics.
    An earlier management question is whether children with high fever and no source for that fever on physical exam should be given prophylactic antibiotics in an effort to prevent possible complications of occult bacteremia such as meningitis, septic shock, or pneumonia. One recent study[15] found no evidence that routine oral use of amoxicillin in children with fever greater than 39°C prevented major focal infectious morbidity associated with bacteremia.

32. When should children with lacerations be given antibiotic prophylaxis?
This is controversial, but a conservative set of guidelines would include:
    1. Lacerations involving cartilaginous exposure of the nose or ear
    2. Wounds of the perineum
    3. "Dirty wounds" (trash sites, farm settings, gravel- or dirt-covered areas)
    4. Animal bites: requiring resuturing for cosmetic reasons; significant deep tear or puncture wounds; or hand wounds.
    5. Lacerations associated with significant crush injury (where deep tissue necrosis may be ongoing)
    6. All human bites, especially from closed-fist injury (may be joint or tendon exposure)

33. What are the recommendations for tetanus toxoid booster in a child with a laceration?

Guidelines for Tetanus Prophylaxis

NO. OF PRIMARY IMMUNIZATIONS	YEARS SINCE LAST BOOSTER	TYPE OF WOUND	RECOMMENDATION*
2	Irrelevant	Low risk	T
		Tetanus prone	T + TIG
3	10	Low risk	T
		Tetanus prone	T
3	5–10	Low risk	No treatment
		Tetanus prone	T
3	5	Low risk	No treatment
		Tetanus prone	No treatment

*T = tetanus toxoid, TIG = human tetanus immune globulin.
From Fleisher G: Infectious disease emergencies. In Fleisher G, Ludwig S (eds): Textbook of Pediatric Emergency Medicine. Baltimore, Williams and Wilkins, 1983, p 409, with permission.

Low-risk wounds include those that are recent (< 6 hours), not infected or contaminated with feces, soil or saliva, superficial enough to permit irrigation and debridement, and surrounded by viable tissue. Typically, these are linear lacerations. Tetanus-prone wounds include those that don't fit the above criteria and wounds typically caused by puncture, crush, injury, burns, or frostbite. (See also chapter on Immunization.)

34. How many days should sutures remain in place?
In general, as the site of laceration proceeds, from head to toe, the length of time of suture placement increases: eyelids—3 days; scalp, face—5 days; trunk and upper extremities—7 days; and lower extremities—10 days.

35. Which lacerations should be repaired by a surgeon?
  Large complex lacerations
  Stellate or flap lacerations
  Lacerations with questions of tissue viability
  Lacerations involving lip margins (vermillion border)
  Deep lacerations with nerve damage
  Lacerations that evoke intention tremors in the medical house officer

36. In what instances are the use of xylocaine with epinephrine contraindicated as an anesthetic?
When there is a question of tissue viability and in any instance in which vasoconstriction might produce ischemic injury to an "end organ" without an alternative blood supply (e.g., tip of nose, margin of ear, tip of finger or toe), xylocaine with epinephrine should not be used.

37. Should human bites be sutured?
Generally, human bites should not be sutured. Because the human mouth is a veritable gutter of organisms compared to the animal mouth, there is a greater risk of infection with human bites. Unless there is a cosmetic need for suturing (e.g., face or neck injuries), human bites should be left open. In either case, they should be observed very carefully for signs of infection.

38. How is a human bite distinguished from a dog bite?
Human bites generally are crush injuries rather than tear injuries. The distance between the two main puncture sites (caused by the "canines" or cuspids) can be helpful. A distance greater than 3 cm suggests a human bite.

39. When should a nerve injury be suspected in a finger laceration?
1. Abnormal testing of sensation (diminished pain or two-point discrimination)
2. Abnormal autonomic function (absence of sweat or lack of wrinkling of skin after soaking in water)
3. Diminished range of motion of finger (may also indicate joint, bone or tendon disruption)
4. Pulsating blood emerging from wound (on flexor aspect, nerve is superficial to digital artery and arterial flow implies nerve damage)

40. What should be done if nerve damage is suspected?
Immediate repair is not essential and this is not a true emergency. Delayed nerve repair is very satisfactory, particularly in younger children. If an operating suite and personnel are not poised to proceed, skin closure can be done and the operation deferred. Care must be taken not to stop the arterial bleeding with a hemostat or other clamp as this may further damage the nerve. Simple pressure, often for extended periods, generally suffices.

41. How should traumatically amputated digits be handled?
The severed digit should be cleansed (with sterile normal saline and not Betadine), wrapped in saline-soaked gauze, kept in a water-tight package, and placed on ice. Successful reimplantations have been performed for fingers up to 24 hours and for arms and hands up to 4 hours. Severe crush injuries cannot be repaired.[2]

42. What are the indications for skull x-rays in children with head trauma?
There are almost no *routine* indications for skull x-rays in the setting of trauma. Skull fractures have been shown to correlate very poorly with intracranial injury. If significant intracranial injury is suspected because of altered mental status or focal neurological exam, a CT scan is indicated. Skull x-rays may be warranted if there is:
1. Suspicion of a depressed skull fracture by palpation or by history such as head injury by a projectile.
2. Suspicion of a basilar skull fracture (e.g., blood in middle ear or CSF discharge from ear or nose).
3. Significant head trauma in an infant with an open fontanel in order to evaluate suture widening.
4. Medico-legal considerations in cases of suspected child abuse.

43. How should children with linear skull fractures be managed?
No therapy or hospitalization is required for an alert child with a simple linear skull fracture and a nonfocal neurologic exam. An exception to this rule might be an infant with an open fontanel who should be hospitalized for observation. There is a theoretical risk that fractures across the grooves of the middle meningeal artery or sagittal sinus will have a higher risk of complications, and these children may warrant hospitalization for observation.

44. What are the clinical signs of acutely increased intracranial pressure?
Early: headache, nausea, vomiting, dizziness, diplopia, unsteady gait
Late: papilledema, deterioration of consciousness, bradycardia, dilation of pupil(s), decerebrate posturing

45. What are the options for medical management of acutely increased intracranial pressure following head trauma?
Intubation with mechanical hyperventilation to lower $PaCO_2$
Gentle tracheal toilet + sedation to minimize intracranial pressure spikes
Maintenance of "adequate" systemic blood pressure (systolic blood pressure exceeding intracranial pressure as measured by an intracranial transducer)
Positioning in a 30° head-up position to facilitate central venous drainage
Avoidance of overhydration

Barbituate coma
Hypothermia
Mannitol and diuretics
Steroids

46. What are the emergency room priorities in the evaluation of a child with a headache?

As with all common presenting symptoms, the emergency room physician's main priority is to rule out diagnostic possibilities that may be life-threatening—the "diagnostic exigencies." The main causes of headache in these categories are (1) malignant hypertension, (2) increased intracranial pressure (e.g., mass lesion and/or acute hydrocephalus), (3) intracranial infections (e.g., meningitis, encephalitis), (4) subarachnoid hemorrhage, (5) stroke, and (6) acute angle closure glaucoma (eye-threatening, but rare in children).

47. What are the initial symptoms of spinal cord compression?

67%—motor weakness (e.g., limp)

50%—pain (may be radicular in distribution with accentuation by cough, spinal flexion or spinal percussion)

33%—sensory disturbances and autonomic disturbances, including bowel and bladder dysfunction

rare—signs of increased intracranial pressure due to hydrocephalus, usually from a high cervical tumor.[1]

48. What are the different degrees of burn injuries?

Classification of Burn Wounds

DEGREE	DEPTH	INCHES	CLINICAL APPEARANCE	CAUSE
1°	Epidermis	0.002	Dry—erythematous	Sunburn, scald
2°	Superficial dermis	0.02	Blisters, moist, erythematous	Scald, immersion, contact
	Deep dermis	0.035	White eschar	Grease, flash fire
3°	Subcutaneous	0.040	Avascular—white or dark, dry, waxy (yellow)	Prolonged immersion, flame, contact, grease, oil
4°	Muscle		Charred, skin surface cracked	Flame

From Coren CV: Burn injuries in children. Pediatr Ann 16:328–329, 1987, with permission.

49. Which burn injuries require hospitalization?

Second degree burns covering more than 10% of body surface area (BSA)

Third degree burns covering more than 2% of BSA

Significant burns involving hands, feet, face, or perineum

Self-inflicted burns

Burns resulting from child abuse

Explosion, inhalation, or chemical burns (where other organ trauma may be involved)

Significant burns in children with chronic metabolic or connective tissue diseases (in whom healing may be compromised with the increased risk of secondary infection)

Significant burns in children younger than age 2 years

50. What are the three most important considerations in children with suspected smoke inhalation?

The questions to ask are:

1. Are there signs of smoke inhalation? Physical exam may reveal carbonaceous sputum, singed nasal hairs, facial burns, or pulmonary abnormalities. These make development of pneumonitis more likely.

2. Are there signs of impending airway obstruction due to mucosal injury and edema? These would include increasing respiratory distress, difficulty in handling secretions or stridor.

3. Are there signs of carbon monoxide poisoning and tissue hypoxia? Possibilities include headache, confusion, irritability, visual changes or other CNS abnormality. Their presence would warrant aggressive oxygen therapy, including consideration of hyperbaric oxygen if available.

51. What is heatstroke?

Heatstroke is a medical emergency of multisystem dysfunction caused by very high fever (usually greater than 41.5°). Profound CNS disturbance—confusion, seizures, loss of consciousness—is the hallmark of the condition. Other problems include (1) hypotension due to volume depletion, peripheral vasodilatation, and myocardial dysfunction, (2) acute tubular necrosis and renal failure with marked electrolyte abnormalities, (3) hepatocellular injury and dysfunction, (4) abnormal hemostasis, often with signs of DIC, and (5) rhabdomyolysis.

52. What is the "critical thermal maximum"?

42°C. This is the body temperature at which cell death begins as physiologic processes unravel. Enzymes denature, lipid membrances liquefy, mitochondria misfire, and protein production fails.[21]

53. What important historical and physical findings are indicators of child abuse?

Historical:
1. Previous multiple hospital visits for injuries
2. History of untreated injuries
3. Cause of trauma not known or inappropriate for age or activity
4. Delay in seeking medical attention
5. History incompatible with injury findings
6. Parents unconcerned about injury or more concerned about unrelated minor problem (e.g., cold, headache)
7. History of abused siblings

Physical Examination:
1. Signs of general neglect, poor hygiene, or failure to thrive
2. Withdrawn or explosive personality
3. Burns, especially cigarette, or immersion burns to buttocks or perineum
4. Genital trauma or venereal infection
5. Signs of excessive corporal punishment (welts, belt or cord marks, bites)
6. Multiple lesions in various stages of resolution
7. Neurologic damage associated with retinal hemorrhages
8. Fractures suggestive of abuse.

From Kottmeier, P: Pediatr Ann 16:343–351, 1987; and Fontana V: Pediatr Ann 13:740, 1984, with permission.

54. What fractures are suggestive of child abuse?

Spinal fractures, posterior and anterior rib fractures, skull fractures, metaphyseal chip fractures, and vertebral, femoral, pelvic, or scapular fractures. These are fractures that commonly result from twisting, throwing, and beating. Metaphyseal chip fractures are the result of the forceful jerking of an extremity. Anterior and posterior rib fractures occur with severe side-to-side compression of the thorax. They are almost never caused by CPR. The description and forcefulness of injury should be consistent with the fracture. One should be especially suspicious if such fractures occur in a child not yet walking.

55. What is the "shaken baby" syndrome?

This syndrome is the most common cause of severe closed head trauma in children less than one year of age. It results from violent shaking of an infant with resultant intracranial hematomas and subarachnoid hemorrhages. The diagnosis is suggested by retinal hemorrhages and bloody or xanthochromic spinal fluid. Confirmation is by CT or MRI scanning. The prognosis is grim for an infant presenting in coma from this abuse. Fifty percent die and nearly half of the survivors have significant neurologic sequelae.

56. What data need to be obtained in the emergency room when caring for the sexually abused child?

The following protocol for children with suspected sexual abuse is used at Children's Hospital of Philadelphia:

Evidence Collection for Sexually Abused Children

TEST	INDICATIONS
1. Gonococcal cultures	History of contact
Pharynx	*or*
Vagina or cervix	Loss of consciousness
Rectum	*or*
	Poor history
2. Urine pregnancy test	Postmenarchal patient
3. Pap smear	If speculum examination is done
4. 2 swabs:	Each body area with seminal secretions by
1 in 0.5 ml saline	history or examination
1 smear on glass slide	
5. Saliva sample: spit; or swabs in 0.5 ml saline	As control for test (4)
	or
	Oral-genital contact
6. Venipuncture	
Rapid plasma reagin test	Same as for (1)
3–5 ml of serum for blood group antigens	As control for (4) and/or (5)
7. Foreign pubic hairs and controls	If present (must be *plucked*)

From Ludwig S: Child abuse. In Fleisher G, Ludwig S (eds): Textbook of Pediatric Emergency Medicine. Baltimore, Williams and Wilkins, 1983, p 1051, with permission.

57. What percent of sexual abuse is committed by individuals known previously by a child or adolescent?

70–80%

58. What are poor prognostic indicators for victims of near-drowning?

Orlowski[25] has categorized five indicators (with one point for each):
   1. Age <3 years
   2. Estimated maximum submersion time longer than 5 minutes
   3. No attempts at resuscitation (i.e., CPR) for at least 10 minutes after rescue
   4. Patient in coma on admission to emergency department
   5. Arterial blood gas pH <7.10

For a score <2, there is a 90% chance of recovery. For a score >3, there is only a 5% chance of recovery.

59. How is the degree of dehydration estimated in a child?

Dehydration in Children: Clinical Signs*

CLINICAL SIGNS	MILD	MODERATE	SEVERE
Activity	Normal	Lethargic	Lethargic to coma
Color	Pale	Gray	Mottled
Urine output	Decreased (<2–3 ml/ kg/hr)	Oliguric (1ml/ kg/hr)	Anuria
Fontanel	Flat	Depressed	Sunken
Mucous membranes	Dry	Very dry	Cracked
Skin turgor	Slight decrease	Marked decrease	Tenting
Pulse	Normal to increased	Increased	Grossly tachycardic
Blood pressure	Normal	Normal	Decreased
Weight loss	5%	10%	15%

*Hypernatremic dehydration may occur with only moderate changes in clinical signs.
From Rogers MC (ed): Textbook of Pediatric Intensive Care. Baltimore, Williams and Wilkins, 1986, p 509, with permission.

60. Are MAST trousers of value in pediatric resuscitation?
Also called pneumatic anti-shock garments (PASGs), the MAST (military anti-shock trousers) suit is a pneumatic device that inflates around the lower extremities and pelvis. There are increasing reports in adults of its positive benefits (augmentation of blood pressure in hypovolemic patients, stabilization of pelvic fractures) and potential negative effects (exacerbation of internal bleeding above the diaphragm, possible compartment syndrome with lower extremity fractures). There is very little literature on its role in pediatrics, although use of the MAST suit in children to augment blood pressure and stabilize pelvic fractures in trauma settings appears to be increasing.

61. When are steroids indicated in the treatment of shock?
The controversy regarding steroids relate to their role in treating septic shock. There are data in animals that steroids given prior to, or concomitantly with, endotoxin can improve survival. In the actual clinical setting, early steroids have not been shown to decrease long-term mortality, although they may be helpful in early reversal of shock. This includes two large recent studies in adults. Less is available relating to their use in pediatrics, and they remain an unproven therapy. Because of the theoretical benefits of steroids, they may be considered in children with shock not responsive to conventional measures. One reason to give steroids in the setting of unexplained shock is the possibility of adrenal insufficiency, such as in overwhelming meningococcal infections (Waterhouse-Friderichsen syndrome).

62. Is colloid or crystalloid better for the treatment of hypotension?
Colloid (blood, fresh frozen plasma or 5% or 25% salt-poor albumin) and crytalloid (Ringer's lactate, normal saline) are equally effective for the treatment of hypovolemic hypotension. In the setting of hypovolemic shock, use whatever product is most readily available. Certain instances might warrant tailoring of the volume expander. Hypotension due to large recent blood loss is best treated with whole blood or packed red blood cells and plasma to correct the anemia. Ringer's lactate would be less appropriate in the setting of hyperkalemia and hypotension because it contains 4 mEq K^+/liter. One should always remember the risks of blood products as volume expanders and the cost of albumin, which is nearly 50–100 times that of normal saline.

63. A large bolus of air has accidently been injected into a 6 year old child. What is the proper treatment?
The main problem is that the air can block the right ventricular outflow tract or main pulmonary artery. This is similar to "vapor lock" in automobiles in which air in the carburetor prevents fuel from flowing and a stall results. The patient should be placed in a steep head-down position with the right side up to trap air in the upper right ventricular chamber and prevent passage to the outflow tract. Therapeutic options include (1) 100% oxygen; (2) careful monitoring, including EKG leads; (3) observation for symptoms or signs of arrhythmia, hypotension, or cardiac arrest; (4) if air is auscultated in the heart, a right ventricular tap should be considered; and (5) if arrest occurs, standard CPR should be initiated, as manual compression may help to dislodge air emboli.

64. Name four true dental emergencies (require immediate evaluation by a dentist).
    1. Tooth fractures involving the pulp of a secondary tooth (hemorrhaging noted from central core of tooth)
    2. Primary or secondary tooth intrusion (tooth pushed into socket)
    3. Secondary tooth extrusion (vertical displacement out of socket)
    4. Secondary tooth avulsion (a tooth that has been knocked out). A dentist should be consulted immediately only if the tooth is available for reimplantation.
    Reference: Nelson L: Dental emergencies. In Fleisher G, Ludwig S (eds): Textbook of Pediatric Emergency Medicine. Baltimore, Williams and Wilkins, 1983, pp 998–1004.

65. How should parents be advised when 4-year-old son's front baby tooth has been knocked out?

If the tooth was completely knocked out, it should not be reimplanted. Pressure at the site to control the bleeding is all that is necessary. No emergency room visit is necessary. The tooth fairy must be notified to provide the customary rate. If part of the tooth remains in the socket, the patient should be brought to the emergency room or a dentist because an intruded tooth (pushed in) may interfere with secondary dentition.

66. What are the indications for diagnostic peritoneal lavage?

Peritoneal lavage, the infusion and aspiration of fluid from the peritoneal cavity, has been used as a diagnostic test for abdominal bleeding and perforation of the intestine. It was most commonly used following blunt abdominal trauma. This test has been very accurate in assessing intraabdominal injury in the past, particularly intraperitoneal hemorrhage (97–98% accuracy). It is being supplanted by abdominal CT scan with and without contract, which can detect hemoperitoneum and pneumoperitoneum, specific organ injuries, and retroperitoneal injuries. Indications now might include (1) rapid assessment of occult intraabdominal hemorrhage in a patient with nonabdominal trauma requiring urgent operative repair (insufficient time for CT), (2) equivocal CT results, and (3) unavailable CT.[4]

67. What is the first diagnostic study indicated in a clinically suspected splenic tear?

If the patient is stable, a CT scan with contrast.

68. A 7-year-old is admitted with an x-ray proven pelvic fracture. What urologic procedure is needed?

The urethra as it passes through the prostate is very close to the pubic bone and is thus susceptible to injury when there is disruption by a pelvic fracture. Urethral damage should be suspected in all patients with pelvic fractures. This is true even without hematuria. The recommended diagnostic procedure is a retrograde urethrogram. Of note, a boggy, high-riding prostate found on rectal exam and/or blood seen at the urethral meatus are clinical signs of possible urethral disruption.

69. In the setting of abdominal trauma, when is an intravenous pyelogram indicated?

1. *Hematuria.* Most significant renal injuries (exceptions below) will have hematuria, although the extent of hematuria does not correlate with the severity of injury. An IVP helps define the type of injury: contusion, superficial cortical laceration, deeper caliceal laceration, complete renal fracture, vascular pedicle injury, or renal artery thrombosis. The IVP can also define congenital or acquired abnormalities that may predispose to hematuria in the setting of even mild trauma. Dipstick analysis for blood without microscopic evaluation is insufficient, as myoglobin from muscular injury can cause a positive reading.

2. *Fracture of twelfth rib or vertebral transverse process.* Because of its close proximity, the kidney is susceptible to lacerations from these fractures.

3. *Palpable flank mass.* If caused by complete renal fracture, pedicle injury, or vascular thrombosis with urine or blood extravasation, the patient usually demonstrates signs of shock. Importantly, pedicle injury or vascular thrombosis often demonstrate no hematuria.

4. *Significant flank pain or nausea.* Either may be a sign of severe renal injury along with possible intraperitoneal or retroperitoneal pathology.

If transport to a radiology department is not possible, the study may be done acutely in the emergency room. Renografin (meglumine diatrizoate) is given at a dose of 3 cc/kg and portable abdominal films are taken at 1 and 15 minutes. This will give good resolution of asymmetric renal filling, renal architecture, and dye extravasation due to injury.[12]

70. What percentage of major abdominal trauma in children is due to penetrating injuries?

Less than 10%, contrasted to 50% in teenagers and adults.

71. What are the three most important considerations in the evaluation of nasal trauma?

1. *Bleeding.* If persistent, bleeding should be controlled with pressure, topical vasoconstrictors, cauterization, and anterior or posterior nasal packing.

2. *Septal hematoma.* If the nasal septum is bulging into the nasal cavity, there is likely a hematoma that must be drained. If no drainage is done, abscess formation or pressure necrosis can result in a cartilaginous septum, leading to a saddle nose deformity.

3. *Watery rhinorrhea.* This may be a sign of cribriform plate, suborbital ethmoid, sphenoid sinus, or frontal sinus fracture with CSF leak. Classically, CSF glucose is high and rhinorrhea from a URI is low, but this distinction is often not present. Confirmation is needed by radioisotope scans or CT scan with metrizamide dye. If positive, hospitalization is warranted for observation and prophylactic antibiotics due to the risk of meningitis.

More extensive facial trauma requires evaluation for many items, especially midface fractures and eye pathology. Determining if the nose is fractured is a lower priority item because: fracture reduction is done only if there is distortion of the nose; distortion usually cannot be properly assessed acutely due to swelling; and reductions can be delayed.

72. How long before a broken nose in a child must be reduced?

If a nasal bone fracture is causing asymmetry, which is noted as the swelling from acute trauma subsides, the fracture should be reduced within 4–5 days because of the rapid rate of healing. A delay longer than this may result in malunion.

73. In which region of the anterior nasal septum do most nosebleeds begin?

Kisselbach's plexus

74. What features suggest gonococcus as the likely cause of pelvic inflammatory disease (PID)?

(1) Onset of symptoms during menstruation, (2) patient lacks previous episode of PID, (3) three or more leukocytes from cervical swab containing gram-negative intracellular diplococci, and (4) sexual partner with gonorrhea.

75. What is the Fitz-Hugh–Curtis syndrome?

A perihepatitis caused by gonococci and less commonly by chlamydia. It is characterized by high fever and right upper quadrant tenderness that may be mistaken for acute hepatitis or cholecystitis. The pathophysiology appears to be direct spread from a pelvic infection along the paracolic gutters to the liver where inflammation and capsular adhesions form (the so-called "violin string" adhesions seen on surgical exploration). The key to making the diagnosis is suspicion the RUQ pain may not be primary. On exam, there is vaginal discharge and adnexal tenderness and lab tests reveal normal or only mildly elevated LFTs and intracellular diplococci on Gram stain of the discharge.

76. What is the differential diagnosis of vaginal bleeding?

At Any Time	After Menarche
Trauma	Dysfunctional uterine bleeding
Tumor	Bleeding diathesis
Before Normal Menarche	Gonorrhea
Hormonal	Birth control pills
1. Neonatal bleeding	Intrauterine device
2. Exogenous estrogen	Ectopic pregnancy
3. Precocious puberty	Spontaneous abortion
Nonhormonal	Placenta previa
1. Urethral prolapse	Abruptio placentae
2. Vaginitis	
3. Foreign body	

From Paradise JE: Vaginal bleeding. In Fleischer G, Ludwig S (eds): Textbook of Pediatric Emergency Medicine. Baltimore, Williams and Wilkins, 1983, p 256, with permission.

77. How do the color changes in an ecchymosis progress?
0–1 day: reddish-blue
1–5 days: purple/blue
(~1 week) 5–7 days: green/yellow
(~1½ weeks) 7–14 days: brown
1½–4 weeks: resolution

78. What is the normal tidal volume of a child?
Approximately 7 cc/kg

79. What cardiovascular changes occur as body temperature falls?
35–32°:   elevated HR, cardiac output, and blood pressure; peripheral vasoconstriction and increased central vascular volume; and normal EKG.
32–28°:   diminished HR, cardiac output, and blood pressure; and EKG irregularities: PVCs, supraventricular arrhythmias, atrial fibrillation, and T wave inversion.
Below 28°: severe myocardial irritability: ventricular fibrillation, usually refractory to electrical defibrillation; often absent pulse or blood pressure; and EKG: "J" waves

80. What are the hazards of rewarming a hypothermic patient too rapidly?
1. Core temperature "afterdrop"—seen especially in external rewarming, which causes peripheral vasodilatation and initially return of cold venous blood to core.
2. Hypotension—peripheral vasodilatation increases total vascular space, and hypothermia is often a hypovolemic state because of cold-induced diuresis and cold-induced renal tubular and concentrating ability dysfunction in the setting of depressed myocardial function.
3. Arrhythmias—rewarming alters acid-base and electrolyte status in the setting of irritable myocardium.
These hazards are more likely to occur if external rewarming techniques (electric blankets, overhead warmers, bath immersion) are used alone rather than with core rewarming techniques (warm IV fluids, peritoneal dialysis or hemodialysis, inhalation rewarming, or extracorporeal blood rewarming).

81. Why do victims of submersion usually suffer from heat loss and clinical hypothermia?
The thermal conductivity of water is 32 times greater than that of air.

82. Why are alkali burns worse than acid burns of the eye?
Alkali burns are caused by lye as in Drano or Liquid Plumr, by lime, and by ammonia among others. They are worse than acid burns because the damage is ongoing. When spilled in the eye, acid is quickly buffered by tissue and limited in penetration by precipitated proteins. Damage is usually limited to the area of contact. Alkali, however, has a more rapid and deeper advancement, causing progressive damage at the cellular level by combining with membrane lipids. This underscores the importance of extended irrigation of the eyes, particularly in alkali burns.

83. What is the difference between hordeolum, sty, and chalazion?
Clinically, very little. For anatomic and pathologic purists, there are moderate differences. The sebaceous and apocrine sweat glands of the eyelid consist of those that drain near the eyelash follicle (glands of Moll and Zeis) and those that drain nearer the conjunctiva (Meibomian glands).

Hordeolum—purulent, usually staphylococcal infection of these glands; external hordeolum on skin side if Moll or Zeis involved and internal hordeolum on conjunctival side if Meibomian; red, swollen, tender—a mini-abscess.

Sty—an external hordeolum

Chalazion—initially a non-inflamed lipogranulomatous swelling in the Meibomian gland which readily can become superinfected; an internal hordeolum; more likely to be chronic and require excision.

No matter what the name, all are treated with warm compresses and topical antibiotic drops and usually resolve within 7 days.

84. What are the most common infectious causes of conjunctivitis by age?

Less than 2 days	Chemical (silver nitrate)
2 days to 2 weeks	*Chlamydia trachomatis* ("inclusion blennorrhea")
	Neisseria gonorrheae
	Escherichia coli and other gram-negative bacilli
2 weeks to 3 months	*C. trachomatis*
	Viral
	N. gonorrheae
	Staphyloccocus aureus
	Streptococcus species
	E. coli and other gram-negative bacilli
Greater than 3 months	Viral
	Allergy
	Bacterial, any above

From Diamond GR: Red eye. In Fleischer G, Ludwig S (eds): Textbook of Pediatric Emergency Medicine. Baltimore, Williams and Wilkins, 1983, p 229, with permission.

85. If complete testicular torsion has occurred, how long before the testis is not surgically resalvageable?

6 hours. However, it is clinically impossible to distinguish partial from complete torsion and thus duration of symptoms should not be used as a gauge for determining viability. Duration of symptoms does correlate with abnormal testicles on follow-up examination, underscoring the need for prompt diagnosis. Two-thirds of patients with testicles salvaged between 12 and 24 hours after the onset of symptoms had palpable evidence of testicular atrophy on followup, compared with only 10% when the diagnosis was made in less than 6 hours.[30]

86. What is Kehr's sign?

A sign of potential trouble. Kehr's sign is left shoulder pain felt after abdominal trauma, often elicited by LUQ palpation or by placing the patient in the Trendelenburg position. It is referred pain caused by diaphragmatic irritation and often by blood, and may be a sign of splenic rupture.

87. What is the difference between a felon and a paronychia?

A paronychia is an inflammation or infection in the soft tissue adjacent to the nail (onyx = nail, Greek). A felon is an infection (often an abscess) in the fat pad spaces (also known as volar pulp) of the distal phalanx.

88. What is the DiFabrizio theorem of medical education?

$$\text{Knowledge} \propto \frac{1}{\text{lecturing ability}}$$

Bibliography

1. Allegretta G, et al: Oncologic emergencies. Pediatr Clin North Am 32:601–611, 1985.
2. Almquist EE: Hand injuries in children. Pediatr Clin North Am 33:1523–1540, 1987.
3. Bone RC, et al: A controlled clinical trial of high-dose methylprednisolone in the treatment of severe sepsis and septic shock. N Engl J Med 317:653–658, 1987.
4. Bresler MJ: Computed tomography vs. peritoneal lavage in blunt abdominal trauma. Topics Emerg Med 10:59–73, 1988.
5. Brunette MG, Lands L, Thibodeau L: Childhood asthma: Prevention of attacks with short-term corticosteroid treatment of upper respiratory tract infection. Pediatrics 81:624–629, 1988.
6. Coren CV: Burn injuries in children. Pediatr Ann 16:328–339, 1987.
7. Emergency Medicine Symposium III. University of California, San Diego. June 20–24, 1988, pp 164–186. (Office of Continuing Medical Education.)
8. Fleisher G, Ludwig S (eds): Textbook of Pediatric Emergency Medicine. Baltimore, Williams and Wilkins, 1983; second edition 1988.
9. Fontana V: The maltreatment syndrome of children. Pediatr Ann 13:740, 1984.
10. Geishel JC, et al: The usefulness of chest radiographs in first asthma attacks. N Engl J Med 1983, 309:336–339, 1983.
11. Greene JW, et al: Management of febrile outpatient neonates. Clin Pediatr 20:375–380, 1981.
12. Hoover DL: Genitourinary trauma. Topics Emerg Med 4:57, 1982.
13. Hughes W, Ruedy J: Should calcium be used in cardiac arrest? Am J Med 81:285–296, 1986.
14. Jaffe AC: Animal bites. Pediatr Clin North Am 30:405–413, 1983.
15. Jaffe DM, et al: Antibiotic administration to treat possible occult bacteremia in febrile children. N Engl J Med 317:1175–1180, 1987.
16. Kernig E, Chernick V: Disorders of the Respiratory Tract in Children. Philadelphia, W.B. Saunders, 1983, pp 18–19.
17. Kottmeier P: The battered child. Pediatr Ann 16:343–351, 1987.
18. Leonidas JC et al: Mild head trauma in children: When is a roentgenogram necessary? Pediatrics 69:139–143, 1982.
19. Losek JD, et al: Prehospital care of the pulseless, nonbreathing pediatric patient. Ann Emerg Med 5:370–374, 1987.
20. Mahoney WJ, et al: Long-term outcome of children with severe head trauma and prolonged coma. Pediatrics 71:756–762, 1983.
21. McElroy CR: Update on heat illness. Topics Emerg Med 2:1–18, 1980.
22. McLellan D, Giebink GS: Perspectives on occult bacteremia in children. J Pediatr 109:1–8, 1986.
23. Nichols D, et al: Factors influencing outcome of cardiopulmonary arrest in children. Crit Care Med 1984, 12:287, 1984.
24. Orlowski JP: Cardiopulmonary resuscitation in children. Pediatr Clin North Am 27:495–512, 1980.
25. Orlowski JP: Drowning, near drowning and ice water submersions. Pediatr Clin North Am 34:87, 1987.
26. Roberts F, Shopfner CE: Plain skull roentgenograms in children with head trauma. AJR 114:230–240, 1972.
27. Rogers MC (ed): Textbook of Pediatric Intensive Care. Baltimore, Williams and Wilkins, 1986.
28. Rossetti V, et al: Difficulty and delay in intravascular access in pediatric arrests. Ann Emerg Med 13:406, 1984.
29. Rushton AR: The role of the chest radiograph in the management of childhood asthma. Clin Pediatr 21:325–328, 1982.
30. Sheldon CA: Undescended testis and testicular torsion. Surg Clin North Am 65:1303–1329, 1985.
31. Spivey WH: Intraosseous infusions. J Pediatr 111:639–643, 1987.
32. Torphy DE, et al: Cardiorespiratory arrest and resuscitation of children. Am J Dis Child 158:1099–1102, 1984.
33. VA Cooperative Study Group: Effect of high-dose glucocorticoid therapy on mortality in patients with clinical signs of systemic sepsis. N Engl J Med 317:659–665, 1987.
34. Weinberger M: Clinical pharmacology of drugs used for asthma. Pediatr Clin North Am 1981, 28:47–69, 1981.

ENDOCRINOLOGY

Daniel E. Hale, M.D.

1. What laboratory tests are indicated in the evaluation of suspected thyroid dysfunction?

Diseases of the thyroid represent a heterogeneous group of disorders. As such, there are no "standard" thyroid function studies appropriate for all children with suspected thyroid disease. Laboratory testing is based on the patient's signs and symptoms. If the clinical findings suggest *hyperthyroidism*, the quantity of circulating thyroxine (T_4) and tri-iodothyronine (T_3) should be determined. Some measure of thyroid hormone binding capacity should also be obtained: a radioactive tri-iodothyronine uptake (RTU, T_3U) or thyroid binding globulin (TBG) is equally useful. Thyrotropin (thyroid stimulating hormone, TSH) should be undetectable in the face of hyperthyroidism; hence, a TSH determination is not a part of the initial evaluation of hyperthyroidism. If the clinical findings are consistent with *hypothyroidism*, the laboratory evaluation consists of the quantitation of T_4 and TSH. A low T_4 and an elevated TSH are diagnostic of hypothyroidism. If *diffuse thyroid enlargement* (goiter) is present, but there are no findings suggestive of hyper- or hypothyroidism, a T_4, TSH, and antithyroidal antibodies (antimicrosomal and anti-thyroglobulin antibodies) should be obtained. Positive antibody studies (titers greater than 1:200) provide strong presumptive evidence of thyroiditis. Lower titers may be seen in many systemic diseases. A *discrete area of enlargement* of the thyroid (thyroid nodule) necessitates both laboratory and radiologic investigations. Laboratory studies should include T_4, TSH and antithyroidal antibodies. An ^{123}I scan will delineate the location of the mass and provide information on both thyroid and nodule function. A nonfunctioning (cold) mass is more likely to be malignant. Ultrasonography may be helpful in the identification of cystic lesions. Surgical exploration is often required as well, but this is predicated on the other investigations.

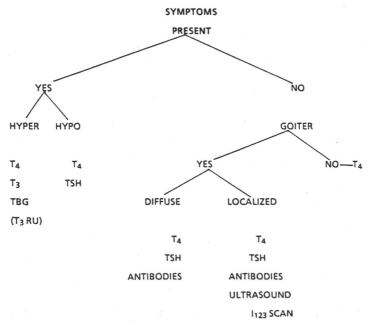

2. What are the causes of acquired hypothyroidism in childhood?
Chronic lymphocytic thyroiditis
  (autoimmune thyroiditis, Hashimoto's)
  Associated with chromosomal abnormalities
    Down, Turner, Klinefelter syndromes
  Associated with other endocrine diseases
    Diabetes mellitus
    Hypoadrenalism (Schmitt syndrome)
  Associated with congenital infection
    Rubella, toxoplasmosis
Subacute thyroiditis (DeQuervain's)
  Post-viral
Goitrogen ingestion
  Iodides, expectorants, thioureas (propylthiouracil, carbimazole)
Thyroid removal
  Surgery
  Radioactive iodine ablation
Infiltrative disease
  Cystinosis, histiocytosis X
Hypothalamic or pituitary disease

"Late onset" congenital (large ectopic)

"Pseudo" hypothyroidism
  TBG deficiency
  Peripheral resistance to thyroid hormone
  "Euthyroid sick" syndrome

3. What are the causes of congenital hypothyroidism?
Primary
  Thyroid agenesis/dysgenesis
    Athyrosis
    Hypoplastic thyroid
    Ectopic thyroid
  Inborn error of thyroid hormone synthesis
    Dyshormonogenesis
Secondary
  Hypopituitarism
  Hypothalamic abnormality
    Septo-optic dysplasia
Other
  "Transient"
  Maternal factors
    Goitrogen ingestion
    Iodide deficiency
    Autoimmune thyroiditis
  "Pseudo"
    TBG deficiency
    Prematurity
    "Euthyroid sick" syndrome

4. What are the signs and symptoms of congenital hypothyroidism?

Symptoms	Signs
Lethargy	Hypotonia, slow reflexes
Poor feeding	Poor weight gain
Prolonged jaundice	Jaundice
Constipation	Distended abdomen
Mottling	Acrocyanosis
Cold extremities	Low body temperature
	Umbilical hernia
	Macroglossia
	Coarse features
	Large fontanels/wide sutures
	Hoarse cry
	Goiter

5. When must therapy begin in congenital hypothyroidism? Why?

As early as possible. Less than 20% of patients will have obvious clinical signs at 3–4 weeks of age. Since prompt initiation of therapy is necessary for optimal outcome, screening is now performed on all newborns in the United States at 2–3 days of age, and most children are started on therapy prior to 1 month of age. The prognosis for intellectual development is directly related to the amount of time from birth to the initiation of therapy. Children started on hormone replacement prior to 30 days of age have a mean IQ of 106; children not treated until 3 to 6 months have a mean IQ of 70.

6. What drug preparation and dosage are recommended for replacement thyroid in children with congenital or acquired hypothyroidism?

L-thyroxine. There is no oral suspension of L-thyroxine; however, the tablets can be readily crushed, dissolved in a small amount (5–15ml) of infant formula, and administered using an oral syringe. L-thyroxine can also be mixed with pureed fruit or cereal. Approximate starting doses are:

Weight (kg)	L-Thyroxine (μg)
<3.5	25
3.5–5.0	37.5
5.0–7.5	50
7.5–10.0	62.5
10.0–20.0	75
20.0–40.0	100

After therapy is started, thyroid tests (T_4, TSH) should be repeated in 3–4 weeks and the dosage adjusted according to test results and clinical findings. The T_4 value should be maintained in the upper half of the normal range for age. Optimally the TSH should be in the normal range as well. Practically, however, this goal is not always achievable without making the child clinically and biochemically hyperthyroid.

7. What are the causes of congenital goiter?

Iodine deficiency or excess
  Medication
Maternal goitrogen ingestion
  Propylthiouracil, methimazole, carbimazole
Congenital hyperthyroidism

Dyshormonogenic defects
  Defective peroxidase activity
  Defective iodotyrosyl coupling
  Defective iodothyronine synthesis
  Defective thyroglobulin
  Defective iodotyrosine deiodination

8. What is Penred's syndrome?

Penred's syndrome is characterized by the unique association of goiter and nerve deafness. It is the most frequently encountered of the inherited defects in thyroxine biosynthesis. The precise enzymatic diagnosis is not known but appears to be defective peroxidase activity. Penred's syndrome is inherited as an autosomal recessive condition and accounts for about 7% of all individuals with congenital deafness. Patients affected are usually euthyroid.

9. What is chronic lymphocytic thyroiditis (CLT) and how is it diagnosed?

CLT, also called Hashimoto's disease or autoimmune thyroiditis, is the most common thyroid problem in children, and is thought to be caused by organ-specific antibodies. Patients with CLT may come to medical attention due to the presence of goiter or clinical findings suggestive of hypo- or hyperthyroidism. The preponderance of patients are asymptomatic with a goiter at the time of presentation. The adequacy of thyroid function can be assessed by measuring the circulating levels of thyroxine (T_4) and thyroid stimulating hormone (TSH). The presence of thyroid antibodies in high titers (greater than 1:200) confirms the diagnosis. The two common antibody titers used are antithyroglobulin antibody and antimicrosomal antibody. Low titers of these antithyroidal antibodies may be found in a variety of other thyroidal diseases, and antibodies may not be detectable in 10–20% of affected individuals.

10. What is the prognosis for children with CLT?

About half of all children who present with euthyroid goiter will have complete resolution of the goiter within 5 to 6 years regardless of whether or not thyroxine replacement is given. It is not possible to predict which children will recover completely, which will remain euthyroid with goiter, and which will become hypothyroid. As a general rule, any child identified with thyroid disease should have T_4 and TSH values obtained yearly.

11. What other autoimmune endocrine diseases are associated with CLT?

Adrenal insufficiency (Schmitt's syndrome), diabetes mellitus, autoimmune polyglandular syndromes (Type II).

12. How is the hyperthyroidism of Graves' disease distinguished from that occasionally found in CLT?

Patients with hyperthyroidism due to CLT may be indistinguishable from those with Graves' disease. The presence of ophthalmologic findings points toward the latter entity, but the absence of exophthalmos does not rule out Graves'. The demonstration of human thyroid stimulating antibodies (HTSI, LATS) is confirmatory of the Graves' diagnosis, but these tests are not readily available. The best test to distinguish between these two entities is the ^{123}I-uptake test performed 6 and 24 hours after the administration of the isotope. Low or normal uptake supports the diagnosis of CLT, whereas elevated uptakes at 6 and 24 hours are more supportive of the diagnosis of Graves'.

13. What is the relationship between CLT and hypothyroidism?

CLT is probably the most common cause of acquired hypothyroidism in children, and may or may not be associated with goiter. The diagnosis of hypothyroidism is confirmed by a low T_4 and an elevated TSH. Sometimes, however, the T_4 is maintained in a normal range and is associated with an elevated TSH (compensated hypothyroidism). This combination of laboratory values is suggestive of a failing thyroid. T_4 production in these individuals is maintained by excess stimulation from pituitary TSH. While positive antibody titers strongly support CLT as the cause of the hypothyroidism, the absence of antibodies does not rule out CLT, since hypothyroidism often occurs late in the course of CLT. Most children who are hypothyroid at the time of diagnosis will need thyroid hormone replacement for life. Treatment with L-thyroxine should be started as soon as the chemical abnormality is confirmed. In those children with goiter and a significantly elevated TSH, initiation of therapy generally results in diminution in the size of the goiter.

14. What is Graves' disease?

Graves' disease is a multisystem disease characterized by thyrotoxicosis, diffuse goiter, infiltrative ophthalmopathy and occasionally an infiltrative dermopathy. The features of this disease may occur singly or in any combination. The full syndrome may never develop. There has been a tendency to use the terms "Graves' disease," "thyrotoxicosis," and "hyperthyroidism" interchangeably; however, there are other causes of hyperthyroidism, which are listed below.

Excess TSH
    TSH producing tumor
    Pituitary resistance to T_4 suppression
Abnormal thyroid stimulation
    TSH receptor antibody
Thyroid autonomy
    Adenoma
    Multinodular goiter

Thyroid inflammation
    Subacute thyroiditis
    Postradiation thyroiditis
Nonthyroidal source of hormone
    Ectopic tissue
    Hormone ingestion

15. What is the cause of Graves' disease?

The current view is that Graves' disease is an autoimmune disorder in which there are TSH receptor antibodies. Binding of the antibody to its antigen (the TSH receptor) results in the stimulation of thyroid hormone production and release, thus producing thyrotoxicosis. All thyroid receptor antibodies identified thus far belong to the IgG class of immunoglobulins. The general name used for these antibodies is human thyroid stimulating immunoglobulin (HTSI). In the older literature some types of HTSI were called long-acting thyroid stimulator (LATS) or LATS-protector (LATS-P).

16. What are the clinical and laboratory findings in Graves' disease?

The onset of symptoms is usually gradual, with increasing emotional lability and deteriorating school performance and behavior as prominent features in most children. Since the onset of Graves' disease and puberty may coincide, many parents initially attribute the psychologic changes to the normal adolescent process. The younger child may simply be thought to be "hyperactive." Sleep disturbances, nervousness, and weight loss may be noted, as well as easy fatigability and heat intolerance. Observation of the child's behavior, while the history is being obtained from the parent, is often instructive. The physical exam provides a number of important clues to diagnosis. Oral temperature may be slightly increased (100°F). Weight may be low for height, and many children will be tall for age and genetic potential at the time of initial evaluation. Some children will have experienced an acceleration in growth rate at the same time that their behavior began to deteriorate. The pulse rate is usually inappropriately high for the age of the child and a widened pulse pressure or elevated blood pressure is often present. Warm, moist hands and feet will usually be found. Prominent eyes are commonly noted, although this is a more variable finding in children than in adults. Fine fasciculations may be noted in the tongue upon extension. Thyroid enlargement is a consistent finding. The thyroid is usually firm, symmetrical, smooth, and nontender. The presence of a discrete node or area of tenderness warrants further investigation. The gland may be two to four times enlarged. A hyperactive precordium may accompany the changes in blood pressure, and functional systolic murmur may be heard. Either delayed or advanced puberty may be found. The bone age will be normal or advanced.

17. How is Graves' disease managed?

The three types of therapy are antithyroid medication, radioactive (^{131}I) ablation, and subtotal thyroidectomy.

Treatment Options for Hyperthyroidism

	MEDICAL	[131]I	SURGICAL
Contraindications	Noncompliance Previous drug reaction	Pregnancy Prepubertal(?)	Inadequate presurgical preparation
Effectiveness	65–95%	90–100%	80–100%
Pretreatment	None	Antithyroidal medications stopped 3–5 days prior to [131]I	Preferably euthyroid with thionamides then iodine treatment for 7–14 days to involute thyroid
Treatment	Dosage based on patient body weight	Dosage based on estimated gland size and I uptake	Removal of all thyroidal tissue except that in close proximity to vital structures
Acute complications	Drug reaction; GI upset; arthralgias; agranulocytosis	Hyperthyroidism; local tenderness	vocal cord paralysis; bleeding at surgical site; hypocalcemia
Long-term complications	Essentially none; complications due to drug resolve when drug is discontinued	Hypothyroidism; ? genetic or radiation damage	Hypothyroidism; hypoparathyroidism; vocal cord paralysis

18. Which drugs are used to treat Graves' disease?

The principal drugs are listed below. The thionamide derivatives, propylthiouracil and methimazole, are the keystones of long-term management; however, their effective onset of action is slow since they block synthesis but not release of thyroid hormone. Propranolol is useful in treating many of the beta-adrenergic effects of hyperthyroidism; hence it is useful in acute management but should be discontinued when the thyroid disease is controlled. Iodide, which can transiently block thyroid hormone release, and glucocorticoids are useful "stop-gap" medications while awaiting the inhibitory effects of the thionamides. They are generally used only when the patient is acutely symptomatic (thyroid storm).

Medications Used in the Treatment of Hyperthyroidism

DRUG	DOSAGE AND ADMINISTRATION	EFFECT	CONTRAIN-DICATIONS	ADVERSE REACTIONS
Propylthiouracil (PTU)	Initial: 6–7 mg/kg/24 hr q 6–8 hr, po	Blocks organification of iodide and peripheral conversion of T_4 to T_3	Past history of drug toxicity; history of noncompliance; dose held to minimum during pregnancy	Agranulocytosis, 1%; All reactions, 5%; reactions include mycoarthralgias, neuritis, hepatitis, skin rashes, urticaria, lupus-like syndrome; loss of taste
Methimazole (Tapezol)	Initial: 0.6–0.7 mg/kg/24 hr q 8–12 hr, po	Blocks organification of iodide	Same as for PTU. Not recommended during pregnancy	Agranulocytosis, 0.2%; all reactions, 10%. Reactions as for PTU.
Propranolol (Inderal)	0.1 mg/kg, q 6 hrs, IV if patient with thyroid storm; 1 mg/kg, q 6 hr po until euthyroid	Decreases adrenergic component of thyrotoxicosis; may also impair peripheral conversion of T_4 to T_3	Heart block; asthma; usage in pregnancy associated with small fetal size and may cause postnatal hypoglycemia or bradycardia	Bradycardia, hypertension; hypoglycemia

Table continued on next page.

Medications Used in the Treatment of Hyperthyroidism *(Continued)*

Iodine (SSKI)	KI (saturated solution contains 1g KI/ml) 2–3 drops q 8 hr, po	Blocks T_4 release by thyroid gland; this is a transient effect but is useful in acute management	Previous reactions to I; not useful for long-term treatment	Acneiform skin rash; drug fevers, conjunctivitis, vasculitides, eosinophilic granulocytosis
Glucocorticoids	Hydrocortisone, 50–60 mg/m²/day, q 4 hours		None; should be used only during the early phase of treatment	

19. Has radioactive iodide fallen into disfavor as a treatment option for Graves' disease? Why or why not?

No. Radioactive iodide (^{131}I) is actually increasing in popularity in the treatment of Graves' disease. Concern has been voiced about the possible risk of thyroid carcinoma, leukemia, thyroid nodules, or genetic mutations. While the numbers of individuals treated during childhood with ^{131}I and followed for prolonged periods of time remain small, the combined experience suggests that children are at no significantly increased risk for these problems. Thionamide medications must be discontinued for 3–5 days prior to treatment with ^{131}I, since these medications interfere with iodide uptake. The dosage of ^{131}I is based on the estimated size of the gland and the rate of uptake of ^{123}I on a preliminary study. Radiation thyroiditis may occur and lead to exacerbation of the hyperthyroidism 10–14 days after radioiodine administration. If this occurs these children can usually be managed with propranolol. Some local tenderness may also be present. Not surprisingly, the most common complication of ^{131}I treatment is hypothyroidism, with 20% of patients becoming hypothyroid by one year, and almost 50% by 15 years. Thus, all patients who are treated with ^{131}I should have T_4 and TSH levels measured frequently during the first year after treatment and at least yearly thereafter.

20. What factors should be considered in the surgical treatment of Graves' disease?

Complete or partial removal of the thyroid gland is the oldest treatment modality for hyperthyroidism. Optimally, the patient should be euthyroid prior to surgery. For this purpose, oral iodide for 7–14 days is the drug of choice since it effectively blocks thyroid synthesis and causes thyroid involution. The complications of surgery include death, vocal cord paralysis, and damage to the parathyroid glands. Each of these problems occurs in less than 5% of adult patients. While similar statistics are not available on large series of children and adolescents, our impression is that mortality is lower than that reported in adults and hypoparathyroidism is more frequent. Permanent hypothyroidism has been reported in as many as 50% of patients, and hyperthyroidism has recurred in as many as 20% of patients. Obviously, the most critical factor is the skill and experience of the surgeon.

21. What endocrine disturbances are associated with Graves' disease?

A great number of endocrinologic functions are altered in thyrotoxicosis; however, only a few of these changes are clinically relevant to children and adolescents.

1. Hyperthyroidism may be associated with either delayed puberty or early puberty. The mechanisms for these are not clear.

2. Post-pubertal females often have menstrual irregularity prior to treatment. The intermenstrual interval may be either prolonged or shortened initially, generally with diminished flow. Frank amenorrhea often is found.

3. Hypercalcemia has been noted in a significant number of patients with hyperthyroidism with an increase in both total and free calcium concentrations. The serum alkaline

phosphatase level is also elevated. These changes are similar to those found in hyperparathyroidism; however PTH levels are low or undetectable. True hyperparathyroidism and Graves' disease may coexist, and should be suspected if the hypercalcemia does not improve as the hyperthyroidism is controlled.

4. The manifestation of thyroid hormone excess—flushing, sweating, tachycardia, gastrointestinal hypermotility—are similar to those seen in carcinoid syndrome; however, the plasma serotonin concentration, the urinary 5-hydroxyindoleacetic acid excretion, and platelet monoamine oxidase activity are normal.

22. What is the pathogenesis of the exophthalmos in Graves' disease?

It is unknown but several facts suggest an autoimmune process: (1) histologic studies reveal lymphocytic infiltration of the retrobulbar muscles, (2) circulating lymphocytes are sensitized to an antigen unique to the retrobulbar tissues, and (3) the thyroglobulin-antithyroglobulin antibody complexes found in patients with Graves' disease bind specifically to the extraorbital muscles.

23. How should a solitary thyroid nodule be evaluated in a child?

Of all children found to have solitary thyroid nodule, about 30–40% will have a carcinoma, 20–30% will have an adenoma, and the remainder will have any of the following: thyroid abscess, thyroid cyst, multinodular goiter, Hashimoto's thyroiditis, subacute thyroiditis, or nonthyroidal neck mass. Given the relatively high incidence of carcinoma, a thyroidal mass demands prompt evaluation. A thorough history to rule out previous irradiation to the head or neck is important, since there is a significantly increased incidence of thyroid carcinoma in such individuals. A family history of thyroid disease increases the likelihood of CLT or Graves' disease. Careful examination of the thyroid is helpful; tenderness of the thyroid suggests subacute thyroiditis. Laboratory tests should include T_4, TSH, and thyroid antibodies. The presence of high antibody titers is suggestive of CLT and rules against a malignant process; however, in all cases, radiologic studies should be undertaken and in many cases, surgical exploration is required. The principal tools used in the investigation of a thyroid mass are ^{123}I-iodide scanning and ultrasound. Ultrasound is useful in delineating the size of the mass, its anatomic relationship to the rest of the thyroid, and the presence of cystic structures. ^{123}I-iodide imaging that reveals a single nonfunctioning mass suggests a carcinoma or adenoma and is a clear indication for surgery. Patchy uptake is more characteristic of CLT, while a poorly functioning lobe may be found in subacute thyroiditis.

24. In what clinical circumstances should hypoparathyroidism be suspected?

Hypoparathyroidism may occur sporadically or as part of a familial syndrome consisting of various combinations of presumptively autoimmune diseases. It may also be associated with thymic aplasia and severe immunologic deficiencies (DiGeorge syndrome) or may result from damage incurred during neck surgery or irradiation.

25. What are the clinical manifestations of hypoparathyroidism?

The clinical manifestations are predominantly those of hypocalcemia, although some findings are more suggestive of hypoparathyroidism. The particular symptoms and signs will depend on the age of the child, the duration of the disease, and the presence of other syndromic or autoimmune phenomena. Lenticular cataracts are common in hypoparathyroidism, but are also associated with longstanding hypocalcemia of any cause. Psychiatric disorders, including depression, paranoia, and frank psychosis, have been noted in association with hypoparathyroidism. Dry scaly skin, psoriasis, and patchy alopecia have been found commonly. Mucocutaneous candidiasis has been associated with the familial form of this disease. Unusually brittle hair and fingernails are often found. Hypoplasia of tooth enamel is expected if the hypoparathyroidism was present at the time of dental development. Intestinal malabsorption and steatorrhea have also been described.

26. What are the polyendocrine disorders and how are they distinguished from each other?

There are two groups of polyendocrine disorders. The first entails the development of pluriglandular neoplasia and is referred to as multiple endocrine neoplasia (MEN) syndrome. There are three distinct subtypes, and each may begin in childhood. The second involves the clustering of multiple endocrine dysfunctions and is autoimmune in nature. It has been referred to as autoimmune polyglandular syndrome (autoimmune polyendocrinopathy, APE). The subtypes of both syndromes are delineated below.

Multiple Endocrine Neoplasia (MEN) Syndrome

	MEN I (Wermer's)	MEN II (Sipple's)	MEN III (multiple mucosal neuroma)
Hyperparathyroid	+ + + +[1]	+ + +[2]	±
Islet cell tumors			
Gastrin producing	+ + +	−	−
Insulin producing	+ +	−	−
Pituitary adenomas	+ +	−	−
Carcinoid tumors	+	−	−
Adrenal adenomas	+	−	−
Thyroid disease	±	−	−
Visceral lipomas	±	−	−
Medullary thyroid carcinoma	−	+ + + +	+ + + +
Pheochromocytoma	−	+ +	+ +
Mucosal neuromas	−	−	+ + + +
Inheritance	AD[3]	AD	—
Incidence	0.02–0.2/1000	—	—
Screening initiated	15 years	5 years	1 year

[1]Hyperplasia. [2]Adenoma or hyperplasia. [3]Autosomal dominant.

Autoimmune Polyendocrinopathy Syndromes

	APE I	APE II
Hyperthyroidism	−	+[2]
Hypothyroidism	+	+[2]
Hypoparathyroidism	+[1]	−
Adrenal insufficiency	+[1]	+[2]
Diabetes mellitus	−	+[2]
Gonadal failure	+	+[2]
Myasthenia gravis	−	+[2]
Mucocutaneous candidiasis	+[1]	−
Alopecia	+	+
Vitiligo	+	+
Pernicious anemia	+	+
Chronic active hepatitis	+	−
Celiac disease	−	+[2]
Malabsorption	+	+
Onset	Childhood	Adulthood
Inheritance	Familial; no HLA association; multiple individuals in a generation; autosomal recessive	Associated with the HLA B8DR3

[1]Classical features of APE I.
[2]Diagnosis of APE II requires that at least 2 of the annotated features be present.

27. What is McCune-Albright syndrome?

This syndrome is the association of polyostotic fibrosis dysplasia, precocious puberty, and café au lait pigmentation. These nevi classically have an irregular border ("coast of Maine"), while the lesions in neurofibromatosis have a more regular border ("coast of California"). The syndrome may occur in either an incomplete (pigmented nevi and bony changes without precocious puberty) or expanded form (the hallmark features plus other findings—gigantism, hyperthyroidism, Cushing's syndrome, and ovarian cysts). It occurs most commonly in females. The syndrome may be due to excess production of hypothalamic releasing hormones or to autonomous function of the involved gland (ovary, adrenal, thyroid).

28. How should children with hypercalcemia be managed?

Acute management depends on the level of calcium and the severity of signs and symptoms, while chronic management depends on identification and treatment of the underlying cause. Calcium in excess of 15 mg/dl or the presence of significant symptoms (vomiting, hypertension) constitutes a medical emergency and requires immediate intervention to lower the serum calcium level. In general, this is accomplished by the concurrent administration of isotonic saline at 2-4 times maintenance rates and furosemide (1 mg/kg, IV q 6 h). Furosemide is a potent diuretic and calciuric agent. Meticulous monitoring of input and output, serum and urinary electrolytes, and serum magnesium is required. Electrocardiographic monitoring is mandatory.

29. What is used to treat hypercalcemia that is resistant to saline and furosemide?

Phosphate (1 mmol/kg body weight given over 6-8 hours IV or oral phosphate 1-2 mmol/kg per day in 4-6 doses) is used to treat hypercalcemia resistant to saline and furosemide. This is almost always effective and the effect can be sustained; however, there is considerable risk of soft tissue calcification. Other therapies have been used acutely, including intravenous EDTA, sodium sulfate, and calcitonin. Hemodialysis has been used on occasion with variable success.

30. How are asymptomatic children with hypercalcemia managed?

When calcium levels are less than 15 mg/dl, management focuses primarily on lowering calcium intake and decreasing gastrointestinal absorption. Vitamin D should be eliminated from the diet and calcium intake should be restricted. Cortisone lowers gastrointestinal absorption of calcium; however, its onset of action is relatively slow. Therefore, it is of limited usefulness in the acute management of hypercalcemia. Plicamycin (25 ug/kg), a cytotoxic substance initially used as a cancer chemotherapeutic agent, is a potent inhibitor of bone resorption and has been used in some cases of hypercalcemia.

31. What are the causes of hypercalcemia?

An easy mnemonic for causes of hypercalcemia is high, 5-I, and T: high (hyperparathyroidism), 5-I (ingestion, infection, immobilization, infantile, idiopathic), and T (tumor).

Hyperparathyroidism
  Isolated
  Syndromic (multiple endocrine
  neoplasia I, II)
Ingestions
  Milk-alkali syndrome
  Vitamin D intoxication
  Vitamin A intoxication
  Thiazide diuretics
Infections
  Sarcoidosis
  Tuberculosis

Immobilization
Infantile
  Subcutaneous fat necrosis
  Secondary to maternal
  hypoparathyroidism
  Idiopathic (Lightwood's)
  Hyperplasia
Idiopathic
Tumors
Familial

32. What are the causes of adrenocortical insufficiency in childhood?
Primary
   Inherited enzymatic defects (Congenital adrenal hyperplasia)
      21-hydroxylase deficiency
      11-hydroxylase deficiency
      3-beta hydroxysteroid dehydrogenase deficiency
      17-hydroxylase deficiency
      Desmolase deficiency
   Autoimmune
      Isolated
      Polyglandular endocrinopathy (APE I, APE II)
   Infectious
      Tuberculosis
      Meningiococcemia
   Surgical
   Trauma
      Bilateral adrenal hemorrhage
   Iatrogenic
   Adrenal atrophy secondary to prolonged steroid therapy
Secondary/Tertiary
   Panhypopituitarism
   Craniopharyngioma
   Other pituitary or hypothalamic tumor
   CNS trauma
   CNS irradiation

33. What are the clinical features of the various forms of congenital adrenal hyperplasia?

Clinical Features of Disorders of Adrenal Steroidogenesis

ENZYME DEFECT	SEXUAL AMBIGUITY		POSTNATAL VIRILIZATION	SALT WASTING	HYPERTENSION
	Female	Male			
21-Hydroxylase					
Salt-wasting	+	0	+	+	0
Simple-virilizing	+	0	+	0	0
Late-onset	0	0	+	0	0
11-Hydroxylase	+	0	+	0	+
17-Hydroxylase	0	+	0	0	+
18-Hydroxylase	0	0	0	+	0
3-β HSD	+	+	+	+	0
Desmolase	0	+	0	+	0

34. Differentiate Cushing's syndrome from Cushing's disease.
Cushing's syndrome refers to the clinical findings associated with adrenocortical hyperfunction while Cushing's disease specifically refers to adrenocorticoid excess secondary to increased pituitary ACTH.

35. What are the causes of Cushing's syndrome in childhood?

Tumor
  Adrenal
    Adenoma
    Carcinoma
  Other
    Ectopic ACTH production
    Pheochromocytoma
    Wilms' tumor

Hypothalamic/pituitary dysfunction
    Pituitary adenoma
  Exogenous cortisol

36. What are the clinical findings in Cushing's syndrome?

1. Accumulation of fat on the trunk and head, resulting in the characteristic "moon facies" and "buffalo hump." The extremities are often disproportionately thin due to muscle catabolism.

2. Capillary fragility resulting in easy bruisability and ecchymosis.

3. Increased translucency of the skin and fragility to trauma; stria are common on the abdomen, thighs, and axilla, and may be violaceous in color.

4. Evidence of virilization may be present including acne, pubic hair, hirsutism and secondary amenorrhea.

5. Growth failure may be the only finding.

6. Hypertension.

37. What are the laboratory findings in Cushing's syndrome?

Elevated hematocrit, low eosinophil count, elevated blood glucose, hypokalemia, and hypochloremic alkalosis. The bone age is retarded but not as profoundly as the height age. Osteoporosis may be present. The most useful screening procedure is the measurement of 17-hydroxysteroid metabolites in a 24-hour urine collection. These must be normalized to either body surface area or to creatinine excretion.

38. How rapidly can the dose of steroid hormone be reduced?

The rapidity with which steroids can be tapered depends on the duration of treatment, the amount and type of glucocorticoid used and the disease process for which the steroids were instituted. As a general rule, the reduction from pharmacologic to physiologic doses is predicated on the underlying disease, whereas the taper from physiologic doses to complete withdrawal is dependent upon the degree of steroid-induced adrenal suppression. It is well documented that modest doses of glucocorticoids given for relatively brief periods of time can interfere with pituitary-adrenal regulation and result in adrenal atrophy. The guidelines presented below are a distillation of recent reviews on this topic. Please note that all recommendations are in milligrams of hydrocortisone.

Protocol for Tapering Steroid Medications

DURATION OF TREATMENT (DAYS)	DOSE	ADRENAL SUPPRESSION	RECOMMENDATIONS
<3	<3x	None	Stop abruptly
	>3x	Unlikely	Reduce by 50% for 2 days then stop
>3 but <10	>1x	Unlikely	Reduce by 50% for 2 days then stop
>10 but <30	>1x	Possible	Reduce by 25% every 4 days until physiologic, then as per protocol (See #3 in answer to question 39)
>30	>1x alternate days	Possible	Taper as per protocol
	>1x every day	Probable	Taper as per protocol

39. What is the protocol for tapering steroids *from* physiologic doses (20 mg/m²/day)?

1. Change to hydrocortisone preparation.

2. Taper to 10 mg/m²/day over 2 weeks. If stressed, dose must be increased to 3x maintenance dose.

3. At the end of the second week, withhold AM hydrocortisone dose and obtain an AM cortisol level.

    a. If plasma AM cortisol is greater than 10 mg/dl, stop supplementation but stress coverage is required until the adequacy of adrenal response to stress (ACTH stimulation test) is determined.

    b. If plasma AM cortisol is less than 10 mg/dl, continue supplementation (10 mg/m²/day). Repeat AM cortisol in one month. Stress coverage must be maintained.

40. What are the relative potencies of the major steroid preparations?

Potencies of Steroid Preparations

CHEMICAL COMPOUND	GLUCOCORTICOID POTENCY	MINERALOCORTICOID POTENCY
Cortisol (Hydrocortisone)	1	+ +
Cortisone	0.8	+ +
Prednisolone	4	+
Predisone	3.5	+
Methylprednisolone	5	0
Fludrocortisone	15	+ + +

41. How is the *adequacy* of adrenal response to stress evaluated?
 1. Perform 1-hour ACTH stimulation test (Cortrosyn Stimulation Test)
    a. Draw initial blood for cortisol.
    b. Administer Cortrosyn (0.25 mg/m^2) IV, push.
    c. Obtain blood at 30 and 60 minutes for cortisol levels.
 2. If increment of plasma cortisol is greater than 6 μg/dl and maximum is greater than 20 μg/dl, no further stress coverage is needed.
 3. If the increment is less than 6 μg/dl and/or the maximum is less than 20 μg/dl, stress coverage should be maintained. Testing should be repeated in 1–2 months.

42. How should an infant with ambiguous genitalia be evaluated?
First, an adequate history must be obtained. This may reveal a history of maternal androgen ingestion (rare now, but common in the 1960's when Provera was used as progestational agent) or a family history of similarly affected infants. The physical examination may be helpful. The presence of a gonadal structure in the labioscrotal fold strongly implies the presence of some Y chromosomal material. Gonads containing both ovarian and testicular components (ovotestes) have been found in the inguinal canals. It is rare, however, to find an ovary in the inguinal canal. In the absence of a palpable gonad, no conclusions can be drawn concerning chromosomal sex. The size of the phallic structure and the location of the urethral meatus provide no information concerning gonadal or chromosomal content; however, phallic size and function are of importance when decisions are made regarding gender-of-rearing. The presence of midline abnormalities (cleft palate) suggests hypothalamic or pituitary dysfunction, while congenital anomalies such as an imperforate anus suggest structural derangements. Digital rectal exam will confirm the patency of the anus and may allow the uterus to be palpated; however, the more useful evaluation of the internal structures is provided by the radiologist. Ultrasound is useful in identifying the uterus, and, on occasion, the ovaries. The absence of a uterus suggests that testes were present early in gestation and produced mullerian inhibiting factor, causing regression of the mullerian-derived ducts, including the uterus. The injection of contrast medium into the urethral opening(s) will often demonstrate a vaginal pouch posterior to the fused labioscrotal folds. Occasionally, the cervix and cervical canal will be highlighted by this study as well. The clinical laboratory is of considerable help. Chromosomal analysis is useful for predicting gonadal content, while measurement of adrenal steroid metabolites is important for recognizing enzymatic disorders of adrenal steroid synthesis.

43. What determines the approach to management of ambiguous genitalia?
Once the infant has been evaluated, two questions must be answered. The first is a diagnostic one—what pathophysiologic mechanism(s) led to the abnormalities demonstrated by the various studies? The second is related to patient management—how will this child best be

able to function sexually and reproductively? The answers to the first question generally guide management if there is no evidence of a Y chromosome. For example, a genetic female who is virilized secondary to 21-hydroxylase deficiency requires corrective surgery and appropriate medication with hydrocortisone and fluorocortisone. The potential for normal sexual and reproductive function is good. If Y chromosomal material is present, the answers to the second question play an important role in management. For example, a genetic male with the 3-beta-hydroxysteroid dehydrogenase deficiency may be markedly undervirilized, with a phallus less than 2 cm in length, hypospadias, and bilaterally undescended testicles. Appropriate medication will relieve the adrenal insufficiency; however, corrective surgery is unlikely to produce a penis of adequate size for sexual function; hence, serious consideration must be given to rearing this child as a female.

44. What laboratory studies are indicated in a child with diabetic ketoacidosis (DKA)?
Initial laboratory values should include a blood glucose, electrolytes (Na^+, K^+, Cl^-, HCO_3^-), blood urea nitrogen, and a blood gas. Subsequently, glucose should be monitored hourly until it is less than 300 mg% and the patient is alert. Electrolytes should be monitored at least every 4 hours until normalized. Monitoring of blood gases and pH is predicated on the severity of the patient's illness and the degree of abnormality on the initial values.

45. How should fluids be managed during an episode of DKA?
The most critical aspect of the management of diabetic ketoacidosis is the provision of adequate fluid. Rapid volume expansion with isotonic saline (20 ml/kg) should be undertaken in the first hour. Repeat bolus (10 ml/kg) may be necessary if the patient remains significantly hypotensive and/or tachycardic after the initial bolus. Subsequent fluid replacement is based on the assumption of 10–15% dehydration at the time of presentation as well as the provision of maintenance fluids. Ongoing urinary loss must also be considered since it will remain high as long as the blood sugar exceeds the renal glucose threshold (160–180 mg%). Glucose is not added to the rehydration solution until the blood glucose falls below 300 mg/dl. As a general rule, approximately half of the deficit is replaced during the initial 8-hour period.

46. Why do potassium levels fall during management of DKA?
(1) Dilutional effects of rehydration, (2) correction of acidosis (less K^+ exchanged out of cell for H^+ as pH rises), (3) insulin administration (increases cellular uptake of K^+), and (4) ongoing urinary losses. Most patients are potassium depleted, although the serum potassium is usually normal or elevated on occasion. A low potassium is thus particularly worrisome for it suggests severe depletion and indicates that the methods of compensation may be failing. If the initial K^+ is greater than 4 mEq/L, 40 mEq/L of potassium should be added to the infusate. If the initial K^+ is less than 4 mEq/L, then 60 mEq/L should be used and the serum K^+ should be closely monitored.

47. How should insulin be administered in children with DKA?
Either continuously intravenously or hourly intramuscularly. Intravenous insulin is infused initially at a rate of 0.1 U/kg/hr. This rate is adjusted to allow blood sugar to fall by about 100 mg/dl per hour. Alternatively, intramuscular insulin can be used with an initial dose of 0.25 U/kg followed by 0.1 U/kg on an hourly basis. Only regular insulin is used. There is no place for intermediate or long-acting insulins in the treatment of diabetic ketoacidosis. Injection of insulin subcutaneously is inappropriate for the management of diabetic ketoacidosis.

48. Should bicarbonate be used in the treatment of children with DKA?
The use of bicarbonate in the treatment of diabetic ketoacidosis in children has been both advocated and denounced. The establishment of an adequate intravascular volume and the provision of sufficient quantities of insulin *are far more important* in the treatment of diabetic ketoacidosis than bicarbonate. The decision to initiate bicarbonate therapy should be based on an arterial blood gas, not a venous blood gas. The three clear indications for bicarbonate therapy are symptomatic hyperkalemia, cardiac instability, and an inadequate ventilatory compensation. Each of these conditions requires admission to an intensive care unit where appropriate monitoring can be undertaken and ventilatory assistance provided if necessary.

Use of Bicarbonate in the Treatment of Diabetic Ketoacidosis

PRO	CON
Improved myocardial contracility and response to catecholamines if pH is less than 7.0	Low cardiac output problems rare in children
Ventilatory response to acidosis blunted when pH is less than 7.0	Ventilatory response well-maintained in children
With usual dosages of bicarbonate no adverse effects on oxygen binding with hemoglobin from children with DKA	Rapid correction of acidosis shifts the hemoglobin-oxygen dissociation curve to the left, thus potentially decreasing tissue oxygenation
Questionable clinical relevance of paradoxical CNS acidosis	Paradoxical CNS acidosis demonstrated in both animals and humans
May be useful in treating the rare patient who is hyperkalemic	Hypokalemia can result from uptake of K+ into cell as acidosis is corrected. Hypokalemia 6 times more common in patients treated with bicarbonate

49. How is the transition made to intermittent insulin therapy in DKA?

The transition from an insulin infusion to intermittent subcutaneous therapy is predicated on three factors:

1. *Normalization of biochemical parameters.* Insulin infusion provides a highly sensitive and effective means of normalizing the blood sugar, thus ending the osmotic diuresis and the consequent need for large volumes of fluid replacement. Furthermore, insulin halts fatty acid mobilization, effectively stopping ketogenesis and the consequent acidosis. Insulin infusions should not be stopped until the blood sugar is less than 300 mg%, the pH is greater than 7.3, and the bicarbonate is greater than 15 mEq/L.

2. *Resumption of oral food intake.* As long as the patient is not eating and is receiving a constant supply of glucose by vein, it is easier to maintain a stable blood sugar using an insulin infusion rather than intermittent subcutaneous insulin. When oral intake is resumed, food is usually provided on an intermittent (bolus) basis; hence, it is reasonable to provide insulin in an intermittent fashion as well.

3. *Convenience/normal schedule.* Patients with diabetes generally are placed on a q.i.d. insulin regimen for the initial 24–36 hour period after an episode of ketoacidosis. Regular insulin is given prior to meals and the bedtime snack. Therefore, it is most convenient to stop the insulin infusion and give an appropriate dose of subcutaneous insulin 20–30 minutes prior to the ingestion of the first substantial meal.

50. What types of insulin are used for controlling diabetes in an outpatient setting?

Types of Insulin Used*

	ONSET OF ACTION (HRS)	PEAK OF ACTION (HRS)	DURATION OF ACTION (HRS)
Regular	½–1	2–4	5–7
Insulin Zinc (Prompt, Semilente)	1–3	2–8	12–16
Isophane (NPH)	3–4	6–8	18–24
Insulin Zinc (Lente)	1–3	8–12	24–28
Protamine Zinc	4–6	14–24	36
Insulin Zinc (Extended, Ultralente)	4–6	18–24	24–36

*Both the short-acting (regular, semilente) and the intermediate-acting (NPH, lente) are available as a beef/pork mixture, pure pork, pure beef, semisynthetic (modified pork), and human (recombinant DNA derived) forms.

51. How is insulin administered?

Insulin is routinely administered subcutaneously. Injections are given in the arm, thigh, buttocks, and abdomen. Most patients are currently on two shots each day. Each injection is a combination of short-acting and intermediate-acting insulins, and most patients receive their shots prior to breakfast and prior to supper. More complex schedules and insulin combinations are used in some circumstances. Patients receive about two-thirds of their total daily insulin in the morning injection and one-third in the evening dose. About two-thirds of the morning dose is of intermediate-strength and one-third is short-acting. In the evening, the amounts of intermediate-acting and short-acting insulin are equal. The distribution may be different depending on food intake and exercise schedules. Prepubertal children beyond the "honeymoon" period generally require between 0.5 and 0.75 U/kg/day of insulin, while postpubertal individuals more commonly require 0.75-1.0 U/kg/day. Athletic individuals or those with a low caloric intake require less insulin.

52. Is there a role for insulin pumps?

Near-normalization of serum glucose can be obtained by the continuous infusion of subcutaneous insulin provided by portable insulin infusion devices. Insulin is infused through a 25 gauge scalp vein needle positioned under the abdominal skin and connected to the pump via a flexible plastic catheter. The complications of pump therapy fall into two general categories: the first is related to the presence of an indwelling catheter; the second is due to the use of a machine that is not able to monitor glucose directly, and is reliant on the patient for feedback. Cutaneous abscesses at the needle site are common and subcutaneous lumps have been frequently reported. The incidence of both of these problems can be reduced by meticulous attention to asepsis and to replacement and repositioning of the needle on a regular basis. The more serious problems are related to the inability of the pump to detect and respond to the blood sugar independent of the patient. This has resulted in numerous cases of hypoglycemia, seizures, and death. Diabetic decompensation has also occurred when insulin delivery was interrupted but not detected.

53. How is blood glucose monitored at home?

Blood is obtained by finger-prick and applied to a chemically-coated strip. The strips can be read visually or with a specific strip reader. A wide range of finger-prick devices, strips, and strip readers are available for these purposes. For optimal maintenance of diabetic control, four or more blood glucose determinations are necessary each day. Blood tests are routinely obtained before meals and preceding the bedtime snack.

54. What is the role of diet and exercise in diabetic children?

Both diet and exercise play an important role in the maintenance of good diabetic control. Consistency with regard to both the simple sugar (glucose, fructose) content and the timing of intake relative to insulin amount and action is critical. The inclusion of complex carbohydrates and fiber may help to prevent wide swings in serum glucose levels. Due to the high incidence of atherosclerosis, fat content has been increasingly limited. Currently, it is thought that the relatively high incidence of renal disease may be partially due to the high protein intake, so that protein intake is usually limited as well.

55. How is diabetic control evaluated?

While blood glucose measurements are the mainstay of diabetic monitoring, these measurements are prone to observer error or misreport; thus, the principal value of a glycohemoglobin determination is that it provides an objective reference point for evaluating diabetic control which is not subject to patient manipulation. Glycohemoglobin is formed nonenzymatically within the cell. Initially an unstable bond is formed between glucose and the hemoglobin molecule. With time, this bond rearranges to form a more stable compound in which glucose is covalently bound to the hemoglobin molecule. The amount of the unstable form may rise rapidly in the presence of a high blood glucose level, while the stable form changes slowly and provides a time-averaged integral of the blood glucose concentration through the 120-day life of the red blood cell. The interpretation of glycohemoglobin levels requires that the physician be familiar with the potential errors of these measurements. First, the analysis of the sample requires that appropriate chemical steps are undertaken to eliminate the unstable form. Failure to do this will result in falsely elevated levels. The reported value may also be affected by various hemoglobinopathies. Sickle cell disease or trait results in falsely low values, while persistent high fetal hemoglobin (thalassemia) results in falsely elevated levels. From a clinical perspective, the glycosylated hemoglobin result can be used either to reinforce good management or to confront patients whose records are inconsistent with their glycohemoglobin levels.

56. What are the long-term complications of diabetes?

Since the availability of insulin and improved methods of metabolic normalization have markedly decreased deaths from the acute metabolic complications of diabetes, there has been a consequent increase in disability and death from degenerative complications of the disease. The effects of diabetes have been divided into macrovascular (stroke, gangrene, myocardial infarction) and microvascular (retinopathy, nephropathy, and neuropathy) complications.

    1. The macrovascular changes are secondary to atherosclerosis. The atherosclerotic risk is greatest in poorly controlled individuals, probably due to the associated hypercholesterolemia and hypertriglyceridemia. Peripheral macrovascular disease is similar to that found in nondiabetic subjects, but it begins at an earlier age, advances more rapidly, and is more common. Leg and foot amputations are five times more common in diabetics than nondiabetics.

    2. The microvascular changes are equally devastating.

        a. Diabetic nephropathy accounts for 25% of patients receiving long-term renal dialysis in the United States. Retrospective studies suggest that as many as 50% of patients with insulin-dependent diabetes diagnosed before the age of 30 will develop end-stage renal disease. Microscopic changes in the glomerular basement membrane are present by 2 years after the diagnosis of diabetes. Microalbuminemia is often present by 10–15 years, followed by a proteinuric period (>0.5 g/24 hours). Beyond this point there is a relentless decline in glomerular function. An azotemic period begins on average by 17 years and frank uremia occurs by 20 years.

        b. Diabetes is the leading cause of adult blindness in the United States. The retinal disease is characterized as either background (simple) or proliferative retinopathy. By 25–30 years of disease 90% of patients with IDDM have demonstrable retinal lesions. The onset of the proliferative form of retinopathy carries a high risk of blindness. Vitreous hemorrhage, scarring, and retinal detachment occur frequently. Approximately 10% of patients develop proliferative retinopathy within 14 years. The disease will proceed to blindness in 43% of IDDM patients within 5 years of the onset of proliferative changes.

        c. Three forms of diabetic neuropathy have been characterized: (1) *mononeuropathy* involving a peripheral or cranial nerve. The usual presentation is the sudden appearance of foot drop, wrist drop, or paralysis of third, fourth, or sixth cranial nerves. Generally, the abnormality subsides in several days. (2) *Symmetrical peripheral polyneuropathy* is a symmetrical sensory loss in the distal lower extremities. Upper extremity involvement and motor deficits are uncommon. Numbness, tingling, and burning of the affected extremities are common and generally are worse at night. The pain may be severe on occasion. Due to the loss of sensory input, injuries may occur which are asymptomatic. Increased surveillance for these injuries in affected patients is required. (3) *Autonomic neuropathy* may result in orthostatic hypotension, sexual dysfunction, and motility disorders of the esophagus, stomach, gallbladder, small intestine, colon, and urinary bladder.

57. Define hypoglycemia.

A serum glucose of less than 50 mg/100 ml; symptoms may or may not be present. Hypoglycemia is a chemical finding and its presence should lead to a thorough search for the underlying pathology.

58. What clinical findings are associated with hypoglycemia?

They are nonspecific and may be attributed to factors other than the chemical abnormality. For example, a child with a temperature of 40°C as part of a viral syndrome may have a seizure. The seizure is likely to be classified as a "febrile seizure." The fact that the child has not eaten for 48 hours and is hypoglycemic may be missed entirely. The clinical findings of hypoglycemia are attributable to both the decreased availability of glucose to the central nervous system and to the adrenergic stimulation caused by a low or falling blood sugar. Neuroglycopenic symptoms include irritability, headache, confusion, unconsciousness, and seizure. Adrenergic signs include tachycardia, tremulousness, diaphoresis, and hunger. Any combination of the above signs and symptoms should lead to the measurement of blood glucose. In addition, a glucose concentration should be obtained from any child presenting to the physician with a seizure or coma. A history of a possible ingestion of propranolol, ethanol, or a hypoglycemic agent, particularly by the young child, should also increase surveillance for hypoglycemia.

59. What are the causes of childhood hypoglycemia?

Increased glucose utilization
  Hyperinsulinism
    Islet cell adenoma, hyperplasia, or nesidioblastosis
    Ingestion of oral hypoglycemic agents
    Exogenous insulin
  Large tumors
    Wilms' tumor
Decreased glucose production
  Inadequate glycogen reserves
    Defects of glycogen synthesis
      Glycogen synthetase deficiency
  Inability to mobilize glycogen
    Glucagon deficiency
    Defects in glycogenolysis
      Debrancher deficiency
  Ineffective gluconeogenesis
    Inadequate substrate
      "Ketotic hypoglycemia"
    Enzymatic defect
Diminished availability of fats
  Depleted fat stores
  Failure to mobilize fats
    Hyperinsulinism
  Defective utilization of fats
    Enzymatic defects in fatty acid oxidation
      Long-chain or medium-chain acyl CoA dehydrogenase deficiency
      Carnitine transport defect
Decreased fuels and fuel stores
  Fasting
  Malnutrition
  Prolonged illness
  Malabsorption

Increased fuel demand
  Fever
  Exercise
Inadequate counterregulatory hormones
  Growth hormone deficiency
  Cortisol deficiency
  Hypopituitarism

60. Are there any laboratory tests that are helpful in determining the cause of the hypoglycemia?

The principal laboratory evaluations include the measurement of the metabolic compounds associated with fasting adaptation as well as the hormones that regulate these processes. Blood obtained at the time the child is hypoglycemic is most helpful in this regard. Specific substances to be measured in blood include beta-hydroxybutyrate and free fatty acids as markers of fatty acid metabolism; lactate, pyruvate, and alanine as markers of the gluconeogenic pathways; and insulin, growth hormone, and cortisol as the principal regulatory hormones. Taken together, these provide valuable clues as to the cause. For example, low levels of ketones and free fatty acids suggest that fat was not appropriately mobilized. As a consequence, ketones were not formed by the liver. This would be seen in hyperinsulinism and would be confirmed by a high level of circulating insulin. Urine obtained around the time of hypoglycemia is also useful because it can be tested for ketones in the emergency setting. It can also be evaluated for drugs and for metabolic by-products (organic acids, amino acids) associated with known causes of hypoglycemia. If appropriate studies are not obtained at the time of presentation, a careful fasting study must be undertaken to evaluate fasting adaptation, since profound hypoglycemia and/or repeated hypoglycemia are associated with significant morbidity and mortality.

61. What is the treatment for hypoglycemia?

1. The principal acute treatment is the provision of glucose either orally or intravenously. If the patient is alert, orange juice or cola (4–8 ounces) may be given. If the patient is obtunded, intravenous glucose (2–3 ml of 10% dextrose/kg of body weight) should be administered. If venous access cannot be achieved relatively promptly, glucose can be provided via a nasogastric tube, since glucose is rapidly absorbed from the gut. The risk of prolonged hypoglycemia far outweighs the risk associated with the passage of a nasogastric tube in the obtunded patient. Subsequently, the blood sugar should be monitored closely, and, if necessary, maintained by the constant infusion of glucose (6–8 mg/kg/min). Larger quantities may be necessary and the blood sugar should be closely followed.

2. Glucagon promotes glycogen breakdown; thus it can effectively raise glucose levels under conditions where glycogen stores have not been depleted (hyperinsulinism).

3. Glucocorticoids have been used in the past for the treatment of hypoglycemia, particularly in the newborn. The only clear indication for their use is adrenal insufficiency (primary or secondary). The empirical use of glucocorticoids in the treatment of hypoglycemia should be undertaken only after a diligent and thorough search for the underlying pathophysiologic mechanism has been completed.

62. What are the frequency, duration, and clinical features of gynecomastia in pubertal males?

Gynecomastia is common in males during puberty, with as many as 65% of boys between the age of 14 and 14.5 years having some breast development. In 27% it will last for longer than 1 year and in 7% for longer than 2 years. It occurs most commonly during Tanner genital stage 3–4. Usually it consists of subareolar enlargement (breast bud) and is bilateral. The breast bud may be tender.

63. How is gynecomastia evaluated?

A simple history and physical examination are usually adequate to rule out pathologic processes. Hormonal or radiologic evaluations are rarely necessary in a midpubertal boy who presents with breast enlargement. In contrast, the prepubertal child warrants more concern, as does the child with chronic complaints suggestive of an intracranial mass or a pubertal age boy with little or no virilization.

64. What are the causes of gynecomastia?

Normal pubertal development
Recovery from chronic disease
Drugs
   Estrogens
   Testosterone
   Phenothiazine
   Meprobamate
   Hydroxyzine
   Reserpine
   Spironolactone
   Digoxin
   Marijuana
Inadequate androgen production
   Klinefelter's syndrome
   Testicular failure
   Isolated LH deficiency (fertile eunuch)
Excessive estrogen production
   Feminizing tumors (usually adrenal)
"Local" disorders or pseudo-gynecomastia
   Carcinoma of the breast
   Neurofibromatosis
   Hemangiomas
   Lipomas
   Abscess
   Bruise
Other
   Pituitary tumor
   Testicular tumor
   Thyroid disease (hyper or hypo)

65. What is the sella turcica and what is the significance of its enlargement on a skull film?

The sella turcica derives its name from the Latin word for Turkish saddle. The name reflects the anatomical shape of the saddle-like prominence on the upper surface of the sphenoid bone in the middle cranial fossa. A variety of conditions can lead to sellar enlargement including tumors of the pituitary or functional hypertrophy of the pituitary, which may occur in primary hypothyroidism or primary hypogonadism. Radiologic techniques for defining pituitary anatomy include skull radiographs, CT, and MRI.

66. What are the clinical manifestations of growth hormone excess?

Prior to puberty, the cardinal manifestations are an increase in growth velocity with minimal bony deformity and soft tissue swelling. This condition is called pituitary gigantism. Hypogonadotrophic hypogonadism and delayed puberty often coexist with the growth hormone excess and affected children exhibit eunuchoid body proportions. If the growth hormone excess occurs after puberty (after epiphyseal closure), coarsening of the facial features and soft tissue swelling of the feet and hands occur.

67. What endocrine tests should be ordered to identify children with acromegaly/gigantism?

The most useful test for growth hormone excess is the measurement of somatomedin-C (IGF-I). This protein, produced in response to growth hormone, is high in nearly all affected patients. Growth hormone levels that are low (less than 5 ng/ml) do not necessarily rule out growth hormone hypersecretion, because growth hormone release into the systemic circulation may be episodic.

68. What is Nelson's syndrome and how is it diagnosed?

One approach to the treatment of Cushing's disease has been bilateral adrenalectomy. Subsequently, demonstrable pituitary tumors develop in as many as one-third of the patients. These tumors may be large enough to produce local pressure symptoms and there is increased pigmentation of the skin and mucosa. This combination of findings is called Nelson's syndrome. The diagnosis is confirmed by a significant elevation of the ACTH level and/or the demonstration of a mass lesion on CT examination of the sella turcica.

69. What systemic disease processes can affect the hypothalamus?

A wide variety of diseases can affect the hypothalamus and pituitary. These can be due to destruction of the pituitary (tumor, infarct), a genetic deficiency of a particular hormone-producing cell type (e.g., isolated LH deficiency), interruption of median eminence-pituitary stalk connection (surgical stalk section), loss of inhibitory or excitatory input from the hypothalamus (e.g., idiopathic precocious puberty), or input from the cerebrum (e.g., psychogenic amenorrhea). A number of systemic diseases may also have effects on the hypothalamic/pituitary axis—some by direct central nervous system invasion and others by uncharacterized means.

70. What are the causes of hypothalamic-pituitary dysfunction?
Intracranial
  Congenital
    Inherited deficiencies—GRF, GnRH
    Syndromic
      Laurence-Moon-Biedl
      Prader-Labhart-Willi
    Craniopharyngioma
    Rathke pouch cyst
    Hemangioma
    Hamartoma

  Infectious
    Meningitis
    Encephalitis

  Tumors
    Glioma
    Dysgerminoma
    Ependymoma

  Trauma
    Subarachnoid hemorrhage
    Intraventricular hemorrhage
    Surgical stalk section

  Idiopathic

Systemic
  CNS Involvement Demonstrable
    Kernicterus
    Congenital infection
    Sarcoidosis
    Eosinophilic granuloma
    Tuberculosis
    Neurofibromatosis
    Leukemia

  CNS Involvement Not Demonstrable
    Anorexia nervosa
    Psychosocial dwarfism
    Chronic illness

71. What clinical signs or symptoms suggest hypothalamic dysfunction?
The signs and symptoms of hypothalamic dysfunction are as variable as the processes controlled by the hypothalamus, ranging from disorders of hormonal production to disturbances of thermoregulation. Either precocious or delayed sexual maturation has been seen, and together represent the most common presentation of hypothalamic abnormality in childhood. Diabetes insipidus, psychic disturbances, and excessive sleepiness are found in about one-third of all patients and may be the first manifestation of disease. Eating disorders (obesity, anorexia, bulimia) are also reported as are convulsions. Dyshydrosis and disturbances of sphincteric control are occasionally seen.

72. What hormonal features are seen in anorexia nervosa?
Amenorrhea is seen in most cases due to hypothalamic pituitary dysfunction with decreased FSH and LH levels. Twenty-five percent experience amenorrhea before weight loss, emphasizing the psychologic effect on physiology. Males are often infertile. Symptoms suggestive of hypothyroidism such as constipation, cold intolerance, dry skin, bradycardia and hair or nail changes are common. Thyroid studies, however, are relatively normal except for a low T_3 and increased rT_3, a less active isomer. The T_3/rT_3 reversal is seen also in conditions associated with weight loss as a means to adopt to a lower energy state. Other abnormalities include a loss of diurnal variation in cortisol, diminished plasma catecholamine levels, normal or increased growth hormone levels, and flattened glucose tolerance curves.

73. What are the causes of short stature?
  1. Familial
  2. Constitutional delay
  3. Chronic disease
        Inflammatory bowel disease
        Chronic renal failure
        Cyanotic heart disease
  4. Chromosomal
        Turner's (45XO)
        Down's (Trisomy 21)
  5. Endocrine
        Hypothyroidism
        Growth hormone deficiency
        Hypopituitarism
        Hypogonadism
        Cushing's syndrome
  6. Other
        Psychosocial
        Primordial dwarfism
        Cranio-spinal irradiation

74. How should children with short stature be evaluated?

The evaluation is based on the differentiation of the child into one of the six categories and the consequent pursuit of the specific site of defect. In most children, this can be accomplished by a thorough history and careful physical examination. Since adult size is primarily genetically determined, a history of familial heights, growth patterns, and ethnic origins is mandatory. The age at which puberty occurred in other family members is often helpful in identifying children with constitutional delay, since this entity tends to run in families, the strongest association being that of father and son. Most women will remember their age at menarche, and this age can be used as a reference for the age at which other pubertal events occurred. The most useful reference point for adult males is the age at which they reached their adult height, since almost all normal males will have reached their adult height by 18 years of age (high school graduation). Significant growth beyond this age suggests a history of pubertal delay. The gestational and birth history are often revealing. About half of small-for-dates infants, while growing at normal rates, remain small throughout childhood. Girls with Turner's syndrome are often short at birth, and many are noted to have edema of the hands and feet in the newborn period.

A review of systems should be undertaken with particular emphasis on systemic disease, intracranial pathology, and medication usage. Growth failure in inflammatory bowel disease may precede the onset of clinical disease by more than a year. Chronic headaches or visual difficulties may presage pituitary or hypothalamic pathology. Frequent use of pharmacologic doses of steroidal hormones may suppress linear growth. Changes in the level of activity, sleeping patterns, or bowel habits can be an early indication of thyroid disease, while failure to change shoe size and excess abdominal obesity suggest a deficiency of growth hormone. An examination of photographs taken of the child and the child's siblings at various ages can be helpful in separating familial changes from clinical problems.

Access to previous growth records is absolutely essential since endocrine diseases affect the rate of linear growth. These records can often be obtained from the school, the family physician, the child's "baby book" or the "door jam" in the family home. If records are not available, it is useful to obtain heights every 3 months over a 6–12 month period prior to the initiation of extensive testing. Since linear growth is the real issue in short children, the primary focus is on obtaining accurate sequential height measurements. It is essential that this process be standardized and that the same observer obtains the measurement.

75. What laboratory studies should be obtained in the evaluation of short stature?

Screening tests for endocrinologic diseases should not be undertaken unless the growth rate is abnormally low. For prepubertal children over the age of three, growth rates in excess of 5 cm per year are adequate to rule out endocrinologic causes of short stature. With lower growth rates, the standard screening tests are a serum thyroxine (T_4) and a somatomedin-C level. Random growth hormone levels are of little value, since even in the normal child, growth hormone levels are low most of the time. Unlike growth hormone, the concentration of somatomedin-C varies minimally on a day-to-day basis, and low values can be distinguished from normal values. Factors other than growth hormone deficiency may lower the level of somatomedin-C, including hypothyroidism, malnutrition, liver disease, or a protein-losing disease such as nephrosis. A low somatomedin-C in the absence of the aforementioned factors is suggestive of growth hormone deficiency. A positive diagnosis depends on the response to provocative testing for the growth hormone. If the child has both a low T_4 and a low somatomedin-C, thyroid hormone replacement should be initiated promptly and a repeat somatomedin-C obtained after the thyroid levels have normalized.

A bone age should also be obtained. The rate of bony maturation corresponds better with physical development than does chronologic age. Generally, a radiograph of the left hand and wrist is obtained and compared with the standards determined by Greulich and Pyle. Occasionally a more complete bone age using the knees, elbows, and ankles is required. A single bone age is of value in differentiating familial short stature (normal bone age) from other causes of shortness. A delayed bone age (greater than 2 S.D. below the mean) that is consistent with the child's height age is suggestive of constitutional delay, while a markedly delayed bone age is suggestive of endocrinologic or chronic disease. Serial bone ages separated by 6 months are often helpful, since in both the normal child and the child with constitutional delay, a bone age will advance in parallel with chronologic age, while in endocrinologic disease, the bone age fails progressively further behind chronologic age. Chromosomal analysis is not part of the initial evaluation of a short child unless there are historical or physical findings suggestive of an abnormality.

76. What is the differential diagnosis for diabetes insipidus in childhood?
Vasopressin deficiency
  Genetic: defective synthesis
  Hypothalamic tumors: glioma, craniopharyngioma, cysts
  Post-traumatic: accidental, neurosurgical
  Inflammatory: meningitis, encephalitis
  Granulomatous disease: tuberculosis, sarcoidosis, Wegener's
  Vascular: aneurysm, thrombosis

Vasopressin resistance
  Genetic: nephrogenic diabetes insipidus, medullary cystic disease
  Pharmacologic: lithuim, demeclocycline, diuretics
  Osmotic diuresis: diabetes mellitus
  Electrolyte abnormalities: hypercalcemia, hypokalemia
  Renal disease: renal tubular acidosis, polynephritis, papillary necrosis
  Hemodynamic: hyperthyroidism
  Other: psychogenic or drug-induced polydipsia, tricyclics, thioridazine

77. How should children with suspected diabetes insipidus be evaluated?
The clinical history provides useful clues. The child who sleeps for 8–12 hours and does not become dehydrated despite the lack of intake is unlikely to have diabetes insipidus. In many instances, the demonstration of a concentrated urine (>800 mOsm/L) in the presence of a normal serum (<290 mOsm/L) after a normal period of fluid abstinence is adequate to rule out the diagnosis of diabetes insipidus. If these results are equivocal, then a more complex water deprivation test must be undertaken. The key to making the diagnosis of diabetes insipidus rests in the demonstration of an inappropriately dilute urine in the presence of concentrated serum. Physical evidence of dehydration (weight loss · 5% of body weight, tachycardia, postural hypotension, loss of skin turgor) consistent with these chemical findings is strongly supportive of the diagnosis.

Water deprivation tests should be performed under well-controlled circumstances with meticulous attention to detail. A basal weight, blood pressure, pulse rate, and serum and urine osmolalities are obtained. Fluids are then withheld. Clinical parameters are followed at least hourly. Urine output is recorded on an hourly basis as well. The frequency with which urine and serum osmolalities are obtained depends on the rapidity of weight loss and/or the volume of urine output, but no less frequently than every 4 hours. The study is generally stopped when the serum osmolality reaches 305 mOsm, when the patient has significant loss (≥ 5%) of body weight, or when the patient demonstrates the ability to conserve water. If the diagnosis is confirmed by the test, the study is ended with synthetic antidiuretic hormone (DDAVP) and the provision of fluids. If urine osmolality rises rapidly while urine volume and serum osmality fall, antidiuretic hormone deficiency is indicated. If there is little or no response, antidiuretic hormone resistance is indicated (nephrogenic diabetes insipidus).

78. What is the Tanner staging system?
It is the standardization of terminology to delineate the normal sequence of events that occur during puberty.

Sex Maturity Stages

STAGE	BOYS	GIRLS
	Pubic Hair	**Pubic Hair**
I	None	None
II	Countable, straight, increased pigmentation and length; at base of penis	Straight, increased pigmentation and length; medial border of labia and mons
III	Darker, begins to curl, increased quantity	Darker, begins to curl, increased quantity
IV	Increased quantity, coarser texture; covers most of pubic area	Coarser; labia and mons well covered
V	Adult distribution; spread to medial thighs and lower abdomen	Adult distribution with feminine triangle and spread to medial thighs
	Genitals	**Breasts**
I	Prepubertal	Prepubertal
II	Slight testicular enlargement (>5 ml); slight rugation and darkening of scrotum	Breast bud present, increased areolar size
III	Further testicular enlargement; penile lengthening	Further enlargement of breast bud; no secondary contour
IV	Further testicular enlargement; increased rugation of scrotum; increased penile breadth	Areola and papilla form secondary mound on breast contour
V	Adult	Mature; areola part of breast contour; nipple projects.

79. What is precocious puberty?

The appearance of physical changes associated with sexual development earlier than normal (3 S.D. from the mean age for that change). In practical terms this means the appearance of breast buds (Tanner Stage II) before 7.5 years, pubic hair (Tanner Stage II) before 7.5 years, or menses before 9.25 years in the female; in the male, the appearance of pubic hair or genital development before 9.5 years is considered abnormal.

80. What are some of the various forms of precocious puberty?

The terms used to describe precocious puberty reflect the fact that normal puberty is an orderly process by which female children are feminized and male children are masculinized. The development of breast tissue but no pubic hair is called *precocious thelarche*. If pubic hair subsequently develops, the term *precocious puberty* is used. If pubic hair develops without breast tissue, the term *precocious pubarche* is used. Since pubic hair development in the female is thought to be due to adrenal androgens, the term *precocious adrenarche* is used as well. If the pubertal changes, though early, proceed in an orderly fashion, beginning with breast budding, followed by pubic hair development, a growth spurt, and finally menstruation, the term *true precocious puberty* is used. The orderly nature suggests that pituitary and/or hypothalamic centers are intact and regulating the pubertal process appropriately. *Pseudo-precocious puberty* is used when some of the changes of puberty are present but their appearance is isolated or out of the normal sequence. For example, menses without breast development would be classified as "pseudo-precocious." When the changes of puberty are consistent with the child's gender, they are referred to (for some odd reason) as heterosexual. (If you have read this far, you now understand why simple description is easier.) The child with 3 cm breast buds bilaterally and no pubic hair could be labeled using any of the following terms: precocious thelarche, "early" precocious puberty, isosexual precocious puberty, etc. It boggles the mind. Furthermore, having a name provides a false sense of security since the name has the aura of a diagnosis yet does not address the underlying cause.

81. How should a child with precocious puberty be evaluated?

This evaluation is often costly and complex, and in most cases a specific cause will not be identified. As a general rule of thumb, the younger the child and the more rapid the onset of the condition, the greater the likelihood of pathology.

1. *History.* Since pubertal changes are affected by the pituitary/hypothalamus, the adrenal and the gonad, the history and physical exam focus on signs and symptoms related to these tissues. Rarely, a gonadotropin or a sex hormone will be produced by a tumor (e.g., a liver hepatoma producing human chorionic gonadotropin). Questions should be asked concerning the intake of estrogenic compounds either from medications (birth control pills, estrogenic creams) or from plant and animal sources. The chronology of the physical changes should be noted as well.

2. *Physical examination.* This should include examination of the optic fundus for evidence of increased intracranial pressure and careful visual fields for evidence of optic nerve compression by hypothalamic or pituitary masses. Note should be made as to whether the child's appearance is consistent with his or her chronologic age. The presence of facial hair and acne suggests increased levels of androgens. Androgens also tend to increase muscle bulk and definition. The presence of breast tissue suggests increased estrogen as does increased size of the areola. The quantity and location of body hair should be noted in detail. In females, the cornification of the vaginal epithelium due to increased estrogen results in a change in the color of the vaginal mucosa from a prepubertal red to a more opalescent pink. The labia minora also becomes more prominent and visible between the labia majora. In the male, the earliest evidence of puberty is testicular enlargement. Pubertal development *without* testicular enlargement usually suggests adrenal pathology. The size of each testicle is easily determined using a Prader orchidometer. Increased rugation of the scrotum and some increase in pigmentation also accompany puberty. The stretched length of the penis can also be compared to normal standards.

3. *Radiologic evaluation.* This focuses on the gonad, the adrenal, and the pituitary. In the female, ultrasound evaluation serves to rule out adrenal and ovarian masses or cysts. Increased echogenicity and increased size of the uterus are suggestive of endometrial proliferation and uterine growth in response to elevated circulating levels of estrogen. In the male, ultrasound is adequate to rule out adrenal masses. CT is the preferred means for investigating the cranial cavity and the pituitary fossa. A bone age is often helpful in determining the duration of exposure to the elevated sex hormone. For example, a child with precocious thelarche secondary to ingestion of several birth control pills is unlikely to have an advanced bone age. In contrast, a child with the non-salt-losing form of the 21-hydroxylase deficiency (congenital adrenal hyperplasia), who has been exposed to excess androgens since birth, will have a bone age far greater than chronologic age.

4. *Laboratory evaluation.* Initial studies should include a determination of luteinizing hormone (LH), follicle stimulating hormone (FSH), estradiol, and testosterone. Adrenal steroid levels (17-hydroxyprogesterone, androstenedione, and cortisol) should also be determined. More extensive studies may be needed in a virilized child if the initial studies are normal. Provocative testing of the pituitary/hypothalamic axis using a synthetic gonadotropin releasing factor (GnRH) or of the adrenal using an ACTH agonist (Cortrosyn) may be needed, especially in the child presenting with slight but progressive pubertal changes.

Bibliography

General Text

1. Hung W, August GP, Glasgow AN: Pediatric Endocrinology. Garden City, Medical Examination Publishing Co., 1978.
2. Kaplan SA: Clinical Pediatric and Adolescent Endocrinology. Philadelphia, W.B. Saunders Co., 1982.

Adrenal Disorders

3. Byyny RL: Withdrawal from glucocorticoid therapy. N Engl J Med 295:30–32, 1976.
4. Christy NP (ed): The Human Adrenal Cortex. New York, Harper and Row, 1971.
5. Fass B: Glucocorticoid therapy for nonendocrine disorders: withdrawal and "coverage." Pediatr Clin N Am 26:251–256, 1979.
6. New MI, Levine LS: Congenital Adrenal Hyperplasia. New York, Springer-Verlag, 1984.

Calcium/Phosphorus Metabolism

7. Root AW: Recent advances in calcium metabolism. J Pediatr 88:1–18, 177–199, 1976.

Diabetes Insipidus

8. Hendricks SA, Lippe B, Kaplan SA, Lee WNP: Differential diagnosis of diabetes insipidus: Use of DDAVP to terminate the seven hour water deprivation test. J Pediatr 98:244–246, 1981.
9. Richman RA, Post EM, Notman DD: Simplifying the diagnosis of diabetes insipidus in children. Am J Dis Child 135:839–842, 1981.

Diabetes Mellitus

10. Foster DW, McGarry JO: The metabolic derangements and treatment of diabetic ketoacidosis. N Engl J Med 309:159–68, 1983.
11. Malleson PN: Diabetic ketoacidosis in children treated by adding low-dose insulin to rehydrating fluid. Arch Dis Child 51:375–376, 1976.

Fasting Adaptation/Hypoglycemia

12. Bier DM, Leake RD, Haymond MW, et al: Measurement of "true" glucose production rates in infancy and childhood with 6,6-dideuteroglucose. Diabetes 26:1016–1023, 1977.
13. Pagliara AS, Karl IE, Haymond M, Kipnis DM: Hypoglycemia in infancy and childhood. J Pediatr 82:365–379, 1973.

McCune-Albright

14. Albright F, Butler AM, Hampton AO, Smith P: Syndrome characterized by osteitis fibrosis disseminata, areas of pigmentation and endocrine dysfunction, with precocious puberty in females. N Engl J Med 216:727–747, 1937.

Multiple Endocrine Neoplasia

15. Newsome HH: Multiple endocrine adenomatosis. Surg Clin North Am 54:307–393, 1974.
16. Sipple IH: The association of pheochromocytoma with carcinoma of the thyroid gland. Am J Med 31:163–166, 1961.
17. Wermer P: Genetic aspects of adenomatosis of endocrine glands. Am J Med 16:363–371, 1954.

Pituitary Disorders

18. Kannan CR (ed): The Pituitary Gland. New York, Plenum Medical Book Co., 1987.

Puberty

19. Prader A: Delayed adolescence. J Clin Endocrinol Metab 4:143–155, 1975.
20. Root AW: Endocrinology of puberty in normal sexual maturation. J Pediatr 83:1–19, 1973.
21. Tanner JM: Growth and Adolescence, 2nd ed. Oxford, Blackwell, 1962.

Thyroid Disease

22. Dussault JH, Walker P (eds): Congenital Hypothyroidism. New York, Marcel Dekker Inc., 1983.
23. Ingbar SH, Braverman LE (eds): The Thyroid. Philadelphia, J.B. Lippincott Co., 1986.

GASTROENTEROLOGY AND NUTRITION

David A. Piccoli, M.D.

1. What are the daily total energy requirements for infants and children?

The nutritional requirements of infants and children depend on age and on the presence of any special circumstances that may increase or decrease demands or losses. Although the body can compensate for a wide range of diets, guidelines have been established for intake.

Daily Energy Requirements Based on Age and Weight

AGE (yr)	CALORIES (per kg/day)
Infants	
0–0.5	117
0.5–1	105
Children	
1–3	100
4–6	85–90
7–10	80–85
11–14	M: 60–64 F: 48–55
15–18	M: 43–49 F: 38–40

From the Food and Nutrition Board, National Research Council Recommended Daily Dietary Allowances, rev 9th ed and 10th ed. Washington, D.C., National Academy of Sciences, 1974, 1979.

2. What happens if calorie intake is inadequate?

To satisfy energy requirements, the diet must contain a balance of protein, carbohydrate, and fat, in addition to water, vitamins, minerals, and trace elements. Each gram of protein or carbohydrate supplies 4 kcal and each gram of fat provides 9 kcal. If caloric intake is inadequate, protein will be diverted from synthetic pathways and converted into energy.

3. What is the calorie-nitrogen ratio?

The relationship between energy and protein intake. Usually a ratio of 150:1 or more is required, but this ratio is modified in states of increased protein utilization or decreased protein metabolism.

4. Why do total energy requirements vary for each individual?

Total energy requirements are calculated to provide sufficient calories for basal metabolism, specific dynamic action, growth, physical activity, fecal losses, urinary losses, and increases of metabolism due to disease states. While guidelines are established for normal infants and children, these must be modified to compensate for special needs. Although most children with nutritional problems have increased caloric requirements, there are children with increased body reserves or decreased physical activity who require significantly fewer calories than normal.

5. What are the requirements for protein, fat, and carbohydrates in infants and children? What percentage of caloric intake should each supply?

Protein should account for 7–15% of caloric intake, and should include a balance of the 11 essential amino acids. Protein requirements range from 0.7–2.5 gm/kg/day. Fats should provide 30–50% of caloric intake. While the majority of these calories are derived from long-chain triglycerides, sterols, medium-chain triglycerides, and fatty acids may be important in certain diets. Linoleic acid and arachidonic acid are essential for tissue membrane synthesis, and approximately 3% of intake must be composed of these triglycerides. The remaining 50–60% of calories should come from carbohydrates. About half of these are contributed by mono- and disaccharides such as sucrose and lactose, and the remainder as starch.

Recommended Protein Intake (gm/day)

	AGE (yr)	WEIGHT (kg)	PROTEIN (gm)
Infants	<0.5	6	$2.2 \times kg$
Infants	0.5–1	9	$2.0 \times kg$
Children	1–3	13	23
	4–6	20	30
	7–10	28	34
Males	11–14	45	45
	15–18	66	56
	19–22	70	56
Females	11–14	46	62
	15–18	55	64
	19–22	55	64
Pregnancy			+30
Lactation			+20

Adapted from the Committee on Dietary Allowances, and Food and Nutrition Board: Recommended Dietary Allowances, rev 9th ed. Washington, D.C., National Academy of Sciences, 1980.

6. How is nutritional status assessed in children?

Nutritional status can be assessed from historical information and the clinical condition of the patient. A retrospective 24-hour dietary recall may provide adequate information, but a precise 72-hour prospective intake record is substantially more accurate. A social and environmental assessment, and in some cases a feeding skills session, is advised to determine the adequacy of the eating environment. This may demonstrate significant abnormalities in the infant or in the maternal interaction. The physical signs of malnutrition occur late in the course of deficiencies, and thus earlier manifestations should be sought.

1. The most easily obtainable information comes from a carefully plotted *growth chart.* Anthropometric data give an estimate of the height, weight, and head circumference of a child, compared to a population standard. Growth curves also provide a plot of weight for height (or stature). At any single point in time, this is a more accurate representation of the current nutritional status of the child. A change in the child's percentile after the first 6–12 months may signify the presence of a nutritional problem or systemic disease.

2. *Compare actual with ideal body weight* (the average weight for height age). The ideal body weight is determined by plotting the child's height on the 50th percentile, and recording the corresponding age. The 50th percentile weight for that age is obtained, and this ideal body weight is divided by the actual weight. The result is expressed as a percentage, the percent ideal body weight. This gives a better stratification of patients with significant malnutrition. A %IBW of >120 is obese, 110–120 is overweight, 90–110 normal, 80–90 mild wasting, 70–80 moderate wasting, and <70 is severe wasting.

3. *Measurement of midarm circumference* provides information about the subcutaneous fat stores, and the midarm-muscle circumference (calculated from the triceps skinfold thickness) estimates the somatic protein or muscle mass. Subscapular skinfold thickness measurements may be preferable in infants. These values can be compared to standards for the patient's age and sex. Nomograms based on these measurements can be used to calculate the percent of body fat in children. Potential errors in calculation arise when there is overhydration or underhydration, extreme obesity, musculoskeletal disorders, and profound mental-motor retardation.

4. *Laboratory assessment* of nutritional status can provide objective data about the patient. Vitamin and mineral status can be directly assayed. Measurements of albumin (half-

life 14–20 days), transferrin (half-life 8–10.5 days), and prealbumin (half life 2–3 days) can provide information about protein synthesis, but each may be affected by certain diseases. The ratio of albumin to globulin may decrease in protein malnutrition. The creatinine height index is a measure of lean body mass which decreases as muscle protein is used as an energy source. Specific measurements of nitrogen balance may be obtained to determine the degree of protein anabolism or catabolism.

7. What are the physical findings associated with malnutrition?

Clinical Signs of Malnutrition

CLINICAL SIGN	NUTRIENT
Epithelial	
Skin	
Xerosis, dry scaling	Essential fatty acids
Hyperkeratosis, plaques around hair follicles	Vitamin A
Ecchymoses, petechiae	Vitamin K, Vitamin C
Hair	
Easily plucked, dyspigmented, lackluster	Protein-calorie
Nails	
Thin, spoon-shaped	Iron
Mucosal	
Mouth, lips, and tongue	B vitamins
Angular stomatitis (inflammation at corners of mouth)	B2 (riboflavin)
Cheilosis (reddened lips with fissures at angles)	B2, B6 (pyridoxine)
Glossitis (inflammation of tongue)	B6, B3 (niacin), B2
Magenta tongue	B2
Edema of tongue, tongue fissures	B3
Spongy, bleeding gums	Vitamin C
Ocular	
Pale conjunctivae secondary to anemia	Iron, folic acid, vitamin B12, copper
Bitot's spots (grayish, yellow, or white foamy spots on the whites of the eye)	Vitamin A
Conjunctival or corneal xerosis, keratomalacia	Vitamin A
Musculoskeletal	
Craniotabes, palpable enlargement of costochondral junctions ("rachitic rosary"); thickening of wrists and ankles	Vitamin D
Scurvy (tenderness of extremities, hemorrhages under periosteum of long bones; enlargement of costochondral junction; cessation of long bone osteogenesis)	Vitamin C
Skeletal lesions	Copper
Muscle wasting	Protein-calorie
General	
Edema	Protein
Pallor—Anemia	Vitamin E (prematures), iron, folic acid, vitamin B12, copper
Neurologic	
Mental confusion	Protein, vitamin B1 (thiamine)
Peripheral neuropathy	Vitamin E

Table continued on next page

Clinical Signs of Malnutrition *(Continued)*

CLINICAL SIGN	NUTRIENT
Cardiovascular	
Beriberi (enlarged heart, congestive heart failure, tachycardia)	Vitamin B1
Tachycardia secondary to anemia	Iron, folic acid, B12, copper, vitamin E in premature infants
Gastrointestinal	
Hepatomegaly	Protein-calorie
Endocrine	
Thyroid enlargement	Iodine

From Kerner JA (ed): Manual of Pediatric Parenteral Nutrition. New York, John Wiley & Sons, 1983, p 22, with permission.

8. How are marasmus and kwashiorkor distinguished clinically?

Although both disorders are due to a deficiency in energy intake, the syndromes differ dramatically because of the available protein sources. Kwashiorkor is edematous malnutrition due to low serum oncotic pressure. The low serum proteins result from a disproportionately low protein intake, compared to the overall caloric intake. These children appear replete or fat, but have dependent edema, hyperkeratosis, and atrophic hair and skin. They generally have severe anorexia, diarrhea, frequent infections, and may have cardiac failure. Marasmus is severe non-edematous malnutrition caused by a mixed deficiency of both protein and calories. Serum protein and albumin levels are usually normal but there is a marked decrease in muscle mass and adipose tissue. Signs are similar to those noted in hypothyroid children, with cold intolerance, listlessness, thin sparse hair, dry skin with decreased turgor, and hypotonia. Diarrhea, anorexia, vomiting, and recurrent infections may be noted.

9. What are the immunologic abnormalities associated with malnutrition?

Increased susceptibility to infection, decreased total circulating lymphocytes ($<2500/mm^3$ in the first 3 months of life and $<1800/mm^3$ later), and anergy or impairment of delayed cutaneous hypersensitivity to skin test antigens. A number of the disease states that result in malnutrition have a direct effect on the immunologic competence of the host.

10. What are the requirements for essential fatty acids in infancy and childhood?

The primary essential fatty acid in humans is linoleic acid. It is converted to longer chain fatty acids with multiple double bonds, which are essential components of membranes. Arachidonic acid is also a component of membranes, but it can be synthesized from linoleic acid. A dietary intake of linoleic acid at a level of 1–2% of dietary calories will prevent both the biochemical and the clinical manifestations of essential fatty acid deficiency in humans. Medium-chain triglycerides do not provide essential fatty acids. Oral fats high in linoleic acid include safflower oil (72%), sunflower oil (61%), and corn oil (54%).

11. During breastfeeding, how long before the breast is emptied?

Breastfeeding varies with each mother-infant pair. Although breastfeeding of at least 15 minutes on the first side and 5–15 minutes on the second is recommended, the majority of the milk is released in the first 5–8 minutes. This varies with the time and completeness of the letdown phase, and the vigor and attention of the baby to the feeding itself.

12. Are supplementary formula and water feedings necessary in breastfed infants?

No

13. When may occasional bottle-feeding be introduced in breastfed infants?

After lactation has been established (approximately 2 weeks postpartum).

14. When does an infant's first appetite spurt occur?
8–10 days of age.

15. When should weaning from breastfeeding be initiated?
The American Academy of Pediatrics recommends breastfeeding for 12 months with the introduction of supplementary foods at 4 to 6 months.

16. May milk be heated in a microwave oven?
No. Microwave heating produces uneven temperatures. Also, human milk is easily damaged by high temperatures.

17. Should breastfeeding be continued throughout most maternal illnesses?
Yes. Exceptions are maternal AIDS, active untreated tuberculosis, herpes of the breast region, and primary herpes.

18. What are the major complications of intravenous hyperalimentation?
Mechanical, infectious, and metabolic.

1. Mechanical complications vary with the type of infusion and the delivery system, and include local or distant site thrombosis, perforation of the vasculature or heart, and accidental breakage or infiltration of the infusate into the subcutaneous, pleural, or pericardial space. Unfortunately, accidental dislodgment or disconnection is all too common in pediatric patients, and an emergency clamp should always be accessible.

2. Line-associated sepsis is a life-threatening complication that is associated with poor line aseptic technique. Any patient with a fever and a central line should have an immediate set of peripheral and "line" cultures and be started on antibiotics pending the initial results. Because sepsis can be seeded by contaminated intravenous solutions, all equipment should be cultured in suspected line sepsis.

3. The metabolic complications of hyperalimentation may be limited by close monitoring of the patient and an understanding of the primary disease process:

Potential Metabolic Complications of TPN

COMPLICATION	POSSIBLE ETIOLOGY
Disorders related to metabolic capacity of the patient	
Congestive heart failure and pulmonary edema	Excessively rapid infusion of TPN solution
Hyperglycemia (with resultant glucosuria, osmotic diuresis, and possible dehydration)	Excessive intake (either excessive dextrose concentration or increased infusion rate)
	Change in metabolic state (e.g., sepsis, surgical stress, use of steroids)
	Common in low birth weight infants if dextrose load exceeds their ability to adapt
Hypoglycemia	Sudden cessation of infusate
Azotemia	Excessive administration of amino acids or protein hydrolysate (excessive nitrogen intake)
Electrolyte disorders	
Mineral disorders	
Vitamin disorders	
Trace element disorders	
Essential fatty acid deficiency	Inadequate intake
Hyperlipidemia (increased triglycerides, cholesterol, and free fatty acids)	Excessive intake of intravenous fat emulsion

Table continued on next page

Potential Metabolic Complications of TPN *(Continued)*

COMPLICATION	POSSIBLE ETIOLOGY
Disorders related to infusate components	
Metabolic acidosis	Use of hydrochloride salts of cationic amino acids
Hyperammonemia	Inadequate arginine intake, ? deficiencies of other urea cycle substrates, ? plasma amino acid imbalance, ? hepatic dysfunction
Abnormal plasma aminograms	Amino acid pattern of infusate
Miscellaneous	
Anemia	Failure to replace blood loss; iron deficiency, folic acid and B1 deficiency; copper deficiency
Demineralization of bone; rickets	Inadequate intake of calcium, inorganic phosphate, and/or vitamin D intake
Hepatic disorders	Prematurity; malnutrition; sepsis,
Cholestasis	? hepatotoxicity due to amino acid
Biochemical and histiopathologic abnormalities	imbalance; exceeding non-nitrogen calorie-nitrogen ratio of 150:1 to 200:1, leading
Cholelithiasis	to excessive glycogen and/or fat deposition
Hepatitis	in the liver; decreased stimulation of bile flow; nonspecific response to refeeding
Eosinophilia	Unknown

Modified from Heird WC: Total parenteral nutrition. In Lebenthal E (ed): Textbook of Gastroenterology and Nutrition in Infancy. New York, Raven Press, 1981, p 662.

19. How frequently and with what laboratory tests should a patient on hyperalimentation be monitored?

Patient Monitoring

All laboratory values should be recorded at the onset of therapy

Every Shift

Temperature and vital signs

Urine dipstick for sugar and specific gravity (until stable)

Daily

Physical examination

Weight

Input and output

Dextrostix as indicated

Weekly

Anthropometrics

Laboratory Monitoring

Daily until stable, then twice per week

Serum glucose, sodium, potassium, chloride, and bicarbonate

BUN and creatinine

Calcium, phosphate, and magnesium

Weekly

Complete blood count with platelets

Bilirubin and liver function tests

Cholesterol and triglycerides

Albumin, total protein, total iron binding capacity

As indicated by disease state

Serum B_{12}, iron, trace elements, serum amino acids

20. Name and describe the three tests that should be included in the diagnostic workup for Hirschsprung's disease.

Anorectal manometry, barium studies, or rectal biopsy.

1. Rectal manometry is performed with a perfused balloon catheter inserted above the sphincter and gradually withdrawn. The balloon is intermittently inflated to induce the normal relaxation response of the sphincter. While this test poses the least risk to the patient, it is sometimes difficult to interpret in infancy and in children with severe chronic constipation.

2. The barium enema may demonstrate a persistent, irregularly contoured narrow segment starting just above the rectal ampulla, which may extend for only a few centimeters or for the entire length of the colon (in total colonic aganglionosis). Dilatation of the bowel is proximal to this segment. There is commonly a shelf or transition zone at this area, but this may not be present early in infancy. Following the study, retention of barium 24 or more hours is suggestive of Hirschsprung's disease or a significant motility disorder. It is important to remember that no bowel preparation should occur before the barium enema, and no rectal examinations or enemas should have been administered within the previous 24 hours. Likewise, the radiologist should be informed of the possibility of Hirschsprung's disease, as a special marked catheter is inserted to evaluate the distal anorectum.

3. Confirmation of the diagnosis requires a rectal biopsy to evaluate the intramural ganglion cells of the submucosal and myenteric plexuses. The presence of ganglion cells excludes the diagnosis. The absence of ganglion cells may be corroborated by special stains but must be interpreted with caution, as the identification relies on the persistence of the pathologist and the adequacy of the specimen.

21. What are the clinical presentations of Hirschsprung's disease?

Aganglionic megacolon is responsible for 20–25% of cases of neonatal intestinal obstruction. Most infants with Hirschsprung's disease have symptoms in the first week of life, which are commonly unrecognized. Neonatal intestinal perforation, obstruction with bilious vomiting, and toxic enterocolitis have significant morbidity and mortality. Recurrent meconium plug syndrome may occur.

Clinical Findings in Neonates with Hirschsprung's Disease

Delay in passage of meconium	95%
Evidence of a lower intestinal obstruction, complete or partial, with abdominal distention, bilious vomiting, respiratory distress	50%
Obstipation with abdominal distention; failure to thrive, followed by vomiting or diarrhea	25%
Intestinal perforation (appendiceal and cecal) with perforation	4%

From Swenson O, Sherman JO, Fisher JH: J Pediatr Surg 8:587–594, 1973, with permission.

22. What findings on physical examination suggest Hirschsprung's disease?

Hirschsprung's disease is four times more common in boys and is frequently associated with Down's syndrome. There is a family history in 7% of cases. The physical examination may show a markedly distended abdomen with a palpable stool mass. The rectal examination is most important in distinguishing Hirschsprung's disease from chronic severe constipation. The anal canal and rectum are usually empty, with no palpable fecal material. The canal itself is fairly tight and narrow, and the sphincter may feel tight as well. If the radiograph demonstrates fecal colonic impaction and the rectum is empty, Hirschsprung's disease is probable. In contrast, a patient with normal functional constipation may have concomitant encopresis (i.e., soiling, which is very unusual in patients with Hirschsprung's disease) and on rectal exam they have a loose sphincter with a patulous rectum, and commonly a hard fecal impaction extending to the sphincter, obstructing full rectal examination.

23. What is the cause of Zollinger-Ellison (ZE) syndrome?
A gastrin-secreting tumor, with resultant severe gastric acid hypersecretion.

24. What are the signs and symptoms of ZE syndrome?
Patients usually present with symptoms secondary to peptic ulcer disease, and nearly all patients with ZE develop ulcers at some time in the course of the disease. In general, these ulcers are more persistent and progressive, and commonly less responsive to treatment. Although the duodenal bulb is the most common location for both ZE and non-ZE associated ulcers, atypical ulcers in the distal duodenum or jejunum are more common in ZE. In children, any ulcer that does not heal after the first course of therapy should be investigated, as should patients with gastric acid hypersecretion and prominent gastric rugae.

25. How is the diagnosis of ZE syndrome confirmed?
A simple screening test is the fasting serum gastrin level, which should be obtained when the patient is not receiving acid blockade (H_2 blockers) or antacids. An elevated level requires prompt further investigation. Usually, the gastrin level is at least three-fold elevated in patients with ZE syndrome. Unfortunately, many patients with an elevated gastrin level do not have ZE. Furthermore, some patients with a normal gastrin level may have a hormone-secreting tumor. When the diagnosis is strongly suspected but the serum gastrin concentration is low, a gastric acid secretion test is useful. Arteriography and CT scanning may be useful in locating a tumor, but in a large number of cases even exploratory laparotomy may not identify the lesion.

26. What are the manifestations of milk protein allergy in childhood?
Milk protein allergy and milk intolerance have been blamed for nearly every symptom in infancy. It is important to distinguish between a milk protein allergy, a lactose intolerance, and the common side effects of significant milk ingestion. True food protein allergy is less common than its diagnosis, but may vary from subacute symptoms to a life-threatening emergency.

    Acute manifestations of milk protein allergy
        Angioedema
        Urticaria
        Acute vomiting and diarrhea
        Anaphylactic shock
        Gastrointestinal bleeding
    Subacute symptoms
        Chronic vomiting
        Intestinal obstruction
        Persistent diarrhea
        Malabsorption
        Protein-losing enteropathy
        Hypoproteinemia with or without edema
        Upper gastrointestinal bleeding
        Lower gastrointestinal bleeding
        Hemoptysis
        Abdominal distention
        Failure to thrive
        Colic

Diarrhea of variable severity is the most common manifestation of a milk protein allergy. Histological abnormalities of the small intestinal mucosa have been documented, with the most severe form seen as a flat villous lesion. Protein-losing enteropathy may result from disruption of the surface epithelium. The stools of children with primary milk protein intolerance often contain blood. At sigmoidoscopy there is an erythematous and friable mucosa, and biopsies demonstrate a cellular infiltration, often with eosinophils, and changes in the surface and glandular epithelium. Heiner's syndrome is hematemesis and hemoptysis with failure to thrive associated with milk allergy.

27. How is the diagnosis of milk allergy confirmed?

A careful history and physical examination are most important. The laboratory tests available are not sensitive or specific enough to fully confirm the diagnosis. Tests of humoral or cellular immune function, RAST tests, intradermal skin testing, and IgE levels have not been diagnostic. Specific assays for serum immunoglobulins directed against individual proteins in milk formulas may be useful. The peroral small bowel biopsy may show signs of superficial damage, but post-enteritis syndrome, celiac disease and other diseases also present with this finding.

The accurate diagnosis of milk protein allergy still relies on the clinical challenge test, evaluated according to the Goldman criteria. Symptoms must resolve upon removal of the offending antigen, and recur on rechallenge. Because so many of the symptoms are subjective or multifactorial, this sequence must be repeated three times in order to confirm the diagnosis. It is important to differentiate symptoms of lactose intolerance from those of milk protein allergy in any rechallenge situation.

28. What are the four varieties of lactose intolerance in childhood?

1. Primary or congenital alactasia is a rare disorder caused by absent or markedly decreased lactase in the small intestine as demonstrated by biopsy specimens. The levels of other surface enzymes are normal. This rare autosomal recessive disorder presents at birth in infants fed a lactose-containing formula, with severe watery diarrhea that resolves when lactose intake is eliminated.

2. Acquired or post-enteritis lactose intolerance is due to the destruction of the superficial mucosa of the small intestine and its resident lactase. Resolution of this syndrome occurs following repair of the microvillus environment.

3. Term and preterm newborns have a limited capacity to hydrolyze lactose in the first few weeks of life. In certain situations this may be clinically important, but in normal breastfed infants it does not justify formula changes. Stool-reducing substances are commonly present in stools of breastfed infants.

4. Late-onset lactose intolerance is due to the progressive decrease in small intestinal lactase activity seen in most mammals during childhood. Fifteen to 80% or more of adults are lactose malabsorbers, and in many ethnic groups this defect is uniform and severe. These patients have distention, bloating, discomfort, nausea, or diarrhea from lactose-containing foods.

29. What are the causes of secondary lactose intolerance?

Any disorder that alters the mucosa of the proximal small intestine may result in secondary lactose intolerance. For this reason, the lactose tolerance test is commonly used as a screening test for intestinal integrity, although this has the disadvantage of concomitantly identifying all primary lactose malabsorbers. Although a combination of factors is present in many disease processes, secondary lactose intolerance can be organized into lesions of the microsurface, total surface, transit time, and site of bacterial colonization in the small bowel.

At the microvillus/brush border
  Post-enteritis
  Bacterial overgrowth
  Inflammatory lesions
    Crohn's disease
At the level of the villus
  Celiac disease
  Allergic enteropathy
  Eosinophilic gastroenteropathy

Bulk intestinal surface area
  Short bowel syndrome
  Bacterial overgrowth in proximal small bowel
  Altered transit with early lactose entry into colon
  Hyperthyroidism
  Dumping syndromes
  Enteroenteral fistulas

30. What are the inherited disorders of carbohydrate malabsorption?

Monosaccharides
  Glucose-galactose malabsorption
Disaccharides
  Congenital alactasia (lactase deficiency)
  Congenital sucrase-isomaltase deficiency
  Trehalase deficiency

Polysaccharides
  Congenital amylase deficiency
Pancreatic insufficiency syndromes
  Shwachman syndrome
  Cystic fibrosis

Glucose-galactose malabsorption is an autosomal recessive disorder of carrier-mediated transport. Patients have a normal ability to absorb fructose. Sucrase-isomaltase deficiency is the most common of the congenital abnormalities of carbohydrate absorption. The combined defect always coexists, and is as high as 10% incidence in some populations. By contrast, congenital lactase deficiency is extremely rare. Trehalase is a brush border enzyme whose only function is to digest trehalose. The source of trehalose is mushrooms, and occasionally gas and diarrhea attributed to rich or spicy foods may be due to this deficiency. Obviously, this disease is of little clinical importance (except to mushroom farmers). Additionally, all humans lack the enzymes to digest stachyose and raffinose, two sugars in high concentration in beans. This explains the "beans syndrome," which for most people is clinically similar to lactose intolerance.

31. What is the pathophysiology of celiac disease?

The relationship of the small intestinal flat villous lesion to celiac disease is well established, but the pathogenesis is still unclear. One theory is that an intestinal enzyme that normally digests gluten is absent, resulting in a toxic reaction that produces changes in the intestinal epithelium. This has been actively sought, but never conclusively proven. A number of immunologic abnormalities have been suggested in celiac patients. Children with celiac disease have circulating antigliadin antibodies (gliadin is an alcohol-soluble protein found in wheat), and there is an increase in IgA- and IgM-containing plasma cells in the lamina propria. The number of intraepithelial lymphocytes is also increased. Each of these phenomena may disappear on a prolonged gluten-free diet. Celiac disease is associated with HLA antigens B8, DR3, and DR7. The lectin hypothesis is based on the theory that a cell surface membrane defect may allow gluten to act as a lectin and the subsequent reaction causes cell toxicity. Other hypotheses have focused on an increased permeability of the mucosal barrier, or precipitation by viral infections.

32. What are the diagnostic criteria for celiac disease?

In order to diagnose celiac disease, multiple small bowel biopsies must be obtained. In a typical sequence, the first biopsy on gluten should show villous atrophy, with increased crypt mitoses and disorganization and flattening of the columnar epithelium. This should resolve fully on the second biopsy after a strict gluten-free diet. In order to assure the diagnosis, and to eliminate the possibility of a coincidental recovery of an infectious enteritis, a third biopsy must be obtained after the patient has again been challenged with gluten. This biopsy again must show the manifestations of the disease. The increasing utility of commercial antigliadin antibodies may shorten the expense and invasiveness of this sequence. In many patients, the titer falls dramatically with treatment, and increases again with challenge. Unfortunately, the currently available tests are not sensitive or specific enough to be used alone for diagnosis.

33. What are the symptoms of celiac disease in children?

Gluten-sensitive enteropathy (GSE, celiac disease) is a relatively common cause of severe diarrhea and malabsorption in infants and children. Children with celiac disease commonly present between the ages of 9 and 24 months with failure to thrive, diarrhea, abdominal distention, muscle wasting, and hypotonia. After several months of diarrhea, growth slows. Weight typically decreases before height. Often these children become irritable and depressed, and display poor intake and symptoms of carbohydrate malabsorption. Vomiting is less common. On examination the growth defect and the distention are commonly striking. There may be a generalized lack of subcutaneous fat, with wasting of the buttocks, shoulder girdle, and thighs. Edema, rickets, and clubbing may also be seen.

34. When do symptoms of celiac disease begin to appear?

Some patients with celiac disease are not diagnosed until after 3 years of age, and others present well into adulthood. In these patients the bowel symptoms and failure to thrive are less obvious, and constipation may be a symptom. The recurrent colicky abdominal pain may be misinterpreted until short stature, iron-deficiency anemia, or vitamin deficiencies ensue. Family studies have demonstrated that some patients with flat villous lesions are entirely asymptomatic. Both treated and untreated patients with celiac disease have an increased incidence of small bowel malignancy in later life.

35. How does the introduction of cereal to the diet affect the presentation of celiac disease?

Cereals are not usually introduced until 5–6 months of age; however, when cereals are introduced during early infancy, they result in the presentation of celiac disease at a younger age, when the infant has less reserves. Vomiting is more frequent in this situation, and the diarrhea more watery. The impression frequently is that of an acute enteritis, and on diet restriction the child may again improve.

36. What is a "celiac crisis"?

This occurs rarely in young patients who may be superinfected with a viral syndrome, and who appear acutely ill, lethargic, dehydrated, and in shock. Hypoglycemia, hypoproteinemia, and electrolyte abnormalities are often seen.

37. How are children with celiac disease managed?

Elimination of all gluten-containing substances in the diet, correction of any nutritional and metabolic abnormalities, and patient education. All wheat- and rye-containing foods and flours are eliminated, and most recommend the elimination of oats and barley as well. Corn, rice, and potato flour are substituted (cookbooks are available for the celiac family). Many prepared foods contain gluten, and a full dietary counseling session is necessary to ensure compliance. Patients may require vitamin and mineral supplementation and may remain lactose intolerant for some time. In general, all catch-up growth should be completed before the child is challenged with gluten. While the development of symptoms may again take years following reintroduction of gluten, evidence of small intestinal injury is usually present early in the challenge. Insidious adolescent linear growth failure may not be evident until closure of the growth plates renders it irreversible.

38. How does secretory diarrhea differ from osmotic diarrhea?

Secretory diarrhea is distinguished from osmotic diarrhea in that osmotic diarrhea stops when the patient is placed on intravenous fluids and fasted. In osmotic diarrhea, the sum of the concentrations of fecal electrolytes is much less than the osmolality of the fecal fluid. If the osmotic diarrhea is driven by carbohydrate malabsorption, the fecal pH is low, with concomitant reducing substances on Clinitest examination. In secretory diarrhea, the sum of the cations doubled should roughly equal the measured stool osmolality. When the patient is fasted, the diarrhea must continue unabated.

$$\text{Osmotic diarrhea: } ([Na^+] + [K^+]) \times 2 < \text{fecal fluid osm}$$
$$\text{Secretory diarrhea: } ([Na^+] + [K^+]) \times 2 = \text{fecal fluid osm}$$

39. What are the pathophysiologic processes involved in secretory diarrhea?

Increased hydrostatic tissue pressure
Secretory agent or toxin associated with activation of adenylate
cyclase-cAMP system
    1. Enterotoxin-producing bacteria (*V. cholerae, E. coli*)
    2. Non-enterotoxin-producing bacteria (Salmonella)
    3. Methylxanthines (theophylline, caffeine)
    4. Prostaglandins
    5. VIP (small intestine and colon)
    6. Dihydroxy bile acids

Secretory agents, not proved to be associated with activation of adenylate cyclase-cAMP
  1. Glucagon
  2. GIP
  3. Secretin
  4. CCK
  5. Calcitonin
  6. Serotonin
  7. Substance P
  8. Cholinergic agents
  9. Laxatives (ricinolic acid, bisacodyl, phenolphthalein, oxyphenisatin, dioctyl sodium sulfosuccinate)
  10. Bacterial enterotoxins (*Shigella dysenteriae* I, *Staphylococcus aureus*, *Clostridium perfringens*, *Pseudomonas aeruginosa*, *Klebsiella pneumoniae*)
  11. Metabolic inhibitors (substituted phenols)
Mucosal injury
  1. Shigella, *E. coli* (non-enterotoxin-producing strains)
  2. Transmissible gastroenteritis virus
  3. Celiac disease
  4. Regional enteritis
  5. Ulcerative colitis
  6. Lymphoma
  7. Ischemia
Chronic diarrheal syndrome associated with intestinal secretion
  1. Pancreatic cholera syndrome
  2. Medullary carcinoma of thyroid
  3. Ganglioneuroma and ganglioneuroblastoma
  4. Zollinger-Ellison syndrome
  5. Carcinoid syndrome
  6. Congenital chloridorrhea
  7. Surreptitious laxative and diuretic ingestion
Miscellaneous
  1. Secretion of nerves to intestinal loop ("paralytic secretion")
  2. Intestinal obstruction
  3. Intestinal distention
Reference: Sleisenger MH, Fordtran JS (eds): Gastrointestinal Disease: Pathophysiology, Diagnosis, Management, 4th ed. Philadelphia, W.B. Saunders Co., 1989, with permission.

40. How should children with secretory diarrhea be managed?

It is important to identify an etiology for secretory diarrhea. After the child is taken off feeds, a vigorous attempt must be initiated to maintain fluid and electrolyte balance. If this is successful, the child should be evaluated for proximal small bowel damage, enteric pathogens, and a baseline malabsorptive workup. If abnormalities of the mucosal integrity are suspected, a small bowel biopsy is performed, and if significantly abnormal the patient may be given parenteral alimentation and gradual refeeding. Electron microscopy may reveal congenital abnormalities of the microvillus membrane and brush border. If the evaluation is negative, hormonal causes of secretory diarrhea (such as a VIPoma, hypergastrinoma, or carcinoid syndrome) must be considered. The list of active gastrointestinal hormones is rapidly expanding, and unusual tumors stimulating diarrhea have been identified. Bacterial overgrowth may cause a secretory process, although usually this diarrhea will abate somewhat with fasting. A number of congenital abnormalities have been identified, and are classified under the diagnosis of intractable diarrhea of infancy. If no etiology is identified, severe protracted disease may occur, and central parenteral alimentation is initiated. Careful monitoring and maintenance of intravenous access are critical because of marked fluid shifts.

41. What are the two types of hepatic failure?

Acute and fulminating, or chronic. Fulminant hepatic failure is an acute impairment of hepatic function, with concomitant encephalopathy in patients who were previously normal. Chronic hepatic failure may be due to a wide variety of infectious, toxic, and metabolic abnormalities.

42. What are the clinical manifestations of chronic hepatic failure?
The patient is jaundiced. There may be spider angiomas, a caput medusae, and palmar erythema. The mental status may be altered, and the patient may be tremulous or demonstrate asterixis. Fetor hepaticus, development of ascites, fluid retention, renal hypoperfusion, and a metabolic alkalosis may occur. Gastrointestinal bleeding may be a fatal complication. Renal failure and bacteremia may complicate a metabolic and electrolyte disaster. Cerebral edema and coma are ominous signs.

43. What is the clinical presentation in acute hepatitis?
In patients with an acute hepatitis, a steady deterioration of hepatic function is the first sign of hepatic failure. There is worsening of the hyperbilirubinemia, with decreased synthetic capacity as evidenced by a deteriorating vitamin K–resistant coagulation profile, decreased fibrinogen, urea and serum albumin. There may be the onset or worsening of encephalopathy, with concomitant increases in serum ammonia. Biochemical deterioration indicated by increasing bilirubin, decreasing transaminases, and receding hepatic size is an ominous sign of hepatic parenchymal collapse. These patients are at risk for spontaneous hypoglycemia.

44. What are the three groups of biochemical assays for hepatic disease?
Those related predominantly to hepatocellular inflammation or turnover, those related to hepatic function, and those indicating obstruction of the biliary tree. Unfortunately, no single test is specific, and commonly panels of tests must be considered simultaneously to determine the hepatic disease process.

45. What are the most sensitive indicators of hepatic function?
The most sensitive indicator of hepatic disease is the fasting serum bile salt assay. Bile salts are synthesized and excreted by the liver to promote fat absorption, and conserved by ileal reabsorption into the enterohepatic circulation. While highly sensitive, this assay is of no use in hepatic failure. Since hepatic failure denotes the impairment of hepatic function, the most clinically useful assays monitor the processes of synthesis, detoxification, excretion, and metabolic regulation. Synthesis of serum proteins, such as albumin, and clotting factors are important indicators of hepatic function, but interpretation can be complicated by infection, disseminated intravascular coagulation, and third space fluid shifts. Other measures of true hepatic function include transamination and urea synthesis, and drug detoxification and elimination. Tests of aminopyrine, methacetin, caffeine, and galactose metabolism have all been recently used in an attempt to quantify hepatic function in a meaningful way.

46. How should children with liver failure be managed?
The management of hepatic failure should focus on current metabolic and physiologic derangements, synthetic support, and prevention or reduction of CNS effects and encephalopathy. Diagnostic testing for treatable diseases and the initial evaluation for liver transplantation should be completed.

Management of Hepatic Failure

Metabolic monitoring
Flow sheet for accurate monitoring of:
- all diagnostic studies and results
- current laboratory studies
- hepatic size and mental status exams
- vital signs, input/output, and daily weights

Monitor glucose and electrolytes daily or more frequently
Hepatic functions and hematologic studies should be obtained several times per week
Glucose should be infused continuously via nasogastric tube or intravenous line
Monitor for hypoglycemia and hyperglycemia

Table continued on next page

Management of Hepatic Failure *(Continued)*

Gastrointestinal hemorrhage
Pass a nasogastric tube to monitor upper hemorrhage in patients with portal hypertension
Daily vitamin K IV (0.2 mg/kg) for 3 days, and continue if response is seen
Judicious administration of fresh frozen plasma for clinical bleeding
Have blood cross-matched at all times; for variceal bleeders, have 40 ml/kg and 0.2 U/kg
　　platelets available
For gastritis or peptic ulceration, treat with cimetidine (30 mg/kg/day) and maintain gastric
　　pH above 5

Hepatic encephalopathy
Limit protein intake to 1–2 gm/kg/day, and use modified hepatic amino acid preparations
Administer lactulose at 1 ml/kg q6h until diarrhea begins, and then titrate to achieve mild
　　diarrhea
Peritoneal dialysis may be indicated in severe coma, and prior to transplant
Intracranial pressure monitoring in advanced cases

Hepatorenal syndrome/renal status
Monitor urine output by shift
Place a central line to monitor central venous pressure in patients with oliguria
Treat with 25 gm% albumin as needed to support blood pressure and urine output
Limit sodium intake to 1–2 mEq/kg/day, including all plasma products, medications, and
　　parenteral alimentation
Fluid restrict as tolerated by patient condition

Other support
Avoid drugs metabolized by the liver
Culture all sites including peritoneal fluid with every episode of fever

Further therapeutic modalities
Identify a transplant center, list patient, and perform pretransplant evaluation
Identify transportation to center, check all insurance and travel arrangements
Prepare support structures for patient and parent

---

47. What are the two types of inflammatory bowel disease (IBD) in children?
Ulcerative colitis and Crohn's disease (regional enteritis). Ulcerative colitis is limited to the
superficial mucosa of the colon. The disease always involves the rectum, and extends
proximally to a variable extent. Limited distal ulcerative colitis has been termed ulcerative
proctitis, and in children may have a better prognosis. Regional enteritis, or Crohn's disease,
is a transmural inflammation of the bowel which may affect the entire gastrointestinal tract
from the mouth to the anus. The syndrome of limited Crohn's colitis may be difficult to
differentiate from ulcerative colitis.

48. Which features differentiate ulcerative colitis from Crohn's disease?

Differential Diagnosis in Ulcerative Colitis and Crohn's Disease

FEATURE	ULCERATIVE COLITIS	CROHN'S DISEASE
Relative incidence of symptoms		
Rectal bleeding (gross)	Common	Rare
Diarrhea	Often severe	Moderate or absent
Pain	Less frequent	Almost always
Anorexia	Mild or moderate	Can be severe

Table continued on next page

Differential Diagnosis in Ulcerative Colitis and Crohn's Disease *(Continued)*

FEATURE	ULCERATIVE COLITIS	CROHN'S DISEASE
Weight loss	Moderate	Severe
Growth retardation	Usually mild	Often pronounced
Extraintestinal manifestations	Common	Common
Involvement		
Small bowel		
Extensive	—	10%
Lower ileum	<5%	90%
Colon	100%	75%
Rectum	95%	50%
Anus	5%	85%
Distribution of lesions	Continuous	Segmental
Roentgenologic features	Superficial ulcers, loss of haustration, no skip areas, shortening	Serpiginous ulcers, thumbprinting, skip areas, string sign
Pathologic changes	Diffuse mucosal	Focal transmural granulomas
Response to treatment		
Steroids and sulfasalazine	75%	25% to 50%
Parenteral nutrition and elemental diets	Poor	Very good to induce a remission
Azathioprine or 6-mercaptopurine	Good in selected cases	Good in selected cases
Surgery	Excellent	Fair or poor
Course		
Remissions	Common	Difficult to define
Relapse after surgery	Common if rectum is not removed	35% to 100%
Cancer risk	High in pancolitis	Slight

From Silverman A, Roy CC: Pediatric Clinical Gastroenterology. St. Louis, C.V. Mosby, 1983, p 354, with permission.

49. What are the symptoms, signs, and laboratory findings in IBD?

Intestinal symptoms
> Diarrhea, often heme positive or grossly bloody but may be heme negative
> Abdominal pain
> Tenesmus
> Peptic symptoms
> Anorexia, nausea
> Vomiting or obstruction
> Abdominal distention
> Increased flatulence

Extraintestinal symptoms
> Weight loss or decrease in weight growth velocity
> Short stature or decrease in linear growth velocity

Abdominal signs
> Abdominal tenderness, rebound, guarding
> Abdominal mass
> Palpable loops of bowel
> Cutaneous fistulization

Extraintestinal signs
> Systemic
>> Fever, spiking or low grade, with or without chills
> Mucosal/cutaneous
>> Mouth sores, aphthous stomatitis
>> Erythema nodosum
>> Pyoderma gangrenosum
> Joint disease
>> Arthralgias or arthritis
>> Ankylosing spondylitis

Extraintestinal signs *(continued)*
    Ocular
        Uveitis
        Episcleritis
        Conjunctivitis
    Hepatic
        Chronic active hepatitis
        Sclerosing cholangitis
        Gallstones
    Perianal disease
        Abscesses
        Perianal fissures or fistulization
        Fistulas to the abdominal wall
        Enterovesical fistulas
        Vaginal fistulas
    Other site
        Dehydration
        Tachycardia
        Clubbing
        Renal (oxalate) stones
        Thrombophlebitis
        Pulmonary disease
Laboratory abnormalities
    Anemia
    Microcytosis
    Thrombocytosis
    Leukocytosis
    Elevated erythrocyte sedimentation rate
    Hypoalbuminemia
    Decreased folate, B_{12}, iron, zinc, copper, magnesium
    Fat malabsorption
    Carbohydrate malabsorption (lactose, xylose)

50. What is the risk of malignancy in children with IBD?

The risk of malignancy has not been systematically studied in pediatric populations with inflammatory bowel disease. The risk in adults depends both on the disease and its duration. After 10 years of ulcerative colitis, the risk rises dramatically (1–2% incidence of malignancy per year). The risk is felt to be higher in patients with pancolitis compared to those with limited left-sided disease. The carcinomas associated with ulcerative colitis are often poorly differentiated and metastasize early. They have a poorer prognosis and are more difficult to identify by radiographic and colonoscopic examinations. Most authors indicate that carcinoma of the bowel is much less common in Crohn's disease, although this has been disputed recently. In addition to the malignancy risk of the primary disease, immunosuppressive therapy such as azathioprine may increase the risk of neoplasia.

51. What are the complications of Crohn's disease and ulcerative colitis?

The complications and presentations of IBD have considerable overlap.

1. *Severe perianal disease* can be a particularly debilitating complication. More prevalent in Crohn's disease, it may range from simple skin tags to total devastation of the perineum. Deep perianal abscesses can interfere with the ability to sit and walk, and open drainage is often necessary. More extensive surgical removal may result in damage to the sphincter and subsequent incontinence. Fistulization to the vagina, bladder, or directly to the skin may occur.

2. In Crohn's disease, *enteroenteral fistulae* may occur and "short-circuit" the absorptive process. The thickened bowel may obstruct or perforate, requiring operation. The recurrence rate is high after surgery, repeated operations are often necessary, and short bowel syndrome may result. In many cases a permanent ostomy is placed, although pouch construction and continent ileostomies have become more common.

3. In ulcerative colitis, the patient may require *surgery* because of the severity or the duration of disease. In the past, most patients had total colectomy and ileostomy, but the current recommended procedure is a subtotal colectomy and an endorectal pullthrough with rectal mucosal stripping. This procedure maintains intestinal continuity, and the patient develops normal rectal continence, although with increased stool frequency.

4. *Toxic megacolon* may occur with either form of IBD, but is much more common with ulcerative colitis. After a progressive course, fever and a decrease in diarrhea usually herald a distended tender and tympanitic abdomen. The profound dilatation of the bowel may be segmental or total, and massive hemorrhage or perforation may ensue. Mortality is high if toxic megacolon is not identified and treated aggressively.

5. *Growth retardation and delayed puberty* are seen in both diseases, but are more common in Crohn's disease. The insidious onset may result in several years of linear growth failure before the correct diagnosis is made. With epiphyseal closure, linear growth is terminated, and short adult stature will be permanent.

6. *Hepatic complications* of IBD include chronic active hepatitis and sclerosing cholangitis, which may require liver transplantation.

7. *Nephrolithiasis* may occur in patients with resections, or patients with steatorrhea, due to increased intestinal absorption of oxalate.

8. Chronic reactive and restrictive *pulmonary disease* has been noted.

9. Arthralgias are common, but destructive *joint disease* is uncommon.

52. What is the treatment for ulcerative colitis in children with mild, moderate, or severe disease?

Treatment varies according to the age of the patient and the duration and severity of the disease. Sulfasalazine (Azulfidine) is the usual first therapy in all cases of ulcerative colitis, except if the patient is G6PD deficient or highly sulfa-allergic. Folate supplementation should be given concomitantly. Steroid or 5-aminosalicylic acid enemas may control distal limited disease. In more severe cases, prednisone (or any of the steroid group) is used to induce remission. When outpatient therapy is unsuccessful, elemental diets or parenteral alimentation are instituted. Long courses of intake restriction and aggressive intravenous nutritional therapy are likely to be efficacious. Immunosuppressive therapy (azathioprine) may have a role in the maintenance of remission. When medical therapy fails, or when toxic megacolon is present, surgical therapy is necessary.

53. What are the main reasons for growth failure in children with Crohn's disease?

Anorexia, inadequate intake, malabsorption (energy sources, micronutrients), increased demands, and increased losses (energy sources, protein).

54. What is the prognosis for children with IBD?

Patients with Crohn's disease can be expected to lead a functional and productive life. However, as many as three fourths will require surgery within 5 years, and only half of those with growth failure will achieve significant catch-up growth. Careful attention to psychologic factors will increase the patient's skills and ability to cope with the unpredictable nature of the disease. The outcome for patients with ulcerative colitis is better unless toxic megacolon or carcinoma develops. In these patients, surgery is curative, and the chronic morbidity depends on the type of surgery employed.

55. What percentage of children with IBD have joint manifestations? Which joints are most commonly affected?

About 20% of patients with Crohn's disease have a history of joint disease at the time of presentation. More than half have joint manifestations sometime in the course of their disease. It is usually mild, asymmetric, migrating, and resolves quickly without deformity. This may appear before the onset of clinical bowel disease. Ankylosing spondylitis is more common with ulcerative colitis, but is exceedingly rare in the pediatric population. The typical attack of arthritis presents acutely, often affecting a single joint in the lower extremity. The knee and ankle are most frequently affected, followed by the proximal interphalangeal, elbow, shoulder, and wrist joints. The attack usually subsides within several weeks. The usual course is complete resolution without residual damage.

56. What are the gastrointestinal and nutritional manifestations of cystic fibrosis?
Intestinal
      In utero perforation—meconium peritonitis
      Meconium ileus or equivalent
      Intestinal atresia
      Intestinal obstruction
      Intussusception
      Abdominal distention
      Rectal prolapse
      Recurrent abdominal pain
      Peptic or duodenal ulcer
Nutritional/Metabolic
      Dehydration
      Diarrhea
      Steatorrhea
      Fat-soluble vitamin deficiencies
      Failure to thrive
      Delayed onset of puberty
      Enhanced appetite
Hepatobiliary
      Neonatal cholestatic jaundice
      Hepatomegaly
          Steatosis
          Focal biliary cirrhosis
      Portal hypertension
      Splenomegaly
      Nonvisualization of the gallbladder
      Cholelithiasis
Other
      Diabetes

57. What are the abnormalities associated with alpha-1-antitrypsin deficiency?
Alpha-1-antitrypsin deficiency was first described in chronic obstructive pulmonary disease in adults. Later it was recognized as an etiologic factor in neonatal cholestasis, hepatomegaly, hepatitis, and cirrhosis with liver failure. Early in the disease, a liver biopsy may demonstrate either bile duct proliferation (as seen in biliary atresia) or bile duct paucity (as seen in arteriohepatic dysplasia). Since alpha-1-antitrypsin is the major inhibitor of neutrophil elastase, it has an important protective function in the lung. There are more than 40 electrophoretic variants of this enzyme, with the M protease inhibitor (pi) type being the most common and the most active. Hepatic disease is associated with the Z phenotype, which has the lowest serum activity. Membranoproliferative glomerulonephritis has been described in Pi Z patients. Cryptogenic cirrhosis in adults is more common in patients with Pi MZ than in the normal population.

58. What is Pi typing?
Since alpha-1-antitrypsin is an acute phase reactant, levels in patients with the deficiency may be artificially elevated, especially if there is chronic inflammation or liver disease. There are over 40 variants of the protein, each with a different electrophoretic mobility. The protease inhibitor typing, or pi typing, takes advantage of these mobilities for identification of the different alleles. The proteins are inherited in a codominant fashion, and thus both genes are expressed in one individual. PiM is most common, with a distribution of about 87%, PiMS

8%, PiMZ 2%, and others less than 1%. The incidence of PiZ ranges between 1:1,700 and 1:5,000.

59. How is ascites diagnosed by physical examination?

When ascites is significant it is commonly visible with viewing the patient at the bedside and in the standing position. Bulging flanks are a sign of chronic ascites. Palpation of the abdomen may reveal a heavy fullness, and a fluid wave can be demonstrated in a cooperative child by tapping sharply on one flank while receiving the wave with a hand on the other flank. The transmission of the wave through fatty tissue should be blocked with a hand in the center of the abdomen. Percussion of the abdomen demonstrates a central area of tympany at the top surrounded by percussion dullness. This dullness shifts when the patient moves laterally or sits up. Cooperative and mobile patients may be examined in the knee–chest position, and the pool of ascites tapped while listening for a change in sound transmission with the stethoscope. This is felt to be the most sensitive sign for ascites, but is clearly not applicable in many patients. Even an experienced physician will not detect small amounts of ascites. Although ascites can be demonstrated on radiographs, the most sensitive and specific test is an abdominal-pelvic ultrasound.

60. What is the differential diagnosis for ascites in infants and children?

Cirrhosis	Neoplastic
Hypoproteinemic	Peritonitis
Nephrosis	Pancreatic
Protein-losing enteropathy	Tuberculous
Malnutrition	Chylous
Cardiac	Iatrogenic
Vascular	Post-ventriculoperitoneal shunt
Budd-Chiari	Post-dialysis

61. Which surgical procedures are used to treat portal hypertension?

Portal decompressive surgery
    Portocaval shunt   Portal vein to inferior vena cava (IVC)
    Mesocaval shunt   Superior mesenteric vein to graft to IVC
    Splenorenal shunt   Splenic vein to renal vein
        With splenectomy
        Without splenectomy
    Other shunts (mesorenal, coronocaval)
Devascularization surgery
    Esophageal transection
Orthotopic hepatic transplantation

62. What are the complications of portocaval shunts in childhood?

Bleeding esophageal varices are a life-threatening complication of portal hypertension. The therapeutic modalities available for incurable liver disease and progressive portal hypertension include medical management, sclerotherapy, esophageal transection, colonic interposition, portosystemic shunts, and liver transplantation. Portosystemic shunts include portocaval, mesocaval, central splenorenal, and distal splenorenal shunts, and each operation has advantages and disadvantages. The experienced surgeon must identify the anatomy preoperatively, and measure the size of feeder vessels to be shunted. Risks in pediatric patients include the development of encephalopathy and the relatively high incidence of shunt closure and thrombosis.

63. What are the clinical findings in portal hypertension?

Obstruction to portal flow is manifest by two physical signs: splenomegaly and increased collateral venous circulations. Collaterals are evident on physical examination in the anus and the abdominal wall, and by special studies in the esophagus. Hemorrhoids may be collaterals, but in older patients are present in high frequency without liver disease, and thus their presence has no predictive value. Dilatation of the paraumbilical veins produces a rosette around the umbilicus (the caput medusae), and the dilated superficial veins of the abdominal wall are visible. A venous hum may be present in the sub-xiphoid region, from varices in the falciform ligament.

64. Clinically, how does one differentiate upper from lower gastrointestinal (GI) bleeding?

Any upper gastrointestinal hemorrhage may present as rectal bleeding or heme-positive stools. The differential diagnosis of GI hemorrhage is extremely large and site specific, and therefore it is important at the outset to define the site of bleeding. The easiest and most straightforward method is to pass a small soft nasogastric tube atraumatically at the time of bleeding. If a lavage is negative, it is unlikely that the bleeding is above the ligament of Treitz, and in any event is not gastric, esophageal, or nasal. The character and quantity of blood may aid in the diagnosis, but may also be misleading. Generally, black or tarry blood has been denatured with acid, and thus likely to have originated above the ligament of Treitz, but this has also been reported in patients with Meckel's diverticulum. Dark maroon or currant jelly stools classically originate from the distal ileum or colon, but with increased transit can come from the proximal bowel. The difficulty is defining the site of bleeding by the magnitude and color of the blood underscores the importance of the initial nasogastric tube insertion.

65. What are the steps in the evaluation of a child with GI hemorrhage?

The initial step is determination of the site and magnitude of bleeding, and whether it is ongoing at the time of the evaluation. If the patient has cardiovascular compromise, an immediate fluid resuscitation is necessary. Blood is crossmatched, and coagulation status and hemoglobin are determined. When the patient is stabilized, a nasogastric tube is passed to determine the site of bleeding. In patients with small amounts of bleeding or with occult blood, the evaluation can proceed as outlined below.

1. **History**
   Manifestation of bleeding, color, character
   Chronicity
   Associated pain
   Syncope, dizziness, tachycardia
   Other systemic diseases
   Family history
   Medication history
   Social history
2. **Physical examination**
   Vital signs
   Acuity or chronicity
   Anthropometric data
   Pallor
   Cutaneous signs
   Abdominal pain or mass
   Hepatosplenomegaly
   Rectal examination
3. **Laboratory studies**
   Complete blood count with platelets
   Reticulocyte count
   Hepatic and renal function tests
   Coagulation profile
   Sample to blood bank for crossmatch

4. **Special studies**
   Nasogastric tube
   Barium studies of the upper or lower bowel
   Upper or lower endoscopy
   Nuclear medicine bleeding scans
   Meckel's scan
   Arteriography
   Exploratory laparotomy
5. **Specific therapeutic measures**
   Replace intravascular volume with crystalloid
   Type and cross for packed cells or whole blood
   Secure airway if necessary
   Establish monitoring, with CVP line
   Gastric lavage to monitor ongoing hemorrhage
   H_2-blockers prophylactically
   Vitamin K as needed
   Endoscopic sclerotherapy
   Endoscopic coagulation (heater probe or laser)
   Sengstaken-Blakemore tube
   Intravenous vasopressin
   Intraarterial embolization
   Emergent surgery

66. What are the major causes of upper GI hemorrhage?

Pharyngeal source

Esophageal varices

Esophagitis

Gastritis

Gastric ulcer, duodenal ulcer

Mallory-Weiss tear

Vascular lesion

Mass lesion or foreign body

67. What are the causes of significant lower GI hemorrhage?

Meckel's diverticulum

Colitis (ulcerative, Crohn's, infectious, radiation/chemotherapy, ischemic, allergic)

Vascular lesion (angiodysplasia, hemangiomas)

Mass lesion (malignancy, duplications, polyposis)

Intussusception

Midgut volvulus

68. What is the management for massive upper GI bleeding?

Massive upper gastrointestinal hemorrhage is a life-threatening emergency, and initial therapy precedes the specific diagnostic evaluation.

Brief history (magnitude and character of bleeding, previous episodes, bleeding disorders)

Vital signs

Intravascular access and serologic studies (CBC, liver function tests, coagulation profile, crossmatch)

Nasogastric tube insertion

Full history and physical examination

Transfusion and intravascular support

Determination of probable etiology

1. Peptic disease

    Diagnostic endoscopy

    Therapeutic endoscopy

    H_2-blockers, antacids, sucralfate

If no resolution,

    Surgical repair of ulcer

    Partial resection

2. Variceal bleeding

    Diagnostic endoscopy

    Therapeutic variceal sclerosis

    Vasopressin

    Sengstaken-Blakemore tube

If no resolution,

    Emergency portosystemic shunt

    Esophageal devascularization

3. Mallory-Weiss tear

4. Superficial vascular anomaly

    Endoscopic ablation

69. What are the causes of intussusception?

Intussusception is caused by one proximal segment of the bowel being invaginated and progressively drawn caudad and encased by the lumen of distal bowel. This causes obstruction, and may occlude the vascular supply of the bowel segment. There is commonly a lead point on the proximal bowel which initiates the process. Lead points have included lymphoid hyperplasia, hypertrophied Peyer's patches, eosinophilic granuloma of the ileum, lymphoma, lymphosarcoma, leiomyosarcoma, leukemic infiltrate, polyps, duplication cysts, ectopic pancreas, Meckel's diverticulum, hematoma, Henoch-Schönlein syndrome, worms, foreign bodies, and appendicitis.

70. What is the most common type of intussusception? What are the less common types?

Ileocolic intussusception (it is also the most common cause of intestinal obstruction in infancy). Cecocecal and colocolic intussusceptions are less common. Gastroduodenal intussusception is rare, and is usually associated with a gastric mass lesion such as a polyp or a leiomyoma. Enteroenteral intussusception is seen after surgery and in patients with Henoch-Schönlein syndrome.

71. What is the most common presentation of intussusception?

Ileocolic intussusception is twice as common in boys, and usually occurs before the second year of life. Half of all cases occur between the third and the ninth months. Most cases do not have any identifiable etiology, but there is a seasonal clustering in the spring and fall which may be related to the increase in respiratory and enteric infections during those times, with resultant reactive intestinal lymphoid tissue. Colicky pain is seen in over 80% of cases but may be absent. It typically lasts 15–30 minutes, and the baby usually sleeps between attacks. In about two-thirds of cases there is blood in the stool (currant jelly stools). Other presentations include massive lower GI bleeding or blood streaking on the stools. The infant may appear quite toxic, dehydrated, or in shock. Fever and tachycardia are common. A right lower quadrant mass may be palpable, or the area may feel surprisingly empty. Distention may accompany decreased bowel sounds. Radiographs typically demonstrate a small bowel obstruction pattern, but the diagnostic study of choice is a barium enema, which should be performed in all children with symptoms less than 48 hours in duration. In 80% of cases the barium enema under fixed hydrostatic pressure will reduce the intussusception. If this is unsuccessful, surgical reduction is necessary.

72. What is the treatment for intussusception?

Proximal intussusceptions require surgical reduction. In 80% of the cases of ileocolic intussusception the barium enema will reduce the intussusception. The barium is elevated to less than 3.5 feet above the patient and the ileum gradually reduced. This approach may cause perforation in rare cases. Other patients will require operative reduction of the intussusception, and resection if significant necrosis has developed.

73. How frequently does intussusception recur?

Idiopathic ileocolic intussusception recurs in about 3% of all cases. Intussusceptions in older children tend to recur at a higher frequency if the causative lesion is not removed. It is important to investigate cases of recurrent intussusception.

74. What is the normal liver span throughout childhood?

Liver size depends on the method used to evaluate it. In general, a combination of percussion and gentle palpation will yield accurate results if a tape measurement is included.

Expected Liver Span of Infants and Children					
Males			Females		
Age, yr	Mean Estimated Liver Span	SEM	Age, yr	Mean Estimated Liver Span	SEM
6 mo	2.4	2.5	6 mo	2.8	2.6
1	2.8	2.0	1	3.1	2.1
2	3.5	1.6	2	3.6	1.7
3	4.0	1.6	3	4.0	1.7
4	4.4	1.6	4	4.3	1.6
5	4.8	1.5	5	4.5	1.6

Table continued on next page

Expected Liver Span of Infants and Children					
Males			Females		
Age, yr	Mean Estimated Liver Span	SEM	Age, yr	Mean Estimated Liver Span	SEM
6	5.1	1.5	6	4.8	1.6
8	5.6	1.5	8	5.1	1.6
10	6.1	1.6	10	5.4	1.7
12	6.5	1.8	12	5.6	1.8
14	6.8	2.0	14	5.8	2.1
16	7.1	2.2	16	6.0	2.3
18	7.4	2.5	18	6.1	2.6
20	7.7	2.8	20	6.3	2.9

From Lawson EE, Grand RJ, Neff RK, Cohen LF: Clinical estimation of liver span in infants and children. Am J Dis Child 132: 474–476, 1978, with permission.

75. How should a normal child with isolated hepatomegaly be evaluated?

All children with isolated hepatomegaly should have a careful history and physical examination. Family history of liver disease, previous exposure to hepatitis, foreign travel, blood transfusions, and drugs or toxins should be determined. One should verify that the liver is indeed large, and not displaced by adjacent structures or hyperinflation. The consistency, character, and tenderness of the liver will provide information about possible etiologies. The spleen should be carefully palpated. Cutaneous signs of chronic liver disease and portal hypertension, lymphadenopathy, retinal pathology, cardiac lesions, and abdominal venous hums may indicate a particular etiology. Isolated hepatomegaly without splenomegaly or central nervous system involvement should be evaluated systematically in order to conserve resources.

76. Which laboratory studies are sensitive indicators of hepatic dysfunction?

Total and direct bilirubin   Gamma glutamyltranspeptidase
Fasting bile salt level   Total protein and albumin
ALT and AST   Coagulation profile
Alkaline phosphatase   Urinalysis
If evidence of transaminase elevations are present, then
Hepatitis A IgM   Alpha-1-antitrypsin level and pi typing
Hepatitis BsAg and anti-core Ab   Sweat test
CMV titers and culture   Urine metabolic screen
EBV titers   24-hour urine copper
Additional evaluation should include
Abdominal ultrasound, with Doppler
of portal vessels
DISIDA scan as needed
Liver spleen scan

77. What is the differential diagnosis for hepatomegaly?

Hepatocytic inflammation
Infectious (bacterial, viral, mycobacterial, fungal, abscess, parasitic)
Non-infectious (toxic, drug-induced, autoimmune, post-obstructive)
Kupffer cell (septicemia/systemic infection, malignancy, granulomatous hepatitis, vitamin A toxicity)
Congestion (congestive heart failure, Budd-Chiari, sickle cell, vascular tumors)
Infiltration
Non-neoplastic (extramedullary hematopoiesis, cysts, benign tumors)
Neoplastic (histiocytosis syndromes, leukemia, lymphoma, metastatic tumors, hepatoblastoma, hepatocellular carcinoma)

Storage (glycogen storage disease, mucopolysaccharidoses, lipidoses, gangliosidoses)

Metabolic (alpha-1-antitrypsin disease, galactosemia, hereditary fructose intolerance, hereditary tyrosinemia, Wilson disease, hemochromatosis, Reye syndrome, fatty-acyl CoA
dehydrogenase deficiency)

Steatosis (malnutrition, hyperalimentation, acute refeeding, steroids)

Portal tract (congenital hepatic fibrosis, idiopathic cirrhosis)

Bile duct abnormalities (arteriohepatic dysplasia, obstruction, biliary atresia, sclerosing
cholangitis)

Miscellaneous (juvenile rheumatoid arthritis, systemic lupus erythematosus, cerebrohepatorenal syndrome, cystic fibrosis, endocrine (hypopituitarism, hypothyroidism,
hypocorticolism)

78. How and when does biliary atresia present?

In classic cases, a term infant develops a recognizable jaundice by the third week of life, with
increasingly dark urine and acholic stools. Usually the child appears well, with good growth.
The skin color sometimes appears somewhat greenish yellow. The spleen becomes palpable
after the third or fourth week, at which time the liver is usually hard and enlarged. In other
cases, the jaundice is clearly present in the conjugated form in the first week of life. There is
also a strong association between the polysplenia syndrome and biliary atresia.

79. What is the Kasai procedure, and what are its complications?

The Kasai procedure is a hepatic portoenterostomy. The remnants of the extrahepatic biliary
tree are identified, and a cholangiogram is performed to verify the diagnosis. Dissection and
resection of the remaining extrahepatic ducts and the fibrous plate present at the porta are then
performed. A Roux-en-Y jejunal limb is constructed to drain bile from the porta, and in some
cases this limb is temporarily exteriorized at a double-barrel ostomy. Postoperative complications include intestinal obstruction, early and late ascending cholangitis, peristomal
breakdown, and stomal varices. In nearly half the cases, the procedure does not establish bile
flow, and in most patients there is ongoing inflammation and the development of portal
hypertension.

80. When should a Kasai procedure be performed?

As soon as possible. Earlier operation results in a dramatically improved outcome. Patients
operated before 70 days of age have increased likelihood of a successful procedure, although
exceptions at both ends of this spectrum are common. Some surgeons now suggest that
infants diagnosed late in the course should have a primary liver transplant rather than a
hepatic portoenterostomy.

81. What is Alagille syndrome?

One of the most common etiologies of neonatal cholestasis and hepatitis is arteriohepatic
dysplasia, or Alagille syndrome. Now formally called syndromic bile duct paucity, it consists
of a constellation of conjugated hyperbilirubinemia and cholestasis, typical triangular facies,
cardiac lesions of pulmonic stenosis, peripheral pulmonic stenosis, or occasionally more
significant lesions, butterfly vertebrae, and eye findings of posterior embryotoxon and
Axenfeld's anomaly, or iris processes. The patient may have extreme cholestasis, with
pruritus and marked hypercholesterolemia. Although some patients have mental deficiency,
the majority are normal. The usual mode of inheritance of Alagille syndrome is autosomal
dominant.

82. What are the most common causes of direct hyperbilirubinemia in an infant?

Biliary atresia, alpha-1-antitrypsin deficiency, arteriohepatic dysplasia, and cholestasis
secondary to TPN or sepsis in the premature infant.

83. How should infants with direct hyperbilirubinemia be evaluated?

An immediate evaluation is necessary to determine if treatable or potentially life-threatening disease is present. The type of bilirubin is most helpful in guiding the evaluation, as the etiologies of conjugated hyperbilirubinemia are in general more significant.

Initial evaluation
  Total and direct bilirubin
  ALT, AST, Alkaline phosphatase
  Gamma glutamyl transpeptidase
  Total protein and albumin
  Coagulation profile
  Complete blood count, reticulocyte count, and Coombs
  Blood and urine bacterial cultures
  Urine and nasopharyngeal viral cultures
  Alpha-1-antitrypsin level and pi type
  TORCH studies in mother and infant
  HIV antibody studies
  Urine metabolic quantitation
  Serum amino acid quantitation
  HBsAg and anti-HBc
  Sweat test
  Galactosemia screen
    Urine Clinitest when the infant is received a lactose-containing formula
    Galactose-1-phosphate uridyl transferase

Secondary evaluation
  Ophthalmology examination
    Posterior embryotoxon, Axenfeld's anomaly, chorioretinitis, cataracts,
  Hepatobiliary ultrasound
  Hepatobiliary scintigraphy—DISIDA excretion study
  Percutaneous liver biopsy
  Intraoperative cholangiogram and biopsy

84. What are the endoscopic and pathologic findings in gastroesophageal reflux (GER)?

Simple reflux has no pathologic correlate. If reflux is complicated by esophagitis, there may be erythema, edema, friability, or frank ulceration of the distal esophagus. Histologically the diseased portion of the esophagus may demonstrate neutrophilic or eosinophilic infiltration into the epithelium, and occasionally ulceration.

85. What does the medical treatment of GER include?

The medical treatment of GER and its complications depends on the extent of disease and status of the patient:

Simple gastroesophageal reflux
  Counseling
  Thickened feeding
  Positional therapy
  Bethanechol
  Metoclopramide
Esophagitis
  Antacids
  Cimetidine, ranitidine, or famotidine
  Sucralfate
Failure to thrive
  Nutritional rehabilitation
  Nasogastric feeding

Apnea
  Monitoring
  Fundoplication, if severe
Recurrent aspiration
  Fundoplication, or
  Jejunal feeding
Failure of medical and nutritional therapy
  Fundoplication

86. What are the indications for fundoplication?

The vast majority of infants with developmental reflux do not require fundoplication. Rather, therapy should be directed toward possible esophagitis and failure to thrive. Developmental reflux will resolve in nearly all infants by 15 months of age. Fundoplication is indicated in patients with recurrent aspiration, refractory or Barrett's esophagitis, reflux-associated apnea, and in reflux-associated failure to thrive that is refractory to medical therapy. Patients with severe reflux and psychomotor retardation should be evaluated for a fundoplication if a feeding gastrostomy is contemplated.

87. What are the common sites for intestinal atresia?

Jejunum/ileum and duodenum. Duodenal atresia is caused by a persistence of the proliferative stage of gut development and a lack of secondary vacuolization and recanalization. It is associated with a high incidence of other early embryonic abnormalities. Extraintestinal anomalies occur in two-thirds of patients. In jejunoileal atresia, the lesion occurs after the establishment of continuity and patency, as evidenced by distal meconium seen in these patients. The etiology is postulated to be a vascular accident, volvulus or mechanical perforation. Jejunoileal atresias are usually not associated with any other systemic abnormality.

88. What are the clinical findings of malrotation of the intestine?

Malrotation of the intestine is due to the abnormal rotation of the intestine around the superior mesenteric artery during embryologic development. Arrest of this counterclockwise rotation may occur at any degree of rotation. The lesion may present with in utero volvulus or may be asymptomatic throughout life. Infants may present with intermittent vomiting or complete obstruction. Any infant with bilious vomiting should be considered emergent, and requires careful evaluation for volvulus and other high-grade surgical obstructions. Recurrent abdominal pain, distention, or lower GI bleeding may result from intermittent volvulus. Full volvulus with arterial compromise results in intestinal necrosis, peritonitis, perforation, and an extremely high incidence of mortality. Because of the extensive nature of the lesion, postoperative short gut syndrome is present in many patients who require resection.

89. What are the x-ray findings associated with malrotation?

The upper gastrointestinal series will show malposition and malfixation of the ligament of Treitz. The proximal small bowel may be located in the right upper quadrant, but this is not always true. The cecum viewed from either the upper GI series or the barium enema may be unfixed or malpositioned. In both malrotation and in volvulus, the plain films may be entirely normal. There may be proximal obstruction with gastroduodenal distention. In volvulus, the barium studies may show an obstruction near the gastroduodenal junction, often with a twisted appearance.

90. What is the common presentation of Meckel's diverticulum?

While a Meckel's diverticulum is present in nearly 2% of the population, it is usually silent throughout life. Meckel's diverticulum results from the failure of the intestinal end of the omphalomesenteric duct to obliterate. Although it may be located throughout the small bowel, it is usually within 100 cm of the ileocecal valve. It is twice as common in males, and commonly presents in the first 2 years of life. The typical presentation is massive painless rectal bleeding in a toddler. The blood is usually red or maroon in color, but may be tarry in 10% of cases. The child may present in shock, or may have had similar but minor episodes in the past. Other presentations include intussusception with obstruction, volvulus or torsion. Diverticulitis may be indistinguishable from appendicitis. The diagnosis is made on clinical grounds, and confirmed by a Meckel's scan (see below). Sigmoidoscopy will show normal rectal mucosa, rather than colitis, which eliminates infectious and inflammatory considerations. Occasionally, the diagnosis is made at laparotomy.

91. What is a Meckel's scan?
Radionuclide imaging of the Meckel diverticulum is possible with ^{99m}Tc-pertechnetate. The tracer is taken up by heterotopic gastric mucosa, and both cimetidine and pentagastrin have been reported to increase the sensitivity of the study. The study does have a false negativity rate, and the decision to operate may be made despite a negative study.

92. What is the reason for rectal bleeding in infants with Meckel's diverticulum?
The diverticulum is usually located on the antimesenteric wall, and may lie free or it may be connected by a fibrous band. Twenty to fifty percent of diverticulae have ectopic tissue, which is most commonly gastric in origin. The gastric mucosa, via acid and pepsin secretion, results in ulceration of the adjacent ileal mucosa with resultant hemorrhage.

93. What infectious organisms are associated with gastroenteritis and arthritis?

Non-infectious etiologies	Infectious etiologies
Ulcerative colitis	Salmonella
Regional enteritis (Crohn's disease)	Shigella
Behçet's syndrome	Yersinia
Henoch-Schönlein syndrome	Tuberculosis
	Adenovirus

94. What are the three D's of pellagra?
Dermatitis, dementia, and diarrhea.

95. What percentage of adolescents are obese?
5% are obese (greater than 20% above ideal body weight); 10–20% are overweight (greater than 10–20% above ideal body weight)

96. What percentage of obese children and adolescents become obese adults?
80%

97. How is the diagnosis of anorexia nervosa made?
Anorexia nervosa constitutes a spectrum of psychologic, behavioral, and medical aspects, but the 1980 DSM-III criteria list five minimum factors:
1. Internal fear of becoming obese not diminished by weight loss
2. Distortion of body image ("feeling" fat when emaciated)
3. Weight loss of 25% from original body weight
4. Refusal to maintain body weight over age/height minimum
5. No known physical illness to account for weight loss

98. What are good and bad prognostic indications for recovery from anorexia?
Good: early age at onset, high educational achievement, improvement in body image after weight gain.

Poor: late age at onset, continued overestimation of body size, self-induced vomiting or bulimia, laxative abuse, male.

99. How is the diagnosis of bulimia made?
Bulimia is a syndrome of voracious high-caloric overeating and forced vomiting (by gagging or ipecac), often done during periods of frustration or psychological stress. Its incidence is much higher than anorexia nervosa and males are very infrequently involved. The diagnosis is made by history. Most bulimics do not develop a weight loss. Medical problems include electrolyte abnormalities from vomiting and laxative abuse, pharyngitis and dental erosion from gastric acidity and psychologic difficulties, most commonly depression.

Bibliography

1. Anderson CM, Burke V, Gracey M (eds): Paediatric Gastroenterology, 2nd ed. London, Blackwell Scientific Publications, 1987.
2. Arneil GC, Metloff J: Pediatric Nutrition. Boston, Butterworth, 1983.
3. Berk, JE (ed): Bockus Gastroenterology. Philadelphia, W.B. Saunders, 1985.
4. Franken EA Jr: Gastrointestinal Imaging in Pediatrics. Philadelphia, Harper and Row, 1987.
5. Gracey M, Falkner F (eds): Nutritional Needs and Assessment of Growth. New York, Nestle Nutrition, Raven Press, 1985.
6. Gryboski J, Walker WA: Gastrointestinal Problems in the Infant, 2nd ed. Philadelphia, W.B. Saunders, Philadelphia, 1983.
7. Kelts DG, Jones EG: Manual of Pediatric Nutrition. Boston, Little, Brown and Co., 1984.
8. Kerner JA Jr (ed): Manual of Pediatric Parenteral Nutrition. New York, John Wiley & Sons Inc., 1983.
9. Lebenthal E: Textbook of Gastroenterology and Nutrition in Infancy. New York, Raven Press, 1981.
10. Lifshitz F: Clinical Disorders in Pediatric Gastroenterology and Nutrition. New York, Marcel Dekker, Inc., 1980.
11. Mowat AP: Liver Disorders, 2nd ed. Boston, Butterworth, 1987.
12. Pereira G (ed): Perinatal Nutrition. Clin Perinatol, vol. 13, no. 1. Philadelphia, W.B. Saunders, 1986.
13. Schiff L, Schiff ER (eds): Diseases of the Liver, 6th ed. Philadelphia, J.B. Lippincott, 1987.
14. Silverman A, Roy CC: Pediatric Clinical Gastroenterology, 3rd ed., St. Louis, C.V. Mosby, 1983.
15. Sleisenger MH, Fordtran JS (eds): Gastrointestinal Disease: Pathophysiology Diagnosis and Management, 4th ed. Philadelphia, W.B. Saunders, 1989.
16. Suskind RM: Textbook of Pediatric Nutrition. New York, Raven Press, 1981.
17. Tsang RC, Nichols BL (eds): Nutrition During Infancy. Philadelphia, Hanley & Belfus, 1988.
18. Walker WA, Watkins JB (eds): Nutrition in Pediatrics: Basic Science and Application. Boston, Little, Brown and Co., 1985.

GENETICS

Alan E. Donnenfeld, M.D.
Elaine H. Zackai, M.D.

1. What are the three most common autosomal trisomies and their features?

Features of Common Autosomal Trisomies

FEATURE	TRISOMY 21	TRISOMY 18	TRISOMY 13
Eponym	Down syndrome	Edward's syndrome	Patau's syndrome
Liveborn incidence	1/800	1/800	1/19,000
Mean birth weight	3000 g	2340 g	2480 g
Tone	Hypotonia	Hypertonia	Hypo- or hypertonia
Cranium/brain	Mild microcephaly, flat occiput, 3 fontanelles	Microcephaly, prominent occiput	Microcephaly, sloping forehead, occipital scalp defects, holoprosencephaly
Eyes	Upslanting, epicanthal folds, speckled iris (Brushfield spots)	Small palpebral fissures, corneal opacity	Micro-ophthalmia, hypotelorism, iris coloboma, retinal dysplasia
Ears	Small, low-set, overfolded upper helix	Low-set, malformed	Low-set, malformed
Facial features	Protruding tongue, large cheeks, low, flat nasal bridge	Small mouth, micrognathia	Cleft lip and palate
Skeletal	Clinodactyly 5th digit, gap between toes 1 and 2, excess nuchal skin, short stature	Clenched hand, absent 5th finger distal crease, hypoplastic nails, short stature, thin ribs	Postaxial polydactyly, hyperconvex fingernails, clenched hand
Cardiac defect	40%	60%	80%
Survival	Long term, excluding those with cardiac defects, of whom many die in infancy	90% die within the first year	82% die within the first year
Other features	Leukemia, Alzheimer's	Rocker bottom feet, polycystic kidneys, dermatoglyphic arch pattern	Genital anomalies, polycystic kidneys, increased nuclear projections in neutrophils

2. What is a simian crease?
A single transverse palmar crease that is present in 50–55% of newborn infants with Down syndrome, is frequent in other trisomies, and is present in approximately 4% of normal individuals. Since Down syndrome occurs 1/800 live births, the chance that a newborn with a simian crease has Down syndrome is only 1 in 60.

3. Are there any signs pathognomonic for Down syndrome?
No. However, some phenotypic characteristics occur very frequently.

Frequency (%) of Positive Phenotypic Findings in Infants with Down Syndrome

Sagittal suture separated	98
Oblique palpebral fissure	98
Wide space between first and second toes	96
False fontanel	95
Plantar crease between first and second toes	94
Hyperflexibility	91
Increased neck tissue	87
Abnormally shaped palate	85
Hypoplastic nose	83
Muscle weakness	81
Hypotonia	77
Brushfield spots	75
Mouth kept open	65
Protruding tongue	58
Epicanthal folds	57
Single palmar crease, left hand	55
Single palmar crease, right hand	52
Brachyclinodactyly, left hand	51
Brachyclinodactyly, right hand	50

Modified from Pueschel SM: The child with Down syndrome. In Levine et al: Developmental-Behavioral Pediatrics. Philadelphia, W.B. Saunders, 1983, p 356, with permission.

4. Why is a maternal age of 35 at delivery chosen as the cutoff for recommending amniocentesis for chromosome analysis?

There is a well-known association between advanced maternal age and trisomies (including XXY,XXX,trisomy 13, 18 and 21).

Maternal Age	Approximate Risk of Down Syndrome
30	1:1000
35	1:365
40	1:100
45	1:50

The majority of cases of Down syndrome involve nondisjunction at meiosis I in the mother. This may be related to the lengthy stage of meiotic arrest between oocyte development in the fetus until ovulation, which may occur as much as 40 years later.

5. Why has the incidence of Down syndrome decreased from 1.6/1000 live births to 1.0–1.2/1000 live births over the past 25 years?

The decrease in incidence is a result of the reduction of births in older women and prenatal diagnosis. The risk for older women has not changed, but at the present time only 20% of children with Down syndrome are born to mothers over 35 years of age, whereas 25 years ago 50% of the children with Down syndrome were born to older mothers.

6. Does advanced paternal age increase the risk of having a child with trisomy 21?

There does not appear to be an increased risk of Down syndrome associated with paternal age until after age 55. Some studies have noted an increased risk of Down syndrome after this age, although others have not. The reports are controversial, and the statistical analysis needed to perform such a study is cumbersome. It is known that approximately 20% of all trisomy 21 cases derive the extra chromosome 21 from the father.

7. Which syndromes are associated with advanced paternal age?

Advanced paternal age is well documented to be associated with new dominant mutations. The assumption is that the increased mutation rate is due to the accumulation of new mutations from many cell divisions. The more cell divisions, the more likely an error (mutation) will occur. The mutation rate in fathers over 50 is 5 times higher than the mutation rate in fathers less than 20 years of age. The four most common new autosomal dominant mutations are: achondroplasia, Apert's syndrome (acrocephalosyndactyly), myositis ossificans, and Marfan syndrome.

8. What is a chromosome translocation?

A chromosome translocation is a transfer of chromosomal material between two (or more) nonhomologous chromosomes. The exchange is usually reciprocal (the two segments trading places). The genetic content of the individual is therefore complete, but rearranged. Robertsonian translocation represents a special variety of chromosome translocation in which the long arms of two acrocentric chromosomes (#13,14,15,21 or 22) fuse at their centromeres. The breaks may occur within, above, or below the centromeres. The short arms are usually lost, but this does not produce an abnormality, since the genetic material on the short arms of acrocentric chromosomes occurs in multiple copies throughout the genome. A phenotypically normal individual with a Robertsonian translocation has only 45 chromosomes inasmuch as the long arms of two acrocentric chromosomes are fused into one.

9. Why is a parent with a 14;21 Robertsonian translocation at risk for having multiple miscarriages and/or children with birth defects?

When a parent with a translocation undergoes gametogenesis, six chromosomally different types of gametes can be formed due to unequal segregation of chromosomes during meiosis. The possible outcomes are trisomy 14 (which will abort), monosomy 14 (which will abort), monosomy 21 (which will abort), normal, trisomy 21 (Down syndrome), and a balanced Robertsonian translocation (just like the parent).

10. What percentage of cases of Down syndrome are due to translocations?

3.3% of all cases of Down syndrome are due to unbalanced Robertsonian translocations in which a third copy of chromosome 21 is present, attached to an acrocentric chromosome. The chance of translocation Down syndrome is two to three times greater in children of younger mothers (6–8% of mothers under 30). One of three infants with translocation Down syndrome will have a parent with a Robertsonian translocation. Two thirds of the time, translocation Down syndrome occurs as a de novo event in the infant.

11. What is the overall recurrence risk of Down syndrome?

In chromosomally normal women under age 40, the recurrence risk for Down syndrome is 1% (assuming the father's chromosomes are also normal). Above the age 40 the risk of having a child with Down syndrome increases, primarily as a function of maternal age. If the mother carries a translocation, the recurrence risk is 10%. If the father carries a translocation, the recurrence risk is 3–5%. One theory for this observed discrepancy between maternal and paternal rates of translocation Down syndrome is hindered motility of chromosomally abnormal sperm.

12. What is the expected intelligence and personality of a child with Down syndrome?

The IQ range is generally between 35 and 65, with a mean reported IQ of 54. Occasionally, the IQ may be higher. Intelligence deteriorates in adulthood, with clinical and pathologic findings consistent with advanced Alzheimer's disease. Autopsy results from brains of deceased adults with Down syndrome reveal both neurofibrillary tangles and senile plaques, the same lesions found in Alzheimer's disease. By age 40, the mean IQ is 24. Children with Down syndrome are generally affectionate and docile. They tend toward mimicry and are noted to usually enjoy music, having a good sense of rhythm. However, 13% have serious emotional problems and coordination is usually poor.

13. Are developmental milestones and self-help skills severely delayed in children with Down syndrome?

The delays in average development can be measured in months, as shown below:

Developmental Milestones and Self-Help Skills in Children with and without Down Syndrome (Ages in Months)

| | CHILDREN WITH DOWN SYNDROME | | "NORMAL" CHILDREN | |
	Average	Range	Average	Range
Developmental Milestones				
Smiling	2	1.5 to 4	1	0.5 to 3
Rolling over	8	4 to 22	5	2 to 10
Sitting alone	10	6 to 28	7	5 to 9
Crawling	12	7 to 21	8	6 to 11
Creeping	15	9 to 27	10	7 to 13
Standing	20	11 to 42	11	8 to 16
Walking	24	12 to 65	13	8 to 18
Talking, words	16	9 to 31	10	6 to 14
Talking, sentences	28	18 to 96	21	14 to 32
Self-Help Skills				
Eating				
Finger feeding	12	8 to 28	8	6 to 16
Using spoon and fork	20	12 to 40	13	8 to 20
Toilet training				
Bladder	48	20 to 95	32	18 to 60
Bowel	42	28 to 90	29 ·	16 to 48
Dressing				
Undressing	40	29 to 72	32	22 to 42
Putting clothes on	58	38 to 98	47	34 to 58

From Pueschel SM: The child with Down syndrome. In Levine et al: Developmental-Behavioral Pediatrics. Philadelphia, W.B. Saunders, 1983, pp 358-359, with permission.

14. What is the value of chromosome banding?

Chromosome banding was introduced in the early 1970s and has revolutionized cytogenetics. Prior to banding, all chromosomes appeared as solid, dark figures and could not be individually identified. Stains such as giemsa and quinacrine can now be used to differentially stain certain chromosome regions, producing a characteristic striped pattern which can accurately identify each chromosome. Even small chromosome fragments can often be identified on the basis of their banding patterns. An analogy between unbanded and banded chromosomes is the difference between a silhouette and a color portrait. A silhouette provides a general shape, whereas a color portrait provides details that permit identification of an individual with certainty.

15. What is mosaicism and what are its consequences?

Mosaicism is the possession of multiple chromosomally different cell lines in a single individual. Most mosaicism involves the sex chromosomes and occurs because of defects in mitosis in an early embryo. Normally, chromosomes duplicate and separate equally in mitotic division. Mosaicism occurs when the chromosomes fail to separate (mitotic nondisjunction) or fail to migrate (anaphase lag). In general, the greater the proportion of abnormal cell lines, the worse the phenotype. The earlier in embryonic development an abnormal cell line is established, the higher the percentage of abnormal cells in that individual.

16 What chromosome abnormality is found in cri du chat syndrome?

Cri du chat syndrome is due to a deletion of material from the short arm of chromosome 5 (5p-). Loss of this genetic material causes many problems, including a characteristic cat-like cry in infancy from which the syndrome derives its name (cri du chat = cry of the cat in

French). In 85% of cases the deletion is a de novo event; in 15% the deletion is due to malsegregation from a balanced parental translocation.

17. Name five features of cri du chat syndrome.

Cat-like cry in infancy
Growth retardation (mean birth wt 2650 gm)
Mental deficiency (mean IQ 20–30)
Hypotonia
Microcephaly

Round "moon"-face
Hypertelorism
Epicanthal folds
Down-slanting palpebral fissures

18. What are the four most common sex chromosome abnormalities and their features? Are all identifiable at birth by physical examination?

(1) XXY (Klinefelter's), (2) XYY, (3) XXX, and (4) XO (Turner's). Only infants with Turner syndrome have physical features identifiable at birth which should lead to suspicion of this disorder and chromosome evaluation for diagnosis. Features of Turner syndrome at birth are:

Dorsal hand and pedal edema
Web neck (pterygium colli)
Broad chest with wide-spaced nipples
Congenital heart disease (20%)

Congenital elbow flexion (cubitus valgus)
Renal anomalies, most commonly horseshoe kidneys
Prominent ears

Sex Chromosome Abnormality Syndromes

	47,XXY	47,XYY	47,XXX	45,X
Frequency of live births	1/2000	1/2000	1/2000	1/8000
Maternal age association	+	−	+	−
Mosaicism	5%–25%	Rare	5%–25%	25%–40%
Phenotype	Tall, eunuchoid habitus, under-developed secondary sexual characteristics, gynecomastia	Tall, severe acne, indistinguishable from normal males	Tall, indistinguishable from normal females	Short stature, web neck, shield chest, pedal edema at birth, coarctation of the aorta
IQ and behavior	80–100; behavioral problems	90–110; behavioral problems, aggressive behavior	90–110; behavioral problems	Mildly deficient to normal intelligence, spatial-perceptual difficulties
Reproductive function	Extremely rare	Common	Common	Extremely rare
Gonad	Hypoplastic testes, Leydig cell hyperplasia, Sertoli cell hypoplasia, seminiferous tubule dysgenesis, few spermatogenic precursors	Normal size testes, normal testicular histology	Normal size ovaries, normal ovarian histology	Streak ovaries with deficient follicles

From Donnenfeld AE, Dunn LK: Common chromosome disorders detected prenatally. Postgrad Obstet Gynecol 6:5, 1986, with permission.

19. What causes webbing of the neck in Turner syndrome?

Most fetuses with Turner syndrome spontaneously abort (close to 98%). In many of these aborted fetuses, large fluid-filled posterior nuchal cysts called cystic hygromas have been noted. Cystic hygromas result from jugular lymphatic obstruction between the cervical lymphatics and the jugular venous system. Trapped lymphatic fluid accumulates, causing massive enlargement of the lymphatic spaces of the posterior aspect of the neck. It is hypothesized that if only a partial or temporary obstruction occurs, egress of lymphatic fluid may be possible and the cystic hygroma will resolve, with only redundant nuchal skin folds remaining. This hypothesis is not uniformly accepted. Others believe that the pathogenesis of web neck is not related to lymphatic obstruction, but occurs as a primary developmental defect due to the chromosome abnormality.

20. Besides 45,X what other chromosome aberrations are common in females with short stature and ovarian dysgenesis?

At least 35% of chromosome abnormalities in individuals with Turner syndrome are mosaics. The most common are: (1) 45,X/46,XX; (2) 45,X/46,XX/47,XXX; and (3) 45,X/46,XY. Whenever a cell line with a Y chromosome is identified in a phenotypic female, gonadectomy is recommended due to a high risk of malignancy in the gonads of these individuals.

21. What are the similarities and differences between Noonan syndrome and Turner syndrome?

Similarities: short stature, web neck, cardiac defects, low posterior hairline, broad chest, wide-spaced nipples, edema of the dorsum of the hands and feet, and cubitus valgus.
Differences:

Turner syndrome	Noonan syndrome
Affects females only	Affects both males and females
Chromosome disorder (45,X)	Normal chromosomes, autosomal dominant disorder
Near normal intelligence	Mental deficiency
Coarctation of the aorta is the most common cardiac defect	Pulmonary stenosis is the most common cardiac defect
Amenorrhea and sterility due to ovarian dysgenesis	Normal menstrual cycles in females

22. What is the fragile X syndrome?

It is the most common inherited form of mental retardation in males. Its inheritance pattern is unknown, but its features appear to be similar to an X-linked recessive disorder with variable expression and decreased penetrance. However, 30% of carrier women are also affected, atypical for an X-linked recessive condition, and unusual inheritance patterns that do not fit with typical mendelian inheritance have been observed. Characteristics of the syndrome include mental retardation, hyperactive behavior, a long face, large ears, hyperextensible joints, and macroorchidism in postpubertal males. The diagnosis is made cytogenetically by observing a gap (fragile site) near the end of the long arm of the X chromosome which occurs in greater than 2% of lymphocytes grown in special folic acid deficient media. Most affected males express the fragile X site in 10–30% of their cells. Empiric data reveal that a carrier female has a 38% chance of having a retarded male and a 16% chance of having a retarded female.

23. What is meant by VATER syndrome?

VATER is an acronym for Vertebral, Anal, Tracheo-Esophageal and Renal or Radial abnormalities. It has been expanded to VACTERL to include Cardiac and Limb anomalies. This is a sporadically inherited condition caused by a developmental field defect. All the malformations seen in VATER and VACTERL occur at approximately the same point in embryogenesis. The defects often occur together, so whenever a newborn with a tracheoesophageal fistula is identified, we recommend renal ultrasound, chest x-ray (to rule out vertebral defects), and evaluation for imperforate anus.

24. What are some other acronyms commonly used in genetics?

1. TORCH infections (Toxoplasmosis, Other [syphilis], Rubella, Cytomegalovirus and Herpes)

But we prefer

2. STARCH infections (Syphilis, Toxoplasmosis, AIDS, Rubella, Cytomegalovirus and Herpes), because congenital AIDS is now a well-recognized congenital infection and occurs more frequently than congenital rubella.

3. CHARGE association (Coloboma, Heart defects, Atresia choanae, Retarded growth, Genital and Ear anomalies)

4. LEOPARD Syndrome (Lentigines, EKG abnormalities, Ocular hypertelorism, Pulmonic stenosis, Abnormalities of the genitalia, Retarded growth and Deafness)

5. MURCS association (MUllerian, Renal and Cervical Somite abnormalities)

6. HAIRY PSALMS (Haven't Any Idea Regarding Your Patient. Send A Lot More Serum)

25. Which drugs are known to be teratogenic?

Drug	Major teratogenic effect
Thalidomide	Limb defects
Lithium	Ebstein's tricuspid valve anomaly
Aminopterin	Craniofacial and limb anomalies
Methotrexate	Craniofacial and limb anomalies
Phenytoin	Facial dysmorphism, dysplastic nails
Trimethadione	Craniofacial dysmorphism, growth retardation
Valproic acid	Neural tube defects
Diethylstilbestrol	Mullerian anomalies, clear cell adenocarcinoma
Androgens	Virilization
Tetracycline	Teeth and bone maldevelopment
Streptomycin	Ototoxicity
Warfarin	Nasal hypoplasia, bone maldevelopment
Penicillamine	Cutis laxa
Accutane (retinoic acid)	Craniofacial and cardiac defects
Propylthiouracil	Goiter
Radioactive iodine	Hypothyroidism

Most teratogenic drugs have a deleterious effect in a minority of exposed fetuses. Exact malformation rates are unavailable due to the inability to statistically evaluate a randomized, controlled population.

26. What are the features of the fetal alcohol syndrome?

Facial Characteristics
   Eyes
      Short palpebral fissures
   Maxilla
      Hypoplastic
   Nose
      Short, upturned
      Hypoplastic philtrum
   Mouth
      Thinned upper vermilion
      Retrognathia in infancy
      Micrognathia or relative prognathia in adolescence

Central Nervous System Dysfunction
    Intellectual
        Mild to moderate mental retardation
    Neurologic
        Microcephaly
        Poor coordination, hypotonia
    Behavioral
        Irritability in infancy
        Hyperactivity in childhood

Growth Deficiency
    Prenatal
        <2 SD for length and weight
    Postnatal
        <2 SD for length and weight
        Disproportionately diminished adipose tissue

Features Associated with Fetal Alcohol Syndrome

AREA	FREQUENT	OCCASIONAL
Eyes	Ptosis, strabismus, epicanthal folds	Myopia, clinical microphthalmia, blepharophimosis
Ears		Poorly formed concha, posterior rotation
Mouth	Prominent lateral palatine ridges	Cleft lip or cleft palate, small teeth with faulty enamel
Cardiac	Murmurs, especially in early childhood, usually atrial septal defect	Ventricular septal defect, great-vessel anomalies, tetralogy of Fallot
Renogenital	Labial hypoplasia	Hypospadias, renal defect
Cutaneous	Hemangiomas	Hirsutism in infancy
Skeletal	Aberrant palmar creases; pectus excavatum	Limited joint movements, especially fingers and elbows, nail hypoplasia, especially fifth polydactyly, radioulnar synostosis, pectus carinatum, bifid xiphoid, Klippel-Feil anomaly, scoliosis
Muscular		Hernias of diaphragm, umbilicus or groin, diastasis recti

27. What genetically inherited disease has the highest known mutation rate per gamete per generation?

Neurofibromatosis. The estimated mutation rate for this disorder is 1×10^{-4} per haploid genome. The clinical features are café au lait spots and axillary freckling in childhood followed by development of neurofibromas in later years. There is approximately a 10% risk of malignancy with this condition and mental deficiency is also common.

28. Name the "fat baby" syndromes.

    1. Prader-Willi (obesity, hypotonia, small hands and feet)
    2. Beckwith-Wiedemann (macrosomia, omphalocele, macroglossia, ear creases)
    3. Sotos (macrosomia, macrocephaly, large hands and feet)
    4. Weaver (macrosomia, accelerated skeletal maturation, camptodactyly)
    5. Laurence-Moon-Biedl (obesity, retinal pigmentation, polydactyly)
    6. Infants of diabetic mothers

29. **Which syndromes are frequently associated with microcephaly? macrocephaly?**
Microcephaly

Intrauterine infections
Fetal alcohol syndrome
Fetal AIDS embryopathy
Dubowitz syndrome
Bloom syndrome
Coffin-Siris syndrome
Johanson-Blizzard syndrome
Langer-Giedion syndrome
Maternal PKU
Meckel-Gruber syndrome
Miller-Dieker syndrome

Chromosome abnormalities
Cornelia de Lange syndrome
Pena-Shokeir syndrome
Ruvalcaba syndrome
Seckel syndrome
Shprintzen syndrome
Smith-Lemli-Optiz syndrome
Williams syndrome
Aniridia-Wilms' tumor association
Roberts syndrome

Macrocephaly

Sotos syndrome
Weaver syndrome
Albers-Schonberg syndrome
Mucopolysaccharidoses
Klippel-Trenaunay-Weber syndrome

Marshall-Smith syndrome
Robinow syndrome
Benign familial macrocephaly
Hydrocephalus syndromes

30. **Which syndromes are associated with preauricular tags or pits?**

Goldenhar syndrome
Treacher Collins syndrome
Melnick-Fraser syndrome
Nager syndrome
Townes syndrome
Coffin-Siris syndrome

Frontonasal dysplasia
Wolf syndrome (4p-)
Cri du chat syndrome (5p-)
Trisomy 4p syndrome
Mosaic trisomy 9
Supernumerary der (22)t(11;22)

31. **What are the characteristic features of fetal hydantoin syndrome? What percentage of fetuses exposed to hydantoin will manifest features of the syndrome?**
Craniofacial

Broad nasal bridge
Wide fontanel
Low set hairline
Broad alveolar ridge
Metopic ridging
Short neck
Ocular hypertelorism

Microcephaly
Cleft lip/palate
Abnormal or low-set ears
Epicanthal folds
Ptosis of eyelids
Coloboma
Coarse scalp hair

Limbs

Small or absent nails
Hypoplasia of distal phalanges
Altered palmar crease

Digital thumb
Dislocated hip

Approximately 10% of infants whose mothers took hydantoin (Dilantin) during pregnancy will have a major malformation; 30% will have minor abnormalities consistent with this teratogenic disorder.

From Briggs GC, Freeman RK, Yaffe SJ: Drugs in Pregnancy and Lactation, 2nd ed. Baltimore, Williams and Wilkins, 1986, p 351, with permission.

32. **What are the most common major congenital anomalies in the U.S.?**

Anencephaly and spina bifida. The combined prevalence is between 0.5 and 2.0 per 1000 live births.

33. Which congenital malformations are associated with the fetal AIDS syndrome?
Growth failure and craniofacial abnormalities.

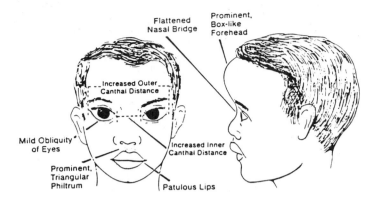

Major facial features noted in human T-cell lymphotropic virus type III embryopathy. Note prominent, box-like forehead; flattened, "scooped-out" appearance of nasal bridge; ocular hypertelorism; prominent palpebral fissure; mild upward obliquity of eyes: flattened columella; prominent, triangular philtrum; and prominent, patulous lips. (From Marion et al: HTLV-III embryopathy. Am J Dis Child 140:639, 1986, with permission.)

34. Which syndromes and malformations are associated with congenital limb hemihypertrophy?

Russell-Silver syndrome
Conradi-Hunermann syndrome
Klippel-Trenaunay-Weber syndrome
Beckwith-Wiedemann syndrome
Wilms' tumor

Hypomelanosis of Ito
CHILD syndrome (Congenital
  Hemidysplasia, Ichthyosiform
  erthyroderma, Limb Defects)
Neurofibromatosis

One of every 32 patients with isolated hemihypertrophy is at risk for developing Wilms' tumor. For this reason renal and abdominal ultrasound should be offered periodically in childhood as a screening device for patients with hemihypertrophy.

35. What are the common symbols used in the construction of a pedigree chart?

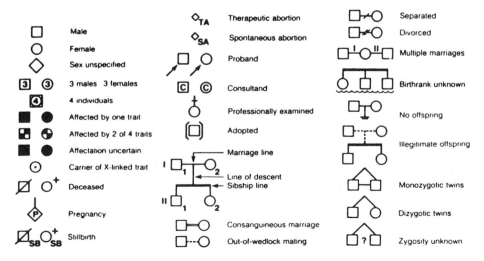

36. What is the Lyon hypothesis?
In any cell only one X chromosome will be functional. Any other X chromosomes present in that cell will be condensed, late replicating, and inactive (called the Barr body). The inactive X may be either paternal or material in origin, but all descendants of a particular cell will have the same parentally derived chromosome inactive. Inactivation is initially random, occurring at the 16-day (blastocyst) stage of embryonic development. For example, in normal females (46,XX) one X chromosome is inactive. In normal males (46,XY) the X is always active, since it is the only one present. In 48, XXXY individuals there will be two inactive X chromosomes per cell. The process of X inactivation allows for gene dosage compensation in females and poly-X males.

37. What is the Haldane hypothesis?
The probability that the mother of a son with an X-linked disease is a carrier when there is no family history of either normal or affected males may be calculated by the formula:

$$m = \frac{(1-f)u}{2u+v}$$

where f = fitness; u = mutation rate in females; v = mutation rate in males. In cases where fitness is zero (virtually no patients reproduce), such as Duchene's muscular dystropy, and the mutation rate of the gene is the same in ova and sperm (u = v), 1/3 of all cases will be new mutants and the probability that the mother is a carrier would be 2/3.

38. What is the significance of dermatoglyphics and what are the three types of patterns found?
Dermal ridge patterns are formed early in embryogenesis. Their pattern is influenced by genetic inheritance, the influence of teratogens, congenital infections, and chromosome abnormalities. The distal phalanges have a variety of dermal ridge patterns that can be classified in three major types: arches, whorls, and loops (see diagram below). Infants with trisomy 18 commonly have a high frequency of arches, an unusual finding in chromosomally normal individuals. In the foot there is a pattern at the base of the great toe. In 50% of patients with trisomy 21, a simple arch pattern (called an open field) will be found. This occurs in less than 1% of controls.

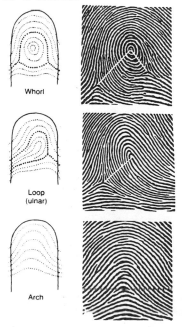

Whorl

Loop
(ulnar)

Arch

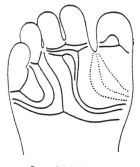

Open field hallucal
dermatoglyphic pattern

From Holt S: The genetics of dermal ridges.
Br Med Bull 17:247, 1961, with permission.

39. Name the syndromes characterized by a senile-like appearance.
1. Progeria (alopecia, atrophy of subcutaneous fat, skeletal dysplasia, early death)
2. Werner syndrome (cataract, thick skin, sparse, gray hair)
3. Cockayne syndrome (growth deficiency, retinal degeneration, impaired hearing, thick skin)
4. Rothmund-Thomson syndrome (poikiloderma, cataract, ectodermal dysplasia)

40. What is a "genetic-lethal" disease?
One that interferes with a person's ability to reproduce as a result of early death (before childbearing age) or impaired sexual function.

41. What is the most common genetic-lethal disease in man?
Cystic fibrosis (CF). CF is the most common autosomal recessive disorder in whites, occurring 1/1600 births, meaning that roughly 1 of every 20 people are heterozygous for this condition. CF is characterized by widespread dysfunction of exocrine glands, chronic pulmonary disease, pancreatic insufficiency, and intestinal obstructions. Males are azospermic. The mean survival is approximately 15–20 years.

42. What is the risk that a couple will have a child with CF if the husband's brother was affected with this disorder? (Assume the husband is healthy and no one in the wife's family has this disease.) Draw the pedigree.

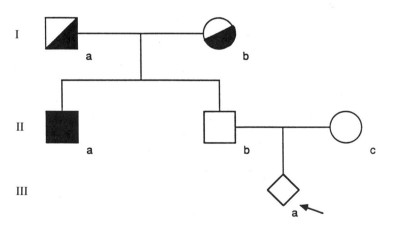

1. Since IIa is affected with CF, both his parents must be carriers.
2. The chance of IIb being a carrier is 2/3, since we know he is not affected by CF.
3. The risk of IIc being a carrier is 1/20 (the population risk).
4. The chance of IIIa being affected is: father's carrier risk × mother's carrier risk × the chance that both will pass on their recessive cystic fibrosis gene to their child; $2/3 \times 1/20 \times 1/4 = 1/120$.

43. What is the proper way to test for low-set ears?
This designation is made when the upper portion of the ear (helix) meets the head at a level below a horizontal line drawn from the lateral aspect of the palpebral fissure. The best way to measure is to align a straight edge between the two inner canthi and determine whether the ears lie completely below this plane as illustrated in the figure. In normal individuals, approximately 10% of the ear will be above this plane.

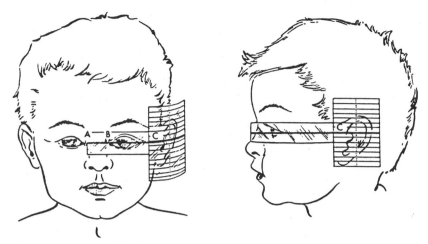

From Feingold M, Bossert WH: Normal values for selected physical parameters: An aid to syndrome delineation. In Bergsma D (ed): The National Foundation-March of Dimes Birth Defects Series 10:9, 1974.

44. What is the difference between a major and a minor malformation?

Major malformations are unusual morphologic features that cause medical, cosmetic, or developmental consequences to the patient. Minor anomalies are features that do not cause medical or cosmetic problems. Approximately 14% of newborn babies will have a minor malformation, whereas only 2–3% of newborns will have a major anomaly.

45. What is the clinical significance of a minor malformation?

Recognition of minor malformations in a newborn may serve as an indicator of altered morphogenesis or may constitute valuable clues to the diagnosis of a specific disorder. The presence of several minor malformations in an individual is unusual and often indicates a serious problem in morphogenesis. For example, when 3 or more minor malformations are discovered in a child, there is a greater than 90% risk of a major malformation also being present. The most common minor malformations involve the face, ears, hands, and feet. Almost any minor defect may occasionally be found as an unusual familial trait.

46. Which syndromes are associated with iris colobomas?

Colobomas of the iris is due to abnormal ocular development and embryogenesis. They are frequently associated with chromosomal syndromes, most commonly trisomy 13, 4p-, 13q-, and triploidy. In addition, they may be commonly found in CHARGE association, Goltz syndrome, and Rieger syndrome. Whenever iris colobomas are noted, chromosome analysis is recommended. The special case of complete absence of the iris (aniridia) is associated with the development of Wilms' tumor and may be caused by an interstitial deletion of the short arm of chromosome 11.

47. Which malformations and syndromes are associated with oligohydramnios? Poly-hydramnios?

In early pregnancy (before 4 months) the majority of amniotic fluid is produced by transudation through the placental membranes and fetal skin. Later in pregnancy, the bulk of amniotic fluid arises as a product of fetal urination. At term, the fetus swallows approximately 500 cc of amniotic fluid per day and urinates an equivalent amount. Fetal urine production increases rapidly from 3.5 ml/hr at 25 weeks to 25 ml/hr at term. Any malformation that leads to impaired urine production will cause oligohydramnios. This includes renal dysplasia, renal agenesis, and bladder outlet obstruction. When uteroplacental insufficiency occurs, the fetus is often faced with poor nutritive and volume support. The fetus will become intravascularly depleted, leading to increased fluid conservation and decreased urine output, causing oligohydramnios. Oligohydramnios is often associated with intrauterine growth retardation.

The etiology of polyhydramnios may be broken down into maternal causes (30%), fetal causes (30%), and idiopathic causes (40%). Maternal disorders such as diabetes, erythroblastosis fetalis, and preeclampsia are often associated with excess amniotic fluid. Fetal disorders that commonly predispose to polyhydramnios are central nervous system anomalies (anencephaly, hydrocephaly, neurologic disorders, etc.), gastrointestinal disorders (tracheoesophageal fistula, duodenal atresia), fetal circulatory disorders, and multiple gestation. The etiology for polyhydramnios in fetuses with central nervous system and upper gastrointestinal anomalies is presumed to be impaired fetal swallowing ability.

48. What is Potter's syndrome and how is it inherited?
Potter's syndrome has come to be synonymous with fetal malformations caused by extreme oligohydramnios. Lack of amniotic fluid leads to fetal compression, a squashed, flat face, clubbing of the feet, pulmonary hypoplasia and, commonly, breech presentation. Normal fetal lung development is dependent on in utero "breathing" and inhalation of amniotic fluid. In the absence of amniotic fluid, pulmonary hypoplasia occurs, and is the cause of death for most fetuses with Potter's syndrome. The underlying mechanism in Potter's syndrome was initially reported to be renal agenesis or renal dysplasia. However, bladder outlet obstruction and prolonged premature rupture of the membranes may also cause this sequence. Some prefer that Potter's syndrome be defined solely as renal agenesis. Renal agenesis is thought to be a sporadic or multifactorial condition, although autosomal dominant inheritance with variable expression (i.e., unilateral renal agenesis in a parent) has also been postulated. For this reason we recommend renal ultrasound in all parents of children with renal agenesis. If the parents have normal renal evaluations, the emipirically determined recurrence risk is approximately 3%. If one of the parents has unilateral renal agenesis, the recurrence risk may be as high as 50% due to a presumed autosomal dominant gene.

49. How is gastroschisis differentiated from omphalocele? What are the features of each?
Both omphalocele and gastroschisis are ventral wall defects, yet their pathogenesis and prognosis differ markedly.

Omphalocele	Gastroschisis
Midline ventral wall defect	Usually defect is to the right of the umbilicus
Umbilical cord inserts into abdominal wall defect	Normal umbilical cord insertion
In 60% of cases, other major malformations are present	In approximately 15% of cases other major malformations are present
Frequently associated with trisomy 18 or other chromosomal abnormalities	Not commonly found in fetuses with chromosomal abnormalities

50. What is the inheritance pattern of bilateral retinoblastoma? Unilateral retinoblastoma?
Bilateral retinoblastoma is a malignant neoplasm of the retina that is inherited in an autosomal dominant fashion with decreased penetrance. The risk to a fetus with one affected parent is 40%. (In 10% of cases where the gene is present, there will be no manifestation of the disorder. This is called decreased penetrance.) A small percentage of patients with unilateral retinoblastoma also inherit the disease in an autosomal dominant fashion. The majority of unilateral retinoblastoma cases are sporadic. A significant proportion of patients with bilateral retinoblastoma will have a cytogenetically identifiable deletion on the long arm of chromosome 13. In other cases, although a deletion may not be visible, linkage analysis with the enzyme esterase D has been useful in determining a genetic defect. The average age at diagnosis is 8 months. Knowledge of the genetics of this disease has guided ophthalmologic surveillance. Eighty-five percent of patients may now expect long-term survival. Early

diagnosis affords more conservative therapy, often simple laser ablation, avoiding enuclea-tion and preservation of sight. In this disease, appropriate genetic counseling is crucial.

51. What is the inheritance pattern of cleft lip and palate?

Most cases of cleft lip and palate are inherited in a polygenic or multifactorial pattern. The male to female ratio is 3:2 and the incidence in the general population is approximately 1/1000. Recurrence risk after 1 affected child is 3–4%; recurrence risk after two affected children is 8–9%.

52. What is the significance of lip pits?

Lip pits derive from small, accessory salivary glands that fistulize on either side of the midline lower lip. This finding is diagnostic of Van der Woude syndrome, whose other features are cleft lip and/or palate and missing second premolars. Inheritance is autosomal dominant, yet variable expression often occurs, and in some cases only the lip pits will be present without the associated cleft lip and/or palate. The chance of an offspring of an individual with Van der Woude syndrome having manifestations of this disorder is 50%.

53. What problems in fetal development are encountered by pregnant women with phenylketonuria (PKU) who have been adequately treated by dietary phenylalanine restriction in childhood?

Dietary restrictions are often liberalized in children with PKU after the risk of mental retardation and neurologic defects have been minimized (about age 10). Mothers who have PKU but have been removed from (or were never on) phenylalanine-restricted diets will experience return to high blood levels of phenylalanine. Hyperphenylalaninemia acts as a teratogen on the fetus, resulting in mental retardation, microcephaly, intrauterine growth retardation, congenital heart defects, and a high spontaneous abortion rate. The implications are staggering. It was once believed that the manifestations of PKU could be entirely prevented by newborn screening and dietary restriction. However, in just one generation, as the fetal effects of maternal hyperphenylalaninemia become more prevalent, PKU-related mental retardation may return to the level it was at prior to mass screening programs. Studies are currently being conducted to determine if phenylalanine-restricted diets started in women prior to conception can minimize these congenital defects. Preliminary evidence suggests this may be helpful.

54. How many forms of dwarfism syndromes are recognizable at birth? What are the two most common types?

There are 21 different skeletal dysplasia syndromes that were classified at The International Nomenclature of Constitutional Diseases of Bone meeting as "recognizable at birth." The most common is thanatophoric dwarfism, a lethal chondrodysplasia characterized by flattened, U-shaped vertebral bodies, telephone-receiver-shaped femurs, macrocephaly, and redundant skin folds, causing a pug-like appearance. Thanatophoric means death-loving (an apt description). The incidence is 1 in 6400 births. Achondroplasia is the most common viable skeletal dysplasia, occurring 1 in 26,000 live births. Its features are small stature (mean adult height 4'2"), macrocephaly, depressed nasal bridge, lordosis, and a trident hand. Some patients develop hydrocephalus due to a small foramen magnum. X-ray findings include narrowing of the interpedicular distance as one proceeds caudally.

55. Why do the sclera of patients with osteogenesis imperfecta appear blue?

Phylogenetically, the sclera are closely related to the skeleton. In many animals, the sclera contains cartilage and osseous material. The primary component of sclera in humans is collagen. It is not surprising that in osteogenesis imperfecta and many other connective tissue diseases the sclera are abnormally thin and transparent, since abnormal collagen formation is the underlying defect in many of these disorders. The bluish color of the sclera in patients with connective tissue (especially collagen) diseases is thought to be due to visualization of the bluish-colored uvea (the eye layer behind the retina) as seen through a more transparent sclera. Uvea literally means grape, the name being derived from the similarity in their colors.

56. What other syndromes are associated with blue sclera?

Ehlers-Danlos syndrome	Marfan syndrome
Roberts syndrome	Hallermann-Streiff syndrome
Russell-Silver syndrome	Incontinentia pigmenti
Marshall-Smith syndrome	

57. Which genetic disorders are associated with hypoplastic left heart syndrome?
While most newborns with hypoplastic left heart syndrome have this defect as an isolated abnormality, several syndromes in which this congenital heart malformation is a component have been identified: Down syndrome, Turner syndrome, Smith-Lemli-Opitz syndrome, trisomy 13, trisomy 18, and Ivemark syndrome. Before extensive reconstructive surgery is attempted, it may be prudent to check the chromosome analysis in cases where dysmorphia is noted.

58. What is a rapid way of assessing hypertelorism?
If an imaginary third eye would fit between the eyes, hypertelorism is possible. Precise measurement involves measuring the distance between the center of each eye's pupil. This is a difficult measurement in newborns and uncooperative patients because of eye movement. In practice, the best way to determine hypotelorism or hypertelorism is to measure the inner and outer canthal distances, then plot these measurements on standardized tables of norms.

Bibliography

1. Jones KL: Smith's Recognizable Patterns of Human Malformation, 4th ed. Philadelphia, W.B. Saunders, 1987.
2. Kaback M: Genetic Issues in Pediatric and Obstetric Practice. Chicago, Year Book Medical Publishers, 1981.
3. Levine MD, et al (eds): Developmental-Behavioral Pediatrics. Philadelphia, W.B. Saunders, 1983.
4. McKusick VA: Mendelian Inheritance in Man, 7th ed. Baltimore, The Johns Hopkins University Press, 1986.
5. Simpson JL, Golbus MS, Martin AO, Sarto GE: Genetics in Obstetrics and Gynecology. New York, Grune and Stratton, 1982.
6. Smith DW, Wilson A: The Child with Down's Syndrome. Philadelphia, W.B. Saunders, 1973.
7. Stanbury JB, et al (eds): The Metabolic Basis of Inherited Disease. New York, McGraw-Hill, 1983.
8. Therman, E: Human Chromosomes, 2nd ed. New York, Springer-Verlag, 1986.
9. Thompson MW, Thompson JS: Genetics in Medicine, 4th ed. Philadelphia, W.B. Saunders, 1986.
10. Vogel F, Motulsky AG: Human Genetics, 2nd ed. Berlin, Springer-Verlag, 1986.
11. Warkany J: Congenital Malformations. Chicago, Year Book Medical Publishers, 1971.

GROWTH, DEVELOPMENT AND BEHAVIOR

Edward B. Charney, M.D.
Mark F. Ditmar, M.D.

Growth and Development

1. What are the three phases of in utero growth and when does maximal growth in body length occur?

Zygote, embryo, and fetus. During the zygote phase, there is an increase in cell organization and differentiation into the three basic cell layers of ectoderm, mesoderm, and endoderm. The embryo phase is marked by major organogenesis up to 8 weeks' gestation. The fetal phase, after 9 weeks' gestation, is marked by a period of incremental linear and weight growth, with linear growth achieving the greatest velocity at mid-fetal life or 4 months.

2. What are the variables that affect in utero growth?

Genetic constitution of the fetus, nutritional status of the mother, placental status, uterine capacity, exposure to infections, or toxic factors (i.e., rubella, alcohol, narcotics).

3. Is length of labor the same for male and female babies?

No. Labor length for boys is about an hour longer than for girls. Although an estimated 120 males are conceived for every 100 females, the fetal and neonatal death rate is greater for males, thereby reducing the sex ratio at birth to just a slight preponderance of males.

4. How many fontanelles are present at birth?

Although there are 6 fontanelles present at birth (2 anterior lateral, 2 posterior lateral, 1 anterior, and 1 posterior), only 2 (the anterior and posterior fontanelles) are usually palpable upon physical examination.

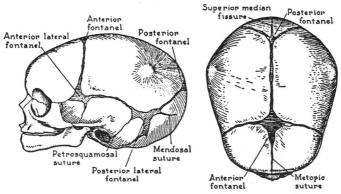

The cranium at birth, showing major sutures and fontanelles. No attempt is made to show molding or overlapping of bones, which sometimes occurs at birth. (From Caffey J: Pediatric X-ray Diagnosis, 6th ed. Chicago, Year Book Medical Publishers, 1972, with permission.)

5. Which conditions are associated with premature or delayed closure of the fontanelle?

Premature closure: microcephaly or small brain, high calcium/vitamin D ratio in pregnancy, craniosynostosis, hyperthyroidism, or it may just be a normal variant. *Delayed closure:* see list below.

Skeletal disorders	Chromosomal abnormalities	Other conditions
Achondroplasia	Down's syndrome	Athyrotic hypothyroidism
Aminopterin-induced syndrome	13 Trisomy syndrome	Hallermann-Streiff syndrome
Apert's syndrome	18 Trisomy syndrome	Malnutrition
Cleidocranial dysostosis		Progeria
Hypophosphatasia		Rubella syndrome
Kenny's syndrome		Russell-Silver syndrome
Osteogenesis imperfecta		
Pyknodysostosis		
Vitamin D deficiency rickets		

References: Popich GA, Smith DW: J Pediatr 80:749, 1972; Barness LA: Manual of Pediatric Physical Diagnosis, 3rd ed. Chicago, Year Book Medical Publishers, 1986, pp 49-50.

6. How does the growth rate of boys and girls differ?

In both boys and girls, the rate or velocity of linear growth begins to decelerate at about 2 years of age. In girls, this deceleration continues until approximately age 11 years, at which time the adolescent growth spurt begins. For boys, the deceleration continues until about 13 years. The peak rate of increase in males occurs at age 14 years.

7. On average, at what age do boys and girls achieve half their adult height?

Girls, 2 years; boys, 2½ years.

8. How do the relative proportions of the head, trunk, and extremities change during childhood?

The relative proportions of the head, trunk and extremities during prenatal and postnatal life are shown below.

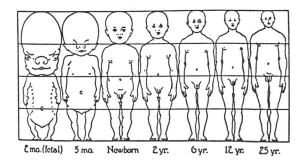

2 mo. (fetal)   5 mo.   Newborn   2 yr.   6 yr.   12 yr.   25 yr.

From Robbins WJ, et al: Growth. New Haven, CT, Yale University Press, 1928, with permission.

9. When do the primitive reflexes in a neonate become extinct?

Primitive or developmental reflexes are normally present at birth and should be extinct by about 6 months of age. Some of these reflexes include Moro, palmar grasp, rooting and tonic neck. Abnormalities in these reflexes include an asymmetric response, absence of expected response, sustained obligatory response, or persistence beyond the age of 6 months.

10. What are the major developmental landmarks for motor skills during the first 3 years of life?

Major *fine motor:* grasp (2–4 months), reaching for an object (3–5 months), transferring objects from hand to hand (5–7 months), fine pincer grasp with index finger and thumb apposition (9–14 months), spontaneous scribbling (12–24 months), copying a circle (2–3 years), and building a tower of 2 cubes (12–20 months) or 4 cubes (16–24 months). Major *gross motor:* steadiness of head when placed in supported sitting (1–4 months), sitting without support (5–8 months), cruising or walking holding on (7–13 months), walking alone (11–15 months), walking up steps (14–22 months), and pedaling tricycle (2–3 years).

11. What historical data should be obtained when evaluating a child with developmental delay? (See also question #13 in Genetics chapter)

Prenatal
  Maternal illness
  Maternal infection
  Maternal malnutrition
  Exposure to toxins
  Exposure to teratogens
  Abnormal fetal movement
  Low birth weight
Perinatal
  Asphyxia
  Abnormal presentation
  Trauma
  Placental dysfunction

Postnatal
  Infection
  Complications of prematurity
  Asphyxia/anoxia
  Seizures
  Presence of congenital defects or
    syndrome
  Hyperbilirubinemia
  Poor nutrition/feeding difficulties
  Abnormal sleep patterns
  CNS trauma

From Levy S: In Schwartz, Charney, Curry, Ludwig: Principles and Practice of Clinical Pediatrics. Chicago, Year Book, 1987, with permission.

12. What are the limitations of the Denver Developmental Screening Test (DDST)?

The DDST is a reliable, economic screening device for detecting children who have a high probability of being developmentally delayed. The real major limitation is its misuse as an IQ test. It is not meant to be a predictor of current or future intellectual ability and is not numerical. To be valid as a screening test, it must be administered in the standardized manner with exact test materials.

13. Do twins develop at a rate comparable to infants of single birth?

Twins exhibit significant verbal and motor delay in the first year of life. The difficulty lies not in the lack of potential but in the relative lack of individual stimulation. In general, children who are more closely spaced in a family have slower acquisition of verbal skills. Twins with significant language delay or with excessive use of "twin language" (language understood only by the twins themselves) may be candidates for interventional therapy.

Reference: Groothuis JR: Twins and twin families. Clin Perinatol 12:467–468, 1985.

14. Should premature infants be scored at chronologic age when assessing development?

Although there is general consensus that some correction factor for prematurity should be used when assessing development, there is not a definite answer to how much correction is indicated and for how long. In general, it is probably appropriate to make a correction during the first year of life by subtracting the number of months the child is premature from the chronologic age. For example, an 8-month-old infant who was 3 months premature should be "scored" on a developmental test as if he or she was 5 months old (8–3). Between 1 and 2 years of age, the amount of correction gets a bit cloudy and an appropriate compromise appears to be a 50% correction factor. For example, the 18-month-old infant who was 2 months premature should be "scored" on testing as if the chronologic age was 17 months. Most would agree that there shouldn't be any correction for prematurity after 2 years of age.

15. What behavioral patterns of early infancy are suspicious for a possible cognitive handicap?
Poor responsiveness to touch, poor eye contact during feeding, diminished spontaneous activity, decreased alertness to voice, irritability, slow feeding. These are particularly worrisome in the setting of higher risks, such as prematurity or early-onset seizures.

Reference: Crocker AC, Nelson RP: Major handicapping conditions. In Levine MD, et al: Developmental-Behavioral Pediatrics. Philadelphia, W.B. Saunders, 1983, p 760, with permission.

16. At what ages do children learn to copy geometric figures?
A child's ability to copy a geometric pattern is an indicator of fine motor control and planning. Significant delay can indicate a problem in vision, attention or neuromuscular control or perception. The skills are acquired at different ages:

3 years—copies circles
4 years—copies cross
4½ years—copies square
5 years—copies triangle

17. How is the intelligence quotient (IQ) determined?
Mental age divided by chronologic age times 100. It is important to note that IQ is not a static phenomenon, but can be changed significantly, depending on the developmental environment.

18. Which tests are most commonly used for IQ measurements in children?
Wechsler Intelligence Scale for Children-Revised (WISC-R) and Stanford-Binet Intelligence Scale.

19. Define mental retardation.
"Mental retardation refers to significantly subaverage general intellectual functioning existing concurrently with deficits in adaptive behavior and manifest during the developmental period." This widely accepted definition encompasses three facets: (1) a quantifiable intelligence test, (2) variable functional deficits in everyday living (inabilities to independently eat, dress, toilet), and (3) onset prior to 18 years of age.

Reference: Warren SA, Taylor RL: Education of children with learning problems. Pediatr Clin North Am 31:332, 1984.

20. What IQ levels correlate with various degrees of retardation?
Borderline retardation, 68–83; mild retardation, 52–67; moderate retardation, 36–51; severe retardation, 20–35; and profound retardation, below 20. Formal classification by the American Association of Mental Deficiency defines retardation as occurring below an IQ of 68. Those with an IQ of 69–83 are not retarded by strict definition, but constitute a group with high likelihood of educational problems and a very high potential for independent functioning.

21. What percentage of retarded individuals are severely or profoundly retarded?
5–10%

22. What is cerebral palsy (CP)?
Cerebral palsy is a disorder of movement and/or posture that results from nonprogressive damage to a developing brain. The damage may occur prenatally (e.g., infection, chromosomal anomaly), perinatally (e.g., prematurity, asphyxia), or postnatally (e.g., head trauma).

23. What are the two major types of CP?
Spastic and nonspastic (e.g., choreoathetosis).

24. How well do Apgar scores correlate with the development of CP?

In a large study of 49,000 infants, low Apgar score correlated poorly with the development of CP. Of term infants with scores of 0–3 at 1 or 5 minutes, 95% did not develop CP. Of those with scores of 0–3 at 10 minutes, 84% did not develop CP. If the 10-minute Apgar improved to 4 or more, the rate for CP was less than 1%. A low Apgar score (0–3) at 20 minutes, however, had an observed CP rate of nearly 60%. Conversely, nearly 75% of patients with CP had 5-minute Apgar scores of 7–10.

Reference: Nelson KB, Ellenberg JH: Apgar scores as predictors of chronic neurologic disability. Pediatrics 68:36–44, 1981.

25. What are some common disabilities associated with CP?

Seizures, mental retardation, learning disability, feeding disorders, and strabismus.

26. What features in an infant suggest a progressive CNS disorder rather than CP as the cause of motor deficit?

1. Abnormally increasing head circumference (possible hydrocephalus, tumor)

2. Eye anomalies such as cataracts, retinal pigmentary degeneration, optic atrophy (possible neurodegenerative disease).

3. Skin abnormalities such as vitiligo, café au lait spots, nevus flammeus (possible Sturge-Weber disease, neurofibromatosis).

4. Hepatomegaly and/or splenomegaly (possible storage disease).

5. Decreased or absent deep tendon reflexes.

6. Sensory abnormalities (loss or diminishment of sense of pain, position, vibration, or light touch).

Reference: Taft LT: Cerebral palsy. Pediatr Rev 6:41, 1984.

27. Do children "outgrow" CP?

In a large collaborative study of children clinically diagnosed at 1 year of age with CP, 55% had no evidence of CP at 7 years of age. Seventy-five percent of those with mild CP outgrew their motor abnormalities, but only 3% of those with severe CP did so. However, those diagnosed with CP at age 1 had a higher likelihood of mental retardation, nonfebrile seizures, or difficulty with speech than the control group.

Reference: Nelson KB, Ellenberg JH: Children who "outgrew" cerebral palsy. Pediatrics 69:529, 1982.

28. When can an infant "taste"?

Taste is present at birth and infants demonstrate a definite preference for sweetness over saltiness or plain water.

29. How good is a newborn infant's vision?

The visual perception system functions in a fairly complex manner at the time of birth and as early as 36 hours after birth many infants can both discriminate a number of facial expressions and imitate them. The human face is the most preferred object of fixation in early infancy. The light sense is one of the most primitive of all visual functions and is present by the seventh fetal month.

30. When do binocular fixation and depth perception develop in children?

Binocularity of vision depends primarily upon adequate coordination of the extraocular muscles and is normally established by 3–6 months of age. At about 6–8 months, early evidence of depth perception is seen, but it is still poorly developed. Depth perception becomes very accurate at 6 or 7 years and continues to improve through the early teens.

31. How does refractive capacity vary with age?

The newborn infant is typically slightly hyperopic (far-sighted). The mild hyperopia actually increases slowly for about the first 8 years; hyperopia then decreases gradually until adolescence, when vision is emmetropic (no refractive error). After 20 years, there is a tendency for myopia (near-sightedness).

32. What is haptic perception?

The acquisition by touch of information about the environment (e.g., objects, spaces). It is a vital process for children with severe visual impairment.

33. When do primary and secondary teeth erupt?

Mandibular teeth usually erupt first. The central incisors appear by 5–7 months and the second molars are in place by 23–30 months. Of the secondary teeth, the central incisors erupt first between 6 and 7 years and the third molars are in place by 17–22 years.

34. What are the first vowel sounds used by an infant?

At about 3 months of age, infants begin to make vowel sounds. Most of these vowel sounds are produced in the low front and mid-center regions of the mouth, producing sounds roughly to [a] as in pat and [e] as in pet. The range of vowels sounds then moves up and back in the mouth until, at about 12 months, virtually the whole range of English vowels is produced.

35. When do children start to "babble"?

Babbling, or the combination of vowel and consonant sounds, begins as early as 3 months and reaches a peak between 9 and 12 months of age. Samuel Johnson referred to babbling as "speech copious with order, and energetic without rule." While babbled noises may sound like they occur in sentence-like sequences, none of it seems interpretable during the early stages. The most frequent consonant sounds in early babbling (3–6 months) are produced in the back of the mouth (such as [g] and [k]), whereas later sounds (such as [b] and [d]) are produced in the front of the mouth. The babbling of infancy appears to be the result of the infant playing with speech production and beginning to gain control over mouth and tongue movements. Babbling begins at about the same time in both deaf and hearing infants. Deaf children stop babbling earlier, probably because of not hearing themselves, and there is not the normal progression to meaningful communicative speech.

36. When does a child say "mama" or "dada"? Which is usually said first?

Between 10 and 15 months of age most children start producing their first clearly identifiable words and often they are reduplicated syllables such as "dada," "baba," or "mama." Most infants usually say "dada" first.

37. What are the warning signs of delayed language development?

Danger Signals of Speech-Language Problems in Preschool Children

By 6 mo:	No response or inconsistent response to sound or voice
By 9 mo:	No response to his/her name
By 12 mo:	Stopped babbling or did not babble yet
By 15 mo:	Does not understand and respond to "no" and "bye-bye"
By 18 mo:	No words other than "mama/dada"
By 2 yr:	No two-word phrases
After 2 yr:	Still jargons or echoes excessively
By 2½ yr:	Speech that is not intelligible to family
By 3 yr:	No simple sentences
By 3½ yr:	Speech that is not intelligible to strangers
By 4 yr:	Consistent articulation errors (besides r, s, l, th)
By 5 yr:	Sentence structure is awkward

Table continued on next page.

Danger Signals of Speech-Language Problems in Preschool Children *(Continued)*

After 5 yr:	Noticeable, persistent dysfluency (stuttering)
By 6 yr:	Unusual confusions, reversals, or word-finding problems in connected speech
After 7 yr:	Any speech errors
Any age	Any persistent hypernasality or hyponasality, monotone pitch, or hoarseness of voice

From Schwartz E: In Schwartz, Charney, Curry, Ludwig: Principles and Practice of Clinical Pediatrics. Chicago, Year Book Medical Publishers, 1987, with permission.

38. What should the workup include for a child with delayed language development?

In-office screening by pediatricians for language development may include: Clinical Linguistic and Auditory Milestone Scale (CLAMS) (Clin Pediatr 1978; 17:847), Bzoch–League Receptive Emergent Language Scale (REEL), or the Peabody Picture Vocabulary Test (PPVT). Failure on one of these screening tests should prompt referral by the pediatrician for an audiologic and complete cognitive assessment. Major conditions in the differential for a child with language delay include hearing impairment or deafness, mental retardation, or autism.

39. What are the causes of stuttering and when does it require treatment?

Stuttering is a common characteristic of the speech of pre-school children. However, the vast majority of children do not persist with stuttering beyond 5 or 6 years of age. Preschoolers at increased risk for persistence of stuttering include those with a positive family history of stuttering and those with anxiety-provoking stress related to talking. A child older than 5 or 6 years who stutters should be referred to a speech-language pathologist for assessment and treatment. The pediatrician can help guide parents of children younger than 5 years of age with stuttering by making the following suggestions:

    1. Do not give the child directives about how to deal with his speech (e.g., "slow down" or "take a breath").

    2. Provide a relaxed, easy speech model in your own manner of speaking to the child.

    3. Reduce the need/expectations for the child to speak to strangers, adults, or authority figures or to compete with others (such as sibs) to be heard.

    4. Listen attentively to the child with patience and without showing concern.

    5. Seek professional guidance if speech is not noticeably more fluent in 2 to 3 months.

Reference: Schwartz E: Speech and language disabilities, In-Principles and Practice of Clinical Pediatrics. Schwartz, Charney, Curry, Ludwig: Chicago, Year Book Medical Publishers, 1987.

40. What are the indications for a formal hearing test?

    1. Parental concern that the child does not hear normally. (This is listed first because although it is often the most reliable early sign of hearing problems, it unfortunately is often overlooked by the pediatrician.)

    2. Birth weight <1500 gm

    3. Family history of childhood hearing impairment

    4. Delay in acquisition of language and/or speech

    5. Congenital perinatal infection (e.g., cytomegalovirus, rubella, herpes, toxoplasmosis, syphilis)

    6. Anatomical malformations involving the head or neck (i.e., microtia, micrognathia, cleft palate)

    7. Hyperbilirubinemia at level exceeding indications for exchange transfusion

    8. Bacterial meningitis

    9. Severe birth asphyxia

    10. Other developmental disabilities (i.e. mental retardation, cerebral palsy)

41. What is autism and how is that diagnosis made?

Autism, a behaviorally defined developmental disorder, has 4 major characteristics: onset before 30 months of age; social indifference or failure to develop normal social responses or interactions with other individuals (social aloneness); absent or abnormal speech and language development; and stereotyped or bizarre responses to objects and other aspects of the environment. Although the majority of autistic children are also mentally retarded, approximately 20% have IQs of 70 or above. There are no consistent physical or laboratory findings—autism is diagnosed by a pattern of abnormal behavior.

42. What are some of the presentations of autism?

1. Avoidance of eye contact during infancy
2. Relating to only part of a person's body (i.e., lap) rather than to whole person
3. Failure to acquire speech or speech acquisition in an unusual manner such as echolalia (repeating another person's speech)
4. Repetition of TV commercials and singing out of context and without communicative purpose
5. Spending long periods of time in repetitive activities and fascination with movement (i.e., spinning records, dripping water)
6. Interest in small visual details or patterns
7. Unusual abilities such as early letter and number recognition
8. Early reading with minimal comprehension

43. How is a child with suspected autism evaluated?

Children with suspected autism should be evaluated for hearing impairment with formal audiologic testing, for mental retardation, and for extreme social deprivation with unusual parental mismanagement and/or overanxiety.

44. Is there biochemical or neurologic basis for autistic behavior?

There is general consensus that the early hypothesis that autism resulted from parental coldness, rejection, or mishandling is incorrect. The current belief is that autistic behavior arises from dysfunction of the central nervous system. Unfortunately, neither the biochemical basis nor the anatomic abnormality responsible for autism is known.

45. When should "toilet training" be started?

When the child is physically and emotionally ready. The physical prerequisite of neurologic maturation of bladder and bowel control usually occurs between 1 and 3 years of age. The child's emotional readiness is often influenced by his or her temperament, parental attitudes, and parent-child interactions. Most, but not all, children begin some emotional readiness by 2 years of age and before 3 years. The "potty chair" should be introduced sometime between 2 and 3 years of age. Most children will achieve daytime bladder and bowel control by 3½ years.

46. Are girls or boys toilet-trained earlier?

On average, girls are toilet-trained earlier than boys. With regard to most other developmental milestones in the first years of life, there do not seem to be significant sex differences (e.g., in walking or running, in sleep patterns, or in verbal ability). Girls do show more rapid bone development.

47. At which Tanner stage do the female and male adolescent growth spurts begin?

Female adolescent growth spurt usually occurs at 12 years of age with Tanner IV breast and pubic hair development. Male adolescent growth spurt usually occurs at 13½ years with Tanner IV genitalia and pubic hair.

48. What is Quetelet's index?

Weight divided by height squared. It is greater at each stage of sexual maturation.

Behavior

49. What are the most common types of behavioral problems in children?
   1. Problems of daily routine (e.g., food refusal, sleep abnormalities, toilet difficulties).
   2. Aggressive-resistant behavior (e.g., temper tantrums, aggressiveness with peers).
   3. Overdependent-withdrawing behavior (e.g., separation upset, fears, shyness).
   4. Hyperactivity.
   5. Undesirable habits (e.g., thumb-sucking, head banging, nail biting, playing with genitals).
   6. School problems.
   Reference: Chamberlin RW: Prevention of behavioral problems in young children. Pediatr Clin North Am 31:332, 1984.

50. What is the difference between a "blue" breathholding spell and a "white" breathholding spell?
Actually, there are far more similarities than differences. Both are syncopal attacks occurring commonly in children ages 6 months to 4 years, peaking between ages 1½ and 3. The blue or cyanotic spell is more common. Distraught crying is provoked by physical or emotional upset, causing anger or frustration. Sudden apnea ensues, followed by cyanosis, opisthotonus, rigidity and later loss of tone. Brief convulsive jerking may occur. The episode lasts from 10 to 60 seconds. A short period of sleepiness may ensue. The white or pallid spell is similar except for skin color. These children on testing demonstrate increased responsiveness to vagal maneuvers. This parasympathetic hypersensitivity may cause cardiac slowing, diminished cardiac output, and diminished arterial pressure, resulting in a pale appearance.

51. When should a diagnosis of seizure disorder be considered rather than a breathholding spell?
   1. Precipitating event is minor or nonexistent.
   2. History of no or minimal crying or breathholding.
   3. Episode lasts longer than 1 minute.
   4. Period of post-episode sleepiness lasts longer than 10 minutes.
   5. Convulsive component of episode is prominent.
   6. Occurs in child less than 6 months or greater than 4 years old.

52. Does thumb-sucking vary with race and culture?
Yes. Various studies found that 45% of American children less than 4 years of age suck their thumbs (boys and girls equally) compared with 30% of Swedish children, 17% of Indian children, and 1% of Eskimo children. Eskimo children probably don't need to suck their thumbs because they are usually carried in their mothers' back packs with a bottle close at hand. Most thumb-sucking stops spontaneously by age 4.
   Reference: Curzon ME: Dental implications of thumb sucking. Pediatrics 54:196, 1974.

53. What is *pavor nocturnus*?
Pavor nocturnus (Latin for fear of the night) is more commonly known as night terrors. These are brief episodes of 30 seconds to 5 minutes in which a child sits up, screams, and appears aroused, often staring and sweating profusely. The child cannot be consoled, rapidly goes back to sleep, and does not recall the episode in the morning. Onset of night terrors in an older child or persistent multiple attacks may indicate more serious psychopathology.
   Reference: Anders TF, Keener MA: Sleep-wake state development and disorders of sleep in infants, children and adolescents. In Levine MD, et al: Developmental-Behavioral Pediatrics. Philadelphia, W.B. Saunders, 1983.

54. What is the difference between night terrors and nightmares?
Nightmares are frightening dreams that occur during REM sleep and may readily be recalled on awakening. Night terrors occur in non-REM stage IV sleep and cannot be recalled.

55. How common is night waking in infancy?
Seventy percent of infants at 3 months of age and 90% of infants at 9 months of age will have uninterrupted sleep between midnight and 5 a.m. Between 9 and 12 months of age, however, the phenomenon of night waking begins and occurs in up to 50% of infants. This declines in the following year, but by age 2 may still occur in up to 20% of infants.
    Reference: Moore T, Ucko C: Night waking in early infancy. Arch Dis Child 33:333–342, 1957.

56. At what age do sleepwalking and sleeptalking occur?
Sleepwalking occurs most commonly between the ages of 5 and 10. As many as 15% of children between the ages of 5 and 12 may have somnambulated once and as many as 10% of 3–10 year old children may sleeptalk regularly. The sleepwalking child is clumsy, noncommunicative, restless, and nonpurposeful. The episode is not remembered. Injury is common during this outing. Sleeptalking is monosyllabic and incomprehensible. Both conditions usually end before age 15. Severe cases may benefit from diazepam or imipramine therapy.

57. Is physical injury a concern in children with head banging?
Although a common problem occurring in 5–15% of normal children, head banging rarely results in physical injury and then usually in autistic or otherwise developmentally abnormal children. Normal children often show signs of bliss as they bang away. The activity usually resolves by 4 years of age. It may resume spontaneously during national board exams.

58. How much do babies normally cry each day?
In Brazelton's oft-quoted study in 1962 of 80 infants, he found that at 2 weeks of age the average crying time was nearly 2 hours per day, increasing to nearly 3 hours at 6 weeks and then declining to about 1 hour at 12 weeks.
    Reference: Brazelton TB: Crying in infancy. Pediatrics 29:579–588, 1962.

59. What are the signs and characteristics of colic in infants?
The principal sign is full-force crying lasting more than 3 hours/day for 3 days in any one week. The crying is paroxysmal in nature during periods of irritability and fussiness. The infant is well fed and healthy but emits considerable flatus. Periods of colic usually occur during the 4 months after the child is brought home from the hospital. The condition should be distinguished from normal crying, which can last almost as long but is usually not as forceful. One must distinguish colic from faulty feeding and other physical problems, including allergies, acute disorders such as otitis media, and other immaturity problems.
    Reference: Carey WB: "Colic" or excessive crying in young infants. In Levine MD, et al: Developmental-Behavioral Pediatrics. Philadelphia, W.B. Saunders, 1983.

60. What are tics and when do they begin to appear?
Tics are sudden, repetitive, involuntary, and purposeless movements that may be motor (e.g., blink, grimace, shrug) or vocal (e.g., clearing of the throat, sniffing, grunting). Most are simple, occur before the age of 6, and peak in the preadolescent years. Progression of tics with increasing complexity can lead to the diagnosis of Tourette's syndrome.
    Reference: Kavanaugh JG, Mattson AKE: Tics. In Friedman SB, Hoekelman RA (eds): Behavioral Pediatrics: Psychosocial Aspects of Child Health Care. New York, McGraw-Hill Book Co., 1980.

61. What is Tourette's syndrome?
More properly called Gilles de la Tourette's syndrome, this is a syndrome complex of five diagnostic features: (1) motor and vocal tics, (2) symptoms waxing and waning over time, (3) symptoms changing in nature over time, (4) occurring between ages 2 and 15, and (5) present

for at least 1 year. When pharmacologic treatment is needed, haloperidol is most commonly used.
   Reference: Barabas G: Tourette's syndrome: an overview. Pediatr Ann 17:391–393, 1988.

62. What percentage of patients with Tourette's syndrome demonstrate coprolalia?
Coprolalia is an irresistible urge to utter profanities, occurring as a phonic tic. Only 20–35% of patients with Tourette's syndrome have this phenomenon and it is not essential for the diagnosis. Of note, 20–50% patients with Tourette's have associated symptoms of attention deficit disorder.

63. What is attention deficit disorder (ADD)?
A central neuropsychiatric disorder of childhood of unknown etiology. It occurs in up to 10% of school-age children. Formerly, it was called hyperactivity syndrome or minimal brain dysfunction. The diagnosis is based on historical and observational criteria of symptoms and signs that demonstrate (1) inattention, (2) impulsivity with or without (3) hyperactivity. The onset must be before age 7 and have persisted for more than 6 months.

64. Is ADD synonymous with "learning disability"?
No. Learning disabilities comprise a large heterogeneous group of presumed central neurodeficiencies that result in difficulties in speaking, listening, writing, reasoning, or mathematics. Many children with ADD have learning disabilities, but many with learning disabilities do not have ADD.

65. What are the major subtypes of ADD?
(1) ADD with hyperactivity (ADDH), (2) ADD without hyperactivity (ADDNoH), and (3) ADD residual type (adolescents diagnosed at an earlier age with ADDH but no longer exhibiting significant hyperactivity).

66. What diagnoses must be excluded when evaluating potential ADD?
Deafness; severe or profound mental retardation (IQ less than 40); other developmental disorders (e.g., autism, childhood schizophrenia); and seizure disorder (petit mal seizures may cause episodic inattention).
   Reference: Shaywitz SE, Shaywitz BA: Diagnosis and management of attention deficit disorder: a pediatric perspective. Pediatr Clin North Am 31:429–457, 1984.

67. How effective are medications for ADD?
Stimulant medications (methylphenidate or Ritalin, amphetamines, pemoline) result in improvement in 70–80% of affected children. The primary benefits occur in improving attention deficiencies and to a lesser extent in diminishing hyperactivity. Benefits in cognition are more controversial. Stimulants appear to work by altering the neurochemical balance of the monoamines (e.g., norepinephrine, dopamine, serotonin) in the central nervous system. Short-term side effects such as sleep disturbances and decreased appetite are common but are usually amenable to dose adjustment. Precipitation of Tourette syndrome may occur. Long-term side effects are under study but may include reduction of both height and weight growth.

68. Why is the designation attention deficit disorder controversial?
Some believe that no coherent syndrome has been demonstrated. Although proponents believe that the signs and symptoms are derived from brain malfunction, some of the characteristics of "ADD," such as low attention span, can come from other causes, such as normal variations in temperament.

69. What is the Feingold diet?
Dr. Benjamin Feingold hypothesized in the early 1970s that hyperactivity in children was due to the ingestion of low molecular weight chemicals, such as salicylates and artificial additives

for color and flavor. He recommended a diet devoid of these substances and claimed up to a 50% improvement in children on such a diet. No controlled studies, however, have been able to demonstrate such an effect.

70. What is the "Damocles syndrome"?

With lengthening survival among children with formerly rapidly fatal diseases (e.g., acute lymphoblastic leukemia), the stresses of uncertainty in long-term life-threatening illnesses have been termed the Damocles syndrome. Such children are at increased risk for developing emotional problems as a result of these stresses.

Reference: Koocher GP, O'Malley JE: The Damocles Syndrome: Psychological Consequences of Surviving Childhood Cancer. New York, McGraw-Hill Book Co., 1981.

71. Is a child aware of his own fatal illness?

Yes, for the most part. Many studies have demonstrated that even young children are cognizant that a medical condition is life-threatening and experience increased levels of anxiety and isolation compared to children with non-fatal illnesses.

Reference: Koocher GP, Berman SJ: Life threatening and terminal illness in childhood. In Levine MD, et al: Developmental-Behavioral Pediatrics. Philadelphia. W.B. Saunders, 1983.

72. Do children comprehend death?

In Levine et al., Koocher and Berman explain the results of studies about this question as follows:

"...studies suggest that egocentrism and magical thinking, which are a part of preoperational thought in young children, dominate concerns about death in early childhood. With the beginning of concrete operational thought at about age six or seven, the child becomes capable of taking the role of another person in the cognitive sense and thereby begins to sense the permanence of death. At this stage, however, the child may still think of death as something that occurs as a consequence of a specific illness or injury rather than as a biologic process. At the time of adolescence with accompanying abstract reasoning capability and formal operational thought, a more complete comprehension of death becomes possible."

Reference: Koocher GP, Berman SJ: Life threatening and terminal illness in childhood. In Levine MD, et al: Developmental-Behavioral Pediatrics. Philadelphia, W.B. Saunders, 1983.

73. What are the signs of sibling deprivation in the presence of a child with a chronic illness?

Depression, rebellion, undue hypochrondria, envy.

74. What are the effects of heavy television watching in children?

The extent of television viewing by children in the U.S. is enormous, with average daily viewing being between three and four hours. TV viewing ranks as the #1 waking activity of the American child. Schorr has summarized seven principal effects:

1. Increased aggressive behavior and acceptance of violence.
2. Difficulty in distinguishing between fantasy and reality.
3. Distorted perceptions of reality (vis-à-vis consumerism, extent of violence, role of minorities).
4. Trivialization of sex and sexuality.
5. Increased passivity and disengagement.
6. Negative effects on cognitive learning.
7. Loss of time and potential to inform and to teach "prosocial" behavior.

From Schorr LB: Environmental deterrents: poverty, affluence, violence and television. In Levine MD, et al (eds): Developmental-Behavioral Pediatrics. Philadelphia, W.B. Saunders, 1983, p. 307, with permission.

75. What are the two types of school refusal?
    1. Anxiety-related: fearful of separation from parents; insecure; more commonly has school phobia with specific fears; girls affected more often than boys; usually good students.
    2. Secondary-gain type: no anxiety about school; prefers ease and comfort of home; boys affected more often than girls; usually poor students.
Reference: Schmitt BD: School refusal. Pediatr Rev 8:99, 1986.

76. What are Erikson's eight life-cycle crises of psychosocial development?
    1. Trust vs. mistrust (infancy)
    2. Autonomy vs. shame and doubt (early childhood)
    3. Initiative vs. guilt (early childhood)
    4. Industry vs. inferiority (school-age)
    5. Identity vs. confusion (adolescents)
    6. Intimacy vs. isolation (young adults)
    7. Generativity vs. stagnation (middle age)
    8. Integrity vs. despair (old age)
Erikson believed that psychodevelopment involves a healthy resolution, balance, or problematic persistence of these alternatives as each stage of life is reached.
Reference: Erikson E: Childhood and Society. New York, W.W. Norton, 1950.

77. What percent of children of divorce remain in the custody of the mother?
90%

78. How do children of different ages vary in their response to parental divorce?
    Preschool (ages 2½–5): most likely to show regression in developmental milestones (e.g., toilet training); increased separation anxiety; sleep disturbances; preoccupation with fear of abandonment; demanding with remaining parent; aggressive with siblings and peers.
    Early school age (6–8): most likely to demonstrate open grieving; preoccupied with fear of rejection and of being replaced; torn by guilt because of conflicting loyalties.
    Later school age (ages 9–12): more likely to demonstrate profound anger at one or both parents; more likely to distinguish one parent as the culprit causing the divorce; deterioration in school performance and peer relationships; sense of loneliness and powerlessness.
    Adolescents: significant potential for acute depression and even suicidal ideation; acting out behavior (substance abuse, truancy, sexual activity); self-doubts about own potential for marital success.
    Generally, children do better when a sense of continuity is established with both parents and when post-divorce parental conflict and bitterness are minimal. However, a very large percentage of children of divorce suffer ongoing psychological distress.
Reference: Wallerstein JS: Separation, divorce and remarriage. In Levine MD, et al: Developmental-Behavioral Pediatrics. Philadelphia, W.B. Saunders, 1983.

79. How common are adolescent suicide attempts?
For each death by suicide, there are 50–200 attempts that fail. This places the number of attempts between 250,000 and 1,000,000 in the U.S. Females attempt more frequently than males (3:1). However, males are more likely to die in an attempt because they use more lethal methods (e.g., knives or guns), as compared with pill ingestion or wrist slashing in females.

80. What are the signs of suicidal tendencies in adolescents?
    1. Signs of depression (fatigue, sadness, loss of appetite, sleep irregularities).
    2. Multiple psychosomatic complaints
    3. "Acting out" behavior (delinquency, truancy, sexual promiscuity, drug or alcohol abuse, running away from home)
    4. History of a previous suicide attempt within 2 years.
    5. Family history of suicide.

81. How common is drug use in adolescents?

A 1985 survey of high school students revealed that two-thirds of students used an illicit drug before finishing high school. Five percent used marijuana on a daily basis and 25% on at least a monthly basis. Stimulant and cocaine use were also high. Sixty-six percent of adolescents use alcohol regularly and 30% of adolescents smoke cigarettes regularly.

82. What are the four types of alcohol and drug use by teenagers?

 1. Experimental—weekend beer or marijuana use at parties.
 2. Recreational—weekday use and progression to harder drugs, liquor.
 3. Problematic—daily use; personality changes noted; difficulties at school and with family.
 4. Addictive—majority of time under the influence of drugs or alcohol; frequent legal problems.

83. When should drug users be referred for professional evaluation and counseling?

Referral or more extensive evaluation depends on the age and development of the adolescent. At any age, the recreational, problematic, or addictive user warrants professional intervention. The younger adolescent may also benefit from evaluation at the experimental stage, if only in an effort to postpone such behavior.

Bibliography

 1. Freidman SB, Hoekelman RA (eds): Behavioral Pediatrics: Psychosocial Aspects of Child Health Care. New York, McGraw-Hill Book Co., 1980.
 2. Levine MD, Carey WB, Crocker AC, Gross RT (eds): Developmental-Behavioral Pediatrics. Philadelphia, W.B. Saunders, 1983.
 3. Zitelli BJ, Davis HW (eds): Atlas of Pediatric Physical Diagnosis. St. Louis, C.V. Mosby Co., 1987.

HEMATOLOGY

Alan R. Cohen, M.D.

1. What infections are noted with increased frequency in patients with sickle cell disease?

Sepsis, meningitis, and osteomyelitis occur more commonly in patients with homozygous or doubly heterozygous sickling disorders (HbSS, HbSC, HbS-β° thal) than in patients who are hematologically normal. Pneumonia probably occurs more commonly in patients with sickling disorders but the extensive overlap between the clinical manifestations of infectious and vaso-occlusive lung disease makes it difficult to sort out the true risk of pneumonia.

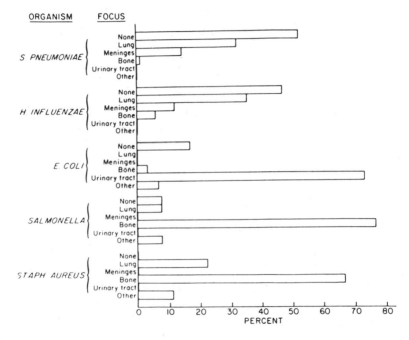

Frequency of focus of infection for specific causes of bacteremia in patients with sickling disorders. (From Zarkowsky HS et al: Bacteremia in sickle hemoglobinopathies. J Pediatr 109:579–585, 1986, with permission.)

2. What are the types of crises in sickle cell disease?

The major types of crises in sickle cell disease are vaso-occlusive (or painful) crisis, aplastic crisis, sequestration crisis and hemolytic crisis.

3. How should a child with a painful crisis be managed?

A painful crisis is one of the most difficult and challenging problems in the treatment of sickle cell disease. The mainstays of treatment are fluid therapy to prevent dehydration (D5/1/4NS or D5/1/2NS at 1.5–2 times maintenance) and analgesia. Approaches to pain control are notoriously varied and untested. The guiding principles are adequate relief of pain, awareness of drug side effects, and close familiarity with a particular drug, including its usual dose and route of administration. For outpatients with an acute painful crisis, acetaminophen or acetaminophen and codeine are reasonable choices. When hospitalization for parenteral analgesic therapy is necessary, drug choices include morphine and meperidine. Continuous infusions of these drugs may provide the most consistent pain relief, but the lack of extensive experience with this mode of therapy in most centers demands careful attention to drug concentration, infusion rate, patient response, and side effects. The treatment of a vaso-occlusive crisis is considerably easier when the physician is familiar with an individual patient's particular pattern of painful episodes and analgesic response. The patient should also be regarded as an excellent source of information regarding what dose of what drug is effective and how long his or her crisis usually lasts. Long-acting oral narcotics and patient-controlled analgesics are two new approaches to the treatment of painful crisis that are being evaluated.

4. What laboratory tests are used to evaluate children with suspected hemoglobin-opathies?

The most important laboratory test is hemoglobin electrophoresis. Unlike a hemoglobin level or "sickle prep," the electrophoresis is definitive. The hemoglobin level may fall within the normal range in some children with sickling disorders, particularly HbSC, diminishing the value of this test for screening purposes. The usual sickle screen fails to distinguish between sickle cell trait and sickle cell disease and therefore will be positive in approximately 8% of black children. Moreover, this test does not identify other abnormal hemoglobins such as HbC or HbD, whose detection may be important in providing accurate genetic counselling for the patient or family. Therefore, for elective evaluation, one should rely upon the hemoglobin electrophoresis for a quick and accurate diagnosis. In an emergency situation when an electrophoresis is not readily available, the CBC and sickle "screen" provide clues within the limitations noted above. The presence of sickle cells on the peripheral smear is, however, a reliable indicator of the presence of sickle cell disease.

Homozygous β-thalassemia is detected by the absence (β^o) or reduction relative to HbF (β^+) in the amount of HbA on electrophoresis. The carrier state for β-thalassemia is characterized by a low mean cell volume (MCV) and, in most instances, an increased level of HbA_2 or HbF. The levels of these two hemoglobins are most accurately measured by column chromatography. Estimation or quantitation from electrophoresis patterns is frequently misleading.

Alpha thalassemia trait remains a diagnosis of exclusion (low MCV in the absence of an identifiable cause) in the clinical laboratory.

Testing For Hemoglobinopathies

Sickling Disorders
    Screen
        Sickledex or other solubility tests
        Shake test
        CBC, reticulocytes, and peripheral smear
    Definitive
        Hemoglobin electrophoresis

Thalassemia Major
    Screen
        CBC and peripheral smear
    Definitive
        Hemoglobin electrophoresis
        Globin chain synthesis

Table continued on next page.

Testing For Hemoglobinopathies *(Continued)*

β-Thalassemia Trait (Thalassemia Minor)
  Screen
    CBC, MCV
  Definitive
    Hemoglobin electrophoresis
    HbA_2
    HbF

α-Thalassemia Trait
  Screen
    CBC, MCV
  Definitive
    α-gene enumeration

---

5. What are the associated morbidities of sickle cell disease and sickle cell trait?

Major causes of morbidity in sickle cell disease include painful crises, infection, severe anemia due to aplasia or sequestration, acute chest syndrome, and cerebral infarct or hemorrhage. Long-term morbidities include renal failure, congestive heart failure, retinal damage, leg ulcers, and aseptic necrosis of the hip. The major clinical problem in sickle cell trait is hematuria. Early recognition of the presence of HbS in a patient with hematuria may help to avert a costly and invasive evaluation. Recent evidence suggests that exhaustive exercise coupled with inadequate fluid replacement may be a cause of sudden death in military recruits with sickle trait. It is presently unknown whether severely ill neonates with sickle trait and hypoxia, acidosis, or fluid imbalance may also be susceptible to increased morbidity and mortality.

6. When does functional asplenia occur in children with sickle cell disease?

It may begin as early as 5 or 6 months of age and may precede the presence of Howell-Jolly bodies in the peripheral smear. Clinical experience indicates that the period of increased risk for serious bacterial infection parallels the development of functional asplenia. Loss of splenic function usually occurs later in patients with HbSC or HbS β$^+$-thalassemia than in patients with HbSS.

7. On routine exam a 13-year-old with sickle cell disease has a palpable spleen. Is this unusual?

The finding of a palpable spleen in a 13-year-old patient with a sickling disorder is a strong clue to the presence of HbSC or HbS β$^+$-thalassemia. In HbSS the spleen is rarely palpable after 5 or 6 years of age.

8. What is the leading cause of death in young children with sickle cell disease?

Bacterial sepsis. This is why evaluation and early treatment of fever in a child with sickle cell disease are so important.

9. What is the incidence of bacterial sepsis in children with sickle cell disease?

In children with HbSS, it is 8 per 100 patient-years in the first 3 years of life; in patients with HbSC it is 3.5 per 100 patient-years in the first 3 years of life.

Age-specific Incidence Rates of Bacteremia in Sickle Cell Anemia and Sickle Cell–Hemoglobin C Disease

	AGE (YR)				
	<3	3–5	6–9	10–19	≥20
Patients with SS					
Number of patients	459	571	630	958	983
Patient-years	752	1025	1333	2843	3480
Number of events	60	26	14	18	30
Events/100 patient-years	7.98[*†]	2.54[*†]	1.05	0.63	0.86[†]
Patients with SC					
Number of patients	177	178	183	277	277
Patient-years	339	305	372	830	1057
Number of events	12	0	1	4	2
Events/100 patient-years	3.54[*]	0	0.27	0.48	0.19

From Zarkowsky HS: Bacteremia in sickle hemoglobinopathies. J Pediatr 109:579–585, 1986, with permission.
[*] Significantly greater than rates in next higher age group (P≥0.01).
[†] Significantly greater than rates in SC patients of corresponding age group (P≥0.01).

10. What is the fatality rate for episodes of bacteremia?
In children less than 3 years of age with HbSS it is approximately 20%, whereas it is much lower in HbSC.

11. What can be done to prevent bacteremia?
The high mortality rate due to bacterial sepsis in young children with sickle cell disease underscores the importance of early diagnosis of the hemoglobinopathy. When neonatal screening reveals sickle cell disease, parents can be counselled regarding the importance of fever and the necessity for early intervention.

12. How should children with sequestration crisis be managed?
Acute sequestration crisis represents a true emergency in sickle cell disease and is the second leading cause of death in young children with this hemoglobinopathy. The clinical problem is primarily one of hypovolemic shock due to pooling of blood in the acutely enlarged spleen. The hemoglobin level may drop as low as 1 or 2 g/dl. The major therapeutic effort should be directed toward replacement of volume with whatever fluid is handy. In most instances, normal saline or colloid solutions will be adequate until properly cross-matched blood is available. Acute sequestration crisis is one of the few instances in sickle cell disease where transfusion with whole blood is appropriate, since the problem is one of hypovolemia and anemia rather than anemia alone. If whole blood is not available, packed red cells alone or packed red cells plus plasma may be an alternative therapy.

13. How effective is the use of prophylactic penicillin and/or pneumococcal vaccine in patients with sickle cell disease?
Both have helped to reduce pneumococcal infection in patients with sickle cell disease. In a recent trial of prophylactic penicillin in patients less than 3 years of age with sickle cell disease, children receiving 125 mg of penicillin VK twice daily had an 84% reduction in pneumococcal infections compared with untreated controls. A new trial will soon establish whether penicillin prophylaxis is equally effective in older children with sickle cell disease. Since most patients with HbSS are functionally asplenic after early childhood, and the rate of pneumococcal infection in older children with sickle cell disease is higher than it is in the normal population (although not as high as in early childhood), there is a strong argument for penicillin prophylaxis. Pneumococcal vaccine should be administered to all children with sickle cell disease who are 2 years of age or older. In some centers the vaccine is administered before 2 years of age, although the serologic response is not as strong at this time. For these children, the vaccine should be re-administered after 2 years of age.

**Penicillin Prophylaxis in Sickle Cell Anemia: Rate of *Streptococcus pneumoniae*
Septicemia per 100 Patient-Years, According to Treatment Group**

AGE (YR)	PENICILLIN	PLACEBO
<1	0.0	20.1
1	2.2	9.1
2	0.0	10.8
3	3.4	3.6
Total	1.5	9.8

Adapted from Gaston M, et al: N Engl J Med 314:1594–1599, 1986.

14. How is splenic function evaluated in children with sickle cell disease?

The absence of splenic function in children with sickle cell disease is most easily detected by the presence of Howell-Jolly bodies in the red cells on the peripheral smear. Measurement of red cell pitting provides an earlier clue to the gradual loss of splenic function, but this test requires special optics and is not available in most routine clinical laboratories. Diminished uptake of radionuclide on spleen scan also indicates the loss of splenic function but requires radiation exposure and does not offer a great deal of information that is not available from the presence or absence of Howell-Jolly bodies.

15. Why are neonates with sickle cell disease asymptomatic?

The presence of large amounts of fetal hemoglobin (HbF) reduces the rate of polymerization of HbS and the sickling of red cells containing this abnormal hemoglobin. As the amount of fetal hemoglobin diminishes after the first 6 months of life, patients with sickle cell disease are increasingly likely to experience their first clinical manifestations. Patients who are doubly heterozygous for HbS and hereditary persistence of fetal hemoglobin (HPFH) never lose the presence of an increased amount of HbF in each red cell. As one might expect from the experience with neonates, these patients have no clinical manifestations related to sickling.

16. What are the hematologic abnormalities associated with Down's syndrome?

Children with Down's syndrome have an increased incidence of leukemia, particularly in the neonatal period. In some patients, a myeloproliferative picture resembling leukemia regresses spontaneously over several months. Down's syndrome is one of the numerous causes of neonatal polycythemia. For unknown reasons, patients with Down's syndrome have an increased MCV, so that this parameter loses most of its value as a test for iron deficiency. Other hematologic manifestations of Down's syndrome are either rare or clinically unimportant, including decreased eosinophils, alterations of platelet biochemistry, and, in the first few months of life, decreased level of HbF.

17. What are the manifestations of idiopathic thrombocytopenic purpura (ITP)?

The most serious is intracranial bleeding. Fortunately, this is rare in childhood ITP, occurring in fewer than 1% of affected patients. However, when intracranial hemorrhage does occur in ITP, the mortality is high, approximately 30 to 50%. Other bleeding manifestations in ITP are relatively mild. Occasionally, mucosal bleeding can be so severe or prolonged as to cause a dramatic fall in hemoglobin level requiring red cell transfusions. However, for most children the only manifestations of ITP are ecchymoses and petechiae.

18. What are the indications for gammaglobulin, steroid therapy, or splenectomy in ITP?

The treatment of a newly diagnosed child with ITP and no serious bleeding remains extremely controversial. Within 2 to 5 days of diagnosis, most children will have less bleeding, even if there is no substantial rise in the platelet count. Approximately 50% of children with acute ITP recover within 2 months. Thus, for most children the disease is mild and self-limited.

   1. *Gammaglobulin.* Intravenous administration of gammaglobulin (1 g/kg/dose) will raise the platelet count in approximately 85% of children with acute ITP. The response occurs

within 24 hours of the infusion and generally lasts approximately 3–4 weeks. Currently, there is no evidence that gammaglobulin alters the natural course of ITP.

2. *Steroids.* Steroids are similarly effective but take a bit longer to work. Some hematologists choose to treat all patients with acute ITP with either gammaglobulin or steroids, despite the high expense of the former and the side effects of the latter. The rationale for treatment is prevention of the rare but catastrophic occurrence of intracranial hemorrhage and the avoidance of limitations of physical activity that might otherwise be imposed on a child with ITP.

3. *Splenectomy.* Splenectomy improves the platelet count in most but not all patients with ITP. For acute ITP, the role of splenectomy should be limited to bleeding that is life-threatening and unresponsive to other measures such as gammaglobulin and steroids. Patients with ITP lasting more than 1 year and continued bleeding or unacceptable restrictions may be reasonable candidates for splenectomy. Regular intravenous administration of gammaglobulin offers an alternative form of therapy.

19. Should a child with ITP receive platelets?

Platelet transfusions usually do not increase the peripheral platelet count in children with ITP because the anti-platelet antibody produced by the patient is as effective against donor platelets as it is against his or her own platelets. Nonetheless, patients with ITP and life-threatening bleeding may benefit from platelet transfusion since there may be a local hemostatic effect even in the absence of a demonstrable effect on the peripheral platelet count.

20. What is the natural history of ITP?

Approximately 50% of children with acute ITP have normal platelet counts within 2 to 3 months of diagnosis, and 75% of children with ITP are well after 6 months. By 1 year, only 10% of children with ITP remain thrombocytopenic. Some of these children with chronic ITP will still improve on their own, sometimes as long as 5–10 years after diagnosis. The benign natural course of ITP should be considered carefully before instituting treatment that is hazardous or irreversible.

21. What are the inherited disorders of platelet function?

Several rare, inherited disorders of platelet function involve membrane receptors or metabolic processes that are important for platelet aggregation and the formation of a primary platelet plug. In more severe disorders such as Glanzmann's thrombasthenia, bleeding usually occurs early in life. Hemorrhagic manifestations include prolonged bleeding from circumcision, sustained gastrointestinal bleeding, and oral mucosal bleeding. Platelet transfusions are effective initially, but over time there is a high risk of alloimmunization to donor platelets.

Congenital Disorders of Platelet Function

Membrane glycoprotein abnormalities
   Bernard-Soulier syndrome
   Glanzmann's thrombasthenia

Granule defects
   Hermansky-Pudlak
   Wiskott-Aldrich
   Chediak-Higashi
   Gray platelet syndrome

Metabolic abnormalities
   Impaired arachidonic acid release
   Cyclooxygenase deficiency

22. Which patient populations are at highest risk for the development of iron-deficiency anemia?

Iron deficiency occurs when dietary intake of iron is inadequate to meet the needs of an expanding red cell mass or to overcome the loss of iron due to bleeding. Therefore, pediatric patients are at greatest risk for iron-deficiency anemia toward the end of the first year of life and again during adolescence. At 1 year of age, growth is rapid and the hemoglobin mass must expand accordingly. If the diet contains an adequate amount of iron, red cell production is not compromised, altough little or no iron is left over for storage purposes. If the baby prefers iron-poor cow's milk to the exclusion of solid foods such as iron-enriched cereals, vegetables, or meats, red cell production falters due to the unavailability of iron. During the pubertal growth spurt, the red cell mass once again expands and iron intake must be adequate to keep up with this need. In teenage girls, the balance of iron is further complicated by the beginning of regular menses, so that iron intake must be sufficient not only to meet the needs of accelerated growth but also to make up for blood loss.

23. In which groups of children is it important to screen for iron deficiency?

For a number of reasons, including the use of iron-fortified formulas, avoidance of whole cow's milk, early introduction of solid foods, and public health measures designed to provide adequate nutritional iron for low-income families, iron-deficiency anemia is less of a problem in young children than it used to be. Whether or not screening all children at 1 year of age is cost-effective is not clear. Certainly all children with a dietary history suggestive of poor iron nutrition should have the hemoglobin or hematocrit checked during the first year of life. Premature infants are born with lower iron stores than full-term infants, and therefore are particularly susceptible to developing iron-deficiency anemia during rapid growth in the first year of life. Premature infants should have the hemoglobin level or hematocrit checked at 6 to 9 months of age.

24. What is the earliest laboratory response to iron therapy?

The reticulocyte count begins to rise 3 to 5 days after the institution of iron therapy in patients with iron-deficiency anemia. The hemoglobin level rises several days later. For patients with mild iron-deficiency anemia, the hemoglobin level should be checked after several weeks of therapy. For patients with more severe anemia, it is often useful to check the hemoglobin level and reticulocyte count after a few days of treatment to make sure that the hemoglobin level has not declined to dangerous levels and that the reticulocyte response is beginning.

25. What is the recommended duration of iron therapy in a child with iron-deficiency anemia?

Patients with iron-deficiency anemia should be treated with ferrous sulfate for 2–3 months. During the first month of treatment, sufficient iron is received to restore the hemoglobin level to normal. Subsequent therapy is designed to replace iron stores. No matter how long treatment is continued, it is important to remember to address the underlying cause of the iron-deficiency anemia. If the child has iron-deficiency anemia because of inadequate iron intake, the diet should be adjusted to provide adequate iron. If abnormal bleeding is the cause of iron deficiency anemia, appropriate diagnostic and therapeutic steps should be taken to alleviate the bleeding.

Treatment of Iron-deficiency Anemia

Drug and Dose	Response
Ferrous sulfate, 6–9 mg/kg/d of elemental iron (ferrous sulfate contains 20% elemental iron)	Increased reticulocyte count at 3–5 days Increased hemoglobin level at 7–10 days
Duration	Other Measures
2–3 months	Restoration of normal diet Prevention of abnormal blood loss

26. What is the mechanism of the physiologic anemia of infancy?

The physiologic anemia of infancy occurs at 8–12 weeks in full-term infants and 6–8 weeks in premature infants. Full-term infants may have hemoglobin levels as low as 10 g/dl at this time and premature infants may have hemoglobin levels as low as 8 g/dl. The mechanism responsible for the decline in hemoglobin level is not clear. In premature infants, erythroid progenitor cells are present in normal numbers and show an appropriate response to erythropoietin. However, the production of erythropoietin in response to tissue hypoxia is somewhat blunted, perhaps contributing to the anemia.

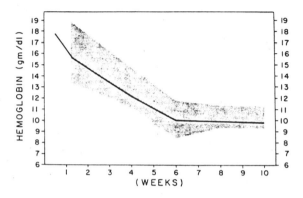

The decline in hemoglobin during the first 10 weeks of life in healthy preterm infants with birth weights of 100 to 1500 g. Shaded area represents the range of values observed. (From Oski FA, Naiman JL: Hematologic Problems in the Newborn. Philadelphia, W.B. Saunders Co., 1982, p 75, with permission.)

27. What is the etiology of the anemia of acute and chronic infection?

Chronic infections and other inflammatory states impair the release of iron from reticuloendothelial cells, thereby decreasing the amount of this necessary ingredient that is available for red cell production. Giving additional iron under these circumstances further increases reticuloendothelial iron stores and does little to help the anemia. Acute infection may cause anemia through a variety of mechanisms including bone marrow suppression, shortened red cell life span, red cell fragmentation, and immune-mediated red cell destruction.

28. What are the sideroblastic anemias?

Sideroblastic anemias are a rare group of disorders in which iron incorporation into the porphyrin ring to form heme is impaired. The result is an accumulation of excessive iron in the mitochondria of the nucleated red cells. These cells, when stained for iron, are known as ringed sideroblasts because of the presence of stainable iron in the mitochondria which encircle the nucleus. Sideroblastic anemia may be inherited in a sex-linked pattern. Acquired sideroblastic anemia may also be an early manifestation of acute myelogenous or myelomonocytic leukemia. Sideroblastic anemias generally are unresponsive to drug therapy, although some patients do improve when given pyridoxine or pyridoxal phosphate.

Major Findings in Sideroblastic Anemia

1. Anemia with hypochromic red cells (most marked in inherited type); macrocytic component with dimorphic blood smear in acquired type
2. Reticulocytes vary from low to 2–3 per cent
3. Serum Fe high, almost saturating TIBC

Table continued on next page.

Major Findings in Sideroblastic Anemia *(Continued)*

4. Bile pigments: mild unconjugated hyperbilirubinemia, fecal urobilinogen increased relative to hemoglobin mass
5. Marrow: erythroid hyperplasia, sometimes "megaloblastoid" (may respond to folate), storage iron typically increased, ringed sideroblasts
6. Red cell survival normal or mildly shortened
7. Ferrokinetics: ineffective erythropoiesis
8. Variable, incomplete response to pyridoxine, folic acid, liver extract, androgens, removal of excess iron
9. Associated findings
   a. Occasional leukopenia, thrombocytopenia, or thrombocytosis (especially acquired type)
   b. Occasional splenomegaly, hepatomegaly
   c. Hemochromatosis (especially in inherited type)
   d. Acute myelogenous or myelomonocytic leukemia (acquired type)

From Nathan DG and Oski FA. Hematology of Infancy and Childhood, WB Saunders Co., Philadelphia, 1987, p 373.

29. What are the common disorders of red cell morphology and how are they inherited?
Hereditary spherocytosis and hereditary elliptocytosis are the two most common. Hereditary spherocytosis is usually inherited in an autosomal dominant pattern. More recently, kindreds with an autosomal recessive form of hereditary spherocytosis have been described. In approximately 30% of children with hereditary spherocytosis, neither parent has anemia or morphologic alterations of the red cells. Some of these cases may represent new mutations in the child, whereas others may represent the autosomal recessive form of the disease. Hereditary elliptocytosis is inherited in an autosomal dominant pattern.

30. What are the immediate and long-term complications of exchange transfusions?
Immediate complications include hypocalcemia due to binding of calcium by citrate, thrombocytopenia due to the removal of platelets and the use of stored blood that may have decreased numbers of platelets, hyperkalemia due to accumulation of potassium in stored blood, hypovolemia due to removal of blood without adequate replacement, and diminished oxygen delivery due to the use of blood stored for more than 5–7 days with a loss of 2,3-DPG. Late complications in the newborn include anemia, which occurs for unknown reasons, and, rarely, graft vs. host disease due to the introduction of donor lymphocytes into a relatively immunocompromised neonatal host.

31. Which infectious diseases are known to cause atypical lymphocytosis?
Atypical lymphocytes are most commonly associated with infectious mononucleosis but may be seen with other viral diseases such as cytomegalovirus, and are also very common in newborns and young infants who are healthy.

32. What is the Mentzer index?
MCV divided by the red cell count. The formula is used to distinguish between the two leading causes of microcytosis, iron deficiency and thalassemia trait. In iron-deficiency anemia, microcytosis is accompanied by a decreased red cell count. On the other hand, patients with thalassemia trait have microcytosis and a high red cell count. Consequently, a Mentzer index greater than 13 is usually associated with iron-deficiency anemia, while a Mentzer index below 13 is more commonly associated with thalassemia trait. Like most formulas, this one is not infallible and should never be used for genetic counselling in the place of specific diagnostic tests.

33. What are the causes of thrombocytosis and when should thrombocytosis be treated?
The major causes are solid tumors and chronic inflammatory states such as infection and collagen vascular diseases. Thrombocytosis is also common in patients with sickle cell disease and in children with hemolytic red cell disorders who have undergone splenectomy.

In contrast with adults, a high platelet count in children does not appear to be a cause of significant morbidity. There is no magic platelet count at which treatment of thrombocytosis is warranted. In some centers, aspirin in doses of 60–300 mg daily is administered when the platelet count exceeds 1–1.5 million per cubic millimeter. Early introduction of aspirin therapy may be more important if the patient has other problems that might contribute to hyperviscosity such as a high white count or hemoglobin level.

34. What causes the coagulation abnormalities in von Willebrand's disease? How are they evaluated?

They result from the reduction in the overall production of the factor VIII molecule or an alteration in the balance of large and small multimers that usually comprise the factor VIII molecule. The platelet itself is not abnormal but its function may be impaired because of its interaction with factor VIII. The resulting laboratory abnormalities may include a prolonged partial thromboplastin time, decreased factor VIII coagulant activity, decreased factor VIII antigen, and decreased ability of patient plasma to induce aggregation of normal platelets in the presence of ristocetin. Analysis of the factor VIII molecule may show an overall decrease in all sizes of multimers or a specific reduction in large multimers, depending on the type of von Willebrand's disease. Bleeding time is usually prolonged. Most importantly, the pattern of positive and negative tests may vary widely from patient to patient. Even the same patient may show some abnormalities on one occasion and other abnormalities when testing is repeated. Thus, testing for von Willebrand's disease can be a tricky business and may require repeated evalutation.

Von Willebrand's Syndrome

GENETIC TRANSMISSION	TYPE I, AUTOSOMAL DOMINANT	TYPE IIa, AUTOSOMAL DOMINANT	TYPE IIb, AUTOSOMAL DOMINANT	TYPE IIc, AUTOSOMAL RECESSIVE	TYPE III, AUTOSOMAL RECESSIVE, HOMOZYGOUS, OR DOUBLY HETEROZYGOUS
Bleeding time	Prolonged	Prolonged	Prolonged	Prolonged	Prolonged
VIII:C	Decreased	Decreased or normal	Decreased or normal	Normal	Markedly decreased
VIII R:Ag	Decreased	Decreased or normal	Decreased or normal	Normal	Absent or minute amounts
VIII R:Rco	Decreased	Markedly decreased	Decreased or normal	Decreased	Absent
Ristocetin-induced agglutination (PRP)	Decreased or normal	Absent or normal	Increased	Decreased	Absent
Crossed immuno-electrophoresis	Normal	Abnormal	Abnormal	Abnormal double peak	Variable—usually abnormal
Plasma multimeric structure	Normal	Large and intermediate forms absent	Large multimers absent	Large multimers absent. Doublet multimer structure	Variable to absent

From Schumacher HR, et al: Introduction to Laboratory Hematology and Hematopathology. New York, Alan R. Liss, Inc., 1984, p 506, with permission.

35. How is a hemophiliac with antibodies to factor VIII managed?

The management of a patient with factor VIII deficiency and a factor VIII inhibitor is usually difficult and should be attempted only in consultation with a hematologist at a hemophilia center. For patients with low-level inhibitors that do not rise with administration of factor VIII, replacement therapy with standard factor VIII products such as cryoprecipitate or concentrate is usually effective if the amounts given are sufficient to overcome the inhibitor. For persons with highter titers of factor VIII inhibitors, minor bleeds such as knee or elbow hemarthroses can usually be managed with factor IX concentrates. The effectiveness of these concentrates is probably a result of the presence of other clotting factors, in particular factors II and VII. When treatment with standard factor IX preparations fail, activated factor IX concentrates such as Autoplex or FEIBA may be effective. Unfortunately, there are no laboratory tests by which to judge the effectiveness of factor IX concentrates for patients with factor VIII deficiency and inhibitors. The clinical response is the only guide. For life-threatening bleeding such as intracranial hemorrhage, the treating physician may not have the luxury of waiting for a clinical response to judge the effectiveness of therapy. Alternative forms of therapy in such situtations include the administration of huge amounts of factor VIII to overcome the high titer of inhibitor or the use of plasmapheresis to reduce the inhibitor load, followed by the administration of factor VIII. While both of these techniques may be initially successful, they have the distinct disadvantage of promoting an anamnestic response approximately 4 to 7 days later, making further factor VIII therapy impossible. Another option for the treatment of serious bleeding in a patient with factor VIII inhibitors is administration of porcine factor VIII, which has little cross-reactivity with human factor VIII.

36. What are the indications for hospital admission of a hemophiliac?

Indications include bleeding in life-threatening areas such as the head or around the airway, bleeding in areas where massive blood loss may occur such as the iliopsoas muscle or the deep thigh, and bleeding that requires repeated therapy and strict bedrest to avoid major complications such as hip hemarthrosis. Patients with significant head trauma such as from a fall from a changing table or down the stairs should usually be admitted for treatment and observation even if there are no neurologic findings when they are first evaluated.

37. What are the most common presentations for hemophilia?

Some children with severe hemophilia will have prolonged bleeding at the time of circumcision, a clinical finding that dates back to biblical times. However, many children with hemophilia, even those with the severe form of the disease, will have little difficulty during the first 6–9 months of life. In these children, hemophilia is often diagnosed only when they begin to cruise or walk and develop bruises that are out of proportion to the degree of trauma. Patients with milder forms of hemophilia may go undetected until they have a dental or surgical procedure that results in prolonged bleeding. This fact provides a rationale for preoperative coagulation testing in children, since an adequate bleeding history may not have had time to develop.

38. What are the advantages and disadvantages of factor VIII concentrates?

Factor VIII concentrates have brought great success as well as great tragedy to patients with hemophilia. When first introduced, they made home therapy a convenient reality and freed patients from repeated trips to the hospital. However, the preparation of these concentrates from the blood of as many as 20,000 paid donors per lot brought forth expected and unexpected consequences related to blood-borne infection. Hepatitis B infection was common in the early years of factor VIII concentrate use, although this problem can now be prevented by the administration of hepatitis B vaccine. Until recently, factor VIII concentrate caused non-A, non-B hepatitis in virtually every recipient. Of course, the major complication of factor VIII concentrates was recognized in the early 1980s when it became clear that the supply of concentrate was contaminated with the human immunodeficiency virus (HIV). Approximately 90% of patients with severe hemophilia who were treated with concentrates between 1978 and 1984 are now infected with HIV. The introduction of dry heat treatment for factor VIII concentrate in 1984 sharply reduced but did not eliminate the transmission of HIV. This process seemed to have little effect on non-A, non-B hepatitis. Newer techniques for reducing the viral load in factor VIII concentrates seem to be much more successful. These include wet heat treatment, exposure to detergent-solvent solutions, and, most recently, preparation using monoclonal antibodies to either the coagulant portion of the factor VIII molecule or the von Willebrand's portion of the molecule. These techniques appear to be extremely effective in preventing transmission of HIV, hepatitis B, and non-A, non-B hepatitis viruses. Studies are currently in progress to help determine the precise risk of virus transmission with these products.

Factor VIII Concentrates

PRODUCT	RISK OF NON-A, NON-B HEPATITIS	RISK OF HIV	COST PER UNIT (MAY 1988)
Untreated concentrate	+ + +	+ + +	.07
Dry heat treated concentrate	+ + +	+[a]	.12
Wet heat treated concentrate	+[b]	−[c]	.38
Detergent-solvent treated concentrate	+[b]	−[c]	.18
Monoclonal concentrate	−[c]	−[c]	.60

[a] Low risk, may be product dependent.
[b] Low risk, studies still in progress.
[c] No reported cases, studies still in progress.

39. How is the dose of factor VIII calculated for a hemophiliac with or without a life-threatening hemorrhage?

For minor hemorrhages, such as knee and elbow bleeds, factor VIII levels should be increased to 20 to 30% of normal. For major bleeding episodes, such as hip bleeds, intracranial hemorrhage, or bleeding around the airway, the factor VIII level should be raised to 70 to 100%. The formula for calculating the factor VIII dose is patient's weight (kg) × desired level of VIII × 0.4. For example, treatment of a simple knee bleed in a patient who weighs 30 kg would be calculated as 30 × 20 × 0.4 for a 20% correction. The total dose would therefore be 240 units. The usual practice is to use the remainder of any vial of factor VIII concentrate that is begun, so that the total administered dose is often somewhat higher than initially calculated.

Calculation of Dose of Factors VIII and IX Concentrates

Factor VIII
    Patient weight (kg) × desired increase (%) × 0.4 = total number of units
    Desired increase
        minor bleed 20–30%
        major bleed 70–100%
Factor IX
    Patient weight (kg) × desired increase (%) × 0.6 = total number of units
    Desired increase
        minor bleed 15–20%
        major bleed 50–100%

40. What are the most common inherited bleeding disorders and what are their inheritance patterns?

Factor VIII and factor IX deficiency are inherited in a sex-linked pattern, so that females are carriers and males are affected. The inheritance of von Willebrand's disease, the most common coagulopathy, is autosomal dominant, as are the other clotting factor deficiencies. In general, heterozygotes for clotting factor deficiencies are not clinically affected. However, recent evidence indicates that some heterozygotes for deficiencies of anticoagulant proteins such as protein C and antithrombin III may have problems related to hypercoagulation such as venous thrombosis.

41. What are the hematologic manifestations of lead toxicity?

The importance and the frequency of hematologic manifestations of lead toxicity have been overstated. Although lead poisoning is generally listed as a cause of microcytic anemia, this hematologic manifestation is rare even in severe lead intoxication. In most instances, microcytic anemia in children with lead poisoning is a result of concomitant iron deficiency. It is not unreasonable to believe that lead would be a cause of microcytic anemia, since lead interferes with several steps in the heme synthesis pathway. Basophilic stippling occurs in the red cells of some patients with lead poisoning, probably due to the inhibition of the enzyme pyrimidine-5'-nucleotidase. However, the absence of basophilic stippling should not be used to rule out the diagnosis of lead poisoning, since most patients will not have this hematologic finding. The reduced amount of pyrimidine-5'-nucleotidase and other unknown factors may contribute to a shortened red cell life span in lead poisoning that occasionally causes a hemolytic anemia.

Incidence of Microcytosis and Anemia According to Classification of Increased Lead Burden

	MICROCYTOSIS	ANEMIA	MICROCYTIC ANEMIA
Class III or IV lead poisoning, n = 58	12 (21%)	7 (12%)	1 (2%)
Blood lead concentration ≥ 50 μg/100 ml n = 26	9 (34%)	3 (12%)	1 (4%)
Erythrocyte protoporphyrin concentration ≥ 110 μg/100 ml n = 55	12 (22%)	7 (13%)	1 (2%)

From Cohen AR, et al: Reassessment of the microcytic anemia of lead poisoning. Pediatrics 67:904–906, 1981, with permission.

42. How can the diagnosis of methemoglobinemia be made at the bedside?

In methemoglobinemia, the inability of the red cell to maintain hemoglobin iron in the ferrous rather than ferric state leads to a loss of oxygen-carrying capacity. When a drop of blood from a patient with methemoglobinemia is placed on a piece of filter paper it generally has a brownish color. When the filter paper is waved in the air, the color of the blood remains brown because the hemoglobin is unable to bind oxygen. In contrast, blood from a normal individual will turn brown to red when the filter paper is waved in the air.

43. What are the causes of methemoglobinemia? How is each variety treated?

The most common causes are oxidant toxins such as antimalarial drugs or nitrates in food or well water, inherited abnormalities of the enzymes that maintain hemoglobin iron in the reduced state, and the M hemoglobins that seem to stabilize hemoglobin in the ferric form. Treatment of methemoglobinemia depends on the cause as well as the severity. When methemoglobinemia is caused by an oxidant toxin and methemoglobin levels are higher than 30%, methylene blue should be administered intravenously as a 1% solution in a dose of 1–2 mg/kg. Patients with inherited enzyme abnormalities or M hemoglobinopathies usually require no specific therapy. However, oral ascorbic acid may occasionally be useful for these patients. Methemoglobinemia has also been found in young infants with acute diarrhea and acidosis. The methemoglobinemia may be related to the lower levels of methemoglobin reductase found during the first year of life. Treatment with intravenously administered methylene blue is appropriate if the methemoglobin level is greater than 30%. Failure to respond to therapy should raise the possibility of G6PD deficiency, which prevents the conversion of methylene blue to the metabolite that is active in the treatment of methemoglobinemia.

Clinical Approach to Methemoglobinemia

SEVERITY (% METHEMOGLOBIN)	SYMPTOMS	TREATMENT
10–30	Cyanosis	None
30–50	Headache, exercise intolerance	Methylene blue, oral: dose determined empirically

Table continued on next page.

Clinical Approach to Methemoglobinemia *(Continued)*

SEVERITY (% METHEMOGLOBIN)	SYMPTOMS	TREATMENT
30–70	Altered consciousness	Methylene blue, 1–2 mg/kg IV push: (a) if improvement, oral methylene blue until oxidant stress eliminated; (b) if no improvement, exchange transfusion (consider hexose monophosphate shunt defect)
> 70	May be rapidly fatal	

From Nathan DG, Oski FA: Hematology of Infancy and Childhood. Philadelphia, W.B. Saunders Co., 1987, p 650, with permission.

44. What is a leukemoid reaction and in what disease states is it noted?

A leukemoid reaction usually refers to a white cell count greater than 50,000/mm³ and an accompanying shift to the left. Causes of leukemoid reactions include bacterial sepsis, tuberculosis, congential syphilis, congenital or acquired toxoplasmosis, and erythroblastosis fetalis. Infants with Down's syndrome may also have a leukemoid reaction that is often confused with acute leukemia during the first year of life.

45. What is the most common cause of epistaxis in childhood?

It is local trauma caused by a penetrating wound from the child's finger, commonly known as nose picking. The investigation of this possibility will be futile if the questioner simply asks the child whether or not he picks his nose. Any child worth his salt and with an ounce of pride will, of course, answer no. Therefore, one must take the child by surprise and simply ask, "Which finger do you use to pick your nose?" Most children will immediately show you the offending finger. Hematologic abnormalities causing epistaxis usually involve platelet disorders. These may be quantitative diseases such as ITP, qualitative disorders such as thrombasthenia, or a disorder such as von Willebrand's disease in which the platelet is an almost innocent bystander.

46. What is the treatment of choice for disseminated intravascular coagulopathy (DIC)?

DIC occurs most commonly in the context of bacterial sepsis and hypotension. The best treatment is reversal of the hypotension through treatment of the infection and appropriate fluid management. If bleeding is severe or if hemorrhage is occurring in a life-threatening location, platelets and fresh frozen plasma should be given to try to make up for the loss of these elements which is occurring from consumption. The idea that administration of these products "fuels the fire," thereby accelerating the thrombotic process, is interesting but clinically of little or no value. If DIC fails to respond to these measures, heparin may be administered in an attempt to interrupt the consumptive process. However, heparin has not been proven to be effective in increasing survival in patients with sepsis and DIC.

47. How is heparin therapy monitored in a child with DIC?

A compelling reason for not using heparin in a child with DIC is the difficulty encountered in monitoring therapy through laboratory studies. Normally, sufficient heparin is given to maintain the PTT at 1.5–2 times the normal level. However, the PTT is usually already prolonged in a child with DIC. A specific measurement of heparin levels is an excellent alternative, but this test is not available in many routine coagulation laboratories. Less prolongation of the PTT, improvement in the platelet count, and decreasing bleeding may be signs of effective heparin therapy or improvement of the DIC.

48. What is the best test for distinguishing between coagulation disturbances secondary to hepatic disease, DIC, and vitamin K deficiency?

Factors II, V, VII, IX, and X are made in the liver, and all of these factors except factor V are vitamin K dependent. Therefore, measurement of factor V is a useful test to distinguish liver disease from vitamin K deficiency, since this factor is reduced in the former and normal in the latter disorder. Factor VIII is reduced in patients with DIC because of the consumptive process, but this factor is normal or increased in liver disease and vitamin K deficiency. Therefore, the factor VIII level is a good test to distinguish DIC from the latter two disorders.

Coagulation Abnormalities in Liver Disease, Vitamin K Deficiency, and DIC

	FACTOR V	FACTOR VII	FACTOR VIII
Liver disease	Low	Low	Normal or increased
Vitamin K deficiency	Normal	Low	Normal
DIC	Low	Low	Low

49. What hematologic abnormality is associated with goat's milk?
Goat's milk contains very little folic acid compared with cow's milk. Infants receiving large amounts of goat's milk may develop megaloblastic anemia due to folic acid deficiency.

50. What is the significance of targeting on an RBC smear?
Red cell targets on a peripheral smear are caused by excessive membrane relative to the amount of hemoglobin. Therefore, target cells are found when the membrane is increased as in patients with liver disease, or when the intracellular hemoglobin is diminished as in patients with iron deficiency or thalassemia trait. Target cells may also be found in patients with certain hemoglobinopathies such as hemoglobin C and hemoglobin S. In these instances, the target cells are caused by aggregation of the abnormal hemoglobin.

51. What are the hematologic manifestations of thyroid disease?
Hypothyroidism causes a normochromic, normocytic anemia that may be a response to the lowered metabolic rate and decreased oxygen requirements found in these patients. Hyperthyroidism is less commonly associated with anemia since thyroid hormone increases erythropoietin production, enhancing erythropoiesis. However, we have made the diagnosis of hyperthyroidism in several children referred to us because of mild anemia and tachycardia that was out of proportion to the degree of anemia. Hypothyroidism has also been associated with qualitative platelet abnormalities and reduction in a variety of clotting factors. However, bleeding is rarely a major clinical problem in this disorder.

52. In what circumstances is it best to transfuse washed RBCs? Why?
When packed red cells are prepared from whole blood and then washed with saline, most of the remaining plasma and white cells are removed from the product. Since nonhemolytic transfusion reactions are usually due to plasma proteins or leukocytes, washed red cells are an ideal product for patients who have experienced febrile or allergic reactions to previous blood transfusions. Washed red cells may also be effective in reducing the transmission of CMV because of the removal of the white cells that normally carry this virus.

53. What laboratory tests are useful in identifying children with hemolytic disorders of the red cell membrane?
Most membrane disorders can be identified by careful analysis of red cell morphology on the peripheral smear. The characteristic spherocytes, elliptocytes, ovalocytes, or stomatocytes are usually readily apparent. The osmotic fragility test is used frequently to confirm the diagnosis of spherocytosis, since spherocytes are more sensitive to osmotic lysis than normal red cells because of their reduced surface to volume ratio. Most membrane disorders are associated with an abnormality in cation and/or water transport across the red cell membrane. Specific studies of intracellular ion and water content may be useful in diagnosing the more unusual varieties of membrane disorders. Additional studies, available only in research laboratories, include analysis of membrane proteins or the genes associated with these proteins.

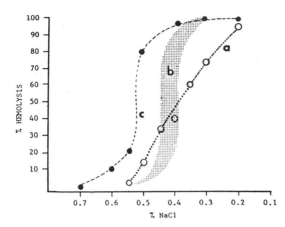

Osmotic fragility test. Curve c is from a patient with hereditary spherocytosis and demonstrates increased osmotic fragility. The shaded area (b) represents the normal range of the test. Curve a is from a patient with thalassemia minor and shows the increased resistance to osmotic lysis found in hypochromic red cell disorders. (From Henry JB: Clinical Diagnosis and Management by Laboratory Methods. Philadelphia, W.B. Saunders Co., 1979, p 1019, with permission.)

54. What are the biochemical variants of G6PD deficiency?

The most common form of G6PD deficiency found in the United States is the Gd^{A-} variant found in approximately 8–10% of black individuals. In this variant, the activity of the enzyme falls rapidly as the red cell ages. The measured G6PD activity is reduced but not absent. The Gd^{Mediterranean} variant has little if any measurable activity. More than 50 other variants of G6PD structure or activity have been described but are rarely identified in patients in the United States.

55. What are the clinical manifestations of G6PD deficiency?

Children with the Gd^{A-} or the Gd^{Mediterranean} variants of G6PD deficiency are usually hematologically normal unless exposed to an oxidant stress. Acute intravascular hemolysis may occur in the face of certain drugs such as the antimalarial agent chloroquine, certain toxins such as naphthalene found in many mothballs, or certain viral infections. These hemolytic episodes are characterized by an abrupt fall in hemoglobin level and a rise in reticulocyte count. Hemoglobinuria may be manifested as a positive test for blood by dipstick in the absence of red cells on microscopic analysis. Jaundice may accompany the hemolysis. The red cells have a characteristic appearance during acute hemolytic episodes. The peripheral smear shows blister cells in which the hemoglobin is pushed to one side of the cell, leaving a clear area beneath the membrane on the opposite side. In the Gd^{A-} variant, the hemolytic episode is usually self-limited since the reticulocytes have a normal complement of enzyme activity and are therefore resistant to the oxidant stress of the drug, toxin, or infection. Recovery usually occurs within 48–72 hours. In the Gd^{Mediterranean} variant, acute hemolysis is more common and more severe due to the lower overall level of enzyme activity.

56. Why do children with pyruvate kinase deficiency tolerate anemia better than children with other anemias?

Levels of 2,3-DPG are increased in the red cells of patients with pyruvate kinase deficiency, shifting the oxygen dissociation curve to the right. As a result of this shift, oxygen is more readily delivered from the red cells to the tissue. This rightward shift of the oxygen dissociation curve is much greater than is ordinarily found in patients with a similar degree of anemia due to other causes. Thus, some of the symptoms normally associated with anemia may be less severe or even absent in patients with pyruvate kinase deficiency.

57. What is the most common red cell enzymopathy of the Embden-Meyerhof pathway?

Pyruvate kinase deficiency is the most common red cell enzymopathy of the Embden-Meyerhof pathway. However, other enzyme deficiencies, including hexokinase deficiency, triose phosphate isomerase deficiency, and glucose phosphate isomerase deficiency, are associated with hemolytic anemia of varying degrees.

58. What are Howell-Jolly bodies?
Howell-Jolly bodies are nuclear remnants found in red cells of patients with reduced or absent splenic function and in patients with megaloblastic anemias. They are occasionally present in the red cells of premature infants. Howell-Jolly bodies are dense, dark, and perfectly round, and their characteristic appearance makes them easily distinguishable from other red cell inclusions and from platelets overlying red cells.

59. Which drugs should be avoided in children with hemoglobin H disease?
Because red cells containing HbH are abnormally sensitive to oxidant stress, drugs such as sulfonamides and antimalarial agents that act as oxidants should be avoided.

60. What is the difference between thalassemia intermedia and thalassemia major?
In thalassemia intermedia, the reduction in beta globin chain production and the resulting imbalance in alpha and beta globin cause a hemolytic anemia, but the anemia is not severe enough to warrant regular red cell transfusions. Affected patients usually are homozygous for beta-thalassemia but may occasionally have a severe form of the heterozygous condition. When patients with thalassemia have an anemia that is severe enough to require red cell transfusions to maintain the hemoglobin level above 7 or 8 g/dl, the condition becomes, by definition, thalassemia major.

61. What are the clinical manifestations of thalassemia intermedia?
The clinical manifestations of thalassemia intermedia can be predicted from the chronic hemolysis and the compensatory increase in red cell production. Linear growth is commonly slowed. Mild jaundice may be present. The liver and spleen are usually enlarged, sometimes to a massive degree. Pubertal development may be delayed. Bone marrow expansion may cause maxillary prominence and frontal bossing, bony changes that produce the Cooley's facies. Older patients with thalassemia intermedia may have manifestations of iron overload from the increased iron absorption that occurs in this disorder. The clinical manifestations of iron overload include cirrhosis, congestive heart failure, cardiac arrhythmias, diabetes mellitus, bronzing of the skin, and a variety of endocrine abnormalities.

62. What are Heinz bodies?
Heinz bodies represent precipitated denatured hemoglobin in the red cell. Heinz bodies occur when the hemoglobin is intrinsically unstable as in Hb Koln or when the enzymes that normally protect hemoglobin from oxidative denaturation are abnormal or deficient as in G6PD deficiency. These inclusions are not visible with a routine Wright-Giemsa stain but can be seen readily with methyl violet or brilliant cresyl blue stains.

63. How are unstable hemoglobins in children identified?
Several methods are available. Many of these hemoglobins can be detected by their abnormal electrophoretic migration. In these instances, it is possible to identify the specific abnormal hemoglobin. Indirect tests include the heat stability test, Heinz body preparation and shake test. The heat stability test takes advantage of the fact that unstable hemoglobins precipitate when they are incubated at 50 degrees for approximately 60 minutes. A variation on this theme is the isopropanol incubation test in which unstable hemoglobins precipitate in the presence of isopropanol. Methyl violet can be used to detect Heinz bodies in the erythrocytes. In the shake test, a hemolysate is made from the patient's blood and shaken vigorously under controlled conditions. Unstable hemoglobins precipitate as does sickle hemoglobin.

64. When does congenital spherocytosis commonly present during childhood?
The time of presentation of hereditary spherocytosis is largely dependent upon the severity of the disease. When hemolysis is brisk, the initial presentation may be jaundice in the neonatal period or signs and symptoms of anemia during early infancy. Some children first present with an aplastic crisis in which the hemoglobin level and reticulocyte count are both low. The latter finding may initially obscure the diagnosis since an elevated reticulocyte count is

expected in a hemolytic disorder. Children with less severe hereditary spherocytosis may not be recognized until a routine blood count reveals a low hemoglobin level or until an enlarged spleen is found on examination. Some children with mild disease will escape detection until they are adults and develop gallstones.

65. What percentage of children with congenital spherocytosis did not inherit an abnormal gene from either parent?
Approximately 30%. In some instances, this pattern may represent an uncommon form of spherocytosis which is inherited in an autosomal recessive fashion. However, most children with hereditary spherocytosis and no affected parent probably represent spontaneous mutations.

66. What is the pathophysiology of the hemolytic anemia in congenital spherocytosis?
In hereditary spherocytosis, an abnormality in the skeletal structure of the red cell membrane allows sodium influx into the red cell followed by water, swelling the cell and decreasing its deformability. This problem is accentuated when the red cell reaches the spleen, where conditions are ideal for the destruction of metabolically incompetent red cells. In this case, the increased rate of glycolysis which is needed to compensate partially for the sodium leak is compromised by the low pH and the small amount of available glucose in the spleen. In addition, the poor deformability of the swollen red cell may lead to trapping of the cell in the cords of the spleen and loss of membrane to the surrounding macrophages. This results in a further reduction in the surface to volume ratio of the red cell, leaving the erythrocyte even less deformable and more vulnerable to a metabolic or mechanical death in its next trip through the spleen. This prominent role of the spleen in the pathophysiology of the hemolytic anemia in hereditary spherocytosis explains why splenectomy is usually curative in this disorder.

67. What is the differential diagnosis for children presenting with splenomegaly and anemia?
The main question is whether the anemia is the cause of the splenomegaly or the splenomegaly is the cause of the anemia. Examples of the first situation include hemolytic anemias in which the spleen plays an active role such as membrane disorders, sickling disorders, and the thalassemia syndromes. The major example of the second situation is hypersplenism due to chronic liver disease and portal hypertension. In this instance, the anemia is a result of sequestration of red cells in the enlarged spleen. Accompanying features usually include mild leukopenia and thrombocytopenia.

Anemia Causing Splenomegaly	Splenomegaly Causing Anemia
Membrane disorders	Cirrhotic liver disease
Hemoglobinopathies	Cavernous transformation of portal vessels
Enzyme abnormalities	Storage diseases
Immune hemolytic anemia	Persistent viral infections

68. What are the clinical and laboratory manifestations of transient erythroblastopenia of childhood (TEC)?
Children with TEC usually present with pallor, lethargy, poor feeding, or irritability. Since the anemia develops slowly due to impaired red cell production, symptoms other than pallor are rarely present until the hemoglobin falls below 6 or 7 g/dl. The laboratory findings include a low hemoglobin level accompanied by inadequate reticulocyte production. In the acute stages of the disease, the bone marrow aspirate shows reduced or absent erythroid activity. During recovery, a wave of early erythroid activity may be seen.

69. What are the clinical and laboratory findings that distinguish TEC from Diamond-Blackfan syndrome?
It is extremely important to be able to distinguish TEC from Diamond-Blackfan syndrome; TEC is a self-limited disorder, whereas Diamond-Blackfan syndrome usually requires life-long treatment. Both are disorders of red cell production that occur in early childhood. While

there is an overlap in the age of presentation, Diamond-Blackfan syndrome commonly causes anemia in the first 6 months of life, whereas TEC occurs more frequently after the age of 1 year. Both disorders are characterized by a low hemoglobin level and an inappropriately low reticulocyte count. The bone marrows may be indistinguishable, showing reduced or absent erythroid activity in both cases. The red cells in patients with Diamond-Blackfan syndrome have fetal characteristics that are useful in distinguishing this disorder from TEC, including increased MCV, elevated level of HbF, and presence of i antigen. Recent studies have suggested that the level of adenine deaminase (ADA) is usually elevated in patients with Diamond-Blackfan syndrome but normal in children with TEC.

Childhood Red Cell Aplasia

FEATURE	DIAMOND-BLACKFAN ANEMIA	TRANSIENT ERYTHROBLASTOPENIA OF CHILDHOOD (TEC)
Number of reported cases	300	160
Age at diagnosis	90% < 1 year	83% ≥1 year
Etiology	Constitutional	Acquired
Antecedent history	None	Viral illness
Physical examination	30% abnormal	Normal
Laboratory:		
Hemoglobin	2–4 g/dl	3–9 g/dl
White cell count	Normal	Normal
Platelet count >450,000/mm^3	60%	34%
MCV increased:		
At diagnosis	30%	0%
During recovery	100%	90%
In remission	100%	0%
Hb F increased:		
At diagnosis	100%	0%
During recovery	100%	100%
In remission	85%	0%
Presence of i antigen:		
At diagnosis	100%	0%
During recovery	100%	60%
In remission	90%	0%

From Nathan DG, Oski FA: Hematology of Infancy and Childhood. Philadelphia, W.B. Saunders Co., 1987, p 205, with permission.

70. What is the treatment for Diamond-Blackfan syndrome?

Diamond-Blackfan syndrome should initially be treated with prednisone at a dose of 2 mg/kg/day. Approximately 75% of patients will respond to steroid therapy, and many of these patients will be able to maintain a normal or nearly normal hemoglobin level with low doses of prednisone. A few patients will have a spontaneous remission during corticosteroid therapy and a few patients will lose steroid responsiveness. Patients who do not respond to corticosteroid therapy usually require regular red cell transfusions. Because of the problems associated with chronic transfusion therapy, bone marrow transplantation has been suggested as an alternative therapy for patients who have a compatible donor.

71. How is the prognosis for Diamond-Blackfan syndrome affected by the age at which therapy is begun?

Several hematologists have suggested that the prognosis is improved when the disorder is diagnosed early in life and corticosteroid therapy is instituted immediately. However, evidence to support this claim is lacking.

72. How are aplastic anemias classified?

Aplastic anemia is usually classified as acquired, constitutional, or preleukemic. The distinction between these forms of the disease is extremely important both in terms of treatment and prognosis.

Classification of Aplastic Anemias

ACQUIRED	CONSTITUTIONAL
Idiopathic	Fanconi's anemia
Drugs	Familial aplastic anemia
Chemotherapeutic	Dyskeratosis congenita
Dose-related	Shwachman-Diamond syndrome
Idiosyncratic	Amegakaryocytic thrombocytopenia
Chemicals and toxins	
Radiation	
Infection	
Hepatitis	
Pregnancy	
Thymoma	
Paroxysmal nocturnal hemoglobinuria	

From Nathan DG, Oski FA: Hematology of Infancy and Childhood. Philadelphia, W.B. Saunders Co., 1987, p 160, with permission.

73. What drugs and conditions have been associated with acquired aplastic anemia?
No cause can be found for most cases of aplastic anemia in children. Although the list of drugs associated with aplastic anemia is quite long, chloramphenicol is far and away the major pharmacologic villain. This drug produces both a dose-dependent aplastic anemia and an idiosyncratic irreversible form of aplastic anemia. The former occurs fairly frequently but resolves when the drug is stopped. The latter is almost always fatal but rarely, if ever, occurs with intravenous administration of chloramphenicol in appropriate doses. Aplastic anemia may also be due to toxins such as benzene or irradiation. Aplastic anemia may also be one component of a congenital or constitutional disorder. In Fanconi's anemia, clinical evidence of bone marrow failure may not appear until 4 or 5 years of age or even later. Shwachman-Diamond syndrome is characterized by pancreatic insufficiency and neutropenia, but thrombocytopenia and anemia may also occur.

74. What preleukemic conditions have been associated with aplastic anemia?
Whether or not aplastic anemia is a preleukemic condition is mainly a matter of definition. Some patients who ultimately turn out to have leukemia may intially present with low peripheral blood counts, a hypoplastic bone marrow and some blasts but not enough to make a conclusive diagnosis of leukemia. However, it is usually obvious from the beginning that these patients do not have the usual type of acquired aplastic anemia that is not associated with an increased number of blasts. Patients with Fanconi's anemia have a propensity to develop leukemia, but the malignancy is probably a result of the underlying chromosomal defects in this disorder rather than the aplastic anemia. Patients with the usual form of acquired aplastic anemia rarely develop leukemia or other malignancies, although this finding may be altered by the use of newer treatments such as antithymocyte globulin and bone marrow transplantation.

75. Which infectious agents are thought to cause aplastic anemia?
Viral hepatitis is the major infectious cause of aplastic anemia. Posthepatitis aplastic anemia tends to be unusually severe. Very few patients survive without treatment. Whether or not antithymocyte globulin (ATG) is as effective for posthepatitis aplastic anemia as it is for other forms of severe aplastic anemia is not entirely clear.

76. What is the outcome for treated and untreated aplastic anemia?
In the absence of treatment, approximately 25% of children with severe acquired aplastic anemia will survive for more than 2 years. With ATG therapy, survival is 50–80% at 2 years.

When a bone marrow transplantation is performed using a histocompatible sibling donor, the 2-year survival rate exceeds 80%. In light of these statistics, the usual approach to the newly diagnosed child with severe acquired aplastic anemia is to perform a bone marrow transplantation if there is a histocompatible sibling to serve as the donor or, in the absence of such a donor, to treat with ATG. Patients who do not respond to ATG therapy have a grim prognosis, although cyclosporine may be effective in some of these children.

77. What are the clinical manifestations of Fanconi's anemia?

Fanconi's anemia, or constitutional aplastic anemia, is a disorder in which numerous physical abnormalities are often present at birth, and aplastic anemia occurs around the age of 5 years. The more common physical abnormalities include hyperpigmentation, anomalies of the thumb and radius, small size, microcephaly, and renal anomalies such as absent, duplicated, or horseshoe kidneys. Mental retardation is found in fewer than one-fourth of affected patients. When patients are recognized early in life on the basis of the physical abnormalities, the early signs of bone marrow failure may be detected before clinical problems related to pancytopenia occur. Increased fetal hemoglobin may be present in the first year of life. Mild thrombocytopenia may occur in infancy or early childhood, but the platelet count may remain only slightly depressed for 4 or 5 years until the usual picture of bone marrow failure occurs.

78. What is the most consistent laboratory finding in Fanconi's anemia?

The presence of chromosomal breaks, gaps, and rearrangements in peripheral blood lymphocytes.

79. What is the normal hemoglobin level and normal mean cell volume (MCV) for infants and children?

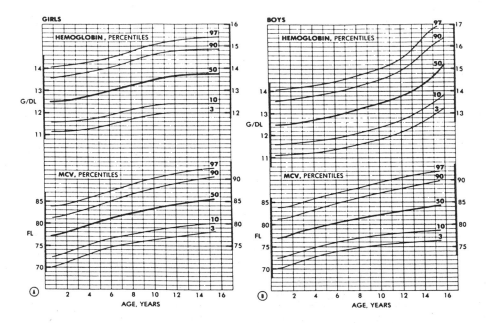

Hemoglobin and MCV percentile curves for girls (A) and boys (B). (From Dallman PR, et al: Percentile curves for hemoglobin and red cell volume in infancy and childhood. J Pediatr 94:26–31, 1979, with permission.)

80. What are the normal leukocyte counts from birth to adulthood?

Normal Leukocyte Counts*

Age	TOTAL LEUKOCYTES		NEUTROPHILS†			LYMPHOCYTES		
	Mean	Range	Mean	Range	%	Mean	Range	%
Birth	—‡	—	4.0	2.0–6.0	—	4.2	2.0–7.3	—
12 hr	—	—	11.0	7.8–14.5	—	4.2	2.0–7.3	—
24 hr	—	—	9.0	7.0–12.0	—	4.2	2.0–7.3	—
1–4 wk	—	—	3.6	1.8–5.4	—	5.6	2.9–9.1	—
6 mo	11.9	6.0–17.5	3.8	1.0–8.5	32	7.3	4.0–13.5	61
1 yr	11.4	6.0–17.5	3.5	1.5–8.5	31	7.0	4.0–10.5	61
2 yr	10.6	6.0–17.0	3.5	1.5–8.5	33	6.3	3.0–9.5	59
4 yr	9.1	5.5–15.5	3.8	1.5–8.5	42	4.5	2.0–8.0	50
6 yr	8.5	5.0–14.5	4.3	1.5–8.0	51	3.5	1.5–7.0	42
8 yr	8.3	4.5–13.5	4.4	1.5–8.0	53	3.3	1.5–6.8	39
10 yr	8.1	4.5–13.5	4.4	1.8–8.0	54	3.1	1.5–6.5	38
16 yr	7.8	4.5–13.0	4.4	1.8–8.0	57	2.8	1.2–5.2	35
21 yr	7.4	4.5–11.0	4.4	1.8–7.7	59	2.5	1.0–4.8	34

Age	MONOCYTES		EOSINOPHILS	
	Mean	%	Mean	%
Birth	0.6	—	0.1	—
12 hr	0.6	—	0.1	—
24 hr	0.6	—	0.1	—
1–4 wk	0.7	—	0.2	—
6 mo	0.6	5	0.3	3
1 yr	0.6	5	0.3	3
2 yr	0.5	5	0.3	3
4 yr	0.5	5	0.3	3
6 yr	0.4	5	0.2	3
8 yr	0.4	4	0.2	2
10 yr	0.4	4	0.2	2
16 yr	0.4	5	0.2	3
21 yr	0.3	4	0.2	3

From Rudolph AM (ed): Pediatrics, 18th ed. Norwalk, CT, Appleton & Lange, 1987, p 1061, with permission.

*Numbers of leukocytes are in thousands per mm^3; ranges are estimates of 95% confidence limits; and percentages refer to differential counts.

†Neutrophils include band cells at all ages and a small number of metamyelocytes and myelocytes in the first few days of life.

‡Insufficient data for a reliable estimate.

(Data on infants under the age of 1 month are derived from Monroe, et al: J Pediatr 95:89, 1979, Weinberg, et al: J Pediatr 106:462, 1985. Other values are from Albritton ED (ed): Standard Value in Blood. Philadelphia, W.B. Saunders, 1952.)

81. What is the average half-life of circulating neutrophils?

Six to seven hours. The half-life may be shortened in patients with acute bacterial infections or anti-neutrophil antibodies.

82. What drugs are known to cause neutropenia?

Drug-induced neutropenia is usually due to interference with normal cellular development or proliferation. Sulfa-containing compounds, thiazides and diphenylhydantoin, phenobarbital and other anticonvulsants may all cause neutropenia by this mechanism. Rarely, drugs may cause an immune neutropenia but this problem is particularly uncommon with the usual therapeutic agents used in pediatrics.

83. What infectious agents are known to cause neutropenia?

Neutropenia can accompany most common viral disorders and is also found in bacterial diseases such as typhoid, paratyphoid, and tuberculosis. Neutropenia is often recognized when a routine blood count and differential are performed during the course of a viral illness such as infectious mononucleosis. Neutropenia found during a viral illness does not pose a significant risk for bacterial infection. As a corollary, when a patient with a typical clinical course for a viral illness is found to be neutropenic, there is no need to begin broad antibiotic coverage as one might in a child with chemotherapy-induced neutropenia and fever. Neutropenia occurs in patients with bacterial sepsis because of depressed bone marrow production and increased peripheral utilization. This type of neutropenia is considered a poor prognostic sign.

84. How frequently do the "cycles" occur in cyclic neutropenia?

The average cycle in cyclic neutropenia is 21 days. However, the length of the cycle varies from patient to patient and may be as short as 14 days or as long as 28 days. The cycle for a particular patient generally remains constant.

85. What are the indications for empiric antimicrobial therapy in the febrile neutropenic child?

When a child with aplastic anemia, cancer, Kostmann's syndrome, or other severe neutropenic disorders develops a fever with an absolute neutrophil count less than 500/mm³, broad-coverage antimicrobial therapy should be instituted after appropriate cultures have been obtained. Similar therapy should be used if the child appears ill but has no fever. When the absolute neutrophil count is 500–1000/mm³, the use of antimicrobial therapy for the febrile child with no specific source of infection can be based upon how ill the child appears. Most importantly, the presence of fever in a child with neutropenia absolutely demands a careful physical examination to determine the degree of toxicity and, when possible, to identify a source for the fever.

86. Of what clinical value is the sedimentation rate?

An elevated erythrocyte sedimentation rate (ESR) is a nonspecific marker for inflammatory disease. The clinical use of the ESR usually exceeds its clinical usefulness. However, the test may be of some value in suggesting the presence of a deep-seated infection or a collagen vascular disease, particularly in patients with a fever of unknown origin. Unfortunately, there are few data to define the predictive value of the ESR in this setting. A better use of the ESR may be the monitoring of the response to therapy in particular infections such as bacterial endocarditis and osteomyelitis. In these conditions, a falling ESR is considered to be a reliable indicator of the resolution of the inflammatory process.

87. What conditions give a low sedimentation rate?

Low erythrocyte sedimentation rates may be due to a reduction in the concentration of large proteins (nephrosis, liver disease, congestive heart failure), abnormal red cell membrane (sickle cell disease), or polycythemia (cyanotic congenital heart disease). A low ESR, however, has little diagnostic value. In fact, it may create confusion by masking the normally increased ESR that is expected during infection in, for example, a patient with nephrotic syndrome and peritonitis or a patient with sickle cell anemia and osteomyelitis.

88. What is the corrected sedimentation rate?

The Wintrobe erythrocyte sedimentation rate is corrected for the hematocrit of the sample. Since anemia by itself may increase the rate at which the red cells fall or sediment in the tube, the result is corrected downward in the anemic patient. A common and still unresolved dilemma is how to interpret an elevated sedimentation rate that corrects to normal in an anemic patient.

89. What is the difference between a Westergren and Wintrobe ESR?

Both the Westergren and the Wintrobe sedimentation rates measure the packing of red cells in a tube at 60 minutes. The Wintrobe column has a length of 100 mm, whereas the Westergren column has a length of 200 mm. The Wintrobe sedimentation rate is considered to be more sensitive in the normal to slightly elevated range, making it a good method for screening. The Westergren method is linear in the moderate to markedly elevated range, enhancing its value for monitoring the activity of an inflammatory disease. The National Committee for Clinical Laboratory Standards has endorsed the Westergren method as the standard for measurement for the erythrocyte sedimentation rate.

90. What is the definition of absolute eosinophilia?

Eosinophils usually account for 1 to 5% of the cells in a white cell differential count. The normal range for the absolute eosinophil count is 100 to 600/mm³. Eosinophilia is usually defined as eosinophils constituting 10% or more of the differential count or as an absolute eosinophil count greater than 1,000–1,500/mm³.

91. What significance can be attributed to an increased eosinophil count?

The most common cause of an increased eosinophil count in children in the United States is an allergic disorder such as asthma, allergic rhinitis, or eczema. Drugs are also a frequent cause of eosinophilia. In foreign countries, an increased eosinophil count is usually due to an invasive parasitic infection. The most common parasitic offender in the United States is visceral larva migrans. Eosinophilia may also occur as a minor component of diseases such as neoplasms, periarteritis nodosa, and cirrhosis. Extremely high eosinophil counts may be seen in a poorly differentiated group of disorders included under the heading of hypereosinophilic syndrome and involving such organs as the heart, lungs, liver, spleen, and CNS.

Causes of Eosinophilia

Causes of Moderate Eosinophilia
    Parasitic infections
        Helminthic: Trichinosis, ascariasis, hookworm disease, strongyloidiasis
        Protozoal: Malaria
        Eosinophilic pneumonia
        Tropical eosinophilia
    Allergic disorders
        Asthma, seasonal pollinosis, urticaria, eczema
    Drug exposure
    Primary hematologic disorders
        Hodgkin's disease
        Fanconi's anemia, thrombocytopenia with absent radius
        Congenital immune deficiency syndromes
        Chronic myeloproliferative states
        Post-splenectomy
    Miscellaneous disorders
        Periarteritis nodosa
        Cirrhosis
        Malignant neoplasms
        Dermatitis herpetiformis
        Radiation therapy
        Peritoneal dialysis
        Congenital heart disease
        Hereditary eosinophilia

Table continued on next page.

Causes of Eosinophilia *(Continued)*

Causes of Exaggerated Eosinophilia
    Visceral larva migrans
    Idiopathic hypereosinophilic syndrome
    Eosinophilic leukemia
    Disorders generally associated with moderate eosinophilia
        Trichinosis, hookworm disease, ascariasis, strongyloidiasis
        Hodgkin's disease
        Periarteritis nodosa
        Drug hypersensitivity

From Lukens JN: Eosinophilia in children. Pediatr Clin North Am 19:969–981, 1972, with permission.

Bibliography

1. Baehner RL (ed): Pediatric Hematology. Pediatr Clin North Am 27(2). Philadelphia, W.B. Saunders Co., 1980.
2. Nathan DG, Oski FA: Hematology of Infancy and Childhood, Vols. I and II, 3rd ed. Philadelphia, W.B. Saunders Co., 1987.
3. Oski FA, Naiman JL (eds): Hematologic Problems in the Newborn, 3rd ed. Philadelphia, W.B. Saunders Co., 1982.
4. Schwartz E (ed): Progress in Pediatric Hematology/Oncology, Vol. III: Hemoglobinopathies in Children. Pochedly C, Miller DR (series eds). Littleton, MA, PSG Publishing Co., Inc., 1980.
5. Stockman JA III, Pochedly C (eds): Developmental and Neonatal Hematology. Pediatric Hematology/Oncology Series, Vol. I. New York, Raven Press, 1988.

IMMUNIZATION

Stephen D. Barbour, M.D., Ph.D.
Adam Finn, M.A., B.M., M.C.R.P. (UK)

1. What is the recommended schedule for active immunization of healthy infants and children?

Recommended Schedule for Active Immunization of Healthy Infants and Children*

RECOMMENDED AGE	IMMUNIZATION(S)	COMMENTS
2 mo	DTP,[1] OPV[2]	Can be initiated as early as 2 wk of age in areas of high endemicity or during epidemics
4 mo	DTP, OPV	2-mo interval desired for OPV to avoid interference from previous dose
6 mo	DTP (OPV)	OPV is optional (may be given in areas with increased risk of polio-virus exposure)
15 mo	Measles, mumps, rubella (MMR)[3]	MMR preferred to individual vaccines; tuberculin testing may be done if indicated
18 mo	DTP,[4,5] OPV,[5] PRP-D[6]	
4–5 yr[7]	DTP, OPV	At or before school entry
14–16 yr	Td[8]	Repeat every 10 yr throughout life

* Adapted, with permission, from the 1986 Red Book. Published by the Committee on Infectious Diseases, American Academy of Pediatrics, Evanston, IL. The changes made relate to new recommendations regarding Hemophilus b conjugate vaccine. For all products used, consult manufacturer's package insert for instructions for storage, handling, and administration. Biologics prepared by different manufacturers may vary, and those of the same manufacturer may change from time to time. Therefore, the physician should be aware of the contents of the package insert.

[1] DTP—Diphtheria and tetanus toxoids with pertussis vaccine.
[2] OPV—Oral poliovirus vaccine contains attenuated poliovirus types 1,2, and 3.
[3] MMR—Live measles, mumps, and rubella viruses in a combined vaccine.
[4] Should be given 6 to 12 months after the third dose.
[5] May be given simultaneously with MMR at 15 months of age.
[6] PRP-D—Hemophilus b conjugate vaccine.
[7] Up to the seventh birthday.
[8] Td—Adult tetanus toxoid (full dose) and diphtheria toxoid (reduced dose) in combination.

2. Is parental permission needed to immunize children?
Yes. Permission should be obtained in the form of verbal informed consent. This means that the parent and patient should be told about the benefits and risks of the vaccination. It is important to make sure that the information given to the parent is understood. When consent is given, a note should be recorded in the patient's chart.

3. Should immunization be delayed in children with minor nonfebrile illnesses?
No.

4. Should immunizations be delayed in children with febrile illnesses?
Yes. Although the child may appear well, the condition may worsen and new symptoms might be blamed on the vaccine administration early in the illness. The child who has a febrile illness at the time immunizations are scheduled should return immediately after the illness has resolved.

5. Should there be any change in the immunization schedule for children with cerebral palsy?
No. This includes immunizations for *Bordetella pertussis,* which should be given at the normal recommended times. If cerebral palsy is associated with a neurologic disorder that is evolving or with seizures, pertussis vaccine should be withheld until the condition is in a stable phase or the seizures are controlled.

6. Should premature babies receive immunization based on post-conceptional age or chronologic age?
Premature babies should be immunized based on postnatal chronological age. If a premature infant is still in the hospital at 2 months of age, then diphtheria, tetanus and pertussis vaccine (DTP) should be given. However, oral poliovirus vaccine (OPV) should be deferred until discharge to minimize the possibility of exposing other infants to a live vaccine that might be spread by stools. The rest of the immunization schedule for premature infants should be the same as for babies delivered at term.

7. Where should intramuscular injections be given?
In infants, the anterior and lateral aspect of the thigh is the preferred site for intramuscular injections. In an older child with sufficient muscle bulk in the deltoid muscle, injections may be given at that site.

8. Is skin preparation needed before an intramuscular or subcutaneous immunization is given?
Prior to immunization, the skin should be cleansed with an antiseptic solution, commonly 70% ethanol, and allowed to dry.

9. Should live virus vaccines be given to children whose mothers are pregnant?
Yes. All live virus vaccines may be given to children even though their mothers are pregnant, provided that the women have normal immunity.

10. What kinds of patients should not receive live virus vaccines?
Live virus vaccines (oral polio, measles, mumps, rubella) are contraindicated in patients with congenital disorders of immune function. Patients with diseases that cause immunosuppression or immune deficiency, or who are on therapy that leads to immunosuppression should not receive live virus vaccines. Immunologically normal siblings or other household contacts of individuals who have immune deficiency should not receive the oral poliovirus vaccine because polio vaccine virus may be transmissible to the immunosuppressed person. Normal household contacts, however, may receive other live virus vaccines, because transmission of those agents to another individual does not occur. Pregnant women should not be given any live vaccines except in special circumstances involving high risk of exposure.

11. Which vaccines may be given during pregnancy?
Diphtheria and tetanus toxoid.

12. What is the risk of local or systemic reactions to pertussis vaccine?
The pertussis component of the DTP vaccine is most commonly associated with these signs and symptoms.

> **Very Common**
> Fretfulness
> Pain at injection site
> Fever > 38°C   } 1 in 2–5 doses
> Drowsiness
> Anorexia

Common
Redness at injection site
Swelling at injection site   } 1 in 11–17 doses
Vomiting
Rare
Persistent screaming (> 3 hours)
High fever (> 40.5°C)   } 1 in 100–1000 doses
Unusual, high-pitched cry
Very Rare
Convulsions   } 1 in 1750 doses
Collapse, shock
Encephalopathy   } 1 in 110,000 doses

13. What is the risk of major neurologic complications or death from pertussis vaccine?
The more serious complications of vaccination are the rarest. Only about 1 in 3 children developing encephalopathy have permanent neurologic deficits (1 in 310,000 doses) and still fewer die. Some of these cases are certainly not caused by the vaccine but occur coincidentally. Although vaccine-associated risks are potentially serious, they must be weighed against the risks faced by the child who gets pertussis during the first year of life: pneumonia, 1 in 5; convulsions, 1 in 40; encephalopathy, 1 in 200; and death, 1 in 140. Infection rates with *Bordetella pertussis* have increased in populations where the immunization rates have diminished. Trials with new acellular pertussis vaccines are in progress and evidence from Japan suggests the vaccine may have equal efficacy and fewer side effects.

14. What age child should not receive pertussis vaccine?
The vaccine should not normally be given to children 7 years of age or older. Although infection occurs in older children and adults, it is usually mild. Effective vaccination of the younger population should control the spread of infection. In exceptional cases, patients over the age of 7 with chronic pulmonary disease who are likely to be exposed to pertussis may be vaccinated. Routine immunization of hospital personnel is not recommended but may be considered during outbreaks. All individuals 7 years of age and older receiving the vaccine should receive half the normal dose (0.25 ml)

15. What should parents be asked prior to their child receiving pertussis vaccine?
The Centers for Disease Control has prepared a comprehensive information sheet for parents about the DTP vaccine. Prior to immunization, the following questions must be asked:
1. Has the child a current febrile illness?
2. Has the child had a previous serious reaction to the vaccine?
3. Has the child ever suffered from fits, delayed development, or any other serious illness?

16. Prior to immunization, what information should be provided to parents?
1. The fully immunized child is unlikely to contract pertussis if exposed, and, if infection occurs, the illness is likely to be mild.
2. Mild local and systemic reactions are common. Serious side effects are rare. If, after vaccination, any of the rare or very rare side effects occur, or if any other parental concerns arise, the child should be seen by a doctor.
3. The parents should be told when the child is due for the next vaccine dose.
4. In many states, full vaccination with DTP vaccine is a requirement for school attendance.

17. What are the absolute and relative contraindications to pertussis immunizations?
Absolute: (1) previous occurrences in the same child of any of the rare adverse side effects: persistent screaming >3 hours; high fever (>40.5 C) in first 2 days; unusual, high-

pitched cry in first 2 days; convulsion in first 3 days; collapse or shock in first 2 days; or encephalopathy in first 7 days; and (2) a prior allergic reaction to the vaccine.

Relative: (1) If a child has had culture-proven pertussis, further vaccination is not necessary (note: this does not apply to tetanus or diphtheria, which may not induce immunity). (2) Children with an intercurrent febrile illness should not routinely receive the vaccine because the fever may represent the beginning of a more serious illness. Under these circumstances, vaccination should be postponed. (3) Children with neurologic disorders that are evolving or associated with seizures and children with progressive developmental delay. (4) Children who have had previous convulsions are more likely to have seizures following vaccination. Such seizures, however, are not thought to have permanent ill effects.

When there is a contraindication to pertussis vaccination, DT vaccine should be given instead of DTP vaccine. Immunosuppressive therapy is not a contraindication to DTP, although vaccination may be postponed until one month after such therapy is stopped, if it is nearly at an end.

18. What kind of vaccine is the diphtheria vaccine?
The vaccine is a toxoid of diphtheria exotoxin inactivated with formalin while retaining antigenic properties. It is usually given as a combined vaccine with pertussis and tetanus toxoid (DTP) or with tetanus toxoid alone (DT) if pertussis vaccine is contraindicated.

19. What is the difference between the pediatric (DT) and adult (Td) types of diphtheria and tetanus toxoid vaccines?
The DT vaccine contains standard doses of diphtheria and tetanus toxoids and should be used to immunize all children less than 7 years old when pertussis vaccination is not required or is contraindicated. The Td vaccine contains a much smaller dose of diphtheria toxoid with a standard tetanus toxoid dose. It should be used to immunize children after their seventh birthday and adults, and is less likely to produce the severe reactions seen in older individuals given the higher dose. Td may be used when tetanus toxoid is required for wound management, as a booster is required every 10 years to ensure continuing diphtheria and tetanus immunity in adulthood.

20. What are the indications for tetanus toxoid vaccine following trauma?
1. *Clean, minor wound.* Immunization is indicated if the primary (three-dose) tetanus immunization is incomplete, if no booster has been given in the previous 10 years, or if immunization history is uncertain.

2. *Other wounds* (e.g., contaminated wounds, crush injuries, burns, frostbite, and other serious injuries). Immunization is indicated if the primary immunization is incomplete, if no booster has been given in previous 5 years, or if immunization history is uncertain.

Td is the preparation of choice in patients aged 7 years of age or older. DTP or DT vaccine should be used in children less than 7 years of age who are not fully immunized. In addition, passive immunization with tetanus immune globulin (250 units) should be given to patients in group 2 who are not known to have had at least three previous doses of tetanus toxoid. It should be given in a separate syringe and at a different site. Whenever appropriate, surgical debridement should be performed and full immunization courses should be completed.

21. What are the contraindications to oral poliovirus vaccine (OPV)?
1. *Pregnancy.* Immunization during pregnancy with oral poliovirus vaccine (OPV) or inactivated polio vaccine (IPV) should be avoided for theoretical reasons unless there is need for immediate protection against polio, in which case OPV is recommended.

2. *Unimmunized adults* at future risk of exposure to polio should receive IPV rather than OPV.

3. *Immunodeficiency.* Patients with an acquired or congenital immunodeficiency should be given IPV rather than OPV, as the inactivated vaccine is safer in these patients and may

provide some protection. Children with symptomatic human immunodeficiency virus (HIV) infection belong to this group.

4. *Household contacts* of individuals who have immunodeficiency disease should be given IPV rather than OPV. Although children infected with HIV who are asymptomatic may be given OPV, it is important to remember that this may jeopardize other family members with symptomatic immunodeficiency. The family situation should be investigated prior to immunization and, where it is uncertain, it is sometimes advisable to be cautious and use IPV. These considerations, together with the rising incidence of HIV infection, make it likely that use of IPV will increase significantly.

22. Does breastfeeding adversely affect the immunogenicity of OPV?

Since breastfeeding does not affect the success of immunization of OPV, no interruption or change in feeding schedule is needed.

23. Is viral gastroenteritis a contraindication to the use of OPV?

A mild gastroenteritis (with infrequent vomiting and diarrhea and without dehydration) is not a contraindication to the use of OPV.

24. What are the relative merits of OPV and IPV?

OPV (or Sabin vaccine) is easy to administer, probably does not need booster doses, and confers immunity to the population at large because it is spread from person to person. OPV has been very effective in virtually eliminating polio from the United States and other countries. Since it may cause disease in immunocompromised individuals, it presents risk to increasing numbers of HIV-infected persons even if not administered to them directly. The current IPV is of enhanced potency. It is given by intramuscular injection and probably requires booster doses. It is a killed vaccine and cannot cause paralytic polio.

25. Should measles, mumps, and rubella (MMR) vaccines be given together or separately?

Measles, mumps, and rubella live virus vaccines given in combination have rates of seroconversion and side effects comparable to administration as separate components. Use of the combined vaccine therefore saves time and expense and increases the likelihood of a child being fully immunized.

26. What is the recommended age for administration of MMR vaccines in the United States?

It is 15 months for all three vaccines. Previous suspected or proven infection with one of the three viruses is not a contraindication to use of the combined vaccine. In addition to the monovalent and trivalent vaccines, bivalent measles-rubella is available.

27. Must a tine or Mantoux test for tuberculosis be done prior to measles vaccination?

Measles infection can worsen the course of tuberculosis. However, the live-virus measles vaccine does not appear to do so. A skin test for tuberculosis is not necessary unless otherwise indicated. If a skin test is placed at the same time as vaccination, it can be read at 48–72 hours in the normal way. If placed afterward, the skin reaction may be suppressed. Thus it is always important to inquire about recent immunizations before performing a tine test.

28. What are the contraindications to MMR vaccination?

These vaccines should not be given either singly or in combination in the following situations:

1. *Intercurrent febrile illness.* The risks of giving the vaccine in such cases are of possibly reduced vaccine efficacy and of false attribution of the evolving illness to the vaccine. Sometimes the risk of poor followup for vaccination may outweigh these considerations. Afebrile upper respiratory symptoms are not considered contraindications.

2. *Pregnancy.* The risks to the fetus are only theoretical.

3. *Immunodeficiency.* This includes primary immunodeficiencies and those associated with malignancies and treatment with immunosuppressive drugs and radiation. It is wise to withhold the vaccines for at least 3 months after cessation of immunosuppressive therapy. The use of these vaccines in children with HIV infection is controversial, although they have not been shown to be dangerous. In the United States they are not currently used in children with symptomatic HIV disease; however, in countries where both HIV and measles infections are common, these vaccines should generally be given.

4. *Allergy.* Previous anaphylactic reactions to eggs or neomycin, which are both present in the vaccine in small amounts, are considered absolute contraindications. Milder allergic reactions are not contraindications.

5. *Passive immunity.* Administration of antibody-containing blood products, such as immune-globulin or whole blood, may suppress immune response to the vaccine. Vaccination should be deferred for 3 months thereafter.

29. Why are children immunized against rubella?
Rubella vaccine is administered to prevent rubella infection in pregnant women and their fetuses. Transplacental congenital rubella infection of the fetus, particularly during the first trimester of pregnancy, often causes devastating handicaps of vision, hearing, and brain function, and congenital heart disease. By contrast, postnatal infection, particularly in children, is usually mild and short-lived. The younger the age at which vaccines become immune, the greater is the impact on spread of the virus in the general population. In addition, it is easier and more effective to include rubella in the vaccination program that all children should receive. Finally, vaccinating pre-pubescent children avoids the theoretical risks of inadvertently administering the vaccine to older patients who might be pregnant.

30. How long after rubella vaccination should pregnancy be avoided? Why?
Three months. The reason is theoretical, and it is important to note that vaccine-associated congenital rubella syndrome has not been observed. Receipt of vaccine before or during pregnancy is not necessarily an indication for therapeutic abortion.

31. Is there a vaccine against chickenpox?
A live chickenpox vaccine was first made in 1974. Since then extensive trials have shown this vaccine to be safe and effective. It is possible that the vaccine will be licensed for use in the United States in the near future when further trials have been completed. Ultimately it may be possible to give children a combined measles, mumps, rubella, and varicella vaccine at 15 months of age.

32. Which vaccine should be used to immunize children against *Hemophilus influenzae* type B?
In December 1987, Hemophilus b conjugate vaccine (diphtheria toxoid–conjugate), also known as PRP-D, was licensed for use in the United States. This new vaccine should now be used in preference to the original Hemophilus vaccine, known as PRP, because of better production of antibodies. PRP may still be used in children aged 24–60 months as a second choice. Other conjugate Hemophilus vaccines are undergoing trials and may soon become available.

33. Which children should be vaccinated against *Hemophilus influenzae* type b and at what age?
1. All children should be immunized with PRP-D when they reach 18 months. (Vaccination of younger children may be recommended in the future.)

2. All unvaccinated children aged 19–60 months should be immunized.

3. PRP-D vaccine should be given to all children less than 61 months of age who have received a single dose of PRP vaccine between ages 18 and 23 months. (Note: There should be

a gap of 2 months between the PRP and PRP-D vaccine doses.) Children given PRP at or beyond 24 months need not be revaccinated.

4. Children aged 5 or more who have functional or anatomic asplenia, including those with sickle cell disease, or who have Hodgkin's disease should also be immunized with PRP-D. In the latter group the vaccine should be given 10–14 days prior to, or 3 or more months after, chemotherapy.

34. Can the Hemophilus vaccine be given with other vaccines?
PRP-D vaccine can be given at the same time as DTP, IPV, meningococcal, and pneumococcal vaccines. This vaccine, however, should be given at different sites with different syringes. Simultaneous administration of OPV or MMR vaccine with PRP-D is not contraindicated, although the size of antibody responses under those circumstances is uncertain.

35. Are Hemophilus vaccines effective and safe?
The vaccines used so far (PRP and PRP-D) have not been associated with any serious adverse reactions, although local reactions and fevers are seen in about 1 in 10 recipients. PRP-D has been shown to be more effective than PRP in inducing antibodies to Hemophilus type b. Trials assessing the efficacy of the vaccines in preventing invasive *H. influenzae* disease in the United States are still in progress.

36. Who should receive the pneumococcal vaccine?
The vaccine is poorly immunogenic in children less than 2 years of age. Therefore only children 2 years of age or older who have increased risk for pneumococcal infection or who are at increased risk for severe disease when infected with pneumococcus should receive the vaccine. High-risk groups include children with sickle cell anemia, asplenia (congenital or splenectomy), nephrotic syndrome, and Hodgkin's disease undergoing therapy. Parents of these children should be aware that the vaccine does not provide complete protection and that these children still require prompt medical attention for febrile illness. There are insufficient data available to assess the need for and efficacy of the vaccine among other high-risk children such as those with organ transplants and chronic disease including heart failure, pulmonary disease, renal failure, diabetes, and immune deficiency. Children in the latter group with immunoglobulin deficiencies are better treated with immunoglobulins. Children 2 years of age or older with human immunodeficiency virus infection are now commonly vaccinated.

37. When and how often should one receive the pneumococcal vaccine?
Children in whom the vaccine is indicated should be immunized at 2 years of age or upon recognition of the disease that places them in the high-risk group. If a therapeutic splenectomy is planned, it is preferable to give the vaccine at least a week prior to operation. The vaccine should be given at least 14 days before chemotherapy for Hodgkin's lymphoma is started. If the vaccine is given during chemotherapy it should be repeated 3 to 4 months after the end of treatment. The length of protection from primary vaccination is unknown. Revaccination, however, is not recommended because some patients may experience severe reactions. Despite the risk of reaction, high-risk children are sometimes revaccinated at 3 to 5 yearly intervals on an empiric basis. The vaccine is not currently recommended for use in normal healthy children and should not be given to pregnant women.

38. Under what circumstances should meningococcal vaccine be given?
Patients who have functional or anatomic asplenia or complement deficiency, or who are 2 years of age or older should be given the vaccine. Revaccination after 2 to 3 years may be useful. The quadrivalent vaccine available in the United States includes antigen from four serogroups: A, C, Y, and W-135. Most infections in children, however, are due to group B meningococci, against which there is no effective vaccine at present. The current vaccine may be used to control outbreaks due to other meningococcal serotypes and can also be used

as an adjunct to chemoprophylaxis of contacts. The vaccine might also be beneficial to persons traveling to areas of epidemic or hyperendemic disease. It is given to all American military recruits.

39. How often should a healthy child have testing for tuberculosis?
The Committee on Infectious Diseases of the American Academy of Pediatrics currently recommends an annual PPD (Mantoux test) for individuals at high risk for tuberculosis. These include children who reside in high prevalence areas or who have family members with tuberculosis. In low-risk groups it is currently thought reasonable to perform skin testing three times during childhood and adolescence at the age of 15 months, prior to school entry at age 4–6 years, and during adolescence at 14–16 years of age. Additionally the tuberculin skin test is indicated for individuals with known exposure to a person with active tuberculosis. If the tuberculin reaction is negative after a known exposure, the test should be repeated in 8–10 weeks because immunologic positivity can take that long to develop.

40. What are the different concentrations of purified protein derivative (PPD) or purified protein derivative tuberculin (PPDT) and when should they be used?
The standard strength of PPD, designated intermediate strength, is five tuberculin units. This strength is used for routine skin test screening (Mantoux test). PPDT is also available in dose strengths of one unit (first strength) or 250 units (second strength). The one tuberculin unit strength is used only in patients who are suspected of having intense tuberculin skin test reactivity. The 250-unit strength is occasionally used in individuals who have skin test negativity with five units where one wants to determine whether reactivity will occur with much higher strength. A positive reaction at 250-unit strength may indicate infection either with *Mycobacterium tuberculosis* or nontuberculous mycobacteria.

41. What are the advantages and disadvantages of the tine test?
The tine test is a multiple puncture skin test using old tuberculin. It is prepackaged, quick, and simple to administer, but it does have several disadvantages. There is poor control of dose of antigen that is actually injected. This means that there will be variability in the amount of test reagent applied. Another problem is potential error in reading the reaction. With this and other multiple puncture tests there is variability in sensitivity and specificity. There is a high rate of both false-positive (20%) and false-negative reactions (up to 10%). All positive reactions to a tine test should be retested using the intermediate-strength purified protein derivative. Because the tine test is associated with false-negative reactions, it should not be used for tuberculin testing of high-risk populations.

42. How are the tine and Mantoux tests administered?
The tine test, containing old tuberculin dried onto a multiple puncture device, is administered by slow, deliberate transdermal injection using the multipuncture device. In the Mantoux test, 0.1 ml of purified protein derivative (PPD) is administered using a No. 26 gauge short beveled needle. PPD antigen should be aspirated into a disposable plastic syringe no more than 1 hour before use. The antigen is injected intradermally on the volar aspect of the forearm producing a 6–10 mm wheal. The Mantoux test is read at 48–72 hours. Measurement of the reaction should be done by touch and measured in millimeters on an arm held with the elbow slightly flexed.

43. When is the Mantoux (PPD) test considered positive?
Reactions of 10 mm or more of induration are considered positive. Smaller areas of induration are often attributed to nontuberculous mycobacterial infection but can be seen with recent infection. Significant positive reactions are often 15 mm or greater. In a child with known contact with an adult with tuberculosis, a zone of 5 mm or larger might be considered positive. In the context of symptoms that are suggestive of tuberculosis, and with an appropriate positive history, the child with a 5–10 mm tuberculin reaction should be evaluated

with a careful physical examination and chest x-ray. The Mantoux test should be repeated after about 4 to 6 weeks.

44. What are the indications and contraindications for Bacille Calmette-Guerin (BCG) vaccination?

BCG vaccination in the United States is rarely used. It is given primarily to tuberculin-negative individuals who are in close contact with active cases of untreated or ineffectively treated pulmonary tuberculosis. It should also be considered for groups with an excessive rate of new infections or when the usual methods of treatment have failed or are not feasible. BCG is a live bacterial vaccine and should never be used in patients with altered immunologic status. It is contraindicated in individuals with cellular or combined immunodeficiencies, including individuals with HIV infection or those who are being treated with immunosuppressive therapy including steroids. It also should not be given to individuals who have burns or skin infections. Vaccination of a pregnant woman is not considered prudent, although there have been no noted adverse effects of BCG on the fetus. Malnutrition itself is not considered a contraindication to BCG. Ideally, BCG should not be administered during treatment with isoniazid. Side effects are uncommon but can be quite severe, including ulceration and abscess at the injection site, dissemination, and death.

45. How does BCG immunization influence tuberculosis skin testing?

BCG immunization leads to skin sensitivity to tuberculin protein, and precludes tuberculin testing as a case finding tool in individuals whose tuberculosis status is unknown.

46. What are the varieties of hepatitis B vaccine?

There are currently two varieties. The older type is a preparation from hepatitis B positive human blood of inactivated hepatitis B surface antigen particles purified by biophysical and biochemical methods. After purification it is inactivated by a three-fold process which destroys representatives of all known classes of virus found in human blood including human immunodeficiency virus. The second newer form of hepatitis B vaccine is a recombinant DNA encoded portion of the hepatitis B envelope protein produced by yeast and purified from that source.

47. Who should receive hepatitis B vaccine?

All individuals who are at high risk for exposure to hepatitis B. Included in this group are infants born to mothers positive for hepatitis B surface antigen and all susceptible household contacts of hepatitis B surface antigen carriers. Infants from high-risk populations (such as Southeast Asians, Haitians, or intravenous drug abusers) should be screened for hepatitis B surface antigen and, if positive, household contacts should be immunized. Patients who are institutionalized or who participate in medical programs involving increased risk (such as renal dialysis) should be vaccinated. Sexual contacts of hepatitis B carriers should receive vaccine as should homosexuals, percutaneous drug users, and individuals who have a large number of heterosexual contacts. Persons with health-care-related jobs who are frequently exposed to blood should be immunized. One milliliter of vaccine should be given IM initially and repeated at 1 month and 6 months. Neonates should receive 0.5 ml of vaccine.

48. What are the recommendations for the administration of hepatitis B immunoglobulin (HBIG)?

HBIG should be used as post-exposure immunoprophylaxis. Immunoprophylaxis with HBIG should be considered for persons who have either accidental percutaneous or mucosal exposure to hepatitis B surface antigen positive blood or body fluids, and individuals who have had sexual contact with a hepatitis B surface antigen positive person. A neonate born to a hepatitis B surface antigen positive mother should be given HBIG as soon as possible, and should begin a series of vaccinations with hepatitis B vaccine. The recommended dose and schedule for neonatal *exposure* are as follows: give HBIG 0.5 ml IM and give hepatitis B vaccine 0.5 ml IM within 7 days and repeat at 1 and 6 months of age.

49. What are the contraindications to hepatitis B vaccine?
The only contraindication is a severe allergic reaction by an individual to prior doses of the vaccine.

50. What is the principal side effect of hepatitis B vaccine?
Soreness at the site of inoculation. Data demonstrate that the hepatitis B vaccine prepared from human blood is safe, does not contain HIV, and has not been associated with any increased risk for development of AIDS-related syndromes in recipients.

51. When should rabies human diploid cell vaccine (HDCV) be administered?
Pre-exposure vaccination is recommended for individuals at high risk for contact with rabies such as veterinarians, animal handlers, cave explorers, hunters exposed to rabid animals, and persons living in or visiting areas of countries where the risk of rabies exposure is high. HDCV is also used as a prophylactic regimen in all persons who have been exposed to rabies; those who have not previously received HDCV should also be given human rabies immune globulin as soon as possible after the exposure.

52. What are the local and systemic reactions to rabies vaccination and how are they treated?
Local reactions occur in 25% of recipients and include pain, erythema, and itching or swelling at the site of vaccination. Mild systemic reactions (headache, nausea, abdominal pain, muscle aches, and dizziness) occur in about 20% of recipients. Reactions of an immune complex nature (arthralgias, arthritis, angioedema, fever), particularly in persons receiving booster doses of HDCV, have been noted. These reactions are generally not life-threatening complications. Mild reactions can usually be managed without treatment or with acetaminophen or aspirin. Rabies prophylaxis generally should not be interrupted because of local or mild systemic reactions or a history of hypersensitivity. Antihistamines may be useful. Anaphylaxis and other life-threatening reactions are extremely rare. Steroids may be employed for severe reactions, but otherwise should not be used, because they increase the risk of rabies in experimentally vaccinated animals.

53. When and to whom should the pediatrician give influenza vaccine?
There are two types of killed influenza vaccine available: the split vaccine should be used for children less than 12 years of age and the whole virus vaccine should be used for older children and adults. Each year in the autumn a new preparation is made, aimed to cover the expected antigenic types for the winter season. Vaccination should be undertaken each year as soon as possible after the vaccine becomes available. When the vaccine is given for the first time, two doses of vaccine are given, one month apart; in subsequent years the same patient should be given only one dose. The vaccine is not recommended for children less than 6 months of age. Children at high risk for severe influenza infection who should be vaccinated include children with: (1) chronic lung diseases, e.g., moderate to severe asthma, bronchopulmonary dysplasia; (2) congenital heart disease causing significant hemodynamic disturbance; (3) hemoglobinopathies including sickle cell disease; and (4) treatment with immunosuppressive drugs. Other groups that should be strongly considered for vaccination include (1) children with chronic renal failure, diabetes mellitus, or other metabolic disorders; (2) children receiving chronic aspirin therapy (who may therefore be at increased risk for developing Reye syndrome following influenza); (3) individuals who are in contact with high-risk children such as household and family members and hospital and nursery personnel (and conversely, children who are in contact with high-risk adults); and (4) children living in institutions, colleges, or boarding schools or attending daycare.

54. What are the recommendations for vaccination against smallpox?
Smallpox is now considered to have been eliminated from the world. Vaccination is no longer recommended in any country. The vaccinia vaccine is highly effective but occasionally causes

serious side effects. Military personnel in both the U.S. and U.S.S.R. still receive the vaccine.

55. Which immunizations can be given together when there has been immunization delay?

When there has been a delay in immunizations, one can simultaneously administer MMR, OPV, and DTP vaccines with excellent results, comparable to separate administration of these vaccines. Protective responses are satisfactory and side effects are not increased. Hemophilus b conjugate vaccine (PRP-D) can be given at the same time as other vaccines, although the antibody responses when given with OPV and MMR have not yet been studied. If return of a patient for further vaccinations is doubtful, simultaneous administration of all vaccines (as appropriate for age and previous vaccination status of the vaccine recipient) is recommended. However, influenza vaccine should not be given within 7 days of immunization with DTP. Injectable vaccines given simultaneously should always be given with different syringes at different sites.

56. What special recommendations regarding vaccination should be made for the child infected with human immunodeficiency virus (HIV)?

Vaccination recommendations for the HIV-infected child include some notable contraindications as well as special indications. The symptomatic HIV-positive child should not receive any live virus vaccines. OPV can be given to the nonsymptomatic HIV-positive child, provided that the child is not in contact with other HIV-positive persons. IPV should be substituted for OPV in symptomatic HIV-positive children or in those who are exposed to other immunosuppressed individuals. MMR vaccine may be given to the asymptomatic HIV-positive child. There is no indication that a person vaccinated with MMR can pass the vaccine viruses to other individuals. *Hemophilus influenzae* b conjugate vaccine should be administered at age 18 months and pneumococcal vaccine at age 2 years or older. Neither BCG nor vaccinia should be administered to the HIV-positive individual, for any reason. DPT vaccinations should proceed at the normal times and doses.

57. What is the recommended immunization schedule for a previously unimmunized patient?

Immunization Schedule for Previously Unimmunized Patients*

RECOMMENDED TIME	IMMUNIZATION(S)	COMMENTS
Less than 7 Years Old		
First visit	DTP, OPV, MMR	MMR if child ≥15 mo old; tuberculin testing may be done if indicated.
Interval after first visit		
1 mo	PRP-D†	For children 18–60 mo
2 mo	DTP, OPV	
4 mo	DTP, OPV	OPV is optional (may be given in areas with increased risk of poliovirus exposure)
10–16 mo	DTP, OPV	OPV is not given if third dose was given earlier
Age 4–6 yr (at or before school entry)	DTP, OPV	DTP is not necessary if the fourth dose was given after the fourth birthday. OPV is not necessary if recommended OPV dose at 10–16 mo following first visit was given after the fourth birthday.
Age 14–16 yr	Td	Repeat every 10 yr throughout life

Table continued on next page.

Immunization Schedule for Previously Unimmunized Patients* *(Continued)*

RECOMMENDED TIME	IMMUNIZATION(S)	COMMENTS
	7 Years Old and Older	
First visit	Td, OPV, MMR	
Interval after first visit		
2 mo	Td, OPV	
8–14 mo	Td, OPV	
Age 14–16 yr	Td	Repeat every 10 yr throughout life

*Adapted, with permission, from the 1986 Red Book. Published by the Committee on Infectious Diseases, American Academy of Pediatrics, Evanston, Il. The changes made related to new recommendations regarding Hemophilus b conjugate vaccine.

†Hemophilus b conjugate vaccine (PRP-D) can be given, if necessary, simultaneously with DTP (at separate sites). The initial three doses of DTP can be given at 1- to 2-month intervals; so, for the child in whom immunization is initiated at 18 months or older, one visit could be eliminated by giving DTP, OPV, MMR at the first visit, DTP and PRP-D at the second visit (1 month later), and DTP and OPV at the third visit (2 months after the first visit). Subsequent DTP and OPV 10 to 16 months after the first visit are still indicated.

58. What are the indications for the vaccines listed in the lefthand column of the table?

Indications for Active Immunization of Children Other Than Routine Vaccination

VACCINE	INDICATIONS
Pertussis vaccine	Children > age 7 years with chronic lung disease and high chance of pertussis exposure
Diphtheria tetanus (DT)	Routine vaccination when pertussis vaccine contraindicated
Adult-type tetanus and diphtheria (Td)	Every 10 years throughout life
	Post-trauma tetanus prophylaxis, age > 7 years
Inactivated polio vaccine (IPV)	Routine childhood vaccination when OPV contraindicated (e.g., immunodeficiency)
Hemophilus b conjugate vaccine (PRP-D)	High-risk and immunocompromised children aged 5 or more (e.g., asplenia, Hodgkin's) (routine for children 18–60 months old)
Pneumococcal vaccine	High-risk and immunocompromised children > age 2 (e.g., asplenia, nephrosis)
Meningococcal vaccine	Asplenia or complement deficiency, given at or after age 2; occasionally used in outbreaks or for case contacts
Bacille Calmette-Guerin (BCG)	Consider for high-risk tuberculin-negative individuals without immune compromise, especially neonates
Hepatitis B vaccine	Infants of HBsAG-positive mothers; children who are household or institution contacts of HBsAg carriers
Rabies human diploid cell vaccine	Children at risk of actual or predicted exposure to potentially rabid animals
Influenza vaccine	Immunocompromised and high-risk children yearly, after age 6 months

Bibliography

1. Barbour SD, Plotkin SA: Immunizations: going beyond the routine recommendations. Diagnosis 10:33–39, 1988.
2. Bart KJ, Orenstein WA, Hinman AR: The virtual elimination of rubella and mumps from the United States and the use of combined measles, mumps and rubella vaccines (MMR) to eliminate measles. Dev Biol Stand 65:45–52, 1986.
3. Centers for Disease Control, DHSS, Atlanta, Georgia: Diphtheria, tetanus and pertussis: guidelines for vaccine prophylaxis and other preventive measures. Ann Intern Med 103:896–905, 1985.
4. Committee on Infectious Diseases, American Academy of Pediatrics: Red Book, 20th ed, 1986.

5. Halsey NA, Henderson DA: HIV infection and immunization against other agents. N Engl J Med 316:683, 1987.
6. Laforce FM: Immunoprophylaxis and chemotherapy to prevent selected infections. JAMA 257:2464–2470, 1987.
7. Plotkin SA, Mortimer EA: Vaccines. Philadelphia, W.B. Saunders Co., 1987.
8. Sixbey JW: Routine immunizations and the immunosuppressed child. Adv Pediatr Infect Dis 2:79–114, 1987.

IMMUNOLOGY

Mary Ellen Conley, M.D.

1. What is the significance of transient hypogammaglobulinemia of infancy?

Transient hypogammaglobulinemia of infancy is not a very useful term. You do not know that it is transient until it is over. Some children who have low concentrations of serum immunoglobulins in the first year of life continue to have abnormalities of immunoglobulin production well into early childhood. An infant who has decreased concentrations of serum immunoglobulins should be carefully followed and the physician should keep an open mind about the possible diagnosis.

2. Are healthy newborns immunodeficient?

All normal babies could be considered immunodeficient when compared with adults. On the surface, all seems well. The newborn has plenty of neutrophils, normal numbers of lymphocytes, even normal numbers of T-helpers and T-suppressors. However, closer scrutiny demonstrates abnormalities in almost every branch of the immune system. Neutrophils exhibit abnormalities in adherence, aggregation, and deformability, and, under stressful conditions, even in phagocytosis and bacterial killing. Natural killer (NK) cell function is decreased. Several complement components are present in decreased concentrations. T-cell suppressor function overrides helper function in assays measuring immunoglobulin production. These are normal congenital immunodeficiencies.

3. How do immunoglobulin levels change during the first year of life?

The normal full-term baby is born with a serum concentration of IgG that is equal to or slightly higher than the mother's. This can be explained by the active transport of IgG across the placenta. However, IgG has a half-life of about 21 days, so that by the time the baby is 3–4 months old, there is very little maternal immunoglobulin left and the baby's serum concentration of IgG reaches a nadir that may be as low as 180–200 mg/dl. In the meantime, the baby has started to make his own antibodies, so that after 3–4 months of age, a slow rise in the concentration of serum IgG becomes evident, which reaches adult levels by 6–10 years of age. IgM is the first immunoglobulin produced in phylogeny and in ontogeny. And, although the normal baby has very low concentrations of IgM at birth, normal adult concentrations are usually achieved by about 1 year of age. IgA is the last immunoglobulin produced, and adult levels are not reached until adolescence. Because delays in production of IgA are not at all unusual, the diagnosis of IgA deficiency is rarely made in a child less than 2 or 3 years of age. IgD and IgE, both of which are present in low concentrations in the newborn, reach 10–40% of adult concentrations by 1 year of age (see figure).

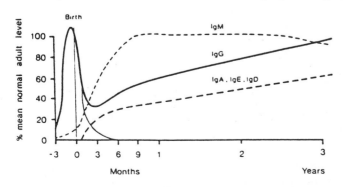

The normal development of serum immunoglobulin levels. (From Hobbs JR: Primary immune paresis. In Adinolfi M (ed): Immunology and Development. Clinics in Developmental Medicine, No. 34. London. Spastics International Medical Publications, in association with William Heinemann Medical Books Ltd., 1969, pp 114–158, with permission.)

191

4. Which children should be suspected of having a possible immunodeficiency?
1. Children whose recurrent or persistent infections result in failure to thrive.
2. Children who have had two or more life-threatening infections.
3. Children who have had an unusual infection with a common organism.
4. Children who have had an opportunistic infection or an infection with an unusual organism.
5. Children with physical findings associated with a particular immunodeficiency (i.e., ataxia and telangiectasia or eczema and bleeding).
6. Children with a family history of immunodeficiency.

5. How common are the primary immunodeficiencies?
There are about 400 new cases annually of primary immunodeficiency for an incidence rate of 1:10,000 (excluding asymptomatic IgA deficiency). The relative prevalences of primary immunodeficiencies are:

B-cell deficiencies	50%
(excluding asymptomatic IgA deficiency)	
T-cell deficiencies	10%
Combined immunodeficiencies	20–25%
Phagocytic deficiencies	15%
Complement deficiencies	Less than 3%

Reference: Stiehm ER (ed): Immunologic Disorders in Infants and Children, 2nd ed. Philadelphia, W.B. Saunders, 1989.

6. What are the B-cell or immunoglobulin deficiencies that might be seen in an immunodeficiency clinic?
Excluding transient hypogammaglobulinemia and IgA deficiency, the most common disorders are common variable immunodeficiency (CVID) and X-linked agammaglobulinemia. CVID may involve T-cells as well as B-cells.

7. What are the primary disorders of T-cells?
This is a harder question. Profound disorders of T-cells result in B-cell defects because most antibody production is T-cell dependent.

8. Is DiGeorge's syndrome a primary disorder of T-cells?
DiGeorge's syndrome, or DiGeorge's anomalad, is abnormal development of the thymus and usually several other facial and anterior neck structures. Because the thymus is required for normal T-cell maturation, these patients may have secondary T-cell defects but the T-cell lineage itself is probably normal.

9. What are the minimal diagnostic criteria for DiGeorge's syndrome?
There are no well-established criteria for DiGeorge's syndrome. Most investigators would agree that a child with DiGeorge's syndrome must have markedly reduced numbers of T-cells (less than 30% of the peripheral blood lymphocytes should be T-cells, with normal being 48–75%). In addition, the child should have either hypocalcemia or cardiac abnormalities. Most affected children also have abnormal facies and many have other congenital anomalies.

10. How do patients with DiGeorge's syndrome usually present?
Most present with cardiac problems. Two unusual cardiac anomalies associated with DiGeorge's syndrome are interrupted aortic arch and truncus arteriosus. Occasionally, hypocalcemia is the first problem. Infection is rarely the presenting complaint. Most children have "partial" DiGeorge's syndrome. The thymus may be very small but some thymic tissue is present. Children with partial DiGeorge's syndrome usually do not have the types of infections seen in children with T-cell deficiencies such as chronic candidal infection or persistent viral pneumonitis or gastroenteritis.

11. What are the modes of inheritance of Bruton's agammaglobulinemia, DiGeorge's syndrome, and severe combined immunodeficiency?

Although there are exceptions with every disorder, Bruton's agammaglobulinemia usually lives up to its alternative name—X-linked agammaglobulinemia. DiGeorge's syndrome is most often sporadic. About half of the patients with severe combined immunodeficiency have inherited autosomal recessive forms of the disease and half have an X-linked disease.

12. How does the age of the patient help in the diagnosis of immunodeficiency?

Patients with T-cell or phagocytic defects often present before 6 months of age. Illnesses beginning around 6 months are more suggestive of B-cell abnormalities. At 6 months, placentally-acquired maternal immunoglobulin has disappeared from the infant's circulation.

13. Name some disorders affecting T-cells and B-cells.

Severe combined immunodeficiency (multiple variants)
Wiskott-Aldrich syndrome
Ataxia-telangiectasia
Common variable immunodeficiency (some cases)
Job's syndrome (probably)
Acquired immunodeficiency syndrome (AIDS)

14. What are the clinical manifestations of T-cell and B-cell deficiencies?

There is much overlap, but generally children with B-cell deficiencies suffer recurrent bacterial infections, including pneumonia and bronchitis, sinusitis, and otitis. Children with T-cell deficiencies have chronic and severe viral and fungal infections, especially from opportunistic pathogens.

15. What are the most common infections seen in children with panhypogammaglobulinemia?

Those caused by *H. influenzae, S. pneumoniae*, and *S. aureus*, including otitis, sinusitis, bronchitis, pneumonia, sepsis, meningitis, cellulitis, septic arthritis, and severe impetigo.

16. What are the common and uncommon manifestations of X-linked agammaglobulinemia?

The most common infections are those described above for children with panhypogammaglobulinemia. The most frequent long-term complications are chronic obstructive pulmonary disease and chronic sinusitis. A few older patients have problems with arthritis. It is not clear whether the arthritis is due to infectious causes or impurities used in early preparations of gammaglobulin. Except for giardia infections, gastrointestinal infections are rare. A relatively rare but devastating complication is chronic enteroviral infection. About 10% of patients develop either chronic polio virus infection from exposure to vaccine polio or chronic echoviral infection manifested as meningoencephalitis, dermatomyositis, and scleroderma. Although high-dose intravenous gammaglobulin may be helpful for this complication, some patients die in spite of this therapy.

17. What in the history or physical examination suggests X-linked agammaglobulinemia?

Infections in children with Bruton's or X-linked agammaglobulinemia begin at about 3–6 months of age, after the loss of maternally acquired antibody. The family history is positive for boys with recurrent infections or early childhood death in about half of patients. When looking for a positive family history, it is helpful to focus on maternal relatives. How many brothers did the maternal grandmother and the maternal great-grandmother have? On physical examination, affected boys have a paucity of lymphoid tissue. Lymph nodes may be palpated but they are not as large as would be expected in view of the child's age and history of infections.

18. Which inherited immunodeficiencies are associated with an increased frequency of malignancy?
Ataxia telangiectasia and Wiskott-Aldrich syndrome.

19. What is the clinical triad for Wiskott-Aldrich syndrome?
Eczema; thrombocytopenia (usually evident at birth with platelet counts ranging from 5,000 to 100,000); and recurrent pyogenic infections, especially otitis media.

20. What is the inheritance pattern of Wiskott-Aldrich syndrome?
X-linked recessive.

21. What are the clinical features of ataxia-telangiectasia?
  Ataxia (beginning as early as 1 year or as late as 6 years)
  Telangiectasias (beginning at 3–6 years of age)
  Recurrent sinus and pulmonary infections (not all patients)
  Delayed secondary sexual characteristics (in some)
  Mental retardation (later in disease)
  Growth failure (later in disease)

22. What are the immunoglobulin abnormalities in the Wiskott-Aldrich syndrome?
Most patients are unable to form antibody against polysaccharide antigens and have markedly elevated IgA and IgE but decreased IgM.

23. What are the major systemic manifestations of selective IgA deficiency?
IgA deficiency is relatively common, occurring with a frequency of about 1/500 to 1/1000. Many individuals with IgA deficiency are completely asymptomatic; however, there is an increased incidence of allergies and upper respiratory tract infections. GI infections and systemic infections are rare. There is also a slightly increased risk of autoimmune disorders in patients with IgA deficiency.

24. What is the pathogenesis of selective IgA deficiency?
It is not at all clear that selective IgA deficiency is a single entity with a single pathogenesis. IgA deficiency may be the last common denominator in a variety of disorders of immune regulation. Defects in the genes for IgA are rarely the problem. B-cells that express surface IgA are almost always present if they are carefully sought, but these B-cells appear to be arrested at an early stage of differentiation. Several investigators have reported either T-cell suppression of IgA production or a lack of T-cell help, but it is unclear whether these findings represent the primary abnormality.

25. What autoimmune disorders are associated with selective deficiency of IgA?
Probably all autoimmune disorders are associated with selective IgA deficiency. About 5–10% of patients with either systemic lupus erythematosus or juvenile rheumatoid arthritis have IgA deficiency, but IgA deficiency is also seen in autoimmune thyroid disease, chronic active hepatitis, and a variety of other autoimmune disorders.

26. What is the mode of inheritance of selective IgA deficiency?
As would be expected for a disorder that may have many different etiologies, IgA deficiency does not follow a single pattern of inheritance. About half of patients with IgA deficiency have family members who have abnormalities of immunoglobulin production, which may include increased production as well as decreased concentrations of a particular immunoglobulin class. The pattern of inheritance may resemble autosomal dominant or autosomal recessive but is more likely to be multifactorial or multigenetic.

27. How should children with selective IgA deficiency be treated?
The problems associated with IgA deficiency are usually rather mild and the affected child should be treated as normally as possible. It is important to avoid making any child an invalid. Although children with IgA deficiency may have more upper respiratory tract infections or problems with allergies than their classmates, they can be treated for their symptoms and should be encouraged to attend school, even when they are not in their best form. The child should be seen by an immunologist once a year so that any complications or questions that arise can be treated early. If surgery is planned, the blood bank should be alerted to ensure that IgA-deficient blood is available.

28. What are the primary phagocytic disorders of childhood and their main functional defects?
Phagocytic disorders are rare. The prototype phagocytic defect is chronic granulomatous disease, a disorder that can occur in both X-linked and autosomal recessive forms. Recently a rare inherited defect in neutrophil adhesion called Mac-1 deficiency, or LFA-1 deficiency, has been reported.

29. What is the metabolic defect in chronic granulomatous disease?
There is a defect in a membrane-associated NADPH oxidase that results in a failure of the neutrophil to produce superoxide radicals that are important in the killing of staphylococcus, gram-negative bacteria, and some fungi.

30. Which types of infections are commonly seen in children with chronic granulomatous disease?
Superficial staphylococcal skin infections, particularly around the nose, eyes, and anus, are seen in almost all affected children who are not receiving therapy. Adenitis is very common. Recurrent pneumonias often lead to chronic pulmonary disease. Indolent osteomyelitis, chronic diarrhea, or intermittent intestinal obstruction may also be seen. A male child with a liver abscess should be considered to have chronic granulomatous disease until proven otherwise.

31. What are phytohemagglutinin (PHA), concanavalin-A (con-A), and pokeweed mitogen (PWM)?
These are plant proteins (lectins) that function both as mitogens and hemagglutinins. Mitogens are agents that promote T-cell and B-cell lymphocyte transformation and vigorous mitotic proliferation. Hemagglutinins, as the name implies, agglutinate red cells. Both properties are useful in tests of lymphocyte function and differentiation. PHA (from the red kidney bean) stimulates T-lymphocytes more than B-lymphocytes. Con-A (from the jack bean) stimulates T-lymphocytes more than B-lymphocytes. Pokeweed (from the North American pokeweed) stimulates B-lymphocytes more than T-lymphocytes.

32. What is Job's syndrome?
Also known as the hyper IgE syndrome, or Buckley's syndrome, Job's syndrome is characterized by: (1) recurrent skin infections—boils or abscesses with reduced amounts of inflammation ("cold abscesses"); (2) recurrent sinopulmonary infections; (3) extremely elevated IgE levels; and (4) eosinophilia. The name derives from the biblical problems of Job. "So went Satan forth from the presence of the Lord and smote Job with boils from the sole of his foot unto his crown."

33. How do patients with complement deficiencies usually present?
Any complement deficiency may result in increased bacterial infections or immune complex disease; however, there is a tendency for early component deficiencies, particularly C2 and

C4 deficiencies, to present with a lupus-like syndrome or recurrent infections with encapsulated bacteria. Late component defects, particularly C5, C6, C7, and C8 deficiencies, most often present with disseminated neisserial infections, i.e., meningococcus or gonococcus.

34. What is the most common neutrophil disorder?
Neutropenia.

35. What is transient neutropenia and how is it treated?
Transient neutropenia usually occurs after a viral infection and generally lasts 3–6 weeks, although it may last up to 6 months. If other hematopoietic cell lines appear to be normal, if the child is not having significant infections, and if the child is otherwise well, transient neutropenia is not a matter of major concern. However, the child should be reevaluated at regular intervals until the neutropenia resolves.

36. What are the appropriate screening tests for a child with suspected immunodeficiency?
The appropriate screening tests depend on why immunodeficiency is suspected. For most children who seem to have had more than their fair share of infections but who are otherwise well, it is sufficient to obtain a complete blood count with differential, platelet count, quantitative immunoglobulins, a total hemolytic complement (CH_{50}), and delayed hypersensitivity tests. To measure antibody responses against specific antigens, anti-blood group substances and anti-tetanus toxoid can be determined.

37. What is the CH_{50}?
This is a screening test that evaluates the function of the classic complement cascade. It assesses the ability of an individual's serum (in varying dilutions) to lyse sheep red blood cells after those cells are sensitized with rabbit IgM anti-sheep antibody. The CH_{50} is an arbitrary unit indicating the quantity of complement necessary for 50% lysis of the red cells in a standardized setting. Test results are usually expressed as a derived reciprocal of the test dilution needed for 50% lysis. The test is relatively insensitive, as major reductions in individual complement components are necessary before the CH_{50} is altered. Therefore, C3 and C4 levels are often included in the initial screening of a child with a suspected complement deficiency.

38. At what age can skin tests be performed safely and accurately?
The risks of delayed hypersensitivity skin testing in young children are minimal. Safety is not a major concern. Skin tests are rarely positive in children less than 5 months of age, in part because of immaturities of the phagocytic system. When testing with tetanus toxoid, candida, and trichophyton antigens, about 90% of children will be positive for at least one antigen by 12–18 months of age.

39. What are the four types of hypersensitivity reactions?
> Type I—IgE mediated; immediate or anaphylactic (e.g., urticaria, allergic rhinitis)
> Type II—Antibody-dependent cytotoxicity (e.g., Goodpasture's syndrome, erythroblastosis fetalis)
> Type III—Immune complex or Arthus reaction (e.g., poststreptococcal glomerulonephritis, serum sickness)
> Type IV—Delayed hypersensitivity (e.g., contact dermatitis, tuberculin skin testing).

40. What is the Rebuck skin window?
It is a test of chemotactic factors and leukocyte mobility which is not often used because it is painful, time-consuming, and leaves a scar. Skin is abraded and coverslips are serially applied to the abrasion over time to collect specimens. On microscopic exam, neutrophils are usually seen by 2 hours and mononuclear cells by 12–24 hours.

41. What is a graft versus host (GVH) reaction?
The immunologic attack by the transplanted or transfused competent lymphoid cells of a donor against the immunoincompetent host. It is most often observed in bone marrow transplant patients but may occur in any immunodeficient host given a transfusion or organ transplant. Clinical manifestations are varied and often begin as early as 6 days. GVH disease frequently presents with a maculopapular rash that coalesces and desquamates. Other features include hepatosplenomegaly, lymphadenopathy, pneumonitis, and diarrhea. A characteristic skin biopsy can establish the diagnosis.

42. How long is the maturation phase of a polymorphonuclear (PMN) cell (from immature myeloblast to mature PMN)?
14 days.

43. What is the half-life of a PMN in blood and in tissue after it has migrated?
Blood, 6 hours; tissue, 1–2 days.

44. What are Kupffer cells?
Fixed tissue macrophages in the liver.

45. What is the distribution of T-cells, B-cells, and NK cells in the peripheral blood of healthy individuals beyond the neonatal period?
Approximately 55–80% of the lymphocytes are T-cells, 5–20% are B-cells, and 5–20% are NK cells. There are usually a small number of cells that cannot be accounted for using the routine typing reagents.

46. What deficiency causes hereditary angioneurotic edema (HANE)?
This is a term no longer used very often that describes an autosomal dominant disorder resulting from a deficiency of C1 esterase inhibitor. C1 esterase inhibitor binds to the C1s subunit of C1, thereby preventing the cleavage of C4 and the activation of the complement cascade.

47. Why are androgens helpful in treating C1 esterase inhibitor deficiency?
Methyltestosterone acts by an unknown mechanism to increase the synthesis of C1 esterase inhibitor. Danazol, an androgenic steroid with more anabolic than masculinizing effects, also increases inhibitor levels and is more commonly the drug of choice.

48. What are the clinical presentations of C1 esterase inhibitor deficiency?
1. Recurrent facial and extremity swelling—acute, circumscribed edema that is not painful, red, or pruritic, clearly distinguishing it from urticaria. Usually self-resolves in 72 hours.
2. Abdominal pain—recurrent, often severe, colicky pain, due to interstitial wall edema with vomiting and/or diarrhea; may be misdiagnosed as an acute abdomen.
3. Hoarseness, stridor—a true emergency, as death by asphyxiation may occur due to laryngeal edema. Epinephrine, hydrocortisone, and antihistamines are often of only limited benefit and tracheostomy is needed if there is progression of symptoms.
The diagnosis is confirmed by direct assay of the inhibitor level.

49. What is the predominant immunoglobulin in breast milk?
IgA.

50. How did the HIV designation for the AIDS virus evolve?
The virus that causes AIDS was isolated in several different laboratories at about the same time. Each laboratory gave the virus a name. In France the virus was called LAV, in Bethesda it was called HTLV-III, and in San Francisco it was called ARV. To reduce confusion, an international panel designated the name human immunodeficiency virus (HIV). HIV is a

retrovirus and bears some similarity to the human T-cell leukemia viruses HTLV-I and HTLV-II, but these viruses do not cause AIDS. Recent studies have suggested that there are other viruses that are very closely related to HIV. The rules for classifying these viruses are not yet clear, so other names are appearing in the literature, including HTLV-IV and HIV-II.

51. Of the pediatric patients in the United States with clinical AIDS, how was the virus acquired?

When pediatric AIDS was first described, about 80% of the patients had acquired the virus from their mothers, during either pregnancy or delivery, and 20% were infected by contaminated blood products. However, because blood products can now be screened, the percentages of children who acquire HIV through transfusions is decreasing.

52. When did testing for HIV blood for transfusion begin?

Spring of 1985. Patients at risk for transfusion-acquired AIDS are those transfused from 1978 to spring, 1985.

53. What is the average age of onset of symptoms in infants with congenitally acquired AIDS?

4–6 months. However, some children have no symptoms until they are over 5 years of age.

54. What immunologic abnormalities are seen in children with HIV disease?

Most patients have elevated serum immunoglobulins; about 10% of patients have hypogammaglobulinemia; failure to make antibodies to specific antigens (e.g., tetanus toxoid, pneumococcal vaccine) is common. In more advanced infection, there is a decreased ratio of helper/suppressor (T4/T8) T-cells, absolute lymphopenia, and decreased in vitro mitogenic responses.

55. What are the most common nonspecific clinical manifestations of children with symptomatic HIV disease?

Lymphadenopathy—90%
Hepatomegaly—80%
Splenomegaly—70%
Poor growth/failure to thrive—60%
Thrush/monilial diaper rash—50%
Recurrent otitis media—45%
Chronic diarrhea—20%

56. What laboratory studies should be obtained in a child suspected of having HIV infection?

In making the diagnosis of HIV infection, the most useful test is HIV serology (e.g., ELISA and Western Blot). About 90% of infected children will have measurable antibody to HIV. However, two caveats must be kept in mind: (1) in a clinically asymptomatic baby less than 9–12 months of age, the antibody may be maternal in origin and may not indicate infection; and (2) some infected babies do not make antibody to HIV. If the clinical suspicion is strong, the mother's serology should be examined. Lymphopenia, abnormal mitogen responses, and inverted T4/T8 ratios are not as common in children with AIDS as they are in adults with AIDS.

57. What is the "Western Blot" test for AIDS?

The Western Blot is the most sensitive and specific test currently available for detection of HIV antibodies. It is more precise than standard enzyme immunoassays which have a higher incidence of false-positive reactions. A current problem, however, is the lack of standardization of the Western Blot among laboratories with resultant variability. The test is also expensive and results may be difficult to interpret. The Western Blot is performed as follows: Purified HIV is separated into protein components by electrophoresis on a gel. These components are transferred from the gel to a nitrocellulose membrane ("the blot"). Serum or plasma is placed over this "blot" and incubated. Antibodies, if present, bind to the antigen. The antibodies are then illuminated by the addition of an enzyme-anti-IgG complex, which binds to the HIV antibody. A substrate is added which is converted to a colored compound in the presence of bound enzyme. The amount of color produced can be quantified.

58. What is AZT?

Azidothymidine (3'-azido-3'-deoxythymidine) is a nucleoside analogue that is effective in slowing the disease process in adult patients with AIDS. Clinical trials are currently under way in the pediatric population. The mechanism of action of AZT is not completely known. AZT inhibits viral reverse transcriptase (the enzyme that allows viral RNA to make copies of itself in DNA) and can incorporate itself into the viral DNA and code for chain termination prematurely.

59. What is lymphocytic interstitial pneumonitis (LIP)?

A chronic pulmonary interstitial disease of lymphocytic and plasma cell infiltration that occurs in about 50% of pediatric AIDS patients. Occasionally there is a concomitant hilar adenopathy. The chest x-ray frequently reveals a noduloreticular pattern. This condition is more commonly seen in patients having generalized lymphadenopathy, salivary gland enlargement, and digital clubbing. Compared to patients with *Pneumocystis carinii* pneumonia, patients with LIP have a considerably longer period of survival.

Reference: Rubenstein A, et al: Pulmonary disease in children with acquired immune deficiency syndrome and AIDS-related complex. J Pediatr 108:498–503, 1986.

60. What is the derivation of the term "serum sickness"?

First described in 1905, serum sickness was the clinical picture of arthritis, vasculitis, and glomerulonephritis that developed in patients given horse serum as an antiserum for diseases such as diphtheria and tetanus. The foreign proteins in the horse serum elicited an antibody response with the formation of immune complexes. These complexes, deposited in varying tissues, caused an inflammatory reaction. Serum sickness is a term now most commonly used to describe delayed drug reactions (e.g., to penicillin or sulfonamides).

61. What is the Raji cell?

The Raji cell, a Burkitt's lymphoma cell (B-lymphoblastoid) obtained from a man named Raji, is used in tests for quantification of immune complexes. It lacks surface IgG and has high affinity for complement and low affinity for IgG. Immune complexes (after being linked to complement) are detected by binding to the Raji cell.

Bibliography

1. Buckley RH: Humoral immunodeficiency. Clin Immunol Immunopathol 40:13–24, 1986.
2. Fallon J, Eddy J, Weiner L, Pizzo P: Human immunodeficiency virus infection in children. J Pediatr 114:1–30, 1989.
3. Fries LF, O'Shea JJ, Frank MM: Inherited deficiencies of complement and complement-related proteins. Clin Immunol Immunopathol 40:37–49, 1986.
4. Lederman HM, Winkelstein JA: X-linked agammaglobulinemia: An analysis of 96 patients. Medicine 64:145–156, 1985.
5. Rogers MF, et al: Acquired immunodeficiency syndrome in children: Report of the Centers for Disease Control National Surveillance, 1982–1985. Pediatrics 79:1008–1014, 1987.
6. Rubenstein A: Pediatric AIDS. Curr Probl Pediatr 16:361–409, 1986.
7. Rubenstein A, et al: Pulmonary disease in children with acquired immune deficiency syndrome and AIDS-related complex. J Pediatr 108:498–503, 1986.
8. Stiehm ER: Clinical and laboratory evaluation of the child with suspected immunodeficiency. Pediatr Rev 7:53–61, 1985.
9. Stiehm ER (ed): Immunologic Disorders in Infants and Children, 2nd ed. Philadelphia, W.B. Saunders Co., 1989.
10. Stites DP, et al (eds): Basic and Clinical Immunology. Los Altos, CA, Lange, 1982.
11. White CJ, Gallin JI: Phagocyte defects. Clin Immunol Immunopathol 40:50–61, 1986.

INBORN ERRORS OF METABOLISM

Richard I. Kelley, M.D., Ph.D.

1. What is the characteristic odor of phenylketonuria (PKU) and what metabolic products are responsible for the odor?
The odor of phenylketonuria is usually described as "musty" or "mousey." Phenylacetic acid is the major metabolite contributing to the odor.

2. What is the "Guthrie bacterial inhibition" test?
In the Guthrie bacterial inhibition test, phenylalanine in a blood specimen directly competes with inhibition of bacterial growth by beta-2-thienylalanine, a phenylalanine analog. Phenylalanine in a blood-soaked filter paper disc diffuses into the bacterial growth medium (agar), reversing the inhibition by beta-2-thienylalanine in a concentration-dependent manner. The amount of bacterial growth surrounding the filter paper disc is proportional to the concentration of phenylalanine in the blood. Excessive bacterial growth around the filter paper disc indicates an abnormally high level of phenylalanine. The development of the Guthrie bacterial inhibition test in 1961 was a major breakthrough that permitted not only widespread inexpensive screening for phenylketonuria, but also the development of screening for other inborn errors of metabolism using the same principles for detection of elevated metabolites.

3. Why is vitamin C given to newborn premature infants with a positive PKU test?
The most common cause of an abnormal PKU blood screening test in premature infants is hyperphenylalaninemia secondary to transient tyrosinemia of the newborn. Transient tyrosinemia appears to be caused by inadequate activity of p-hydroxyphenylpyruvic acid dioxygenase, a vitamin C-dependent enzyme in the tyrosine degradative pathway. Administration of vitamin C increases the activity of the enzyme and facilitates metabolism of both tyrosine and its precursor, phenylalanine.

4. What are the varieties of hyperphenylalaninemia?

Types of Hyperphenylalanemia

DISORDER	BLOOD PHENYLALANINE LEVEL (MG/DL)	ENZYME DEFECT	THERAPY
Classic phenylketonuria	>20	Phenylalanine hydroxylase	Diet
Atypical phenylketonuria	12–20	Phenylalanine hydroxylase	Diet
Persistent mild hyper-phenylalaninemia	2–12	Phenylalanine hydroxylase	Diet
Transient hyper-phenylalaninemia	2–20	Unknown	None
Transient tyrosinemia	2–12	? p-OH-phenylpyruvic acid dioxygenase def. ? secondary to low vit. C	Vitamin C, low-protein formula
Dihydropteridine reductase deficiency	12–20	Dihydropteridine reductase ⎫	
Biopterin synthesis defects	12–20	Dihydrobiopterin synthetase, GTP-cyclohydrolase ⎬	DOPA, OH-tryptophan, tetrahydrobiopterin

5. What is the clinical significance of transient tyrosinemia in the newborn infant?
Neonates (mostly premature) with transient tyrosinemia appear to be more lethargic than
normal infants and feed poorly. There remains debate about the long-term significance of
transient tyrosinemia and the need for treatment by vitamin C and/or protein restriction.
Some studies have suggested mild neurologic and developmental abnormalities during later
childhood in infants who had transient tyrosinemia, whereas other studies show no effect. A
bias of ascertainment (i.e., sick prematures) may explain some of the poor development. A
reasonable attempt should be made to restore the tyrosine and phenylalanine levels to normal
with vitamin C and/or protein restriction.

6. Name the inborn errors of metabolism that cause the renal Fanconi syndrome.

Cystinosis	Wilson's disease
Galactosemia	Glycogen storage disease (one rare
Hereditary fructose intolerance	variant)
Tyrosinemia	Cytochrome C oxidase deficiency
	(some)

There are other rare inherited diseases associated with the complete Fanconi syndrome
(glycosuria, aminoaciduria, phosphaturia, and bicarbonaturia) such as Lowe syndrome,
which may have a "metabolic" basis, but which are poorly understood biochemically at this
time.

7. What are the characteristic clinical signs of alkaptonuria?
Dark urine on exposure to air (e.g., in diaper)
Ochronosis (grayish discoloration of connective tissue)
Degenerative arthritis
Valvulitis and aortic degeneration

**8. What types of malignancies do individuals with albinism have a propensity to
develop?**
Because of the lack of ultraviolet shielding afforded by melanin in normal individuals, albinos
are at risk of malignancies associated with increased sun exposure. The most common lesions
are squamous cell carcinomas arising out of solar keratoses. Other malignancies whose
incidence is increased by solar radiation, such basal cell carcinomas and malignant
melanomas, are relatively uncommon. In one rare form of partial albinism, Hermansky-
Pudlak syndrome, there is an unexplained high incidence of lymphoreticular malignancy.

9. What enzyme deficiency causes albinism?
There are many different, genetically distinct types of albinism, only one of which has been
enzymatically characterized as a deficiency of melanocytic tyrosinase, the enzyme that
initiates the conversion of tyrosine into melanin. So-called "tyrosinase-negative" individuals
have no detectable enzyme activity and never develop cutaneous or ocular pigment.
"Tyrosinase-positive" patients may be completely albinotic at birth but eventually acquire
some pigment.

**10. Which metabolic abnormalities can be detected with a ferric chloride test and what
color reactions are produced?**
The ferric chloride test is one of the oldest urine metabolic tests, yet remains a useful
screening test in this day of sophisticated micro-analytical quantitative methods because of its
simplicity, speed, and differential color reactions.

Positive Reactions for Urine Ferric Chloride Test

DISORDER	MAJOR REACTANT	METABOLITE SOURCE	REACTION
Phenylketonuria	Phenylpyruvic acid	Phenylalanine	Green
Hypertyrosinemia syndromes, severe liver disease	p-OH-phenylpyruvic acid	Tyrosine	Green (fades rapidly)
Histidinemia	Imidazolepyruvic acid	Histidine	Olive-green
Alkaptonuria	Homogentisic acid	Tyrosine	Blue or green (fades rapidly)
Formininotransferase deficiency	Imidazole carboxamide	Histidine	Gray
Ketoacidosis (severe)	Acetoacetate	Fatty acid oxidation	Cherry red
Congenital lactic acidosis	Pyruvate	Amino acids Glucose	Green-gold
Drug ingestion	Salicylates	Aspirin, oil of wintergreen	Purple
	Phenothiazines	Antihistamines Antidepressants Antipsychotics	Purple-pink
	Cyanates		Red
	Aminosalicylic acid	Anti-TB drug	Red-brown

11. Which tests comprise a "urine metabolic screen"?

Common Urine Metabolic Screening Tests*

TEST	SUBSTANCES DETECTED	PRINCIPAL DISORDERS DETECTED
Liquid Tests		
Ferric chloride	See question 10	See question 10
Cyanide nitroprusside	Disulfides	Homocystinuria; cystinuria
Nitrosonaphthol	Tyrosine; p-hydroxyphenyl compounds	Tyrosinemias; malabsorption; intestinal infection
2,4-Dinitrophenyl-hydrazine	Branched-chain ketoacids; pyruvate; acetoacetate	Maple syrup urine disease; lactic acidoses; ketosis
Cetylpyridinium chloride	Mucopolysaccharides	Mucopolysaccharidoses
Reducing substances	Glucose; galactose; fructose	Fanconi syndrome diabetes, etc.; galactosemia; fructose intolerance
Thiosulfate	Thiosulfate	Sulfite oxidase deficiency; molybdenum defects
Chromatography		
Amino acid paper or column chromatography	Amino acids and other ninhydrin-positive substances	Many amino acid disorders; Renal Fanconi syndrome
Organic acid gas chromatography	Organic acids, free and conjugated	Many organic acidurias; lactic acidoses

Table continued on next page.

Common Urine Metabolic Screening Tests* *(Continued)*

TEST	SUBSTANCES DETECTED	PRINCIPAL DISORDERS DETECTED
Oligosaccharide thin-layer chromatography	Oligosaccharides; sialyloigosaccharides	Sialic acid defects; MPS disorders; fucosidosis; other lysosomal storage diseases

*Additional "screening" tests on blood or plasma not usually obtained as "routine" blood chemistries include lactate determination for diagnosis of congenital lactic acidoses, blood ammonia for detection of urea cycle defects and certain organic acidurias, and a qualitative test for galactose-1-phosphate uridyltransferase to rule out galactosemia. Because of the variability and intermittent nature of many metabolic diseases, a normal metabolic screen should never be assumed to have ruled out metabolic disease as a cause of a child's illness. Similarly, because pathologic metabolites may clear from the urine within hours of starting general supportive therapy, "acute" urine specimens should be sent for testing.

12. Which inherited metabolic disorders cause a "sweaty feet" odor?

Isovaleric acid is the principal metabolite causing the "sweaty feet" odor in isovaleric acidemia, an inborn error of leucine catabolism caused by a deficiency of isovaleryl-coenzyme A dehydrogenase. Isovaleryl-coenzyme A dehydrogenase is also one of several enzymes functionally deficient in type II glutaric aciduria (multiple acyl-CoA dehydrogenase deficiency). Both glutaric aciduria type II and isovaleric acidemia may present as a catastrophic neonatal illness, which is often mistaken for sepsis. The recognition of the odor may be lifesaving for these children, many of whom will have treatable defects.

13. What is the blue diaper syndrome?

Blue discoloration of the diaper is caused by intestinal malabsorption of the amino acid tryptophan, which has been reported as an apparently isolated defect of intestinal amino acid transport. Malabsorbed tryptophan is converted by colonic bacteria to indican, which causes blue staining of the diaper on exposure to air. Curiously, patients with Hartnup disease, an inborn error of intestinal and renal transport of all neutral amino acids including tryptophan, do not develop the blue diaper syndrome despite intestinal malabsorption of tryptophan and conversion to indican and other indoles. Bluish discoloration of diapers also has several nonmetabolic causes—methylene blue administration, food colorings, amitriptyline or triamterene ingestion, copper poisoning, and pseudomonas urinary tract infections (bluish green).

14. Which inborn errors of metabolism are considered vitamin responsive?

Many disorders of amino acid metabolism and catabolism have been found to be responsive to pharmacologic doses of vitamins or vitamin-like enzyme cofactors, such as carnitine and betaine. For some treatments, such as biotin for biotinidase deficiency, essentially all patients respond. For others, such as thiamine for maple syrup urine disease, very few are responsive.

Vitamin-responsive Metabolic Diseases

Thiamine
    Pyruvate dehydrogenase deficiency
    Alpha-ketoglutarate dehydrogenase deficiency
    Thiamine-responsive maple syrup urine disease
    *Leigh's disease (occasional)
Riboflavin
    Glutaric aciduria types I and II (occasional)
    NADH-ubiquinone oxidoreductase deficiency

Table continued on next page.

Vitamin-responsive Metabolic Diseases *(Continued)*

Pyridoxine
    Homocystinuria
    Oxaluria
    Cystathioninuria
    Pyridoxine-dependent seizures (possible deficiency of glutamate decarboxylase)
    Beta-alaninemia
Vitamin B12
    Methylmalonic aciduria
    Homocystinuria secondary to defects of cobalamin metabolism
    Transcobalamin II deficiency
    Other defects of cobalamin metabolism
Ascorbic acid
    Transient tyrosinemia (some cases)
Vitamin D
    *Pseudohypoparathyroidism
    Vitamin D-dependent rickets
    *Familial hypophosphatemic rickets
Folic acid
    Hereditary folate malabsorption
    *Homocystinuria (partial response through alternate pathway)
    Formiminotransferase deficiency (possible partial response)
    Dihydrofolate reductase deficiency
    Tetrahydrofolate methyltransferase deficiency
    Nonketotic hyperglycinemia (occasional partial response)
Niacin
    *Hartnup's disease
Biotin
    Holocarboxylase deficiency
    Biotinidase deficiency
    Propionic acidemia (in vitro, ? clinical response in a few cases)
    Methylcrotonyl-CoA-carboxylase deficiency (reported but doubtful)
Lipoic acid
    Lipoamide dehydrogenase deficiency (mixed alpha-ketoacid dehydrogenase deficiency)
Betaine
    *Homocystinuria
Carnitine
    †Systemic carnitine deficiency (as primary defect)
    *Various defects of fatty acid oxidation and organic acid metabolism

---

*In these disorders, the primary metabolic defect is not directly affected by cofactor therapy. Instead, a compensatory metabolic pathway is enhanced, such as increased intestinal phosphate absorption by 1,25 di-OH vitamin D3 to treat hypophosphatemic rickets.
†Most reported cases of "systemic carnitine deficiency" are not primary defects of carnitine metabolism, but rather defects of fatty acid or organic acid metabolism in which serum carnitine levels are secondarily depressed by unknown mechanisms. Some patients with secondary carnitine deficiency will benefit from carnitine administration. Carnitine is synthesized in man from trimethyllysine but may be a true vitamin in some situations.

15. Which inborn errors of metabolism commonly cause acidosis during the neonatal period?

Severe metabolic acidosis in the neonatal period is more commonly caused by sepsis and cardiac defects than inborn errors of metabolism. However, an inborn error of metabolism causing neonatal acidosis is more often than not misdiagnosed as cardiac or infectious disease. Disorders of pyruvate metabolism, gluconeogenic defects, and inborn errors of branched-chain amino acid catablism are the most common inherited metabolic diseases causing metabolic acidosis in the newborn period. *Ketonuria* with acidosis in the newborn period is an especially important sign of an inborn error of metabolism.

Not all of the diagnoses given below have been made in the newborn period, but are listed here because the metabolic stress of childbirth and initial poorer feeding could theoretically precipitate an acidotic crisis.

Metabolic Acidosis in the Newborn Period

Disorders of Pyruvate Metabolism
    Pyruvate dehydrogenase deficiency
    Pyruvate carboxylase deficiency
    Cytochrome c oxidase deficiency and other electron chain transport defects
Gluconeogenic Defects
    Glucose-6-phosphatase deficiency (type I glycogen storage disease)
    Phosphoenolpyruvate carboxykinase deficiency
    Fructose-1-6-diphosphatase deficiency
    Pyruvate carboxylase deficiency
Organic acidemias (most common)
    Methylmalonic aciduria
    Isovaleric acidemia
    Propionic acidemia
    Holocarboxylase synthetase deficiency
    Beta-ketothiolase deficiency
    Methylcrotonyl-CoA-carboxylase deficiency
    Glutaric aciduira—types I and II
Defective renal bicarbonate transport
    Inborn errors of pyruvate metabolism
    Defects of electron transport
    Renal Fanconi syndrome

16. Which metabolic defect produces the odor of cat urine?
Methylcrotonylglycinuria (methylcrotonyl-CoA carboxylase deficiency).

17. What features on physical examination are helpful in differentiating homocystinuria from Marfan's disease?

Differentiation of Homocystinuria from Marfan's Disease

CHARACTERISTIC	MARFAN SYNDROME	HOMOCYSTINURIA
Lens dislocation	Usually upward	Usually downward
Cornea, sclera	Flattened cornea; bluish sclera	Normal
Body habitus and skeleton	Tall; arachnodactyly; pectus	Tall; arachnodactyly; pectus
Joints	Markedly hyperextensible	Most normal or mildly contracted; ankle eversion
Skin	Hyperextensible; striae	Eczema; malar flush; livedo reticularis
Hair	Normal	Thin; dry; reddish
Heart	Mitral valve prolapse + aortic regurgitation murmurs common	Mitral valve prolapse in some
Peripheral vasculature	Often severe varicosities	Diabetic-like peripheral vascular disease
Intelligence	Normal	Mental defect in 50–60%; frank psychosis in some
Family members affected	Autosomal dominant; sibs, one parent, and other generations affected	Autosomal recessive; parents unaffected but may be consanguineous
Other	Emphysema; pneumothorax; hernias	Hepatomegaly

18. What is the presumed pathophysiology for the thrombotic phenomena in homocystinuria?

Most evidence points to direct endothelial damage by homocysteine, exposing surfaces that activate platelet aggregation and thrombus formation. Homocysteine forms disulfide adducts with free cysteine and interferes with the formation of cysteine-cysteine disulfide bonds in proteins such as the endothelial basement membrane proteins and suspensory connective tissue of the lens. The functions of many other different proteins, such as coagulation factor VII, are also affected and may contribute to the thrombotic-hemorrhagic arterial and venous lesions that often develop in this disease.

19. What is the recommended therapy for cystinuria?

Therapy for cystinuria is directed at decreasing the precipitation of the amino acid, cystine (a cysteine disulfide dimer), in the kidney. This is achieved by forced water diuresis and the use of D-penicillamine (dimethylcysteine). D-penicillamine is itself a sulfhydryl-containing amino acid and forms excretable disulfides with free cysteine, thereby decreasing the concentration of cystine in the urine.

20. What is the difference between cystinuria and cystinosis?

Cystinuria is a defect of renal tubular and (in some) intestinal transport of dibasic amino acids (cystine, lysine, arginine, ornithine) named for the formation of renal stones from the least soluble amino acid, cystine. Clinical symptoms are essentially limited to those caused by chronic renal lithiasis—recurrent infection, obstruction, renal colic, hypertension, and renal failure.

Cystinosis is a lysomal storage disease caused by a defect in a lysosomal cystine transport system. In classic infantile nephropathic cystinosis, most clinical abnormalities are attributable to the renal Fanconi syndrome present in almost all affected individuals. Biochemically there is hyperchloremic metabolic acidosis from excessive bicarbonaturia, hypophosphatemia, glucosuria, and generalized aminoaciduria. The presenting clinical problems are growth failure, rickets, and photophobia associated with corneal cystine deposition and a "salt-and-pepper" retinopathy. Eventually, glomerular dysfunction progresses to renal failure, usually by age 10 in the classic form. Milder adolescent and adult forms of cystinosis are also known.

21. What are the inheritance pattern and clinical manifestations of Lesch-Nyhan syndrome?

Lesch-Nyhan syndrome is caused by an X-linked recessive deficiency of hypoxanthine-guanine phosphoribosyltransferase and characterized by overproduction of uric acid. Although affected infants, always males, are usually normal at birth, hypotonia, frequent vomiting, and delayed motor development usually are usually recognized in the first few months. Evidence of extrapyramidal dysfunction—dystonia, chorea, and athetosis—usually appear in the second half of the first year. Between the first and second year, the evolution of spasticity, dysarthria, and lack of ambulation often suggest the diagnosis of "cerebral palsy." After 18 months, the classic compulsive self-destructive behavior usually evolves, most commonly lip mutilation, finger-biting, and head-banging. Although serum uric acid may occasionally be normal in infancy, the urine uric acid/creatinine ratio is pathologically elevated in affected children. Milder deficiencies of the enzyme may present as only spasticity and/or extrapyramidal disease without the classical self-mutilation.

22. What are the most common clinical findings in children with galactosemia?

  Acute
   Poor feeding, vomiting, diarrhea
   Jaundice, severe or prolonged, mostly conjugated but sometimes predominantly unconjugated
     bilirubin
   Liver dysfunction—coagulopathy and elevated serum transaminases
   Hypoglycemia
   Cataracts
   Escherichia coli sepsis (50%)

Chronic
    Developmental disability, especially language
    Acute gastrointestinal symptoms with lactose ingestion
    Ovarian failure or hypofunction

23. What is the earliest metabolic derangement and cause of symptoms in hereditary fructose intolerance?

Hypophosphatemia is the most characteristic metabolic derangement in hereditary fructose intolerance. It can occur within a few minutes of ingestion of fructose and before clinical symptoms appear. Simultaneous with the hypophosphatemia, but somewhat slower in evolution, are hypoglycemia and severe gastrointestinal distress. Although rapid hepatic uptake of inorganic phosphate for phosphorylation of fructose is probably the major factor causing the hypophosphatemia, other factors, such as marked phosphaturia, may have a significant role in causing the hypophosphatemia. A similar hypophosphatemia is characteristic of patients with fructose-1,6-diphosphatase deficiency when fasting.

24. Which inherited metabolic disorders are commonly associated with hypoglycemia?

Inborn errors of metabolism associated with significant hypoglycemia can be grouped according to (1) primary errors of glucose synthesis and release, i.e., gluconeogenesis and glycogenolysis; (2) defects of fatty acid oxidation and ketogenesis, which provide the main sources of fuel for gluconeogenesis; and (3) defects causing "metabolic poisoning" of glucose metabolism, principally the organic acidurias.

Defects of Glucose Synthesis or Release
    Primary Defects of Gluconeogenesis
        Glucose-6-phosphatase deficiency (Type I glycogen storage disease)
        Pyruvate carboxylase deficiency (hypoglycemia uncommon)
        Phosphoenolpyruvate carboxykinase deficiency
        Fructose-1,6-diphosphatase deficiency
    Glycogen storage diseases and other carbohydrate defects
        Type 0—glycogen synthetase deficiency (rare)
        Type Ia—glucose-6-phosphatase deficiency
        Type Ib—microsomal glucose-6-phosphate transport defect
        Type III—amylo-1,6-glucosidase ("debrancher") deficiency
        Glycogen storage disease wth Fanconi syndrome (rare)
        Hereditary fructose intolerance (fructose-1-phosphate aldolase def.)

Defects of Fatty Acid and Ketone Body Metabolism
    Medium- and long-chain acyl-CoA dehydrogenase deficiencies
    Beta-ketothiolase deficiency
    Hydroxymethylglutaryl CoA lyase deficiency
    Glutaric aciduria type II (multiple acyl-CoA dehydrogenase def.)
    Systemic carnitine deficiency (primary defect)
    Hepatic palmitoyl carnitine transferase deficiency

Defects of Organic Acid and Amino Acid Metabolism (most common)
    Methylmalonic aciduria
    Isovaleric acidemia
    Propionic acidemia
    Tyrosinemia
    Maple syrup urine disease (branched-chain ketoacid dehydrogenase def.)
    Glutaric aciduria types I and II
    Pyruvate dehydrogenase deficiency (several enzymatic forms)
    Congenital lactic acidoses secondary to mitochondrial electron transport chain defects or other
        mitochondrial defects

25. What are the clinical findings and metabolic abnormalities in the glycogen storage diseases?

Glycogen Storage Diseases

| TYPE | COMMON NAME | ENZYME DEFICIENCY | CLINICAL AND BIOCHEMICAL ABNORMALITIES | | | |
			Major organ Involvement	Hypogly-cemia	Ketosis	Other
O	—	Glycogen synthetase	Liver + + +	+ +	+ + +	Prolonged hyper-glycemia after feedings
Ia	von Gierke	Glucose-6-phosphatase	Liver + + + kidney + +	+ + +	+	Lactic acidosis; hyperlipemia; hyperuricemia; growth retarda-tion; "doll-like" facies
Ib	—	Defective micro-somal transport of Glu-6-P	Liver + + + kidney + +	+ + +	+	Essentially same as Ia but also neutropenia
IIa	Pompe (infantile)	Lysosomal acid maltese (α-glucosidase)	Muscle + + + heart + + +	—	—	Severe hypotonia and cardio-megaly in early infancy; death by 1 year in most
IIb	Pompe (late juvenile-adult)	Lysosomal acid maltase (α-glucosidase)	Muscle + + liver +/−	—	—	Hypotonia and cardiomegaly; spinal muscular atrophy in some adults
III	Debrancher deficiency	Amylo-1,6-glucosidase	Liver + + + muscle + heart +	+ +	+ +	Growth retarda-tion; late onset myopathy and cardiomyopathy
IV	Brancher deficiency	Amylo-1,4→1,6-transglucosidase	Liver	—	—	Cirrhosis; liver failure; abnor-mal glycogen structure; death in early childhood
V	McArdle	Muscle phosphorylase	Muscle + +	—	—	Muscle weakness and cramping after exercise; lack of lactate rise after exercise
VI	—	Liver phosphorylase	Liver + + +	+/−	—	Marked hepatomegaly; mild growth retardation
VII	—	Phosphofructo-kinase	Muscle + +	—	—	Similar to GSD V
VIII	—	Unknown (very rare)	Liver + + brain + +	—	—	Truncal ataxia; psychomotor deterioration and death

Table continued on next page.

Glycogen Storage Diseases *(Continued)*

| | | | CLINICAL AND BIOCHEMICAL ABNORMALITIES | | | |
TYPE	COMMON NAME	ENZYME DEFICIENCY	Major organ Involvement	Hypogly-cemia	Ketosis	Other
IXa IXb IXc	—	Phosphorylase kinase (defects of phosphorylase activation)	Liver + + +	—	—	Hepatomegaly; mild growth retarda-tion; X-linked recessive inheri-tance in some
X	—	Cyclic 3'5'-AMP dependent kinase	Liver + + + muscle +	—	—	Hepatomegaly and possible muscle weakness, only, reported
XI	—	Unknown	Liver + + + kidney + + +	+ + +	+ + +	Rickets and growth failure secondary to renal Fanconi syndrome; resembles type I; no lactic acidosis

26. Why do patients with von Gierke's disease (type I glycogen storage disease) develop bleeding tendencies?

A platelet defect, presumably secondary, occurs in many patients with type I glycogen storage disease (glucose-6-phosphatase deficiency). Platelets from GSD I patients show impaired release of ADP in vitro in response to collagen and epinephrine. The cause is not known but may be related to secondary changes in platelet cholesterol or phospholipids.

27. What are the characteristic ECG findings in Pompe's disease (type II glycogen storage disease)?

Gigantic QRS complexes in all leads and abnormally short P-R interval.

28. What is the most common hyperlipidemia in childhood?

The common familial hyperlipidemias do not cause major clinical disease during childhood in their typical heterozygous or polygenic forms. However, type I hyperlipidemia commonly causes recurrent abdominal pain and hepatosplenomegaly in the first five years of life, and the even rarer patient with homozygous type II hyperlipidemia (1/1,000,000 births) may suffer from xanthomata and coronary artery disease in the first decade.

29. How are the primary genetic hyperlipidemias classified?

Classification of Primary Genetic Hyperlipidemias

FREDERICK-SON TYPE	LIPIDS ELEVATED	LIPOPROTEIN ELEVATION	PREVALENCE	CLINICAL FINDINGS*
I	Triglyceride	Chylomicrons	Rare	Eruptive xanthomas; pancreatitis; recurrent abdominal pain; lipemia retinalis; hepatosplenomegaly
IIa	Cholesterol	LDL	Common	Tendon xanthomas; PVD
IIb	Cholesterol, triglyceride	LDL + VLDL	Uncommon	PVD; no xanthomas
III	Cholesterol, triglyceride	VLDL remnants	Rare	PVD; yellow palm creases; hyperglycemia
IV	Triglyceride	VLDL	Uncommon	PVD; xanthomas; hyperglycemia
V	Triglyceride, cholesterol	VLDL + Chylomicrons	Very rare	pancreatitis; lipemia retinalis; xanthomas; hyperglycemia

LDL, low-density lipoprotein; VLDL, very low-density lipoprotein; PVD, premature vascular disease; GTT, glucose tolerance test.
*Most not manifest in childhood.

30. What are causes of secondary hyperlipidemia in childhood?
Obesity
Hypothyroidism
Diabetes mellitis
Autoimmune diseases
Lipodystrophies
Sphingolipidoses
Acute intermittent porphyria
Nephrotic syndrome; chronic renal failure
Glycogen storage disease (mostly type I)
Hepatitis, biliary atresia, and other biliary disorders
Congenital lactic acidoses, mitochondrial encephalomyopathies (some)
Progeria, Werner syndrome, Klinefelter syndrome, idiopathic hypercalcemia
Drugs: alcohol, oral contraceptives, thiazide diuretics, beta-adrenergic blocking agents

31. What is the treatment of choice for familial hypercholesterolemia?
Dietary restriction of cholesterol and fat plus a lipid-lowering resin such as cholestyramine.
Cholestyramine and the related resin, colestipol, lower plasma cholesterol by trapping bile
acids in the gut, causing more cholesterol to be shunted to bile acid synthesis. Nicotinic acid
(unknown mechanism) and plasmapheresis have also been used. Homozygous familial
hypercholesterolemia has been treated successfully in a few cases with orthotopic liver
transplantation. Inhibitors of the rate-limiting enzyme of cholesterol synthesis, hydroxymethyl glutaryl CoA reductase, are also available but not yet approved for use in children.
However, these will most likely have a major role in future therapy of hypercholesterolemia.

32. What are the indications for screening for hyperlipidemia in children?
Family history of hyperlipidemia, myocardial infarction or sudden unexplained death before
age 50, premature stroke, or skin xanthomas. Other softer indications include recurrent,
unexplained abdominal pain, unexplained persistent postprandial irritability in an infant, and
abnormally increased weight for height. Because the hyperlipidemias are, in sum, common
diseases (total incidence at least 1/100) in which much damage has been done by the time
clinical signs or symptoms appear, some advocate screening all children, at least in the early
post-pubertal years. However, normal plasma lipid levels in childhood do not rule out a
genetic hyperlipidemia, some of which may not be biochemically manifest until the third or
fourth decade.

33. What are the clinical features of the porphyrias?
A variety of neurovisceral symptoms and/or skin photosensitivity occur in acute attacks.
However, the combination and severity of clinical characteristics are not reliably disease-
specific. Rather, the clinical syndrome serves as a guide to selection of supplementary
diagnostic biochemical studies, and, ultimately, enzymatic assays in patients and other family
members. Because almost all of the porphyrias are inherited, many as autosomal dominant
defects with quite variable penetrance and expression, obtaining a detailed family history
when the disease is suspected is very important.

Neurovisceral Symptoms	Photosensitivity Skin Reactions
Abdominal pain and vomiting	Acute
Constipation, occas. diarrhea	Edematous skin plaques
Muscle weakness	Bullae and vesicle formation
Mental status changes	Urticaria
Peripheral nerve disease	Purpura
Hypertension and/or tachycardia	Chronic
Convulsions	Scarring, erosions, thickening
Bulbar paralysis	Hypertrichosis
Fever	Sensitivity to trauma
	Hyperpigmentation

Clinical Classification of the Major Porphyrias

DISEASE	NEUROVISCERAL ATTACKS	PHOTO-SENSITIVITY	HEPATIC DISEASE	HEMOLYTIC ANEMIA	AGE ONSET	INHERI-TANCE
Erythropoietic Porphyrias						
Erythropoietic porphyria	—	+ + + +	—	+ +	Childhood	AR
Erythropoietic protoporphyria	—	+ +	+ / −	—	Childhood	AD
Hepatic Porphyrias						
Acute intermittent porphyria	+ + + +	—	+	—	Post-pubertal	AD
Porphyria variegata	+ +	+ +	−	—	Post-pubertal	AD
Hereditary copro-porphyria	+ +	+	+ / − *	—	Post-pubertal	AD
Porphyria cutanea tarda	—	+ + +	+ + *	—	Adult	sporadic, some AD

AR, autosomal recessive; AD, autosomal dominant
*Probably a contributing cause (e.g., alcoholic liver disease) rather than primary manifestation of porphyria.

34. What is the metabolic defect and inheritance pattern in Wilson's disease?

Wilson's disease is an autosomal recessive defect of copper metabolism for which the primary biochemical lesion remains unknown. The major biochemical abnormalities include low serum ceruloplasmin, increased urinary copper excretion, decreased incorporation of copper into ceruloplasmin, and markedly increased levels of copper in, most notably, liver, basal ganglia, and cornea (Kayser-Fleischer ring).

35. What are the common clinical presentations of Wilson's disease?

Hepatic
      Jaundice and hepatitis
      Cirrhosis
      Fulminant hepatic failure
Hematologic
      Hemolytic anemia
Neurologic
      Psychiatric disturbance
      Extrapyramidal movement disorder
      Intellectual and behavioral deterioration
      Convulsions

36. How is the diagnosis of Wilson's disease confirmed?

The combination of markedly increased copper levels in a liver biopsy specimen (> 400 μg/gm wet weight), low serum ceruloplasmin, and increased urinary copper excretion is strongly suggestive of classic Wilson's disease, but not absolutely diagnostic. The additional finding of Kayser-Fleischer rings is nearly pathognomonic of Wilson's disease, but their absence, especially in children, does not rule out the disease. The most specific diagnostic test is the demonstration of the slow rate of disappearance of radiolabelled copper from the bloodstream. Newer methods include measurement of radioactive copper uptake and retention by cultured fibroblasts, which is increased in Wilson's disease.

37. What is the treatment of choice for Wilson's disease?

D-penicillamine, a copper-chelating agent. Another copper-chelating drug, trientine, has successfully treated patients with Wilson's disease who have discontinued penicillamine because of hypersensitivity reactions. Zinc sulfate, which inhibits intestinal copper absorption, has also been used for therapy of Wilson's disease.

38. What is the most commonly encountered lipid storage disorder in man?
Gaucher's disease, or glucosyl ceramide lipidosis, which is caused by a deficiency of β-glucocerebrosidase. The incidence varies from 1/100,000 in non-Jewish populations to 1/2500 in Ashkenazi Jews.

39. What lipid storage disorder should be suspected in patients with unexplained proteinuria?
Fabry's disease (alpha-galactosidase deficiency). Proteinuria is also a characteristic of several types of sialic acid storage disease presenting in the newborn period with nephrotic syndrome, coarse facial features, organomegaly, and other physical characteristics of lysosomal storage disorders.

40. What are the treatments of choice for urea cycle disorders?
Acute
> Peritoneal dialysis or hemodialysis
> Induced anabolism with high concentration glucose infusions
> Correction of amino acid deficiencies to prevent secondary catabolism
> Sodium benzoate and phenylacetate to increase ammonia excretion via alternate pathways
> Arginine for ammonia excretion as argininosuccinic acid in argininosuccinic aciduria

Maintenance
> Low-protein diet with supplemental essential amino acids
> Avoidance of fasting, fevers, or other catabolic stress
> Sodium benzoate, phenylacetate
> Supplementation with specific urea-cycle amino acids to prevent deficiency state (and subsequent catabolism) or to enhance ammonia excretion (e.g., arginine in argininosuccinic aciduria)

41. Other than urea cycle defects, what group of metabolic defects can cause neonatal hyperammonemia?
The organic acidemias, especially those often grouped as the "ketotic hyperglycinemias," are commonly associated with hyperammonemia during periods of metabolic decompensation. Defects of fatty acid oxidation, in particular medium- and long-chain acyl-CoA dehydrogenase deficiencies, may present as Reye-like syndromes in the neonatal period, but more commonly present in an older infant at the time of the first major infection. Transient, severe hyperammonemia without known cause is also seen in some premature neonates with respiratory distress.

42. Name the common causes of a false-positive test for urine-reducing substances.
Radiologic contrast dyes, stool contamination, antibiotics (especially ampicillin), pentosuria from pentose-enriched fruits (true positive but nonpathologic), and p-hydroxyphenylpyruvic acid (tyrosinemia).

43. What are the peroxisomal disorders?
Zellweger (cerebrohepatorenal) syndrome, a genetic multiple malformation syndrome, was the first disorder ascribed to a (generalized) defect of the peroxisome, a small intracellular organelle containing a variety of oxidative and synthetic pathways, mostly for lipid metabolism. Extensive studies of peroxisomal biochemistry in many neurologic and genetic diseases have since identified several other apparent primary defects of peroxisomal metabolism. These disorders are characterized by various combinations of hepatic, renal, adrenal, ophthalmologic, and neurologic abnormalities, and specific abnormalities of peroxisomal metabolism. The nosology of the diseases is very complicated and subject to revision. The primary metabolic defect is unknown in most. The following table lists the principal biochemical and clinical characteristics of the major peroxisomal disorders known. Leber's congenital amaurosis, Conradi-Hunermann chondrodysplasia, and isolated deficien-

cies of peroxisomal beta-ketothiolase and acyl CoA oxidase deficiency have been described as possible new peroxisomal diseases, but in too few cases to allow generalization about the clinical and biochemical characteristics or to be certain about their differentiation from existing categories.

Biochemical and Clinical Characteristics in the Peroxisomal Disorders

	Zellweger syndrome	Pseudo-Zellweger syndrome	Neonatal Adrenoleuko-dystrophy	X-linked Adrenoleuko-dystrophy	Infantile Refsum syndrome	Adult Refsum disease	Rhizomelic chondro-dysplasia punctata
Biochemical Abnormalities							
Metabolic Level							
Increased very long-chain fatty acids	+ + +	+ + +	+ + +	+ +	+ +	−	−
Increased urinary pipecolic acid	+ + +	+ + +	+ +	−	+ +	−	−
Increased plasma pipecolic acid	+	+	+ + +	−	+ +	−	−
Decreased tissue plasmalogens	+ + +	−	+ +	−	+ +	−	+ + +
Increased plasma phytanic acid	+	−	+	−	+ +	+ + +	+ +
Increased plasma bile acid intermediates	+ + +	+ + +	+ + +	−	+ + +		−
Clinical and Pathologic Characteristics							
Characteristic							
Abnormal facies	+ + +	+ +	+	−	+	−	+ + +
Congenital hypotonia	+ + +	+ + +	+ +	−	+ +	−	−
Neonatal seizures	+ +	+	+ +	−	+	−	−
Mental retardation	+ + +	+ + +	+ +	dementia	+ +	−	+ + +
Pigmentary retinopathy	+ +	#	+ +	−	+ +	+ + +	−
Sensory deafness	+ +	#	+ +	acquired	+ + +	+ +	−
Absent or diminished hepatic peroxisomes	+ + +	−	+	−	+	−	−
Hepatic fibrosis/cirrhosis	+ + +	+	+	−	+	−	−
Adrenal lipid inclusions and/or dysfunction	+	+ +	+ +	+ + +	#	−	−
Polycystic kidneys	+ + +	+ +	−	−	−	−	−
Epiphyseal or apophyseal calcific stippling	+ +	#	−	−	−	−	+ + +
Growth retardation	+ + +	+ + +	+	−	+	−	+ + +
Mean survival (yr)	0.6	0.9	3.0	9	>5	adult	1.0

= insufficient data.

Bibliography

1. Bondy PK, Rosenberg LE: Metabolic Control and Disease, 8th ed. Philadelphia, W. B. Saunders, 1980.
2. Cohn RM, Roth K: Metabolic Disease: A Guide to Early Recognition. Philadelphia, W. B. Saunders, 1983.
3. Cornblath M, Schwartz R: Disorders of Carbohydrate Metabolism in Infancy, 2nd ed. Philadelphia, W. B. Saunders, 1976.
4. DeGroot LA: Endocrinology, 2nd ed. Philadelphia, W. B. Saunders, 1988.
5. Felig P, et al: Endocrinology and Metabolism, 2nd ed. New York, McGraw-Hill, 1984.
6. Harrison HE, Harrison HC: Disorders of Calcium and Phosphate Metabolism in Childhood and Adolescence. Philadelphia, W. B. Saunders, 1979.
7. Nyhan WL, Sakati NA: Diagnostic Recognition of Genetic Disease. Philadelphia, Lea & Febiger, 1987.
8. Stanbury JB, et al.: The Metabolic Basis of Inherited Disease, 5th ed. New York, McGraw-Hill, 1983.

INFECTIOUS DISEASES

David S. Hodes, M.D.
Asher Barzilai, M.D.
Alexander C. Hyatt, M.D.
Mark F. Ditmar, M.D.

1. Why do serum iron levels fall significantly during the course of infections in children?

In most infections, serum iron levels decrease as iron is transferred from serum binding proteins to intracellular storage sites in the form of hemosiderin in reticuloendothelial cells. The added intracellular iron may aid in bacterial killing. Release is blocked until the infection has abated. Viral hepatitis is an exception. In viral hepatitis, serum iron may be normal or increased because of decreased uptake capability by hepatic reticuloendothelial cells and/or increased intracellular iron release by damaged hepatocytes.

Reference: Beisel WR: Metabolic response of heat to infections. In Feigin RD, Cherry JD (eds): Textbook of Pediatric Infectious Diseases, 2nd ed. Philadelphia, W.B. Saunders, 1987.

2. Does a viral infection respond better to antipyretic therapy than a bacterial infection?

Traditional theory had been that a viral illness should respond better to antipyretics (e.g., acetaminophen) than a bacterial infection. However, there is little difference in the pattern of response, and it is of no clinical help.

3. What is the differential diagnosis for children with recurrent or chronic sinusitis?

A common cause of recurrent or chronic sinusitis is damage to the sinusoidal mucosa resulting from acute infection. In this situation squamous metaplasia may occur, resulting in inadequate bacterial clearance from the sinuses and bacterial overgrowth. Exacerbations of disease may be looked upon as local inflammatory processes whose etiology is only circumstantially linked with such pathogens as *S. pneumoniae* and *H. influenzae*. Allergic causes and local and systemic immune defects such as immotile cilia syndrome, cystic fibrosis, agammaglobulinemia, and chronic granulomatous disease should also be sought. It is important that surgically resectable anatomic causes be excluded. Thus the patient should be examined for the presence of nasal polyps, foreign bodies, septal defects, and tumors.

4. How sensitive and specific are sinus films for diagnosing sinusitis?

For the older child and adult, x-ray studies provide an extremely sensitive and specific test for acute sinusitis. In children under 1 year of age and in all cases of chronic sinusitis, the utility of x-rays is quite limited. If the sinuses are completely opacified, transillumination can be virtually diagnostic. The utility of ultrasonography is currently under investigation.

5. How often is sinus tenderness elicited in radiologically proven cases of sinusitis?

In acute sinusitis, sinus tenderness is demonstrable only 20% of the time, and in chronic sinusitis, almost never.

6. Which organisms are responsible for acute and chronic sinusitis and mastoiditis in the pediatric age group?

In acute, uncomplicated sinusitis, the etiologic organisms closely parallel those associated with acute otitis media: *S. pneumoniae*, *H. influenzae*, and *B. catarrhalis*. *S. aureus* is rather rare. In nosocomial infections, gram-negative organisms are frequently recovered, whereas in the child with dental disease, anaerobes must be considered because of the proximity of the alveoli to the maxillary sinuses. Mucormycosis is also a concern in the immunosuppressed patient. Pseudomonas must always be considered in the patient with cystic fibrosis. While viruses may be responsible for the initiation of sinusitis, symptoms are invariably associated with bacterial superinfection. The precise role of bacterial infection in chronic sinusitis is unknown. Where studies have been done, the same bacteria implicated in acute infection have been found.

7. What are the indications for sinus drainage during the course of sinusitis?
Surgical intervention is seldom needed in uncomplicated cases of sinusitis. It is usually reserved for cases in which neurologic involvement has developed or appears imminent. Surgery may be required in patients with underlying immune disorders or anatomic obstructions, and should be considered as an option when appropriate medical management has failed to halt the disease process.

8. What are the indications for operative intervention in children with mastoiditis?
Most children with mastoiditis will need a conduit for pus to drain. The surgical approach to establishing such a conduit may be as simple as a tympanostomy tube. Posterior auricular fluctuance should be drained, and the procedure should be hastened if signs of neurologic involvement are detected.

9. How commonly does cerumen obscure the diagnosis of otitis media?
Secreted by sebaceous and apocrine glands at the base of hair follicles in the outer third of the ear, cerumen comes in all forms—wet and brown in blacks and whites, and dry and flaky in Orientals. Surprisingly, as many as 50% of white children have no obvious cerumen seen on inspection. When otitis media is part of a differential diagnosis (as in unexplained fever), cerumen must be removed to allow visualization of the tympanic membrane. As many as 30% of cases of otitis media are obscured by this waxy roadblock. Unfortunately, lack of pain is not a helpful clue in diagnosis in that 15–20% of children with otitis media do not have ear pain. The old tale of otitis media being associated with soft wax (from melting by the "hot ear") is unfounded, with that finding occurring in only 10% of cases.
   Reference: Schwartz RH, et al: Cerumen removal: How necessary is it to diagnose acute otitis media? Am J Dis Child 137:1065–1068, 1983.

10. What are the immediate and long-term complications of otitis media?
The most dangerous immediate complications of acute otitis media involve local suppurative spread to structures within the temporal bone and beyond into other compartments of the cranial vault. These include mastoiditis, labyrinthitis, facial nerve paralysis, osteomyelitis, epidural abscess, lateral sinus thrombosis, otic hydrocephalus, meningitis, and brain abscess. Fortunately, in the antibiotic era, these complications have become rare. Other complications include perforation of the tympanic membrane, tympanosclerosis, fixation of the ossicles, cholesteatoma, chronic otitis media, and hearing loss. There is evidence that repeated bouts of otitis media may have adverse effects on the development of speech.

11. What are the indications for prophylactic antibiotics in children with recurrent otitis media?
The minimal criterion for the initiation of antibiotic prophylaxis is three episodes of otitis in 6 months or four within a year.

12. Is there a role for decongestants in the management of children with otitis media?
Clinical trials have shown decongestants to be of no use.

13. How should children with serous otitis media be managed?
The traditional combination of decongestants and antihistamines has been found ineffective in clinical studies. This leaves a trial of antibiotics as the only rational (although unproven)

alternative. Antimicrobial agents similar to those used for acute otitis media are commonly used. Even this approach should be used with caution because the majority of middle ear effusions clear spontaneously within 2–3 months. An effusion present for more than 3 months which is unresponsive to antibiotics should prompt referral to an otolaryngologist.

14. What are the indications for tympanocentesis?

Experts have recommended tympanocentesis in the following situations: (1) the "toxic" appearing child; (2) unsatisfactory response to antibiotics; (3) any suppurative complication; (4) the immunosuppressed host; and (5) the newborn infant, in whom the usual pathogens (*S. pneumoniae, H. influenzae, B. catarrhalis*) may not be the causative agents.

15. What percentage of otitis media is caused by ampicillin-resistant organisms? How should these infections be treated?

At present, about 25% of *H. influenzae* and (from more limited data) 75% of *B. catarrhalis* infections have been shown to produce beta-lactamases (subject to local variation). Thus it can be estimated that about 20% of cases of otitis media, in an average location, will be resistant to ampicillin. Precise knowledge of local resistance patterns is a far better guide. Alternative therapies to ampicillin include cefaclor, trimethoprim-sulfamethoxazole, amoxicillin clavulanate, or erythromycin-sulfonamide.

16. What is quinsy?

Peritonsillar abscess (from Lower Latin for an inflammation of the throat).

17. How is peritonsillar abscess distinguished from peritonsillar cellulitis?

A peritonsillar abscess is diagnosed when a discrete mass is palpated. The bulging abscess causes displacement of the uvula. Trismus more commonly occurs in the setting of abscess than simple diffuse cellulitis, which is characterized by signs of diffuse inflammation only.

18. An intensely erythematous but nontender submandibular or tonsillar node is most suggestive of what infectious process?

Nontuberculous mycobacterium.

19. What are three absolute indications for tonsillectomy and adenoidectomy?

(1) Upper airway obstruction with sleep apnea and associated hypoxemia, carbon dioxide retention, pulmonary hypertension, or cor pulmonale; (2) chronic or recurrent peritonsillar abscess; and (3) suspected or proven tonsillar malignancy.

20. Can group A streptococcal pharyngitis be diagnosed clinically?

Streptococcal pharyngitis is a disease with variable clinical manifestations. Clues suggesting streptococcal disease include the abrupt onset of headache, fever, and sore throat with subsequent physical findings of tender cervical lymph nodes and exudate over the tonsils. The presence of concurrent conjunctivitis, rhinitis, and cough suggests a viral process. The physical findings are by no means diagnostic. Even the most skilled clinician cannot exceed an accuracy rate of about 75%. A throat culture is essential for confirming streptococcal infection.

   Reference: Breese BB, Hall CB: Beta Hemolytic Streptococcal Diseases. Boston, Houghton Mifflin, 1978.

21. What is the rationale for treatment of group A streptococcal pharyngitis?

The primary goal of treatment of group A streptococcal pharyngitis is to prevent acute rheumatic fever. Even with the marked decline in incidence of acute rheumatic fever in the United States, it is still prevalent in much of the world. It has also been found that, in comparison with placebo, penicillin can shorten the course of illness, relieve headache and sore throat, and reduce the frequency of tender cervical lymph nodes. An additional reason for treating streptococcal pharyngitis is to reduce the spread of infection and to prevent suppurative complications. Some cases of acute glomerulonephritis may also be prevented.

22. Should all children with a positive culture for group A streptococcus be treated?
Symptomatic children whose throat cultures yield group A beta hemolytic streptococci should be treated. There is a growing conviction among experts that asymptomatic children who are merely carrying streptococci should not be treated. An easy way to avoid the quandary is not to culture such children and sow the seeds of "streptococcal neurosis" in the family. This policy precludes the reculturing of asymptomatic children who have completed treatment for sore throats. An exception to the general rule of leaving asymptomatic carriers alone is the case of a carrier in household contact with a patient with rheumatic fever.
   Reference: Breese BB, Denny FW, Dillon HC, et al: Consensus: Difficult management problems in children with streptococcal pharyngitis. Pediatr Infect Dis 4:10–13, 1985.

23. What are the acceptable alternative therapies for streptococcal pharyngitis?
The alternatives are numerous. One popular regimen is IM benzathine penicillin, which has the advantage of guaranteed compliance but the disadvantage of being painful. Oral penicillin VK for 10 days is a good alternative. Erythromycin is the most widely recommended agent for penicillin-allergic patients, although many such patients will tolerate cephalosporins. Lincomycin and clindamycin are also acceptable. Sulfa drugs and tetracycline are not appropriate.

24. How long after the development of streptococcal pharyngitis can treatment be initiated and still effectively prevent rheumatic fever?
Treatment should be started as soon as possible, but little is lost in waiting for throat culture results to establish the diagnosis. Although such a delay is not desirable, significant reduction in the occurrence of rheumatic fever can still be achieved when therapy is delayed as long as 1 week.
   Reference: Markowitz M, Gordis L: Rheumatic Fever. Philadelphia, W.B. Saunders, 1972.

25. How should suspected pharyngitis in children under the age of three be managed?
Rheumatic fever in children under the age of three is rare, and therapy is principally aimed at preventing other complications. The rationale for culturing and treating described earlier applies to the younger age group as well.

26. How should febrile infants <3 months and 3–24 months be evaluated and managed?
In all age groups the evaluation should begin with a history (with particular emphasis on infectious illnesses in contacts) and a physical examination. If these investigations are unrevealing, we suggest the following:
   General
         Blood cultures (x2)
         Complete blood count
         Urinalysis and urine culture
         Lumbar puncture (may be omitted in a child ≥ 6 months of age who is not "toxic" and who has no meningeal signs)
   Less than 3 months of age
         If studies do not reveal a focal infection, admit to hospital and administer ampicillin and gentamicin, pending results of cultures.
   3–24 months of age
         If child does not appear toxic and the parents are reliable, observe at home; if either of these conditions is not met, admit to hospital and treat with cefuroxime or ceftriaxone, pending culture results.
   All children with fever over 104°F and WBC counts over 15,000/mm³ should be admitted. (At present teaching hospital–based pediatricians tend to hospitalize febrile infants more often than do private pediatricians, owing in large part to the latter's certainty of continued follow-up.)

27. Is there a risk in performing a lumbar puncture in a bacteremic infant?

A definitive estimate of this risk in humans is not available. Such an estimate would require a systematic study, taking into account such variables as the magnitude of the bacteremia, the amount of blood introduced into the CSF, and the patient's immune status. It is unlikely that such a study could ever be performed, and even if it were, its application to individual cases would be impossible. Suffice to say that the risk is small and would never outweigh the risk of not doing a lumbar puncture.

Reference: Klein JO, Feigin RD, McCracken GH: Report of the task force on the diagnosis and treatment of meningitis. Pediatrics 78:959–982, 1986.

28. What are the causes of lymphadenitis in normal, otherwise healthy children?

In order of frequency of occurrence: (1) *Staphylococcus aureus,* (2) group A beta hemolytic streptococci, (3) *M. tuberculosis,* and (4) atypical mycobacteria.

29. What are the indications for lymph node biopsy or aspiration in a child with adenopathy/adenitis?

Tissue diagnosis should be sought when:
  malignancy is a consideration, i.e.:
      in all children with supraclavicular adenopathy
      in all children with nodes fixed to skin or deep tissue
      in children with persistent fever and weight loss without a specific diagnosis
  atypical mycobacteria are suspected
  a patient fails to respond to antimicrobial agents specific for the common etiologic
      agents
Many authorities suggest biopsy of all nodes remaining enlarged after 3 months of observation. Earlier biopsy can be done if the nodes demonstrate continued growth.

Reference: Knight PJ, Mulne AF, Vassy LE: When is lymph node biopsy indicated in children with enlarged peripheral nodes? Pediatrics 69:341, 1982.

30. What therapy is recommended for children with acute lymphadenitis?

For a healthy child with adenopathy in whom tuberculosis is ruled out, a trial of a penicillinase-resistant penicillin such as oxacillin should be started.

31. How is orbital cellulitis distinguished from periorbital (or preseptal) cellulitis?

Periorbital cellulitis is inflammation/infection in the tissues anterior to the eyelid septum. Orbital cellulitis is a deeper and more dangerous extension into the orbit which may lead to abscess formation and/or cavernous sinus thrombosis. Clinically, the most important evaluations are ocular mobility (e.g., extraocular muscle function), pupillary reflex, visual acuity, and changes in globe position (e.g., proptosis). In periorbital cellulitis, these aspects are normal. Abnormalities in any of these four areas suggests the deeper infection of orbital cellulitis, mandating radiologic evaluation (usually CT scan of the orbit) and possible surgical drainage. Significant eyelid swelling may occur in both types, making visualization of the globe difficult. However, an adequate exam usually can be obtained using eyelid retractors. Although most cases are unilateral (90%), evaluation of the unaffected eye may be helpful. Occasionally, a reflex sympathetic response of abnormal ocular mobility occurs in the unaffected eye, suggesting the deeper infection.

32. Which agents are known to cause food poisoning in children? How can these agents be distinguished by history and clinical presentation?

Food poisoning is best defined as a gastrointestinal upset resulting in nausea, vomiting, and diarrhea, with or without fever, and appearing within 72 hours of ingestion of food contaminated by microorganisms or toxins. The likely offending agents vary according to the nature and time of onset of symptoms after the ingestion.

  Onset within 1–6 hours, nausea and vomiting, no fever
      Staphylococcus aureus toxin
      Bacillus cereus

Continued on next page.

Abdominal cramps and diarrhea within 8–16 hours
  Clostridium perfringens
  Bacillus cereus
Fever, abdominal cramps, diarrhea within 16–48 hours
  Salmonella
  Shigella
  Vibrio parahemolyticus
  Invasive *E. coli*
  Campylobacter jejuni
Abdominal cramps, watery diarrhea within 16–72 hours
  Enterotoxigenic *E. coli*
  Vibrio parahemolyticus
  Vibrio cholerae, non-OI
  Vibrio cholerae, OI (endemic area)
Fever, abdominal cramps within 16–48 hours
  Yersinia enterocolitica
Nausea, vomiting, paralysis within 18–36 hours
  Clostridium botulinum

Reference: Mandell GL, Douglas RG, Bennett JE (eds): Principles and Practice of Infectious Diseases, 2nd ed. New York, John Wiley and Sons, 1985, pp. 681–682, with permission.

33. What bacterial and viral agents are known to cause diarrhea in the pediatric age group? What are the distinguishing characteristics of the diseases caused by these pathogens?

Three Types of Enteric Infection

	I	II	III
Mechanism:	Noninflammatory (enterotoxin)	Inflammatory (invasion, ?cytotoxin)	Penetrating
Location:	Proximal small bowel	Colon	Distal small bowel
Illness:	Watery diarrhea	Dysentery	Enteric fever
Stool exam:	No fecal leukocytes	Fecal polymorphonuclear leukocytes	Fecal mononuclear leukocytes
Examples:	*V. cholerae*	Shigella	*S. typhi*
	E. coli (LT)	Invasive *E. coli*	*Y. enterocolitica*
	E. coli (ST)	*S. enteritidis*	?*C. fetus*
	?Salmonella	*V. parahemolyticus*	
	?*V. parahemolyticus*	*C. difficile*	
	Giardia lamblia	?*C. jejuni*	
	Rotavirus	*E. histolytica*	
	Norwalk-like viruses		
	Cryptosporidia		

From Mandell GL, Douglas RG, Bennett JE (eds): Principles and Practice of Infectious Diseases, 2nd ed. New York, John Wiley and Sons, 1985, p 641, with permission.

34. How is the diagnosis of pseudomembranous colitis made? Which antibiotics are most commonly associated with this disease?

Pseudomembranous colitis is a severe condition seen in patients undergoing intensive antibiotic therapy. It is associated with profuse diarrhea, which may be watery or mucoid, and is usually green, foul-smelling, and often bloody, and is accompanied by abdominal cramps. Fever and leukocytosis are common, and stool smears frequently show leukocytes. Diagnosis is made by sigmoidoscopy, which reveals pseudomembranous plaques or nodules. The causative agent is toxin-producing *C. difficile*. Pseudomembranous colitis occurs most frequently after treatment with cephalosporin, ampicillin, and clindamycin, but many antibiotics may predispose to the condition.

35. What are the therapeutic alternatives for treatment of pseudomembranous colitis?

If the disease is not severe, children may be treated with withdrawal of antibiotics and good supportive care. More severely ill children should be treated with oral vancomycin or metronidazole. Some clinicians have advocated cholestyramine to bind *C. difficile* toxin.

36. How common is asymptomatic *Clostridium difficile* carriage?

C. difficile is the agent most often implicated in antibiotic-associated colitis. Fever, abdominal pain, and bloody diarrhea begin as early as a few days after starting antibiotics (especially clindamycin, ampicillin, cephalosporins). The diagnosis in infancy is more difficult because the carriage rate for *C. difficile* is relatively high. Neonates have a colonization rate of about 20%, infants 30–40%, older children 10%, and adolescents 5%. Toxin assays are more indicative of *C. difficile*-associated disease than culture. However, the toxin may be present without any symptoms, especially in infants.

37. Which bacterial causes of gastroenteritis respond to antimicrobial therapy?

Antimicrobial Therapy for Gastroenteritis

ENTEROPATHOGEN	ANTIBIOTIC
Shigella	TMP-SMX (as 10 mg TMP/kg/day PO or IV q12h for 5 days) or ampicillin if sensitive (100 mg/kg/day PO, IV or IM in divided doses q6h for 5 days)
Campylobacter jejuni	Erythromycin PO will reduce shedding (40 mg/kg/day in divided doses q6h for 5–7 days). For severe illness: erythromycin, aminoglycoside or chloramphenicol IV

Salmonella	Treat:
	    Infants <6–12 months
	    Bacteremia
	    Metastatic foci (e.g., osteomyelitis)
	    Children with specific underlying illnesses
	        Ampicillin or TMP-SMX as for *Shigella*
	        Amoxicillin, 50 mg/kg/day PO in divided doses q8h for 5–7 days
	        Chloramphenicol, 75 mg/kg/day PO or IV in divided doses q6h for 5–7days

Escherichia coli	Neonates
	    EPEC (enteropathogenic): gentamicin (≤7 days old, 5 mg/kg/day q12h) (>7 days old, 7.5 mg/kg/day q8h) (or neomycin)
	Invasive
	    EIEC (enteroinvasive): same as *Shigella*
	    ETEC (enterotoxigenic): none or TMP-SMX (same as Shigella or bismuth subsalicylate*)

Yersinia enterocolitica	Gastroenteritis: none Sepsis: gentamicin (same as for *Escherichia coli*), chloramphenicol (same as for Salmonella) or TMP-SMX (same as for Shigella)
Clostridium difficile	Vancomycin, 10–40 mg/kg/day PO in divided doses q6h for 7 days Metronidazole, 15–40 mg/kg/day PO in divided doses q8h for 7 days
Aeromonas hydrophila	Same as *Shigella* ?Efficacy

From Williams EK, Lohr, JA, Guerradt RL: Acute infectious diarrhea. II. Diagnosis, treatment and prevention. Pediatr Infect Dis J 5:463, 1986.
*Risk of salicylate overdose.
TMP-SMX, trimethoprim-sulfamethoxazole; PO, orally; qxh, every x hours.

38. When should children with Salmonella gastroenteritis be treated?

Consensus management plan for an infant less than 1 year of age with diarrhea who does not require hospitalization at the initial evaluation

I. First evaluation		
A. Colitis (dysentery, fecal leukocytes)	0–12 months	Stool culture Blood culture if <3 months
B. No colitis Diarrhea <5 days	0–12 months	No stool culture Evaluate for nonbacterial causes if indicated
C. History of exposure to Salmonella	0–3 months	Stool culture Blood culture
II. Follow-up evaluation		
A. Diarrhea ≥5 days	0–12 months	Stool culture
B. Stool culture positive Blood culture positive	0–12 months	Admit* Blood culture (repeat) Antibiotics†
C. Stool culture positive; blood culture negative		
1. Toxic, ill, immunocompromised	0–12 months	Admit* Blood culture Antibiotics†
2. Febrile	≤3 months	Admit* Blood culture Antibiotics†
3. Febrile	>3 months	Admit* Blood culture Withhold antibiotics pending blood culture results
4. Afebrile, improving	0–12 months	Reexamine; observe at home
D. Stool culture positive, blood culture not obtained at first visit		See Category C, II

From St. Geme JW III, Hodes HL, Marcy SM, et al: Consensus: management of *Salmonella* infection in the first year of life. Pediatr Infect Dis J 7:615–621, 1988, with permission.
*Includes evaluation for focal infection of meninges, bone, urinary tract, or other sites.
†Cefotaxime, ceftriaxone.

39. How is giardiasis diagnosed?

Identification of cysts in stool specimens is the most common clue to diagnosis; however, this is difficult because excretion may be inconsistent. More than one stool specimen must be examined. Employing Lugol iodine on the stool specimen may help in identifying trophozoites. An alternative diagnostic method is the swallowing of a weighted string (entero test). This allows for the examination of duodenal mucus. Jejunal biopsy is currently believed to be the most sensitive method of diagnosis but it is the most invasive.

40. What clinical features are suggestive of giardiasis?

Most infants and children infected with Giardia are asymptomatic. In the acute form of giardiasis, patients may have diarrhea (93%), weight loss (73%), abdominal cramps (77%), abdominal distention (62%), nausea, and vomiting. Chronic giardiasis is associated with a chronic malabsorption syndrome, which includes protuberance of the abdomen, spindly extremities, and growth retardation. Peripheral or generalized edema and pallor may also occur.

41. Which drugs are effective in eradicating Giardia?

Atabrine (quinacrine) is the drug of choice and can be given orally in a dose of 6 mg/kg/day for 10 days. The daily dose should not exceed 300 mg. Furoxone (furazolidone) in a dose of 8 mg/kg/day for 10 days is also very effective. Flagyl (metronidazole) 15 mg/kg/day also has been recommended for children.

42. How can the WHO oral electrolyte (rehydration) solution be duplicated?

The WHO solution is 2% glucose, 20 mEq K^+/L, 90 mEq Na^+/L, 80 mEq Cl^-/L and 30 mEq bicarbonate/L. This solution is approximated by adding ¾ teaspoon of salt, 1 teaspoon of baking soda, 1 cup of orange juice (for KCl), and 8 teaspoons of sugar to a liter of water.

43. What are the common presentations for Epstein-Barr virus (EBV) infections?

EBV infections are frequently asymptomatic in young children. In adolescents and young adults the exact ratio of symptomatic to asymptomatic infections is unclear, but the classic illness is that of infectious mononucleosis. The symptoms and signs vary in individual cases and the following tables present a summary. Neurologic symptoms are rare but may include encephalitis, meningitis, myelitis, Guillain-Barré syndrome, or cranial or peripheral neuropathies. In children with X-linked lymphoproliferative syndrome, EBV infection may be life-threatening or may induce malignancy or hypogammaglobulinemia.

Manifestations of EBV-Induced Infectious Mononucleosis

Clinical
    Fever
    Sore throat
    Lymphadenopathy
Hematologic
    More than 50 percent mononuclear cells
    More than 10 percent atypical lymphocytes
Serologic
    Transient appearance of heterophile antibodies
    Permanent emergence of antibodies to EBV

Signs of Infectious Mononucleosis

SIGN	RATE	PERCENT	RANGE (%)
Lymphadenopathy	495/526	94	93–100
Pharyngitis	444/526	84	69–91
Fever	399/526	76	63–100
Splenomegaly	244/470	52	50–63
Hepatomegaly	34/370	9	6–14
Palatal enanthem	18/156	11	5–13
Jaundice	37/426	9	4–10
Rash	49/470	10	0–15

Symptoms of Infectious Mononucleosis

SYMPTOM	RATE	PERCENT	RANGE (%)
Sore throat	409/502	82	70–88
Malaise	243/426	57	43–76
Headache	216/426	51	37–55
Anorexia	117/546	21	10–27
Myalgias	66/326	20	12–22
Chills	54/326	16	9–18
Nausea	18/156	12	2–17
Abdominal discomfort	37/426	9	2–14
Cough	3/56	5	5
Vomiting	3/56	5	5
Arthralgias	1/56	2	2

Tables from Mandell GL, Douglas RG, Bennett JE (eds): Principles and Practice of Infectious Diseases, 2nd ed. New York, John Wiley and Sons, 1985, p 974, with permission.

44. What are the clinical signs and serologic findings of chronic EBV infection?

The syndrome of chronic EBV infection has aroused considerable controversy. The syndrome is described as consisting of at least 2 months of persistent or relapsing fatigue, necessitating cessation of normal activities. Also seen are myalgias, intermittent fevers, sore throat, arthralgias, and headache. It has been most commonly described in adult women. In some studies the patients' serologies were marked by elevated titers against early antigen D, and high levels of IgG directed against the viral capsid antibody. Palpable splenomegaly was often noted. Clear delineation of the syndrome and the role of EBV in producing it has been complicated by the fact that asymptomatic individuals may also exhibit the "characteristic" antibody pattern and by the vagueness of the symptoms.

45. What is the differential diagnosis for a positive heterophile test?

Heterophile antibodies are those that react to multiple antigens of varying genetic flavor. EBV infections elicit these antibodies, which cross-react with beef RBCs but not guinea pig kidney cells, even though the antigen is not coded for by the EBV genome. Using various absorptions, a positive heterophile test is highly specific for infectious mononucleosis.

Unabsorbed heterophile	Heterophile after absorption with beef RBCs	Heterophile after absorption with guinea pig kidney	Interpretation
+	−	+	infectious mononucleosis
+	+	−	normal variant
+	−	−	serum sickness

46. What are the indications for the use of steroids in children with EBV infection?

Steroids are indicated in EBV infection for the relief of respiratory obstruction due to swollen tonsils. Some authorities have advocated their use in severe autoimmune hemolytic anemia and for neurologic complications.

47. What are the serologic responses to EBV infection?

Patients make serologic responses to viral capsid antigens, early antigens (D and R), nuclear antigen, and soluble complement-fixing antigen. Neutralizing antibodies are also synthesized but few laboratories measure them.

Serologic Responses to EBV

ANTIBODY SPECIFICITY	TIME OF APPEARANCE IN INFECTIOUS MONONUCLEOSIS	PERCENTAGE OF EBV-INDUCED MONONUCLEOSIS CASES WITH ANTIBODY	PERSISTENCE	COMMENTS
Viral capsid antigen				
IgM VCA	At clinical presentation	100	4–8 weeks	Highly sensitive and specific but difficult to perform
IgG VCA	At clinical presentation	100	Lifelong	Higher titer at presentation and lifelong persistence make IgG VCA more useful as epidemiologic tool than in diagnosis of individual case
Early antigen (EA)				
Anti-D	Peaks at 3–4 weeks after onset	70	3–6 months	Correlated with severe disease; also seen in nasopharyngeal carcinoma
Anti-R	2 weeks to several months after onset	Low	2 months to >3 years	Occasionally seen with unusually severe or protracted illness; also seen in African Burkitt's lymphoma

Table continued on next page.

Serologic Responses to EBV *(Continued)*

ANTIBODY SPECIFICITY	TIME OF APPEARANCE IN INFECTIOUS MONONUCLEOSIS	PERCENTAGE OF EBV-INDUCED MONONUCLEOSIS CASES WITH ANTIBODY	PERSISTENCE	COMMENTS
Epstein-Barr nuclear antigen (EBNA)	3–4 weeks after onset	100	Lifelong	Late appearance helpful in diagnosis of heterophile-negative cases
Soluble complement-fixing antigen (anti-S)	3–4 weeks after onset	100	Lifelong	Late appearance helpful in diagnosis of heterophile-negative cases
Neutralizing antibodies	3–4 weeks after onset	100	Lifelong	Technically difficult to perform

From Mandell GL, Douglas RG, and Bennett JE (eds): Principles and Practice of Infectious Diseases, 2nd ed. New York, John Wiley and Sons, 1985, p 977, with permission.

48. What are the most common agents responsible for bacterial meningitis?

Common Agents Causing Bacterial Meningitis

0–2 MONTHS	2 MONTHS–6 YEARS	6–18 YEARS
E. coli	*H. influenzae*	*S. pneumoniae*
Group B streptococci	*S. pneumoniae*	*N. meningitidis*
Listeria monocytogenes	*N. meningitidis*	
Miscellaneous Enterobacteriaceae		

49. Children of what age are more susceptible to bacterial meningitis?
Ninety percent of cases occur in children between 1 month and 5 years of age. Children between 6 and 12 months are at greatest risk. One must recall that certain children constitute special cases and are susceptible to unusual organisms. For example, the child who has had a neurosurgical apparatus inserted is prone to staphylococcal meningitis. The child exposed to older individuals under crowded living conditions may develop tuberculous meningitis.

50. How commonly is *H. influenzae* type b isolated from throat cultures of normal children?
Carriage of *H. influenzae* type b in the throats of normal children is relatively rare—3–4% is a common estimate. Nasopharyngeal carriage of *H. influenzae* type b strains averages 3–5%. In "closed" populations of young children (e.g., day care centers) the rates can be as high as 50%.

51. Why is *H. influenzae* type b more virulent than nontypable Hemophilus strains?
Typable *H. influenzae* exhibits a polysaccharide capsule. This is thought to enhance virulence by inhibiting phagocytosis, but it is likely that other factors are involved in determining the virulence of *H. influenzae* as well.

52. What effects do phenobarbital and phenytoin have on chloramphenicol blood levels?
Chloramphenicol may potentiate the effect of barbiturates, whereas barbiturates may decrease the effectiveness of chloramphenicol by promoting glucuronidation. The effects are of marginal clinical significance. Chloramphenicol produces a clinically significant enhancement of phenytoin toxicity, often inducing nystagmus and ataxia.

53. How should the dose of chloramphenicol be readjusted when the route of administration is switched from intravenous to oral?
Chloramphenicol is extremely well absorbed by the oral route, and blood levels closely approximate those achieved by IV infusion. A total dose of 50–100 mg/kg/day in 3–4 divided

doses is appropriate for both modes of administration. Neonates should receive 25–50 mg/kg, depending on their size and age.

54. How often should chloramphenicol levels be monitored?

In neonates chloramphenicol toxicity manifested by circulatory collapse ("gray baby syndrome") occurs because hepatic metabolism of the drug is poor. It is necessary to determine serum levels frequently (daily to every other day) to anticipate this complication. The serum chloramphenicol level should be maintained between 10–25 μg/ml. In older children, this syndrome is not seen and the only common side effect is a reversible bone marrow depression that is seldom clinically significant. Monitoring of serum drug levels is unnecessary. Twice weekly blood counts suffice. The fatal aplastic anemia that follows chloramphenicol treatment in 1 in every 20,000–40,000 cases is apparently idiosyncratic, non-dose dependent, and cannot be avoided by drug level monitoring.

55. What are the drugs of choice for meningitis due to *H. influenzae* type b, *S. pneumoniae*, *N. meningitidis*, *L. monocytogenes*, *S. agalactae*, and *E. coli*?

Drugs of Choice for Meningitis

ORGANISM	DRUGS OF CHOICE
H. influenzae type b	Third generation cephalosporins
	Chloramphenicol
S. pneumoniae	Penicillin, vancomycin,* chloramphenicol*
N. meninigitidis	Third-generation cephalosporins
	Penicillin
L. monocytogenes	Ampicillin plus aminoglycoside
S. agalactae	Penicillin, ampicillin
E. coli	Third-generation cephalosporins, imipenem

*For relatively resistant organisms.

56. How long should children with bacterial meningitis be treated?

Recent investigations suggest that 7 days is probably sufficient for children beyond the newborn period. Surveys of pediatric infectious disease specialists reveal that their treatments average 10 days in length. For newborn infants, 3 weeks is recommended. Pediatricians would do well to consider each case individually. If the child is younger and more ill-appearing or if an unusual organism is involved, antibiotics should be given for a longer duration.

57. What are the classic sites of metastatic spread of infection with *H. influenzae* type b bacteremia?

H. influenzae typically spreads to the skin, lungs, epiglottis, joints, and meninges.

58. What are the indications for antimicrobial prophylaxis for *N. meningitidis* infections? How should the contacts be managed?

Antibiotic prophylaxis (rifampin or, if the isolate is know to be sensitive, sulfonamide) is indicated in household, day care, or nursery school contacts of active cases. Only those medical personnel who have had intimate contact with the patient (e.g., through intubation or mouth-to-mouth resuscitation) need to receive antibiotic prophylaxis. Surveillance cultures of contacts should not determine the need for prophylaxis. The most important aspect of prophylaxis is close clinical surveillance of the contacts for fever or malaise.

59. What are the common side effects of rifampin?

It turns the urine red and may permanently stain soft contact lenses.

60. What are the recommendations for rifampin prophylaxis after diagnosis of *H. influenzae* type b infection in a young child?

Rifampin is recommended for contacts in households with young children. Household contacts include those who spent 4 hours or more with the patient in at least 5 of the 7 days preceding the illness. More specifically, prophylaxis is suggested for all those in households where at least one of the patient's contacts is less than 2 years of age and has not been effectively immunized against *H. influenzae*. Prophylaxis for pregnant women is not recommended. The index case should also receive prophylaxis during the latter part of the hospital course. This reduces *H. influenzae* carriage. There is no consensus concerning prophylaxis in day care and nursery school settings.

61. How long after treatment has been initiated must individuals with meningitis remain in respiratory isolation?

24 hours.

62. What are the Damrosch criteria?

The Damrosch criteria define a poor prognosis for patients with meningococcal infection:
  1. Presence of petechiae for less than 12 hours prior to admission
  2. Shock
  3. Absence of meningitis (fewer than 20 WBCs in CSF)
  4. Normal or low peripheral WBC count
  5. Low or normal ESR

The presence of 3 or more criteria indicate a poor prognosis.

Reference: Stiehm ER, Damrosch DS: Factors in the prognosis of meningococcal infection. J. Pediatr 68:457–467, 1966.

63. How quickly is the CSF sterilized in children with meningitis?

In successful therapy, CSF is usually sterile within 36–48 hours of initiation of antibiotics.

Reference: Kagan BM: Antimicrobial Therapy, 3rd ed. Philadelphia, W.B. Saunders, 1980.

64. What are the causes of prolonged or secondary fever in children with bacterial meningitis?

In many cases, particularly those involving *H. influenzae,* prolonged fever may be considered part of the "natural" history of the treated disease. Fevers lasting 8–9 days are not uncommon. If a repeat lumbar puncture early in the course of therapy reveals sterile CSF, the physician can be reassured. Suppurative CNS complications such as subdural empyema are extremely rare and will usually be accompanied by a rocky clinical course. Other sites of infection, such as joints and lung, should be sought. Drug fever is a diagnosis of exclusion. Secondary fevers in children with meningitis are common, usually brief, and most commonly unexplained. In cases where the specific etiology is determined, intercurrent viral infections and phlebitis are the most common diagnoses. The demonstration of a sterile CSF early in the course of therapy is always reassuring.

65. How common are subdural effusions noted in bacterial meningitis? How should they be managed?

Subdural effusions are common in bacterial meningitis and should be considered part and parcel of the disease rather than a complication of it. Estimates of the incidence of subdural effusions vary from 10 to 50%. The incidence is highest in younger infants and in patients with *H. influenzae* meningitis. Most authorities now agree that routine tapping of subdural effusions is unnecessary. Removal of fluid is reserved for patients showing signs of increased intracranial pressure or focal neurologic signs.

Reference: Feigin RD, Cherry JD (eds): Textbook of Pediatric Infectious Diseases, 2nd ed. Philadelphia, W.B. Saunders Co., 1987, p 446.

66. What is the neurologic outcome in children with bacterial meningitis?

In children beyond the newborn period, the incidence of sequelae is about 10–15%, including persistent paralysis, abnormal tone, ataxia, and visual and hearing disorders. Hydrocephalus is very rare. Careful follow-up is needed in assessing estimates, since many deficits present on discharge will resolve with time. The effect of bacterial meningitis on IQ is difficult to assess, but the presence of neurologic abnormalities in the initial illness indicates a poor prognosis.

67. Which bacterial meningitides are more likely to cause permanent hearing loss?

A prospective study of 185 patients with meningitis who were followed for 5 years found that *S. pneumoniae* infections were associated with the greatest likelihood of persistent unilateral or bilateral hearing loss. The percentage of each group developing hearing loss was: *S. pneumoniae*, 31%; *N. meningitidis*, 10%, and *H. influenzae*, 6%.

Reference: Dodge PR, et al: Prospective evaluation of hearing impairment as a sequelae of acute bacterial meningitis. N Engl J Med 311:869–874, 1984.

68. What are the indications for retapping a child with bacterial meningitis?

It is widely agreed that the child who shows no clinical response to therapy in 24–48 hours should be retapped. Some physicians retap all children at this point and some retap at the end of therapy.

69. What are the clinical presentations of acquired cytomegalovirus (CMV) infection?

When it is symptomatic, acquired CMV infection in normal hosts produces fever, malaise, and nonspecific aches and pains. The peripheral blood smear reveals an absolute lymphocytosis and many atypical lymphocytes. In contrast to EBV-infectious mononucleosis, lymphadenopathy and tonsillitis are not prominent. Liver involvement is very common and liver function tests reveal abnormalities. Like EBV disease, CMV mononucleosis can persist for several weeks.

70. What are the means of vertical transmission of CMV from mother to infant?

Vertical transmission of CMV from mother to child can occur transplacentally, natally, or postnatally. The first route of transmission is associated with more severe complications, but the latter two are probably 5–10 times as common. Natally, maternal cervical secretions are the likely source of infection, whereas postnatally breast milk is probably the most important source of infection, with saliva and possibly urine also being important routes of transmission.

71. What is the long-term morbidity of pre- and postnatally acquired CMV?

Prenatally acquired CMV infection, in its severest form, presents with microcephaly, intracranial calcifications, hepatitis, splenomegaly, pneumonia, chorioretinitis, anemia, and thrombocytopenia. The outlook in this situation is grim, with many babies dying and virtually all the rest showing brain damage. Even children with occult, prenatally acquired CMV are at risk for sensorineural hearing defects and learning problems. Although acquired CMV infection produces life-threatening systemic infection in immunosuppressed hosts and transplant patients, it produces only self-limited disease in normal children.

72. Are any antiviral agents effective in eradicating CMV?

No currently available antiviral agent is effective. Gancyclovir, an experimental drug, may be licensed in the near future.

73. What are the most sensitive and specific ways to identify children with CMV infections?

Diagnostic Criteria for CMV Infection

CLINICAL SETTING	CULTURE	IgG ANTIBODY	IgM ANTIBODY	CYTOLOGY	ANTIGEN DETECTION
Congenital	+ + + + (if positive within 1–2 weeks of birth)	+	±	+	−
Perinatal	+ + + + (if negative at birth and positive 3–4 weeks postnatally)	+	±	±	−
Healthy	+ +	+ + + +	+ + + (if seroconversion demonstrated)	±	−
Immunocompromised	+	+	+	±	+ + +

From Drew WL: Diagnosis of cytomegalovirus infection. Rev Infect Dis 10 (Suppl. 3):S468–474, 1988, with permission.

Note: The diagnostic utility of results is given from + to + + + +, the higher the value the greater the utility; ± = false-positives and/or false-negatives possible.

74. When is a fever considered a fever of unknown origin (FUO)?

The definition of FUO, for clinical purposes, is the presence of fever for 8 or more days in a child in whom a careful and thorough history and physical examination and preliminary laboratory data fail to reveal the probable cause of the fever.

75. How should a child with FUO be evaluated?

The most common causes of FUO in children are infectious diseases, connective tissue diseases, and neoplasms. In about 10–20% of cases, a definitive diagnosis is never established. FUO is more likely to be an unusual presentation of a common disorder rather than a common presentation of a rare disorder. After a complete and detailed history and physical examination, the pediatrician should avoid indiscriminately ordering a large battery of tests. The laboratory studies should be directed as much as possible toward the most likely diagnostic possibilities.

76. What are the principal diagnostic criteria for Kawasaki disease?

The diagnosis of mucocutaneous lymph node syndrome, or Kawasaki disease, is a clinical diagnosis. Characteristically there is a combination of prolonged high fevers, erythema multiforme–like rashes, stomatitis, conjunctivitis, palmar erythema, indurative edema of the hands and feet, and cervical lymphadenopathy.

77. What are the clinical stages of Kawasaki disease? What are the pathologic findings in each stage?

Kawasaki Syndrome: Disease Phases, Complications, and Degree of Arteritis

	ACUTE (duration 1–11 days)	SUBACUTE (duration 11–21 days)	CONVALESCENT (duration 21–60 days)	CHRONIC (duration ? years)
Clinical findings:	Fever, conjunctivitis oral changes, extremity changes, irritability	Irritability persists; prolongation of fever may occur; normalization of most clinical findings; palpable aneurysms may develop	Most clinical findings resolve; aneurysmal dilatation of peripheral vessels may persist; conjunctivitis may persist	
Arterial correlates:	Perivasculitis, vasculitis of capillaries, arterioles, and venules; inflammation of intima of medium and larger arteries	Aneurysms, thrombi, stenosis of medium-sized arteries, panvasculitis, and edema of vessel wall; myocarditis less prominent	Vascular inflammation decreases	Scar formation; intimal thickening

From Hicks RV, Melish ME: Kawasaki syndrome. Pediatr Clin North Am 33:1151–1175, 1986, with permission.

78. What etiologic agents have been suggested in Kawasaki's disease?
Although there has been considerable progress in understanding the pathogenesis of Kawasaki syndrome, the inciting agent remains undiscovered. Toxic agents such as mercury and lead, and allergic and immunologic causes have been studied as potential causative factors. Numerous case reports and clinical series report infectious agents associated with Kawasaki disease, including rickettsiae, *Klebsiella pneumoniae,* Escherichia species, para-influenza virus, Epstein-Barr virus, and rotavirus. The association between Kawasaki disease and shampooing or spot-cleaning rugs or carpets has been studied as well as the importance of mites. Recent studies have focused on *Propionibacterium acnes* and retroviruses.

79. What are the recommended primary and secondary therapies for Kawasaki disease?
Intravenous administration of immunoglobulin (400 mg/kg per day for 5 days) early in the course of the disease has been shown to ameliorate symptoms, significantly improve laboratory measures of inflammation, and decrease the prevalence of coronary artery abnormalities. Aspirin should also be used early in the treatment of Kawasaki disease. Doses of 80–100 mg/kg/day should be given in order to achieve serum salicylate levels of 15–25 mg/dl. The dosage should be reduced to less than 10 mg/kg/day after the fever is controlled and the sedimentation rate has returned to normal. If aneurysms have developed, low-dose aspirin may be given indefinitely.

80. Does salicylate therapy change the long-term outcome in Kawasaki disease?
Although widespread use of salicylates has been associated with a decrease of mortality related to Kawasaki disease, as yet there is no absolute proof of its efficacy in affecting the basic pathology of the disease. The only definite effect that can be measured is the reduction

in the duration of fever. Low doses of aspirin are theoretically more effective in the prevention of platelet aggregation and intravascular thrombus formation.

81. How common are rashes related to ampicillin?
Minor reactions to ampicillin are manifested by a morbilliform, erythematous, papular rash that appears about 3 days after initiation of therapy. These rashes are common (7% of ampicillin courses) and are thought to be due to IgM complexes formed with penicilloyl antigens. They resolve spontaneously as IgG-blocking antibodies are formed. Clinical resolution occurs even though ampicillin therapy is continued. Ampicillin rashes should be distinguished from immediate, IgE-mediated hypersensitivity reactions. The latter are rare (1 in every 20,000 courses of drug) and occasionally life-threatening, being manifested by an urticarial rash, shock, bronchospasm, and laryngeal edema. Usually this form of reaction follows immediately upon exposure to the drug, but a mild form may be delayed from a few hours to a few days.

82. What is the average number of upper respiratory infections per year for an infant less than 1 year of age?
3–8 per year.

83. What are the characteristic manifestations of acute epiglottitis?
In acute epiglottitis the child is toxic, febrile, and has difficulty breathing. Inspiratory stridor and a barking cough are rarely noted. The child is usually anxious. Since he cannot handle oral secretions, he is characteristically upright and leaning forward, with head extended, and drooling. If the pharynx is visualized, a cherry-red epiglottis may be seen. The white blood count is usually elevated.

84. What are the etiologic agents of acute epiglottitis? How should children with epiglottitis be managed?
Acute epiglottitis is characteristically caused by *H. influenzae*. Because ampicillin-resistant *H. influenzae* is not a rarity in most locations, this drug (and amoxicillin) cannot be considered reliable in this life-threatening condition. Chloramphenicol is an old standby, but it is rapidly being replaced by the second-generation cephalosporin, cefuroxime, and by third-generation cephalosporins. Acute epiglottitis is a medical emergency. It requires admission to an intensive care unit, and many authorities urge either elective intubation or elective tracheostomy, depending on local expertise.

85. How is epiglottitis differentiated clinically from croup?
Epiglottitis occurs more commonly in older children (3–7 years) and croup in younger children (6 months to 3 years). Epiglottitis has a more rapid onset, evolving to significant stridor in 8–12 hours. Croup develops over 24–72 hours. Children with epiglottitis are more ill-appearing and drool more than those with croup. The latter more frequently have a barking cough, hoarseness, and rhinitis.

86. Are steroids efficacious in croup?
The question of a benefit from steroids in croup has never been answered definitively due to imperfections in the published studies. It is fair to say, however, that in all studies in which a claim of efficacy has been supported, this efficacy has been of little clinical significance.

87. How should infants with croup be managed?
Croup (laryngotracheitis) is almost always a viral disease, with parainfluenza, influenza, respiratory syncytial, and adenoviruses being the most commonly isolated agents. Patients with severe croup require hospitalization. The cornerstones of therapy are mist, oxygen, and a quiet environment. The child should be calmed (by light sedation if absolutely necessary)

and closely observed. Examinations and invasive tests should be minimized, as agitation of the patient should be avoided. Arterial blood gas determinations are generally not indicated. The dreaded complication is complete respiratory obstruction. Depending on local expertise, this must be circumvented either by tracheostomy or endotracheal intubation. These procedures are far better done electively than emergently, and appropriate consultants should participate in the child's management from the time of admission. Steroids and antibiotics are not indicated. Racemic epinephrine can produce dangerous rebound reactions and is usually reserved as adjunctive therapy in those in whom tracheostomy or intubation is imminent.

88. What are the common bacterial and viral agents responsible for pneumonia in the pediatric age group?

Newborn	2–6 months	6 months–5 years	School Age
Group B streptococci	RSV	RSV	*Mycoplasma pneumoniae*
Gram-negative bacilli	Parainfluenza	Parainfluenza viruses	*S. pneumoniae*
S. aureus	Influenza viruses	Influenza viruses	Influenza viruses
CMV	Chlamydia	*S. pneumoniae*	
?Ureoplasma	*S. pneumoniae*	*H. influenzae*	
	H. influenzae	*S. aureus*	

89. Pleural effusions are most commonly associated with which agents?
S. pneumoniae, H. influenzae, S. aureus, M. tuberculosis, and Coxsackie viruses (in epidemic pleurodynia).

90. Pleural fluid with a glucose less than 60 is usually seen in what conditions?
Infected bacterial parapneumonic effusions, tuberculosis, malignancy, and rheumatic disease.
        Reference: Brown RG, Weinstein L: Pleural effusion. In Feigin RD, Cherry JD (eds): Textbook of Pediatric Infectious Diseases, 2nd ed. Philadelphia, W.B. Saunders, 1987.

91. What is the value of blood or throat cultures in children with pneumonia?
Blood cultures provide specific bacteriologic diagnosis. Most patients with pneumococcal pneumonia have bacteremia at some time during their illness. In children in whom the chest roentgenogram shows segmental alveolar consolidation and/or pleural effusion, the isolation of bacterial pathogens from the blood is usually high. Bacterial throat cultures are useful in the diagnosis of group A streptococcal pharyngitis but are of little use in determining the etiology of infection in the lung. As a rule, the correlation of throat and lung bacterial growth is poor and, in an individual case, no conclusions can be drawn. *B. pertussis* is an exception. By contrast, viral and mycoplasmal throat cultures are highly informative.

92. When should a child with pneumonia be hospitalized?
It is advisable to hospitalize all children under 1 year of age, all those with *S. aureus* pneumonia, all those who appear toxic or are hypoxic, all who cannot tolerate oral medications, and all whose family situation is of unclear stability.

93. What percentage of infants born to mothers with positive cervical cultures for chlamydia will develop chlamydial pneumonia during the first 3 months of life?
3–20%.

94. What are the clinical characteristics of chlamydial pneumonia in infants?
        93% of affected children are less than 8 weeks of age
        45% have conjunctivitis
        The presentation is usually subacute with symptoms of more than 1 week
        Little or no fever is present
        Staccato cough and diffuse rales are common (usually good breath sounds)
        Wheezing is unusual

Chest x-ray: demonstrates hyperexpansion, bilateral interstitial infiltrates
70% have absolute eosinophilia (greater than 300 eosinophils/mm^3)
Serum immunoglobulins are elevated
Reference: Tipple MA, Beem MD, Saxon EM: Clinical characteristics of the afebrile pneumonia associated with *Chlamydia trachomatis* infection in infants less than six months of age. Pediatrics 63: 192–197, 1979.

95. What is the most common auscultatory finding in mycoplasmal pneumonia?
Dry rales (crackles)—80%. These may persist 2 weeks or more along with cough and sputum production. Wheezing is heard in less than 50% of patients.

96. What is the radiologic picture of mycoplasmal pneumonia?
The chest x-ray is variable and nonspecific. Most findings are unilateral (up to 85%) and occur in one of the lower lobes. Early in the course of illness, the picture is one of increased interstitial markings with a reticulonodular pattern. Frequently, this progresses to patchy, segmental, or even lobar areas of consolidation. Hilar adenopathy occurs in up to one-third of patients. Pleural effusions, as demonstrated by lateral decubitus views, may occur in up to 20% of children.
Reference: Broughton RA: *Mycoplasma pneumoniae* infections in childhood. Pediatr Infect Dis J 5:71–84, 1986.

97. What is the bedside cold agglutinin test for mycoplasmal infections?
Seventy-five percent of patients with mycoplasmal infections will develop cold agglutinins, which are IgM auto-antibodies that agglutinate human red blood cells at 4°C. The cold agglutinins begin to develop at the end of the first week of illness. The bedside cold agglutinin test involves placing a few drops (about 0.3 cc) into a tube containing sodium citrate or EDTA. The blood and sodium citrate should be present in approximately equal volumes. The mixture is placed on ice for about a minute and the fluid is observed by rolling the tube on its side. Coarsely flocculating red blood cells constitute a positive test. A positive test correlates with a cold agglutinin titer of >1:64. There are many false-negatives, especially early in the disease when cold agglutinin titers are lower. Cold agglutinins may also be seen in infections due to adenovirus, cytomegalovirus, Epstein-Barr virus, influenza, rubella, chlamydia, and listeria.
Reference: Broughton RA: *Mycoplasma pneumoniae* infections in childhood. Pediatr Infect Dis J 5:71–84, 1986.

98. What are the three types of pulmonary aspergillus infections?
  1. Allergic bronchopulmonary aspergillosis: hypersensitivity reactions to aspergillus spores and antigens
  2. Aspergilloma: fungal ball (mycetoma)
  3. Invasive disease: usually in an immunocompromised host

99. What percent of patients with invasive pulmonary disease from aspergillosis will have positive sputum studies (mycelial elements on wet mount or a positive culture)?
15%. Lung biopsy and tissue examination are far more definitive.

100. What clinical features are suggestive of *Pneumocystis carinii* pneumonia?
In the setting of immunocompromise or chronic illness, the patient is often very tachypneic (rate of 70–100), cyanotic, and dyspneic with retractions and nasal flaring. Hypoxemia accompanied by a mild respiratory alkalosis is seen early in the disease. The most striking auscultatory feature is a lack of adventitious sounds (e.g., rales, rhonchi). In infants (2–6 months), the disease may evolve insidiously over weeks after an early afebrile course of mild cough and tachypnea.

101. What are the side effects of pentamidine when used as a treatment for *Pneumocystis carinii* infections?

15–25%:	impaired renal function
	local irritation at injection site
5–10%:	abnormal liver function
	hypoglycemia
	hypotension
	hematologic abnormalities
Less than 5%:	hypocalcemia
	skin rash

Reference: Walter PD, et al: *Pneumocystis carinii* pneumonia in the United States. Ann Intern Med 80:83–93, 1974.

102. What are the three stages of pertussis infections?
1. Catarrhal (1–2 weeks): upper respiratory tract symptoms
2. Paroxysmal (2–4 weeks): severe cough, onset of inspiratory "whoop"
3. Convalescent (1–2 weeks): resolution of symptoms

103. What is the most common cause of death in children with pertussis infections?
Ninety percent of deaths are attributable to pneumonia, most of which are secondarily infected bacterial pneumonias. These can be easily missed in the paroxysmal phase when respiratory symptoms are so prominent and usually attributed solely to pertussis. A new spiking fever should prompt a careful search for an evolving pneumonia.

Reference: Feigin RD, Cherry JD: Pertussis. In Feigin RD, Cherry JD (eds): Textbook of Pediatric Infectious Diseases, 2nd ed. Philadelphia, W.B. Saunders, 1987, p 2134.

104. What is the value of erythromycin in pertussis infections?
If used in the first 14 days of illness or before the paroxysmal stage, erythromycin may eliminate or lessen the severity of symptoms in the paroxysmal stage. If the diagnosis is made after that point, erythromycin should still be given, as it eliminates pertussis carriage in the nasopharynx and may limit the spread of disease. The dose is 50 mg/kg per day for 14 days, not to exceed a total daily dose of 1 gm.

105. What is Bornholm disease?
Known more commonly as epidemic pleurodynia, this is a condition of severe, sharp, spasmodic, pleuritic chest pain or upper abdominal pain that is muscular in origin and occurs in variable periods over days to weeks. It can be very incapacitating. Coxsackie B virus is the most common etiologic agent.

106. In which patients should the use of trimethoprim-sulfamethoxazole (Bactrim, Septra) be avoided or used with caution?
Trimethoprim-sulfamethoxazole acts by sequentially inhibiting steps in the folic acid pathway of bacteria. Disruption of human folic acid synthesis may occur, affecting rapidly replicating cells, especially in the bone marrow and skin. Avoidance or cautious use is suggested in the following settings:

1. Patients who have not received folate supplementation and are known to be or expected to be deficient in folate, including:
   a. Phenytoin use
   b. Therapy with other folate antagonist
   c. Protein-calorie malnutrition
   d. Prematurity
2. Pregnancy
3. Fragile X syndrome
4. Known sensitivity to any sulfonamide
5. Infancy ≤ 2 months of age
6. Skin rash that develops while receiving TMP-SMX
7. G-6-PD deficiency

From Gutman LT: The use of trimethoprim-sulfamethoxazole in children. A review of adverse reactions and indications. Pediatr Infect Dis J 3:355, 1984, with permission.

107. What are the clinical indications for first-, second-, and third-generation cephalosporins?

First-generation cephalosporins

    1. Alternative drugs for patients who cannot tolerate penicillins, although there is a 5–10% risk of cross-reactivity. Liquid suspensions of Keflex are widely accepted by children because of good taste.

    2. Prophylaxis in orthopedic and other surgery.

    3. As empiric drugs in treating fever in the immunocompromised host.

Second-generation cephalosporins

    1. Cefuroxime and cefaclor can be used when *H. influenzae* is a suspected pathogen.

    2. Cefoxitin is a good alternative treatment for children with anaerobic infections.

Third-generation cephalosporins

    1. Alternatives in invasive gram-negative infections.

    2. Ceftriaxone may have a role in outpatient therapy because of its convenient 1 dose/day regimen intramuscularly. When ceftriaxone is given twice per day intramuscularly, excellent blood levels are achieved and this drug may be of use in the child with difficult intravenous access.

108. What is periodontitis?

The periodontium consists of the gingiva, alveolar bone, and the periodontal ligament that connects the two. Periodontitis is the triad of hypertrophied gingiva, loose teeth (due to loss of alveolar bone), and purulent exudate. It is rare in children but may be seen in adolescents with chronically poor periodontal hygiene. Juvenile periodontitis is a disease of rapid alveolar bone loss due to colonization by bacteria pathogenic to the periodontium. It is mainly seen in children with disorders of neutrophil function (e.g., Chediak-Higashi syndrome, cyclic neutropenia).

109. What is gingivitis? How common is it?

Gingivitis is extremely common, affecting nearly 50% of children. The disorder is usually painless and is manifested by bluish-red discoloration of gums, which are swollen and bleed easily. The cause: bacteria in plaque deposits between teeth. The cure: improved dental hygiene and daily flossing.

110. What is Ludwig's angina?

It is an acute diffuse infection (usually bacterial) of the submandibular and sublingual spaces with brawny induration of the floor of the mouth and tongue. Airway obstruction may occur. The infections usually follow oral cavity injuries or dental complications (e.g., extractions, impactions).

111. What is herpangina?

Herpangina is a common viral infection during summer and fall characterized by posterior pharyngeal, buccal, and palatal vesicles and ulcers. Coxsackie A and B viruses and echoviruses are the most common causative agents. In young children, it is often accompanied by a high fever (103–104°). It is distinguished from herpes simplex infections of the mouth, which are more anterior and involve the lips, tongue, and gingiva.

112. What is the difference between Osler's nodes and Janeway lesions?

Both types of lesions are noted in individuals with bacterial endocarditis. Pain is a key discriminator. Osler's nodes are painful, tender nodules found primarily on the pads of the fingers and toes. Janeway's lesions are painless, nontender, hemorrhagic nodular lesions seen on the palms and soles, especially on thenar and hypothenar eminences. Both lesions are rare in children with endocarditis.

    Reference: Farrior JB, Silverman ME: A consideration of the differences between a Janeway's lesion and an Osler's node in infectious endocarditis. Chest 70:239–243, 1976.

113. What are the reasons that properly collected blood cultures may be negative in the setting of clinically suspected bacterial endocarditis?
   1. The bacterial endocarditis may be right-sided
   2. Prior antibiotic use
   3. Nonbacterial infection: fungal (e.g., aspergillosis, candida); unusual organism (e.g., rickettsiae, chlamydia)
   4. Unusual bacterial infection: slow-growing organisms or anaerobes
   5. Lesions are mural, nonvalvular (less likely to be hematogenously seeded)
   6. Nonbacterial thrombotic endocarditis (sterile platelet–fibrin thrombus formations following endocardial injury)
   7. Incorrect diagnosis
   Reference: Starke JR: Infectious endocarditis. In Feigin RD, Cherry JD (eds): Textbook of Pediatric Infectious Diseases, 2nd ed. Philadelphia, W.B. Saunders, 1987, p 1616.

114. What is Chagas' disease?
American trypanosomiasis. This protozoan infection is the most common cause of acute and chronic myocarditis in Central and South America.

115. What is the Romaña sign?
Seen in approximately one-quarter of patients in endemic areas with early Chagas' disease, it is unilateral, painless, palpebral edema often accompanied by conjunctivitis. The swelling occurs near the bite site of the parasitic vector, the Triatoma bug.

116. What is the incubation period for wound botulism?
4–14 days.

117. Why are antibiotics and antitoxins not used in cases of infant botulism?
   • By the time the diagnosis is made, most patients with infant botulism are usually stable or improving.
   • Antibiotics may result in bacterial death with the potential for release of additional toxin.
   • Risk of serum sickness and anaphylaxis.
   • Circulating unbound toxin is not found in ongoing disease.
   • Previously bound toxin is irreversibly bound (recovery based on growth of new nerve sprouts).
   • Excellent prognosis with aggressive supportive care alone.
   Reference: Finegold SM, Arnon SS: Clostridial intoxication and infection. In Feigin RD, Cherry JD (eds): Textbook of Pediatric Infectious Diseases, 2nd ed. Philadelphia, W.B. Saunders, 1987, p 1121.

118. What is "risus sardonicus"?
It is the "sardonic smile" seen in patients suffering from tetanus due to spasm of facial muscles.

119. What are the biphasic features of leptospiral infection?
Both anicteric and icteric cases of leptospirosis have two phases:
   First phase: fever, headache, conjunctivitis, myalgia, abdominal pain; leptospires found in CSF and blood; lasts 4–7 days.
   Second phase: phase of immunologic response; leptospires found in urine; anicteric type (90%): rash, meningitis, uveitis; icteric type (10%): jaundice, myocarditis, hemorrhage, renal dysfunction; lasts 4–30 days.

120. What is the eponym for icteric leptospirosis?
Weil's disease.

121. What area of the body harbors leptospires the longest in a recovering patient?
The aqueous humor. Regions of the eye serve as an immunologic barrier, allowing chronic carriage for months. Some affected patients have recurrent uveitis.

122. What percentage of patients with encephalitis do not have an etiologic agent identified?
60–70%.

123. In the setting of clinical signs and symptoms of an encephalitis, what EEG pattern is suggestive of herpes simplex disease?
Periodic lateralized epileptiform discharges (PLEDs). PLEDs may be seen in other (rarer) causes of encephalitis, such as Epstein-Barr virus and slow viral disease (i.e., Jacob-Creutzfeldt disease and subacute sclerosing panencephalitis).

124. What is restriction analysis?
This is a means of identifying viruses by eliciting an electrophoretic "fingerprint." The viral DNA or RNA is cleaved at specific points by various enzymes (endonucleases) and the resulting fragments are dispersed on a gel revealing a characteristic pattern.

125. When was inactivated (killed) measles vaccine used?
1963–1968. About 1.8 million doses were given.

126. What is "atypical" about atypical measles?
1. Occurs primarily in patients who have received inactivated measles vaccine.
2. Koplik spots are unusual.
3. Rash begins on distal extremities and spreads toward head (in typical measles, the exanthem spreads from head to feet).
4. Conjunctivitis and coryza are not part of prodrome.
5. Hepatosplenomegaly is more common.
Reference: Cherry JD: Measles. In Feigin RD, Cherry JD (eds): Textbook of Pediatric Infectious Diseases, 2nd ed. Philadelphia, W.B. Saunders, 1987, p 1616.

127. Why is post-measles blindness so common in underdeveloped countries?
As many as 1% of all cases of measles in underdeveloped regions result in blindness. In contrast, measles keratitis in developed countries is usually self-limited and benign. There are two principal reasons:
1. Vitamin A deficiency—Vitamin A is needed for corneal stromal repair, and a deficiency allows epithelial damage to persist or worsen. Many malnourished children have accompanying vitamin A deficiency, and vitamin A supplements may be of benefit during active illness.
2. Malnutrition may predispose to corneal superinfection with *Herpes simplex*.

128. Following exposure to chickenpox (varicella), when do symptoms develop?
99% develop symptoms between 11 and 20 days following exposure.

129. Erythema infectiosum (fifth disease) is caused by which virus?
Human parvovirus.

130. What is the traditional numbering of the "original" six exanthematous illnesses?

First disease	measles
Second disease	scarlet fever
Third disease	rubella
Fourth disease	Duke's disease (described in 1900 and was felt to be a scarlatiniform type of rubella; no longer used)
Fifth disease	erythema infectiosum
Sixth disease	roseola subitum (exanthem subitum)

131. When did the World Health Organization certify that smallpox had been globally eradicated?
1980

132. What is the characteristic rash of Rocky Mountain spotted fever (RMSF)?
- usually seen by third day of illness (from 5–11 days after tick bite)
- initially blanching red macules which become petechial
- begins on wrists and ankles and spreads to extremities and trunk within hours
- involves palms and soles

133. What is the Weil-Felix test?
A screening test for RMSF which utilizes the fact that rickettsiae and some Proteus strains (especially OX-19, OX-2, OX-K) share common antigens. Rising titers or a titer greater than 1:160 of these Proteus strains suggest RMSF in the appropriate clinical setting.

134. Sternal edema is classically the sign of what infection?
Mumps

135. What was the original derivation of the term "C-reactive protein"?
This positive acute phase reactant was originally found (and named) because it precipitated with the C-polysaccharide of pneumococcus in the presence of calcium.

136. What are the most common presenting signs and symptoms of toxic shock syndrome?

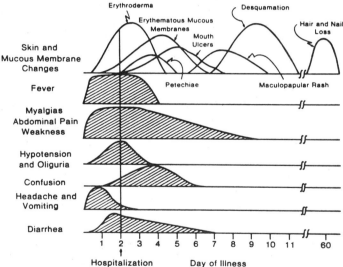

Composite drawing of major systemic skin and mucous membrane manifestations of toxic shock syndrome. (From Chesney PJ, Davis JP, Purdy WK, et al: JAMA 246:741–748, 1981, with permission.)

137. What is the etiologic agent and treatment of choice for toxic shock syndrome?
Toxic shock syndrome is caused by toxins of *S. aureus*. No clear-cut rationale for antibiotic therapy has been established; however, most physicians employ a penicillinase-resistant penicillin.

138. What are "clue cells"?
Clue cells are vaginal epithelial cells to which are attached many bacteria. They are best visualized in saline, wet-mount preparations. They are associated with *Gardnerella vaginalis* infections, which are characterized by leukocyte-free, thick, white material, little vulvar or vaginal inflammation, and a vaginal pH between 5 and 6.

139. What is the value of oral acyclovir in the treatment of genital herpes infections in immunocompetent hosts?
- useful mainly in primary disease
- lessens duration of pain and itching
- lessens number of new lesions
- hastens crusting of old lesions
- shortens viral shedding (and thus many shorten period of contagion)
- delays and reduces frequency of recurrences while on therapy

Long-term studies of its toxicity from chronic use have not been done. Thus, chronic administration should not be used for prophylaxis in individuals who have mild disease. Topical therapy also provides similar benefits for individuals with primary disease; however, it does not reduce the frequency of recurrences. It is also less effective for symptoms of recurrent disease.

140. What is the cause of condylomata acuminata?
These "venereal warts" are caused by the human papilloma virus.

141. What is the clinical triad of Behçet's syndrome?
(1) Recurrent aphthous stomatitis, (2) vulvar ulcerations (painless, but may lead to marked scarring), and (3) ocular inflammation (especially uveitis). Etiology is unclear, but an autoimmune basis is suspected.

142. What is the difference between chancroid and chancre?
Both are acute ulcerative diseases of the external genitalia. Chancroid is painful and caused by *H. ducreyi*. Chancres are painless and caused by *T. pallidum* (syphilis).

143. What is Hutchinson's triad for late congenital syphilis?
(1) Hutchinson's teeth (screwdriver, peg-shaped teeth), (2) interstitial keratitis, and (3) eighth nerve deafness.

144. What are increased risk factors for neonatal herpes infections in mothers with positive cervical cultures?
1. Primary maternal infection during the third trimester. Up to 30–40% of mothers with primary disease will have infants with herpetic disease, but only 3% of infants of mothers with recurrent disease will develop the infection.
2. Rupture of membranes longer than six hours prior to birth.
3. Vaginal delivery.
Reference: Whitley RJ: Neonatal herpes simplex virus infections. Pediatr Rev 7:119–126,1985.

145. How helpful is a Tzanck prep in the diagnosis of neonatal herpes?
The Tzanck prep for multinucleated giant cells has a very high false-negative rate—up to 50%. Cultures, if available, are more reliable.

146. What pathogens should be considered in a dog or cat bite? What is the treatment of choice?
The most frequently isolated pathogens in dog bites are *Pasteurella multocida, Staphylococcus aureus,* and coagulase-negative staphylococci. Anaerobic bacteria that are frequently isolated include Bacteroides and Fusobacterium. *Pasteurella multocida* is the most common pathogen associated with cat bite; tularemia has also been transmitted by cat bites. The wounds from dog or cat bites should be thoroughly cleaned with sterile solution. Debris should be removed and skin tags and devitalized tissue should be surgically debrided. Bites that are seen after 24 hours with or without signs of infection should not be surgically closed. The question of whether to close clean bites surgically that are seen in the first 24 hours is controversial. Penicillin or ampicillin is the drug of choice. Tetracycline is an alternative for penicillin-allergic patients above 9 years of age. Tetanus toxoid should be administered to patients requiring a booster.

147. Swollen, tender pectoral nodes are most suggestive of what infection?
Cat-scratch disease.

148. What causes visceral larval migrans?
Toxocara canis, a dog or cat ascarid, causes this infiltrative granulomatous disease. There is a variety of clinical features, including fever, hepatomegaly, anemia, myocardial involvement, retinal disease, and pneumonitis.

149. Other than definitive serologic tests, what two laboratory tests are most suggestive of Toxocara infection?
(1) Marked eosinophilia (20–90% of peripheral white blood cells), and (2) markedly elevated isohemagglutinin titers (i.e., anti-A and/or anti-B titers in individuals who are not blood type A or B).

150. In what animal is rabies most commonly reported?
Skunks. In 1982, 4480 cases occurred in skunks compared with 850 in bats, 480 in raccoons, 200 in cats, and 150 in dogs.

151. What are the six types of tularemia?
Ulceroglandular, glandular, oculoglandular, typhoidal, oropharyngeal, pneumonic. The most common form of this uncommon disease is ulceroglandular, where a superficial skin ulcer may persist for weeks. The illness is usually transmitted by ticks or deerflies or by the handling of infected animals, especially rabbits.

152. What diseases are transmitted by ticks?

Disease	Agent
Relapsing fever	*Borrelia duttonii*
Q fever	*Coxiella burnetti*
Tularemia	*Francisella tularensis*
Queensland tick typhus	*Rickettsia australis*
Fièvre boutonneuse	*R. conorii*
Rocky Mountain spotted fever	*R. rickettsii*
Asian tick typhus	*R. sibirica*
Colorado tick fever	Arbovirus
Encephalitis	Arbovirus
Lyme disease	Spirochete

From Kaplan SL: Arthropoda. In Feigin RD, Cherry JD (eds): Textbook of Pediatric Infectious Diseases, Philadelphia, W.B. Saunders, 1987, p 2134, with permission.

153. What was the last word correctly spelled in the 1987 National Spelling Bee Championship?
Staphylococci.

Bibliography

1. Bluestone CD, Klein JO: Otitis Media in Infants and Children, Philadelphia, W.B. Saunders, 1987.
2. Davies P, Gothefors L: Bacterial Infections in the Fetus and Newborn Infant. Philadelphia, W.B. Saunders, 1984.
3. Feigin RD, Cherry JD (eds): Textbook of Pediatric Infectious Diseases, 2nd ed. Philadelphia, W.B. Saunders, 1987.
4. Hanshaw JB, Dudgeon JA: Viral Diseases of the Fetus and Newborn, 2nd ed. Philadelphia, W.B. Saunders, 1985.
5. Mandell GL, Douglas RG, Bennett JE (eds): Principles and Practice of Infectious Diseases, 2nd ed. New York, John Wiley and Sons, 1985.
6. Moffet HL: Pediatric Infectious Diseases, 3rd ed. Philadelphia, J.B. Lippincott, 1989.
7. Remington JS, Klein JO: Infectious Diseases of the Fetus and Newborn Infant, 2nd ed. Philadelphia, W.B. Saunders, 1983.

NEONATOLOGY

Mary Catherine Harris, M.D.
Philip Roth, M.D., Ph.D.

General

1. How is gestational age estimated prenatally?

Gestational age may be estimated prenatally in a variety of ways:

1. Menstrual dating: The estimated date of confinement (EDC) can be determined by adding 7 days to the first day of the last menstrual period and counting back 3 months ("Nagele's rule"). This method is fraught with inaccuracies due to the frequent occurrence of irregular menses.

2. Pelvic examination can offer information on gestational age by assessing uterine size. This technique, however, depends on the skill of the examiner as well as the difficulty in examining a particular patient (e.g., obese patient).

3. The ability to detect fetal heart tones usually indicates a gestational age of at least 17–20 weeks.

4. Ultrasound examination is probably the most accurate method for assessing gestational age. In the first trimester, gestational age based on crown-rump length is accurate to within 3 days. From the second trimester on, measurement of the biparietal diameter is most helpful and, up until 34 weeks' gestation, is accurate within 10 days. Useful adjunctive measurements are the femur length, average body diameter (anterior-posterior + lateral ÷ 2), and abdominal circumference.

2. How is gestational age determined postnatally?

Postnatal estimation of gestational age can be determined in one of six ways:

1. Physical assessment
2. Neurologic assessment
3. Combined physical and neurologic assessment
4. Examination of the lens of the eye
5. EEG
6. Nerve conduction velocity

The clinical method used most often is the Ballard modification of the Dubowitz examination using seven physical and six neurologic criteria to define gestational age with an accuracy of ± 2 weeks. However, in order to be accurate, the neurologic assessment must be performed in an alert, rested infant, which is often difficult in the sick, preterm neonate. A typical scoring system is shown on the next page.

Neuromuscular Maturity

	0	1	2	3	4	5
Posture						
Square Window (wrist)	90°	60°	45°	30°	0°	
Arm Recoil	180°		100°-180°	90°-100°	<90°	
Popliteal Angle	180°	160°	130°	110°	90°	<90°
Scarf Sign						
Heel to Ear						

Maturity Rating

SCORE	WEEKS
5	26
10	28
15	30
20	32
25	34
30	36
35	38
40	40
45	42
50	44

Physical Maturity

Skin	gelatinous red, trans-parent	smooth pink, visible veins	superficial peeling, &/or rash few veins	cracking pale area rare veins	parchment deep cracking no vessels	leathery cracked wrinkled
Lanugo	none	abundant	thinning	bald areas	mostly bald	
Plantar Creases	no crease	faint red marks	anterior transverse crease only	creases ant. 2/3	creases cover entire sole.	
Breast	barely percept.	flat areola no bud	stippled areola 1-2mm bud	raised areola 3-4mm bud	full areola 5-10mm bud	
Ear	pinna flat, stays folded	sl. curved pinna; soft c̄ slow recoil	well-curv. pinna; soft but ready recoil	formed & firm c̄ instant recoil	thick cartilage ear stiff	
Genitals ♂	scrotom empty no rugae		testes descend-ing few rugae	testes down good rugae	testes pendulous deep rugae	
Genitals ♀	prominent clitoris & labia minora		majora & minora equally prominent	majora large minora small	clitoris & minora completely covered	

From Dubowitz LMS, Dubowitz V: Gestational Age of the Newborn: A Clinical Manual. Reading, MA, Addison Wesley, 1977, with permission.

3. What are normal vital signs for healthy neonates?

The normal respiratory rate for spontaneously breathing newborns is 40–60 breaths per minute. The heart rate for newborns is generally between 120 and 180 beats per minute. Blood pressure and pulse vary with both postnatal and gestational age and weight, as shown in the figure.

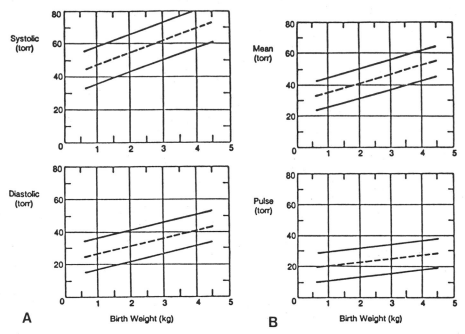

Pressures obtained by direct measurement through umbilical artery catheter in healthy newborn infants during first 12 hours of life. Broken lines represent linear regressions; solid lines represent 95% confidence limits. *A,* Systolic pressure *(top)* and diastolic pressure *(bottom). B,* Mean aortic pressure *(top)* and pulse pressure (systolic-diastolic pressure amplitude) *(bottom).* (From Versmold HT, Kitterman JA, Phibbs RH, et al: Aortic blood pressure during the first 12 hours of life in infants with birth weight 610 to 4220 grams. Pediatrics 67:5:611, 1981; copyright © American Academy of Pediatrics, 1981, with permission.)

4. When should hypertension be treated in the neonate?

Hypertension is defined as a blood pressure greater than 90/60 torr in term neonates and greater than 80/45 torr in preterm infants. A sustained systolic blood pressure greater than 100 torr in the neonate should be investigated and treated.

5. How are initial maintenance fluid requirements determined for the neonate? Subsequent requirements?

Initial approximate fluid requirements for maintenance are:

Weight (gm)	Fluid (cc/kg/day)
<800	80–100
800–1500	60–80
>1500	60

Subsequent fluid requirements should be based on clinical assessment of hydration and laboratory studies (sodium, potassium, chloride, calcium, blood urea nitrogen, urine output and specific gravity, and hematocrit).

6. When should sodium, potassium, and calcium be given to a neonate?

Calcium should be included in the very first intravenous solutions of preterm infants, infants of diabetic mothers, and asphyxiated newborns. Traditionally sodium and potassium are added as a matter of course at 24 hours of age.

7. How is shock in the neonate identified?

Shock is *not* identified by a blood pressure reading, but rather by a constellation of features: decreased arterial pulses, tachycardia, tachypnea, poor capillary refill, mottled blue-white skin, metabolic acidosis, anuria or oliguria, and cool extremities.

8. How is shock treated?

In neonates with septic or hypovolemic shock, vascular access must be rapidly established and large volumes of colloid or blood (if available) should be administered. If central venous pressure (CVP) monitoring is available, it may be used to guide volume administration; however, the absolute CVP reading is less helpful than the rate of rise from a baseline value. Most neonates require *at least* 30 cc/kg of fluid to "fill" their intravascular space. The volume of fluid should be administered over a 1½ hour time period. Some infants will require additional volume expansion. If the intravascular compartment is thought to be adequately repleted and the infant is still in shock, inotropic agents such as dopamine and dobutamine should be started. In addition, acidosis should be treated with ventilation and/or sodium bicarbonate. Where clinically indicated, cultures should be taken and broad-spectrum antibiotic therapy initiated. In dying infants, corticosteroids may be given, although their usage is controversial.

9. What are the best ways to warm a hypothermic infant?

There is much debate as to whether rapid or slow rewarming is preferable, but no good controlled studies exist to answer this question. A general approach consists of placing the infant in a heat-gaining environment to prevent further losses. This can best be achieved by placing the infant in a convectively heated incubator at 36°C with a heat shield to reduce radiant losses and increased humidity to decrease evaporative losses. Under these conditions the air temperature is approximately equal to the environmental temperature in the incubator. Air temperature should be monitored along with skin temperature, which should not exceed rectal temperature by more than 1°C. If the patient's temperature does not stabilize or increase, the incubator temperature should be increased to 37°C and the patient's temperature observed for 15 minutes. If there is still no improvement, the temperature should be increased to 38°C. If temperatures greater than 38°C are necessary, an overhead warmer may need to be placed over the incubator in order to warm its walls and achieve the desired effect.

10. Why don't preterm infants sweat?

The failure of infants born prior to 30 weeks' gestation to sweat is probably the result of incomplete development and differentiation of sweat glands. In term babies, where more data are available, the maximal sweat response to thermal stimuli is one-third that of adults, despite a density of sweat glands which is six times higher.

11. How do you make an infant shiver?

Controversy exists as to whether newborn infants shiver. In some reports, shivering was observed only at temperatures below 22–24°C. In general, thermogenesis in infants may be achieved in large part through muscular activity without shivering and through catecholamine-mediated breakdown of triglycerides in "brown fat."

12. What is brown fat?

Brown fat is the site of non-shivering thermogenesis in response to cold stress in newborn infants. Heat generated at these sites by metabolism of triglycerides is used to warm blood that is returning from the periphery. The major sites are: (1) a thin sheath between the scapulae, (2) small masses around the muscles and blood vessels of the neck, (3) the axillae, (4) the mediastinum between the esophagus and trachea and around the internal mammary vessels, and (5) around the kidneys and adrenals.

13. Should isolettes be run "wet" or "dry"?
Ideally, the relative humidity in the isolette should be maintained at 30–60% to avoid increased water and heat losses. However, this practice is not routinely used because of the increased risk of contamination with water-borne organisms.

14. After a "traumatic" delivery, what are the commonly injured systems?
1. Cranial injuries: caput succedaneum, subconjunctival hemorrhage, cephalhematoma, skull fractures, intracranial hemorrhage, and cerebral edema.
2. Spinal injuries: spinal cord transection.
3. Peripheral nerve injuries: brachial palsy (Erb-Duchenne paralysis, Klumpke's paralysis), phrenic nerve and facial nerve paralysis.
4. Viscera: liver rupture or hematoma, splenic rupture, and adrenal hemorrhage.
5. Skeletal injuries: fractures of the clavicle, femur, and humerus.

15. What is the most frequently fractured bone in the newborn infant?
The bone most frequently fractured during labor and delivery is the clavicle. This injury, which stems from excessive traction, generally results in a greenstick type fracture.

16. What is Throgmorton's sign?
Throgmorton's sign is the extension of the suspensory ligament of the penis prior to micturition in newborn infants. However, thousands of house officers have come to believe that this sign relates to the radiographic finding in a male in which the penis points to the side of pathology.

17. Which babies should have routine ophthalmologic screening examinations for retinopathy of prematurity, and when?
The following guidelines may be used to determine the need for an ophthalmology exam prior to discharge: (1) Birthweight $\leq$ 1750 gm regardless of need for oxygen; and (2) gestational age $\leq$ 37 weeks and need for supplemental oxygen $>$ 18 hours. In the case of twins, if one of the twins fits the criteria for examination, both should be examined. All infants with birthweights $\leq$ 1500 gm should be examined at 5–6 weeks of age (without exception by 7 weeks). Changes associated with retinopathy of prematurity are unlikely to be detected prior to 4 weeks postnatal age. Infants discharged before 4 weeks of age should receive ophthalmologic screening as outpatients.

18. Who were Cheng and Eng?
The original "Siamese twins."

19. What are Spitzer's Laws of Neonatology?

Spitzer's Laws of Neonatology

1. The more stable a baby appears to be, the more likely he will "crump" that day.
2. The distance that you have to go for a transport is directly proportional to the degree of illness of the baby.
3. The incidence of transport calls is inversely proportional to the number of available beds.
4. The nicer the parents, the sicker the baby.
5. The incidence of neonatal problems increases dramatically if either parent is a physician or a nurse.
6. Endotracheal tubes are designed to fall out (become plugged, etc.) at the most critical moment.
7. The milder the RDS, the sooner the infant will find himself in 100% oxygen and maximal ventilatory support.

8. The likelihood of BPD is directly proportional to the number of physicians involved in the care of that baby.

9. The longer a patient is discussed on rounds, the more certain it is that no one has the faintest idea what's going on or what to do.

10. The patient who is glossed over quickly on rounds is the most likely to crump that day.

11. The sickest infant in the nursery can always be discerned by the fact that he is being cared for by the newest, most inexperienced nursing orientee.

12. The surest way to have an infant linger interminably is to inform the parents that death is imminent.

13. The more miraculous the "save," the more likely that you'll be sued for something totally inconsequential.

14. The probability of infection is directly proportional to the number of antibiotics that an infant is already receiving.

15. If it ain't CHD, it's PFC (or vice versa).

16. If they're not breathin', they may be seizin'.

17. Lasix® (vitamin L) will squeeze urine out of bricks. Unfortunately, it doesn't always work as well in babies.

18. Antibiotics should always be continued for _____ days. (Fill in the blank with any number from 1 to 21.)

19. If you can't figure out what's going on with a baby, call the surgeons. They won't figure it out either, but they'll sure as hell do something about it.

20. The month you are on service always has three times as many days as any other month on the calendar.

Reference: Clin Pediatr vol. 20, no. 9, Sept. 1981.

Growth

20. Which fetal hormones are known to affect intrauterine growth?

Insulin, growth hormone, thyroid hormone, and epidermal, fibroblast, and nerve growth factors. Insulin has been called the "growth hormone of the fetus," and stimulates fetal deposition of adipose and glycogen stores, and protein synthesis in muscle. Growth hormone may influence fetal growth, but does not have a critical role during the intrauterine period. The fetal thyroid hormones are essential for the development of the central nervous system, but are probably not important for overall fetal growth. Additional growth hormones such as fibroblast growth factor, nerve growth factor, and epidermal growth factor may promote growth of specific organs. Nerve growth factor stimulates the development of the sympathetic nervous system, while epidermal growth factor has a role in both lung and secondary palate growth and differentiation.

21. How is fetal growth assessed prenatally?

It is assessed by serial exams of fundal height, which are then correlated with dates and fetal heart tones. If there is a size-dates discrepancy, further clarification can be obtained with ultrasound to give estimates of fetal body measurements and weight. An estimation of total uterine volume may also be helpful. Serial biparietal diameters may reliably diagnose abnormal growth patterns, although head sparing frequently occurs. The ratio of head circumference to abdominal circumference may be the best indicator of IUGR, particularly during the third trimester.

22. What factors are associated with intrauterine growth retardation (IUGR)?

Optimal fetal growth depends on: (1) the inherent growth potential of the fetus, and (2) the environment for growth as provided by the placenta and the mother. Epidemiologic factors associated with impaired fetal growth are shown in the table.

Risk Factors for Low Birth Weight*

Pre-pregnancy
  Low weight for height
  Short stature
  Chronic medical illness
  Poor nutrition
  Low maternal weight at mother's birth
  Previous low birth weight infant
  Uterine or cervical anomalies
  Parity (none or more than five)
 	
Pregnancy
  Multiple gestation
  Birth order
  Anemia
  Elevated hemoglobin concentration (inadequate plasma
    volume expansion?)
  Fetal disease
  Preeclampsia and hypertension
  Infections
  Placental problems
  Premature rupture of membranes
	Demographic
	  Race (black)
	  Present low socioeconomic status
	  Socioeconomic status of infant's
	    grandparents
	
	Behavioral (maternal choices)
	  Low educational status
	  Smoking
	  No care or inadequate prenatal care
	  Poor weight gain during pregnancy
	  Alcohol abuse
	  Illicit and prescription drugs
	  Short interpregnancy interval (less than 6
	    months)
	  Age (less than 16 or over 35)
	  Unmarried
	  Stress (physical and psychological)

Modified from Committee to Study the Prevention of Low Birthweight: Prevention of Low Birthweight, Washington, D.C., 1985, Institute of Medicine, National Academy Press.
* Many of these variables are risk factors for both IUGR and prematurity, and are not necessarily univariant risk factors, but rather interact in a complex relationship. Only a few factors exert an independent effect. The relationship between black race and low birthweight remains a significant factor, with a twofold increase in the incidence of prematurity and IUGR when controlled for other risk.

23. What is the ponderal index and how is it used to classify growth-retarded babies?

The ponderal index (PI) is: $\dfrac{\text{weight (g)}}{(\text{length (cm)})^3} \times 100$

This index has been used to estimate the adequacy of intrauterine fetal nutrition. Values less than 2.0 between 29 and 37 weeks' gestation and 2.2 beyond 37 weeks have been associated with fetal malnutrition. Growth-retarded infants with low ponderal indices also appear to be at increased risk for the development of neonatal hypoglycemia. Maternal conditions associated with a low ponderal index (fetal malnutrition) include poor maternal weight gain, lack of prenatal care, preeclampsia, and chronic maternal illness.

24. What morbidities (short- and long-term) are known to occur more frequently in growth-retarded babies?
Short-term morbidities include perinatal asphyxia, meconium aspiration, fasting hypoglycemia, alimented hypoglycemia, polycythemia-hyperviscosity, immunodeficiency.
Long-term morbidities include poor developmental outcome and altered postnatal growth. Most studies demonstrate normal intelligence and developmental quotients in SGA infants, although there seems to be a higher incidence of behavioral and learning problems. The presence or absence of severe perinatal asphyxia is extremely important in predicting later intellectual and neurologic function.

25. What is the oligohydramnios sequence?
The oligohydramnios sequence occurs in infants delivered to mothers with very little amniotic fluid and consists of facial anomalies, limb positioning defects, pulmonary hypoplasia, defects of urinary output, and fetal growth deficiency.

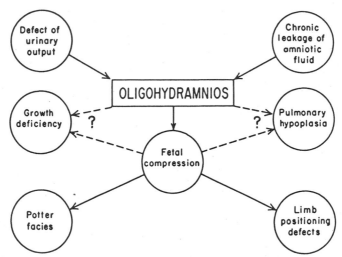

Depiction of the origin and effects of oligohydramnios. The oligohydramnios sequence is implied to be secondary to fetal compression. (From Smith DW: Recognizable Patterns of Human Malformation. Philadelphia, W.B. Saunders Co., 1982, p 484, with permission.)

26. What is the formula for determining size of the anterior fontanelle?

(Length + width)/2, where length = anterior − posterior dimension and width = transverse dimension.

27. When is an anterior fontanelle too big?

Although there is wide variability in the normal size range of the anterior fontanelle, designation of normal upper limits is helpful in identifying disorders in which a large fontanelle may be a feature.

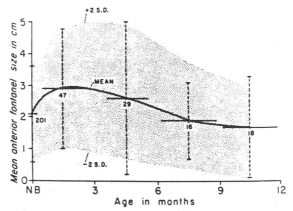

Mean anterior fontanelle size ± 2 S.D. during the first postnatal year. Beyond the newborn period (NB), the data are averaged at 3-month intervals with the number of individuals in each group indicated. (From Popich GA, Smith DW: J Pediatr 80:749, 1982, with permission.)

Nutrition and Feeding

28. How many calories are required for growth in a healthy, growing, preterm infant?

Preterm infants need approximately 120 calories/kg/day. About 45% of the caloric intake should be carbohydrate, 45% fat, and 10% protein. Infants who expend increased calories (e.g., those with chronic lung disease, fever, cold stress, etc.) may need up to 150 calories/kg/day.

29. How quickly should a preterm infant grow?
Preterm infants receiving adequate calories generally gain 15–30 gm/day.

30. What is the optimal protein intake for preterm and term infants?
Preterm infants: 2.7–3.5 gm/kg/day. Term infants: 2.0–2.5 gm/kg/day.

31. What are the essential fatty acids for a newborn infant? Which amino acids are essential for the neonate but not the adult?
Linoleic and arachidonic acid. There are no amino acids specifically essential for the neonate but not the adult; however, cystine, taurine, histidine, and tyrosine may be essential amino acids for preterm infants.

32. What are the recommended dietary allowances for vitamins?

Vitamin A — 1000 IU
Vitamin B_1 — 0.1 mg
Vitamin B_2 — 0.1 mg
Vitamin B_6 — 0.25 mg
Vitamin B_{12} — 0.25 μg
Niacin — 6.6 mg/1000 kcal
Folic acid — 50 μg
Vitamin C — 35 mg
Vitamin D — 400 IU
Vitamin E — 4 mg
Vitamin K — 5 μg

33. What is osteopenia of prematurity? How is it diagnosed and treated?
During the period of rapid growth, many preterm infants exhibit under-mineralization of bone (rickets of prematurity). This condition primarily results from an insufficient intake of calcium and phosphorus, although vitamin D insufficiency, aluminum toxicity, or liver disease may be contributing factors. Infants with this disorder have demineralized bones, despite maintaining a normal serum calcium and phosphorus until late in the disease. The condition is generally diagnosed by routine x-rays and may be treated with calcium (200 mg/kg/day), phosphorus (113 mg/kg/day), and vitamin D supplementation (400 IU/day).

34. What are the manifestations of vitamin E deficiency in the neonate?
Anemia, thrombocytosis, reticulocytosis, and peripheral edema. The Committee on Nutrition of the American Academy of Pediatrics has recommended that 0.7 IU of vitamin E/100 kcal be present in feedings for preterm infants.

35. What are the indications for adding vitamin E to the diet?
Preterm infants have diminished stores of vitamin E at birth, and have impaired absorption of fat-soluble vitamins from the GI tract. Normal vitamin E levels can generally be maintained in preterm infants if they are fed formulas designed for them. If the vitamin E level falls below 1 μg/ml, additional vitamin E, usually 25 IU/day, can be added to the diet. The role of vitamin E in the prevention of retinopathy of prematurity, bronchopulmonary dysplasia, and intraventricular hemorrhage is controversial.

36. What is the E/PUFA ratio?
Vitamin E is a fat-soluble vitamin (antioxidant) that prevents peroxidation of the lipid components (polyunsaturated fatty acids, PUFAs) of the red cell membrane. As the dietary intake of PUFAs increases, the requirements for vitamin E also increase. Inadequate vitamin E intake, increased PUFA intake, or superimposed oxidant stress from substances like iron may cause red cell hemolysis. The American Academy of Pediatrics recommends a ratio of 1 mg of vitamin E for each gram of PUFA in the diet.

37. What are the requirements for fluoride supplementation in newborn infants?
Fluoride supplementation should be provided in infants who are breastfeeding or in areas where the fluoride concentration in drinking water is inadequate.

Supplemental Fluoride Dosage Schedule (mg/day*)

AGE	CONCENTRATION OF FLUORIDE IN DRINKING WATER (PPM)		
	0.3	0.3 to 0.7	0.7
2 weeks to 2 years	0.25	0	0
2 to 3 years	0.50	0.25	0
3 to 16 years	1.00	0.50	0

Adapted from Committee on Nutrition and the Pediatric Nutrition Handbook, American Academy of Pediatrics, Evanston, Illinois, 1985.
*2.2 mg of sodium fluoride contains 1 mg of fluoride.

38. When should newborn infants receive iron?
In the term infant born with a normal hemoglobin concentration, iron supplementation is not needed until 4–6 months of age. In the preterm infant with a normal hemoglobin concentration, iron supplementation is often begun by the time the birth weight has doubled, or at the time of discharge.

39. What are the manifestations of zinc and copper deficiency in the neonate?
Zinc deficiency: dry skin, growth retardation, hepatosplenomegaly, impaired wound healing, hair loss, perioral and perianal rashes, and decreased resistance to infection.
Copper deficiency: hypochromic microcytic anemia, neutropenia, and bony abnormalities.

40. How does the composition of breast milk differ in mothers of preterm infants versus mothers of term infants?
Protein levels as well as sodium and chloride are significantly higher in "preterm" milk, whereas lactose levels are lower. To quote Dr. Frank Oski: "Cow's milk is for calves, human milk is for humans and preterm human milk is for preterm humans."

Differences and Similarities Between Mature and Preterm Human Milk During Early Lactation (0 to 4 weeks)

	MATURE MILK RANGES (per 100 ml)	VS	PRETERM MILK RANGES (per 100 ml)	OVERALL CONSENSUS FROM MULTIPLE STUDIES
Energy (kcal)	70.2–73.6		73.0–76.0	Preterm > Mature
Protein (g)	1.3–1.8		1.5–2.1	Preterm > Mature
Fat (g)	2.9–3.4		3.2–3.6	Preterm ≥ Mature
Carbohydrate (g)	6.4–7.1		6.3–7.2	Preterm < Mature
Na (mg)	15.4–21.8		21.8–39.1	Preterm > Mature
Cl (mg)	36.4–58.8		38.5–63.0	Preterm > Mature
K (mg)	50.7–65.5		53.4–67.0	Preterm = Mature
Ca (mg)	26.7–29.3		26.6–31.4	Preterm ≤ Mature
P (mg)	13.8–16.9		12.9–13.8	Preterm ≥ Mature
Mg (mg)	2.7–3.1		3.0–3.6	Preterm ≥ Mature
Cu (μg)	57.0–73.0		63.0–83.0	Preterm = Mature
Fe (μg)	81.0–111.0		90.0–110.0	Preterm ≥ Mature
Zn (μg)	260.0–535.0		392.0–530.0	Preterm = Mature

From Pereira GR, Barbosa NMM: Pediatr Clin North Am 33:76, 1986, with permission.

41. Which nutrients are inadequate in breast milk?
Breast milk is the ideal feeding source for term infants, and has been recommended as the sole source of nutrition for the first 4–6 months of life by the American Academy of Pediatrics. Iron should be supplemented when solid foods are started, and vitamin D should be added when exposure to sunlight is reduced. The nutritional adequacy of breast milk for preterm infants is controversial. In tiny preterm infants, calcium, phosphorus, sodium, copper, zinc, and vitamin D should be supplemented as soon as feedings are adequately established. The addition of prepackaged "fortifiers" to human milk is an easy way to provide these nutrients and to increase caloric intake.

42. Which viruses can be transmitted in breast milk?
Cytomegalovirus, hepatitis B, rubella, and herpes virus.

43. Does breastfeeding protect the neonate from necrotizing enterocolitis?
Previously, breast milk was thought to decrease the incidence of necrotizing enterocolitis, but recent studies have failed to demonstrate any protective effect.

44. Does breastfeeding offer any protection against infections?
Several specific and nonspecific factors in human milk may help protect the neonate from infection (see table below). Even though all the immunoglobulin classes can enter breast milk, secretory IgA is present in greatest quantities and has the ability to adhere to mucosal epithelium and prevent the attachment and invasion of infectious agents. Lactoferrin binds free iron and limits iron availability to pathogenic gastrointestinal flora. Lysozyme catalyzes the hydrolysis of bacterial cell walls. Recent studies suggest that breast milk may actively stimulate the production of selected immune factors by the infant, including secretory IgA and lactoferrin.

Protective Elements in Human Milk

COMPONENT	COMMENT
Cellular factors	
Macrophage	Phagocytosis
	Produces lysozyme, lactoferrin, and complement
	May regulate B-lymphocyte immunoglobulin production
Lymphocyte	
B-cells	Humoral immunity; IgA synthesis
T-cells	Cellular immunity
	Partially regulate humoral immunity
Growth-promoting factors	
DNA synthesis and cell division in vitro	Functional in both animal and human fibroblasts
DNA synthesis and growth by mucosal cells	Described in laboratory animals
Bifidus factor	Nitrogen-containing polysaccharides that specifically enhance the growth of *Lactobacillus bifidus*
Lactoperoxidase	Functions in conjunction with hydrogen peroxide and cyanide to form an in vitro antibacterial system

From Polmar SH, Manthe ZU: Immunology. In Fanaroff AA, Martin RJ (eds): Neonatal-Perinatal Medicine: Diseases of the Fetus and Infant, 4th ed. St. Louis, C.V. Mosby Co., 1987, p 752, with permission.

45. What is breast milk jaundice?
Breast milk jaundice is a syndrome characterized by an elevated unconjugated bilirubin concentration occurring beyond the first week of postnatal life in breastfed infants.

46. What causes breast milk jaundice?

The etiology is currently unknown, although two general mechanisms have been suggested: (1) competitive inhibition of glucuronyl transferase activity by non-esterified long-chain fatty acids or metabolities of progesterone; and (2) increased enteric absorption of unconjugated bilirubin facilitated by high concentrations of beta glucuronidase found in some breast milk samples.

47. What is the accepted treatment of breast milk jaundice?

Once treatable causes of prolonged unconjugated hyperbilirubinemia have been ruled out (sepsis, hemolytic disease, hypothyroidism, etc.), and the infant is vigorous and healthy on physical examination, the preferred treatment is observation. No cases of kernicterus have been described secondary to breast milk jaundice, although most physicians do not let bilirubin levels exceed 20 mg/dl. When serum bilirubin concentration nears 20 mg/dl, breastfeeding may be stopped for 24–48 hours. This generally results in 30–50% decline of serum bilirubin values.

48. Which drugs excreted in breast milk are considered contraindications to breast-feeding?

Oral anticoagulants (Coumadin), which may produce coagulopathies; tetracycline, which may produce dental staining; thiouracil drugs, which achieve significant blood levels and may inhibit the infant's thyroid activity; and cimetidine, which achieves higher levels in milk than in maternal serum. Other drugs include antineoplastic agents, radioactive drugs, lithium, chloramphenicol, atropine, and ergot alkaloids.

49. How much formula should an average infant drink per day?

A healthy term newborn in the first 1–2 days of life may drink only 0.5–1 oz. every 3–4 hours. Once feedings are well established, infants may ingest 200 cc/kg/day or greater.

50. What are the advantages of a 60/40 whey/casein ratio in infant formulas?

The term 60/40 refers to the percentage of whey (lactalbumin) and casein in human milk or cow's milk formulas. This ratio makes for small curds and therefore easy digestibility by the infant. The 60/40 ratio is of particular advantage in the preterm infant because it is associated with lower levels of serum ammonia and a decreased incidence of metabolic acidosis. Only human milk or formulas that supply protein in this ratio provide adequate amounts of the amino acids, cystine and taurine, which may be essential for the preterm infant.

51. What is the rationale for starting with dilute formula for feeding the preterm infant?

The preterm infant is often started on formula feeds that are one-quarter or one-half strength. Although there are no data to support this clinical practice, many neonatologists believe that starting with dilute formula lessens the likelihood of feeding intolerance and possibly avoids serious complications such as necrotizing enterocolitis. The osmolality of the formula used may be a key determinant of the rapidity of gastric emptying.

52. What are the nutritional advantages of formulas designed for preterm babies?

Advantages of Formulas Designed for Preterm Babies

FEEDING COMPONENT	ADVANTAGE
Protein: 60/40 whey casein	Improved digestion; increased amounts of cystine, taurine
Carbohydrate: glucose polymers + lactose	Glucose polymers are better absorbed than lactose because of decreased production of intestinal lactase in the preterm infant

Table continued on next page.

Advantages of Formulas Designed for Preterm Babies (Continued)

FEEDING COMPONENT	ADVANTAGE
Fats: medium chain triglycerides (MCTs), corn/coconut	MCTs are absorbed directly into portal vein, and are less dependent on bile salts for emulsification and micelle formation
Minerals: increased calcium, phosphorus	Improved bone mineralization
Calories: 24 calories/oz	Increased growth

53. What are the advantages of transpyloric feedings vs. intermittent gavage?

There are no real advantages of transpyloric feedings in neonates. In theory, it was thought that these feeds would overcome problems such as gastroesophageal reflux and delayed gastric emptying. However, studies have demonstrated no difference in volumes of formulas tolerated or weight gain achieved by the two methods. Currently, transpyloric feedings are reserved for neonates who have failed other methods of nutrient delivery. The indications for and complications of various feeding regimens for preterm infants are summarized below.

Methods of Feeding Preterm Infants

METHOD	INDICATIONS	COMPLICATIONS	MANAGEMENT
Continuous Jejunal (NJ)	Premature ($<$ 1000 gm) Severe respiratory distress Intolerance to intermittent gavage	Stiffened feeding tube: GI peforation Inability to remove feeding tubes Decreased fat and potassium absorption	Change feeding tubes every 5 days

Use formula with medium-chain fat; monitor serum electrolytes |
| Intermittent Gastric (gavage) | Inadequate sucking and swallowing mechanism Premature (1000 to 1500 gm) Neurologic disorders Severe respiratory distress | Vomiting and aspiration | Measure gastric residuals prior to each feeding |
| Oral (nipple) | Premature $>$ 1500 gm Normal sucking and swallowing mechanism | Fatigue Increased energy expenditure associated with sucking | Gradual transition from tube to oral feedings Maximal nippling time per feeding: 20 min; give remainder of feed by tube |

From Pereira GR: Feeding the newborn infant. In Polin RA, Burg RD (eds): Workbook in Practical Neonatology. Philadelphia, W.B. Saunders Co., 1983, p 204, with permission.

54. Should intralipid usage be curtailed in the infant with hyperbilirubinemia or respiratory distress?

During lipid hydrolysis, free fatty acids are generated which may compete with bilirubin for binding to albumin. However, to date, no studies suggest a higher incidence of kernicterus in infants receiving intralipid. Lipid deposits have been noted at autopsy in alveolar macrophages and capillaries following intralipid administration. The adverse effects of intralipid on pulmonary function and bilirubin binding are related both to the dose and rate of infusion. A lipid dose of 1 gm/kg administered over 15 hours is safe for any size newborn infant. Therefore, hyperbilirubinemia and respiratory distress are not contraindications to the use of intralipid. In an infant nearing the point of exchange transfusion or receiving 100% oxygen, lipid emulsions should be used with caution.

55. How should lipid infusions be monitored?

Intralipid infusions should be monitored by measuring weekly triglyceride and cholesterol levels. Visible clearing from the serum may also be measured through a capillary tube, but this technique is probably much less reliable. Glucose levels should also be followed, as lipids cause enhanced gluconeogenesis secondary to increased fatty acid oxidation.

Digestive System

56. What is the classic presentation of pyloric stenosis?
An infant 3–6 weeks of age presents with progressive nonbilious projectile vomiting leading to dehydration with hypochloremic, hypokalemic, metabolic alkalosis. On physical exam a pyloric "olive" is palpable and peristaltic waves are visible.

57. What is the best way to palpate a pyloric "olive"?
The examination should be carried out with the infant's stomach empty. The examiner stands to the left of the infant and palpates the right upper quadrant gently.

58. How is pyloric stenosis diagnosed?
If the classic signs and symptoms of pyloric stenosis are present in association with the typical blood chemistry findings (hypochloremic, hypokalemic, metabolic alkalosis), the diagnosis can be made on clinical grounds. If the diagnosis is in doubt, ultrasound can be used to visualize the hypertrophic pyloric musculature. Upper GI contrast studies demonstrate pyloric obstruction with the characteristic "string sign" and enlarged "shoulders" bordering the elongated and obstructed pyloric channel.

59. What is the epidemiology of pyloric stenosis?
Pyloric stenosis is most prevalent in males (M:F ratio of 4:1), occurs most often in first-born children, and is associated with blood types O and B.

60. What special care should be provided to infants who pass meconium prenatally?
Meconium passage *in utero* generally signifies the occurrence of an asphyxial episode, which may result in aspiration of meconium into the lungs. Therefore all infants who have passed meconium should undergo laryngoscopy with suctioning of the pharynx under direct visualization, as well as intubation and suctioning of meconium from the trachea via the endotracheal tube. An infant who has passed minimal amounts of meconium and who is not neurologically depressed need not be suctioned.

61. Differentiate meconium ileus from meconium plug syndrome.
Meconium ileus is one of the most common presentations of cystic fibrosis during the newborn period. In meconium ileus, obstruction of the distal ileum occurs secondary to thick tenacious concretions of inspissated meconium. A barium enema may reveal a microcolon, and 25% of cases have associated intestinal atresia due to intrauterine obstruction. Calcifications suggest antenatal perforation and peritonitis. Meconium plug syndrome presents as either delayed passage of meconium or intestinal obstruction. Barium enema usually demonstrates a normal caliber colon with multiple filling defects. Small preterm infants, infants of diabetic mothers, and infants born to mothers who received magnesium sulfate are especially likely to develop meconium plug syndrome.

62. What is the relationship between formula feedings and necrotizing enterocolitis (NEC)?
Although the majority of infants with NEC have been fed prior to the development of signs, early institution of feedings is standard practice for most intensive care nurseries. Controversy surrounding feeding practices has centered around three areas: the time of initiation of the first feeding, the feeding volume, and the feeding composition. Feedings may contribute to the development of NEC by providing the substrate necessary for bacterial growth and for the production of hydrogen gas. The volume of feedings administered by nasogastric or nasojejunal tubes should be increased gradually to ensure the greatest success of enteral feedings. Although some investigators have suggested a relationship between rapid advancement of feeding volumes and the development of NEC, this remains controversial. Most importantly, as the volume of formula is increased, the amount of residual formula in the stomach must be checked periodically. If the volume of residual formula in the stomach

suddenly increases, feedings should be curtailed or completely stopped. The osmolality of the formula should be considered whenever feedings are begun. Hypertonic feedings can directly injure the intestinal mucosa and have been associated with the development of NEC in both experimental animals and human newborn infants. Hyperosmolar formulas should be specifically avoided whenever transpyloric feedings are used.

63. Which pathogens are thought to cause NEC?
The etiologic relationship between intestinal colonization with specific bacterial pathogens and the development of NEC is unknown, but up to one-third of infants with proven NEC have positive blood cultures. Epidemics of NEC have been associated with a variety of organisms including *E. coli,* Klebsiella, Pseudomonas, Salmonella, and Clostridium. It has been suggested that isolation of proven or suspected cases may help to control these epidemics. Of the many pathogens that have been isolated from children with proven NEC, clostridial species have recently been suggested as primary etiologic agents. Most neonates become colonized with clostridia during the first postnatal day. Clostridia organisms have the propensity to invade ischemic tissue and produce hydrogen gas and toxin.

64. What are the clinical signs of NEC? How should these infants be evaluated?
The clinical signs of necrotizing enterocolitis and suggested workup are shown below. Minimal workup is indicated if signs A or B are present without any other signs. Presence of NEC should be highly suspected if signs A or B are associated with D, E, F, or G. NEC is proven radiographically or at surgery.

Clinical Signs and Evaluation of Necrotizing Enterocolitis

SIGNS	DIAGNOSTIC EVALUATION

Early
A. Increased volume of gastric aspirate, vomiting, abdominal distention
	Suspicion of NEC (minimal workup)
	  Complete blood count and differential
	  Abdominal x-rays, repeat as needed
	  Platelet count
	  Check stools for blood and reducing substances

B. Hematest positive stools	High suspicion of NEC

C. Clinitest positive stools	Complete blood count and differential
	  Abdominal x-rays at least once per 8 hr shift
	  Platelet count 1 to 2 times per day
	  If platelets decreased, obtain PT and PTT
	  Arterial blood gas determination once or twice

D. Lethargy (septic appearance), hypothermia, apnea, etc.	daily for detection of acidosis Measurement of electrolyte levels

Late
E. Abdominal tenderness or erythema
	Proven NEC
	  Complete blood count and differential
	  Abdominal x-rays at least once every 6 hr during acute disease

F. Gross gastrointestinal bleeding	Platelet count two times per day and PT, PTT if decreased Arterial blood gas determination once or twice daily for detection of acidosis
G. Septic appearance with shock	Electrolyte levels

From Polin RA, Burg FD: Necrotizing enterocolitis. In Polin RA, Burg FD (eds): Workbook in Practical Neonatology. Philadelphia, W.B. Saunders, 1983, p 232, with permission.

65. What is considered acceptable medical treatment for NEC?
Therapy should be individualized according to whether there is low suspicion, high suspicion, or proven disease.

Therapy for Necrotizing Enterocolitis

1. Suspicion of necrotizing enterocolitis
   Nothing by mouth for short period of time until symptoms resolve
   Consider peripheral intravenous alimentation in preterm infants
2. High suspicion of necrotizing enterocolitis
   Nothing by mouth for a minimum of one week
   Intravenous alimentation mandatory for all infants
   Nasogastric tube for drainage
   Parenteral antibiotics
   Oral antibiotic therapy (optional)
   Surgical consultation
3. Proven necrotizing enterocolitis*
   Nothing by mouth for a minimum of 2 weeks
   Intravenous alimentation mandatory for all infants
   Consider central venous alimentation for preterm infants
   Nasogastric tube for drainage
   Platelet transfusion if count is less than 25,000/m^3
   Plasma transfusion and vitamin K for correction of other coagulation disorders
   Increased fluid intake during acute disease to account for third space loss
   Surgery is indicated if infant's clinical condition deteriorates, thrombocytopenia or acidosis is
      unremitting, or intestinal perforation or peritonitis develops
   Parenteral antibiotics (oral antibiotics optional)

From Polin RA, Burg FD: Necrotizing enterocolitis. In Polin RA, Burg FD (eds): Workbook in Practical Neonatology. W.B. Saunders Co., 1983, p 235, with permission.
*Proven radiographically or at surgery.

66. What are the indications for surgery in infants with NEC?
Indications include free intraperitoneal air, unrelenting metabolic acidosis, and clinical deterioration despite aggressive management. Because several studies have indicated that early intervention does not improve outcome in neonatal NEC, many surgeons prefer to postpone surgery until the above clinical signs are present.

67. How much bowel can be safely resected in a neonate?
Infants who retain 20 cm of small bowel measured from the ligament of Treitz can survive if the ileocecal valve is intact. If the ileocecal valve has been removed, the infant requires a minimum of 30 cm of bowel to survive.

68. How long should infants with NEC be kept NPO?
Infants with true NEC (radiographic or surgical evidence) should remain NPO for a minimum of 2–3 weeks. Infants in whom the diagnosis is suspected but not proven should be treated conservatively. Many of these infants may be fed after 3–7 days.

69. Is there evidence that oral antibiotics prevent NEC?
In two small studies of high-risk, low birthweight infants, the administration of oral kanamycin/gentamicin was effective in preventing NEC. However, study infants became colonized with organisms resistant to these antibiotics. More recent studies have failed to show a decreased incidence of NEC following prophylactic oral antibiotics. Therefore, antibiotic prophylaxis is not indicated for the prevention of NEC.

70. How does epidemic NEC differ from endemic NEC?

In most nurseries, there is a low background (endemic) incidence of NEC in which no single pathogenic organism is isolated. Many nurseries, however, have experienced clusters or epidemics of NEC, during which there is an unexpectedly high incidence of disease caused by a single pathogen. Infants with epidemic NEC have a lower risk of intestinal perforation and a more favorable outcome than those with the endemic variety.

71. What bowel diseases besides NEC demonstrate pneumatosis?

Pneumatosis intestinalis is not pathognomonic for NEC. Intestinal diseases other than NEC that may present with pneumatosis include Hirschprung's disease, pseudomembranous enterocolitis, neonatal ulcerative colitis, and ischemic bowel disease.

72. What is Pig-Bel?

Pig-Bel is an NEC-like disease afflicting infants and adults in Papua, New Guinea. It is caused by ingestion of *C. perfringens* type C enterotoxin.

73. What is the diving seal reflex?

The diving reflex is a physiologic adaptation to submersion noted in native pearl divers of Australia and other diving mammals. During a sustained dive, cardiac output is directed preferentially to vital organs (brain, adrenals, and heart), and shunted away from other nonvital organs such as the intestines and splanchnic circulations. There is a suggestion that this reflex is present in human newborn infants. In NEC, intestinal ischemic injury may occur secondary to this phenomenon.

74. When does the newborn infant's stomach secrete acid?

The pH of gastric fluid in newborns is usually neutral or slightly acid and decreases shortly after birth. pH values are less than 3 by 6–8 hours of age, and then increase again during the second week of life. Preterm infants frequently demonstrate gastric pH values above 7.

75. Which disaccharidases are slowest to develop prenatally?

The disaccharidases are detectable with low activity at about 12–14 weeks of gestation, and by 24 weeks sucrase, maltase, and isomaltase generally achieve significant levels of activity. Lactase activity lags behind and is frequently not detected until 28–30 weeks of gestation. Many preterm and term infants demonstrate lactose intolerance when measured by breath hydrogen analysis; however, the clinical significance of subclinical lactose intolerance is controversial.

76. Why do newborn infants absorb fat poorly?

Although normal term neonates absorb 90% of the fats ingested, preterm infants absorb significantly less. The major reasons for fat malabsorption include decreased pancreatic lipase activity, decreased uptake and synthesis of bile salts, and impaired bile salt resorption by the terminal ileum. Human milk fat with palmitic acid in the two position is absorbed better than the butterfat found in cow's milk.

77. What is the best position for an infant with reflux?

The infant with reflux should be maintained in an upright (prone) position during and following feedings. Some infants require a 60-degree upright position during most of the day. Infants with reflux should not be placed in an "infant seat" following feedings, as this may increase intra-abdominal pressure and promote reflux.

78. What are the manifestations of peptic ulcer disease in the neonate?

Peptic ulcers in the neonate occur in both the stomach and duodenum and commonly present with GI bleeding. The infant may vomit blood, have blood present in nasogastric aspirates, or pass stools positive for occult blood. Signs and symptoms of hypovolemia may occur due to blood loss, and blood must be vigorously replaced. Intestinal perforation is a rare complication of ulcer disease.

79. What causes gastrointestinal (GI) bleeding in the neonate? (See also questions 65–68 on pp. 110 and 111.)

Gastrointestinal bleeding in the neonate can be divided into two broad categories with several diagnostic possibilities in each:

Etiology of Upper GI Bleeding

Bleeding diathesis
Hemorrhagic gastritis
Stress ulcer
Swallowed maternal blood

Esophagitis
Foreign body irritation
   (nasogastric tube)
Vascular malformations
Duplication

Etiology of Lower GI Bleeding

Well Infant
   Swallowed maternal blood
   Infectious colitis
   Milk allergy
   Hemorrhagic disease
   Duplication of bowel
   Meckel's diverticulum

Sick Infant
   Necrotizing enterocolitis
   Infectious colitis
   Disseminated coagulopathy
   Midgut volvulus
   Intussusception
   Congestive heart failure

From Fleisher G, Ludwig S (eds): Textbook of Pediatric Emergency Medicine. Baltimore, Williams and Wilkins, 1983, pp 161, 165, with permission.

80. How should infants with GI bleeding be evaluated?

Evaluation should include a careful history and physical examination, focusing on other signs and symptoms of systemic illness and/or bleeding as well as the presence of localized sources of bleeding (e.g., fissures). In addition, passage of nasogastric tube to localize bleeding to the upper GI tract versus the lower GI tract is essential. Laboratory evaluation should include a complete blood count, Apt test to rule out swallowed maternal blood, stool culture for bacterial and viral pathogens, and an abdominal x-ray to rule out obstructive processes and necrotizing enterocolitis. In infants with life-threatening upper GI hemorrhage, endoscopy can be performed either immediately, or 12–24 hours after presentation. Air contrast barium radiography can also provide useful information in neonates with upper GI hemorrhage. If all the above studies do not provide a diagnosis and bleeding remains a problem, additional studies should include a Meckel's scan, a technetium scan and/or angiography.

81. What is the differential diagnosis of ascites in the neonate?

Obstructive uropathy
Meconium peritonitis
Chylous ascites
Bile ascites
Intraperitoneal cysts
Hydrometrocolpos
Acute peritonitis with or without fetal or neonatal hepatitis
   Bacterial infection, including syphilis
   Viral infection (cytomegalovirus)
   Toxoplasmosis
Associated with generalized edema or anasarca
   Hemolytic disease of the newborn
   α-Thalassemia (homozygous)
   Twin-twin or fetal-maternal hemorrhage
   Severe cardiopulmonary malformations
      Pulmonary lymphangiectasia
      Cystic adenomatoid malformation of the lung
   Congenital nephrosis
   Chorioangioma of the placenta
   Infantile Gaucher's disease

Syndrome of hyperplacentosis
  Hydramnios
  Edematous placenta
  Hydrops fetalis
  Toxemia of pregnancy
From Sunshine et al: In Fanaroff AA, Martin RF (eds): Neonatal-Perinatal Medicine: Diseases of the Fetus and Infant. St. Louis, C.V. Mosby Co., 1983, p 533, with permission.

82. What are the clinical presentations of tracheoesophageal fistula (TEF) with or without esophageal atresia?

The most common (approximately 85%) form of TEF consists of esophageal atresia with distal TEF. Isolated esophageal atresia without TEF and "H-type" TEF without esophageal atresia each comprise approximately 5–7% of cases. Esophageal atresia with proximal TEF or with both proximal and distal TEF is rare. Clinically, patients with esophageal atresia present with signs of esophageal obstruction, including coughing and choking on secretions and "mucousy" respirations. Additionally, patients with TEF demonstrate secondary respiratory complications, including intermittent cyanosis and aspiration pneumonia. Patients with pure atresia or the absence of distal TEF will have scaphoid gasless abdomens, whereas those with distal TEF will have abdominal distention.

83. How is gastroschisis differentiated from omphalocele in the newborn infant?

Comparative Clinical Features of Gastroschisis and Omphalocele

	GASTROSCHISIS	OMPHALOCELE
Incidence	1/50,000 births	1/5,000 births
Location of defect	Right paraumbilical	Central abdominal
Umbilical cord insertion	Normal	Apex of sac
Herniation of the liver	Rare	Common
Extraintestinal anomalies	Rare	Common

84. What is the differential diagnosis of an abdominal mass in the neonate?

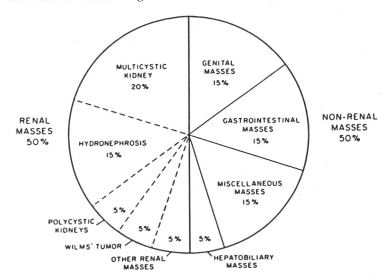

As shown, nearly 50% of these masses are renal in origin. (From Sunshine, et al. In Fanaroff AA, Martin RF (eds): Behrman's Neonatal-Perinatal Medicine: Diseases of the Fetus and Infant. St. Louis, C.V. Mosby Co., 1983, p 531, with permission.)

85. When is the best time for repair of inguinal hernias?
Inguinal hernia repair is performed during the first year of life unless the infant's clinical condition makes surgery unsafe. This repair should obviously be performed earlier in the event of signs or symptoms of incarceration.

Liver and Biliary System

86. Which physiologic factors contribute to the rise in serum bilirubin in the newborn infant?

Possible Mechanisms Involved in Physiologic Jaundice

Increased Bilirubin Load on the Liver Cell
  ↑ Red blood cell volume
  ↓ Red blood cell survival
  ↑ Early-labeled bilirubin
  ↑ Enterohepatic circulation of bilirubin
Defective Hepatic Uptake of Bilirubin from the Plasma
  ↓ Ligandin (Y protein)
    Binding of Y and Z proteins by other anions
  ↓ Relative hepatic uptake deficiency (phase II)
Defective Bilirubin Conjugation
  ↓ UDP glucuronyl transferase activity
  ↓ UDP glucose dehydrogenase activity
Defective Bilirubin Excretion
  Excretion impaired but not rate limiting
Hepatic Circulation
  ↓ Oxygen supply to the liver when umbilical cord clamped
    Portal blood flow bypassing liver sinusoids if ductus venosus patent

From Maisels MJ: Neonatal jaundice. In Avery GB (ed): Neonatology: Pathophysiology and Management of the Newborn. Philadelphia, J.B. Lippincott, 1987, p 556, with permission.

87. What are the kinetics of bilirubin rise and fall in the term and preterm infant?
In the term infant with physiologic jaundice, bilirubin values rise from a level of approximately 2 mg/dl to a mean of 6 mg/dl at 3 days of age (12.9 mg/dl is 2 SD above the mean). Bilirubin levels then fall rapidly by the fifth day of life. In the preterm infant with physiologic jaundice, bilirubin levels peak later and higher. Mean peak concentrations reach 10–15 mg/dl by day 5 of life and then decline slowly over the subsequent 7–14 days.

88. What is the statistical definition of physiologic hyperbilirubinemia in the newborn infant?
During the first few days of life, nearly all infants demonstrate a rise in the serum bilirubin concentration. By definition, physiologic hyperbilirubinemia should not be associated with serum bilirubin concentrations ≥ 12 mg/dl in the term infant or ≥ 15 mg/dl in the preterm infant.

89. What is the minimal workup for all jaundiced infants?
Both direct and total serum bilirubin determinations, a complete blood count with examination of the peripheral smear for red cell morphology, reticulocyte count, and blood type, Rh, and Coombs' determinations.

90. Is phenobarbital or phototherapy more effective for reducing the serum bilirubin concentration in the neonate?
Phototherapy is extremely effective in reducing serum unconjugated bilirubin concentrations in newborn infants. In infants with nonhemolytic, physiologic jaundice, it has nearly eliminated the need for exchange transfusion. In infants with hemolytic processes it will reduce but not eliminate the need for exchange transfusion. In contrast, phenobarbital is

effective in enhancing bilirubin excretion and is useful for the treatment of conjugated hyperbilirubinemia. Phenobarbital is not as effective as phototherapy for reducing serum bilirubin concentrations in infants with unconjugated hyperbilirubinemia.

91. What guidelines are used for exchange transfusion or phototherapy in the jaundiced neonate?
Criteria for exchange transfusion are shown in the table. Phototherapy should be started 4–5 mg/dl below exchange levels.

Serum Bilirubin Level (mg/dl) as Criterion for Exchange Transfusion

	BIRTH WEIGHT (g)				
RISK	<1,250	1,250–1,499	1,500–1,999	2,000–2,499	≥2,500
Standard Risk	13	15	17	18	20
High Risk*	10	13	15	17	18

From Keenan WJ, Novak KK, Sutherland JM, et al: Morbidity and mortality associated with exchange transfusion. Pediatrics 75(Suppl):417, 1985, with permission.
*High risk criteria are met when one or more of the following apply: birth weight less than 1000 g, 5-minute Apgar score less than 3, PaO2 < 40 mmHg for more than 2 hours, pH <7.15 for more than 1 hour, rectal temperature <35°C for more than 4 hours, serum total protein value less than 4 gm/dlx2, serum albumin level less than 2.5 gm/dlx2, hemolysis, or clinical deterioration.

92. Should calcium be given during an exchange transfusion?
It is common practice to administer calcium during an exchange transfusion with ACD or CPD anticoagulated blood. The citrate in these preparations can bind calcium and magnesium and thus produce a significant decrease in these ions. However, administration of calcium during exchange transfusions does not appear to have a significant effect on serum ionized calcium levels, and adverse effects have not been described when calcium has not been administered.

93. What are the indications for albumin in the neonate about to receive an exchange transfusion?
Albumin infusion has been advocated 1–2 hours before exchange transfusion in an attempt to increase the amount of bilirubin removed by the exchange. Albumin may draw tissue-bound bilirubin into the circulation and has been reported to increase bilirubin removed by 40%. Albumin should be administered with caution in infants with respiratory distress and congestive heart failure, and is not used routinely in most nurseries.

94. What is vigintiphobia?
Vigintiphobia, translated from the Latin, is "fear of twenty." In many nurseries, it is common practice to exchange infants without evidence of isoimmunization at bilirubin levels of 20 mg/dl to prevent kernicterus. However, critical bilirubin levels have not been determined for infants with nonhemolytic hyperbilirubinemia. Therefore this common management practice is without scientific support and is termed "vigintiphobia."

95. What percentage of blood volume is removed in a one, two, and three volume exchange transfusion?

Blood Volume Exchanged*	Blood Volume Removed and Replaced by Exchange
1.0	63%
2.0	87%
3.0	95%

*A two volume exchange is usually used, and the exchange transfusion is completed in about 1 hour.

96. How quickly does the bilirubin rebound following an exchange transfusion?
Although 87% of the infant's bilirubin is removed in a two-volume exchange, the serum bilirubin concentration is only reduced to 45% of the pre-exchange level. Equilibration is complete by 30 minutes, at which time the bilirubin rises to 60% of the pre-exchange value.

97. How can the risk of transfusion-acquired cytomegalovirus (CMV) infections be minimized?
It can be minimized by screening blood components for CMV antibody and administering only seronegative blood. However, because of the high prevalence of CMV positivity in the general population, alternative methods have been studied. Frozen deglycerolized red blood cells virtually eliminate transfusion-associated CMV infection, although this method requires 1–2 hours of preparation time and may not be cost effective, particularly in smaller centers.

98. What are the theoretical advantages and disadvantages of the "continuous" exchange transfusion?
The continuous exchange transfusion technique uses two central catheters: one appropriately positioned in the umbilical vein and the other in the umbilical artery. Blood is transfused by constant pump infusion into the umbilical vein, while blood is withdrawn continuously from the arterial catheter by syringe. This method avoids intermittent pressure fluctuations in the central arterial or venous circulations, and may avoid vascular compromise to the gastrointestinal tract, kidneys, and CNS associated with the "push-pull" technique. The disadvantage of this technique is that it requires the placement of two central catheters, which may increase the risk of catheter-related complications.

99. Who was Sister Ward?
In the early 1950s, Sister Ward was the nurse in charge of the unit for premature infants at Rochford General Hospital in Essex, England. On warm summer days, Sister Ward would take her infants to the courtyard to give them a little fresh air and sunshine. It was following such an afternoon of sunshine that Sister Ward observed that sunlight was able to "bleach" the skin of jaundiced human neonates. Here is the account of her discovery as recorded by R. H. Dobbs:

> One particularly fine summer's day in 1956, during a ward routine, Sister Ward diffidently showed us a premature baby, carefully undressed and with fully exposed abdomen. The infant was pale yellow except for a strongly demarcated triangle of skin very much yellower than the rest of the body. I asked her, "Sister, what did you paint it with—iodine or flavine, and why?" But she replied that she thought it must have been the sun. "What do you mean Sister? Sun tan takes days to develop after the erythema has faded." Sister Ward looked increasingly uncomfortable, and explained that she thought it was a jaundiced baby, much darker where a corner of the sheet had covered the area. "It's the rest of the body that seems to have faded." We left it at that, and as the infant did well and went home, fresh air treatment of prematurity continued.

100. What dose and wavelength of light are most effective for reducing the serum bilirubin concentration?
Phototherapy is most effective in the spectral range between 460 and 500 nm. The minimal irradiance (μwatts/cm^2/nm measured at 450 nm) that is effective for reducing the serum bilirubin concentration is 4 μwatts/cm^2/nm. The irradiance at which the maximal decrement in serum bilirubin occurs has not been clearly determined; however, in our nursery doses greater than 12 μwatts/cm^2/nm are not used.

101. Where does phototherapy photoisomerize bilirubin?
Phototherapy is thought to modify bilirubin deposited within the first few millimeters of the skin surface. It is thought to be a two-step process. The photoisomerization process occurs in nanoseconds, whereas the slower, rate-limiting step is the migration of bilirubin (or its isomers) to and from the skin.

102. What is lumirubin?
Lumirubin is a structural isomer of bilirubin formed by the action of phototherapy on the bilirubin molecule. In this reaction, there is a structural rearrangement of atoms in which the vinyl ($-CH=CH_2$) group on carbon 3 forms a new bond with carbon 7.

103. What is Z-E bilirubin?
Z-E bilirubin is a configurational isomer formed by the action of light on the bilirubin molecule. This reaction is a 180° rotation of one of the outer rings around a double bond, and is equivalent to a cis-trans isomerization. Recent experiments suggest that this configurational isomerism is *not* the major mechanism of action of phototherapy. Instead, it is felt that the formation of structural isomers (lumirubin) represents the principal pathway for bilirubin elimination in the neonate.

104. Why is native bilirubin called ZZ bilirubin?
Native bilirubin (bilirubin IXα) is composed of four pyrrole rings joined by three carbon bridges. The outer two rings are joined to the central rings by exocyclic double bonds. At both of the double bonds, two different configurations of atoms are possible (Z and E). The letter Z stands for the German word zusammen, meaning together, and E represents the German word for opposite (entgegen). Therefore, Z and E are equivalent to cis and trans respectively. Native bilirubin has both halves of the molecule in the cis or ZZ configuration.

105. Where does bilirubin go when you turn on the lights?
In the newborn infant, structural isomerization (lumirubin formation) is the principal pathway of bilirubin elimination. Lumirubin is rapidly excreted in the bile, with a half-life of about 2 hours.

106. What are the adverse effects of phototherapy?
Diarrhea, increased insensible water loss and increased skin blood flow, skin rashes, increased platelet turnover, and hemolysis of red blood cells *in vitro*. The bronze baby syndrome, which is a gray-brown discoloration of the skin, serum, and urine, has also been reported in association with phototherapy. *In vitro* experiments with phototherapy have demonstrated mutations in bacteria and impaired reproductive capacities in sea urchin gametes. However, to date, this cell damage has not been demonstrated in newborn infants.

107. How should infants with phototherapy-induced diarrhea be fed?
Loose green stools are a common complication of phototherapy. Studies have found diminished intestinal lactase activity in jaundiced infants undergoing phototherapy, which normalizes when phototherapy is discontinued. As a result, infants with phototherapy-induced diarrhea should be fed a lactose-free diet until the phototherapy is stopped or the symptoms resolve.

108. What is the mechanism of the light-induced increase in insensible water loss (IWL)?
Some investigators have suggested that the increased IWL observed with phototherapy could be due to increased radiant power delivery to the infant. Recent studies, however, have determined that there is no significant difference in radiant power delivered with or without phototherapy (i.e., the increased IWL secondary to phototherapy *cannot* be explained by increased radiant power delivery). Alternatively, the light may directly dilate skin arterioles producing vasodilatation and transcutaneous water loss, or affect central temperature control mechanisms which results in peripheral vasodilatation and water loss.

109. What is the bronze baby syndrome?

The bronze baby syndrome refers to the development of a bronze-black coloration of the skin, serum, and urine of infants receiving phototherapy. Infants who develop bronze baby syndrome typically have an elevated direct serum bilirubin. Bronze baby syndrome occurs secondary to retention of lumirubin that cannot be excreted in the bile. Most infants appear to recover without complications, although a single infant dying with bronze baby syndrome was reported to have kernicterus at autopsy. Although this condition is generally assumed to be benign, it is important that concentrations of direct bilirubin be measured before starting phototherapy. In infants with significant conjugated hyperbilirubinemia, phototherapy should not be used.

110. What are the contraindications to phototherapy?

Infants with a significantly elevated direct-reacting bilirubin or a family history of light-sensitive porphyria should not receive phototherapy.

111. Why should infants receiving phototherapy wear eye patches?

Studies in animals have demonstrated the potential toxic effects of light on the retina, although similar findings have not been demonstrated in human infants. These changes are similar to those of premature aging with loss of rod and cone cells in the exposed areas of the retinas. Despite the lack of human data, it would seem important to continue to shield the eyes of all infants receiving phototherapy.

112. How has the American sea urchin contributed to research in phototherapy?

Speck and Rosenkranz studied the effects of phototherapy on the fertilization and embryogenesis of the American sea urchin. They removed gametes from mature sea urchins and exposed unfertilized oocytes and spermatozoa to phototherapy to determine its effect on post-irradiation fertilization and embryonic development. Light treatment revealed dose-dependent abnormalities in fertilization and subsequent embryonic development.

113. What are the manifestations of kernicterus in the neonate?

The classic manifestations include lethargy, rigidity, ophisthotonus, high-pitched cry, fever, and seizures. These symptoms develop progressively over a period of 24 hours, usually by the third to fourth day of life. Survivors frequently demonstrate choreoathetoid cerebral palsy, hearing loss, and sometimes mental retardation. A paralysis of upward gaze and dental dysplasia have also been described following bilirubin encephalopathy.

114. What clinical factors are known to increase the risk of kernicterus?

Hypoxia, hypoglycemia, acidosis, sepsis, hypothermia, hemolysis, hypoalbuminemia, and defective bilirubin-albumin binding.

115. How much potential bilirubin is there in meconium?

Analysis of meconium stools from both preterm and term infants indicates that there is 1 mg bilirubin/g wet weight and that 50% is unconjugated. At birth the amount of meconium in the gut is estimated to be between 100 and 200 g.

116. What are Liley's Zones I, II, and III?

In classic work originally published by Liley in 1961, it was demonstrated that antenatal determinations of amniotic fluid bilirubin could be used to predict the severity of Rh hemolytic disease. The absorbance of amniotic fluid bilirubin at 450 nm (OD 450) was plotted on a graph versus gestational age, and divided into three prognostic zones: Zone 1, the low zone, indicates unaffected or only mildly affected fetuses; Zone 3, the upper zone, indicates severely affected fetuses; and Zone 2, the mid-zone, is associated with a range of pregnancy outcomes, depending on the trends in amniotic fluid bilirubin values.

117. What is the mechanism of hyperalimentation-induced cholestasis?

The mechanism remains uncertain, although amino acid toxicity has been frequently implicated. Dextrose infusions may also be hepatotoxic, but intralipid administration is probably not causative in this syndrome. Vileisis demonstrated that infants fed a high-protein regimen (3–6 g/kg/day) developed a higher level of direct bilirubin at an earlier time than infants receiving a lower protein load. Other possible etiologies include (1) decreased bile flow and gut motility secondary to the lack of oral alimentation and immaturity of the enterohepatic circulation; (2) cholestasis secondary to absorption of bacterial toxins from the gut during bowel stasis; or (3) amino acid deficiency in hyperalimentation mixtures.

Reference Vileisis: J Pediatr 96:893, 1980.

118. What is the value of calculating the calorie/nitrogen ratio in infants fed intravenously?

A calorie/nitrogen ratio (cal/N) in excess of 200 should be avoided in infants with evidence of hyperalimentation-induced cholestasis. Remember: 6.25 g protein = 1 g nitrogen. For a 1 kg infant receiving 4 g protein/kg/day and 120 nonprotein calories/day, the following calculations can be made:

$$\frac{6.25 \text{ g protein}}{4 \text{ g protein/day}} = \frac{1 \text{ g nitrogen}}{X}$$

$$X = .66 \text{ g nitrogen/day}$$

and

$$\frac{120 \text{ non-protein calories}}{.66 \text{ g nitrogen}} = 200 \text{ cal/N}$$

119. What is the treatment for hyperalimentation-induced cholestasis?

The preferred treatment is to stop intravenous hyperalimentation and begin enteral feedings. If intravenous hyperalimentation cannot be discontinued, the amount of protein infused should be reduced to 2 g/kg/day and cal/N ratio kept below 200. In most infants, the condition is transient and resolves without further therapy. In infants with severe intrahepatic cholestasis, phenobarbital has been shown to stimulate bile secretion and lower serum bilirubin levels.

Metabolism/Endocrine System

120. What are the manifestations of neonatal cold injury?

Neonatal cold injury is primarily seen in low birthweight infants but may also be seen in full-term infants with CNS malformations. Characteristics of this syndrome include poor feeding, lethargy, and coldness to touch associated with core temperatures of $\leq 32.2°C$. Despite the presence of a bright red skin color, which is secondary to decreased dissociation of oxyhemoglobin, these infants display central cyanosis. Respirations are shallow, irregular, and sometimes associated with grunting, and bradycardia as a function of the degree of temperature depression may also be seen. Other findings include CNS depression with decreased responsiveness, abdominal distention with vomiting, and edema of the skin and face which may progress to sclerema. Concomitant metabolic disturbances include metabolic acidosis, hypoglycemia, hyperkalemia, and azotemia.

121. What are the manifestations of hypocalcemia in the neonate?

The major manifestations of hypocalcemia in the neonate are jitteriness and seizures. Additional signs such as high-pitched cry, laryngospasm, Chvostek's sign (facial muscle twitching on tapping) and Trousseau's sign (carpopedal spasm) may be present, but more commonly are absent during the neonatal period.

122. When and how should hypocalcemia be treated in the neonate?
Hypocalcemia should be treated when it is associated with signs or symptoms, or when the serum calcium level is < 7.0 mg/dl. The first line of therapy generally consists of increasing the amount of calcium in the intravenous infusion to achieve 75 mg of elemental calcium/kg/day, and following serum levels every 6–8 hours. Infusion of bolus intravenous calcium (10% calcium gluconate, 2 cc/kg) over 10 minutes should be reserved for the infant with seizures. In the asymptomatic infant, hypocalcemia most frequently resolves spontaneously without any need for further therapy.

123. What is the differential diagnosis of hypocalcemia/hypercalcemia in the neonate?
The causes of hypocalcemia are outlined below. Hypercalcemia, which occurs much less commonly, is noted in infants with primary or secondary hyperparathyroidism, idiopathic hypercalcemia (with or without the associated features of Williams' syndrome), subcutaneous fat necrosis, paraneoplastic syndromes (principally nephroblastoma), those receiving excessive calcium intake, and infants with severe infantile hypophosphatasia, familial hypocalciuric hypercalcemia, or the congenital hypokalemia, hypercalcemia syndrome.

Differential Diagnosis of Hypocalcemia

A. Early neonatal hypocalcemia (first 3 days of life)
   1. Premature infants
   2. Infants with birth asphyxia
   3. Infants of diabetic mothers
B. Late neonatal hypocalcemia (after end of first week)
   1. High phosphate cow's milk formula
   2. Intestinal malabsorption
   3. Postdiarrheal acidosis
   4. Hypomagnesemia
   5. Neonatal hypoparathyroidism
   6. Rickets
C. Decreased ionized fraction of calcium
   1. Citrate (exchange transfusion)
   2. Increased free fatty acid (Intralipid)
   3. Alkalosis

---

124. What is classical neonatal tetany?
Classic neonatal tetany commonly presents toward the end of the first week of life and is related to the ingestion of milk with a high phosphate content. The serum calcium level is generally below 7–8 mg/dl and the serum phosphorus concentration is elevated. Inadequate vitamin D intake during pregnancy may be an additional associated factor.

125. When should serum magnesium concentration be measured in a neonate?
It should be measured in any hypocalcemic infant not responding to calcium therapy, hypotonic infants born to mothers who received magnesium sulfate therapy prior to delivery, and infants with seizures of unknown etiology.

126. How is hypomagnesemia treated?
Hypomagnesemic infants should be treated with 0.25 ml/kg of a 50% solution (100 mg of elemental magnesium/ml) given intramuscularly. Magnesium levels are followed and the dosage repeated if necessary.

127. What are the manifestations of drug withdrawal in the neonate?
The signs and symptoms of drug withdrawal in the neonate can be remembered by using the mnemonic "withdrawal."

W = Wakefulness
I = Irritability
T = Tremulousness, temperature variation, tachypnea
H = Hyperactivity, high-pitched persistent cry, hyperacusia, hyperreflexia, hypertonus
D = Diarrhea, diaphoresis, disorganized suck
R = Rub marks, respiratory distress, rhinorrhea
A = Apneic attacks, autonomic dysfunction
W = Weight loss or failure to gain weight
A = Alkalosis (respiratory)
L = Lacrimation
    From The Committee on Drugs 1982–1983, Albert Pruitt Chairman, Neonatal Drug Withdrawal, Pediatrics 72:896, 1983, with permission.

128. How should drug withdrawal in neonates be treated?
The drugs most commonly used to treat withdrawal symptoms are summarized in the table below.

Treatment of Drug Withdrawal in Neonates

DRUG*	DOSE	COMMENTS
Paregoric	0.2–0.5 ml per dose q 3–4 hr until the symptoms are controlled (term infant)	Contains a high concentration of alcohol, anise oil, and benzoic acid
Diazepam	0.3–0.5 mg/kg/day. Initial dose should be IM followed by PO q 8 hrs	Parenteral diazepam contains 10% ethyl alcohol and 40% propylene glycol
Phenobarbital	20 mg/kg loading dose (IM) then 5 mg/kg/day PO	Phenobarbital is a CNS depressant and may impair bonding and feeding
Methadone	0.1–0.5 mg/kg/day PO q 4–12 hr	$T\frac{1}{2}$ = 26 hours

*These drugs are generally continued for 4–6 weeks, then tapered and stopped.

129. How is the dose of sodium bicarbonate needed to treat metabolic acidosis in the neonate calculated?

$$HCO_3 \text{ (mEq)} = \text{Base deficit (mEq/L)} \times 0.3 \text{ L/kg} \times \text{Body wt (kg)}$$

Generally, it is safest to correct half the base deficit initially, and then reassess acid base status to determine if further correction is necessary.

130. When should THAM be used?
Tris (hydroxymethyl) aminomethane (THAM) is an alkali (like sodium bicarbonate) that offers the advantages of no sodium load, penetration into the cell, and lowering of PCO_2. THAM, however, may cause respiratory center depression and respiratory distress as well as local tissue injury. On a molar basis, THAM offers 50% less buffering activity than bicarbonate. Therefore, THAM is not used during the newborn period.

131. What is Penred's syndrome?
Penred's syndrome is an iodide organification defect in which an iodide transferase is lacking, producing a small goiter and hypothyroidism. This disorder is frequently associated with congenital deafness, despite normal intelligence. Penred's syndrome is transmitted in an autosomal recessive fashion.

132. How is true hypothyroidism differentiated from transient hypothyroxinemia in a neonate?

Stressed or sick preterm infants may demonstrate a transient hypothyroxinemia during the newborn period. These infants present with low serum thyroxine and normal serum TSH values, which will distinguish them from infants with true hypothyroidism (low T_4, elevated TSH).

133. What clinical findings are associated with neonatal hypothyroidism?

They include lethargy, hypotonia, large anterior and posterior fontanels, feeding difficulty, respiratory distress, pallor, constipation, hoarse cry, and perioral cyanosis. Prolonged physiologic jaundice may also occur. The classic features of cretinism typically occur after 6 weeks of life.

134. How is neonatal hyperthyroidism treated?

It is treated with iodine (Lugol's solution), propylthiouracil or methimazole. Iodine inhibits both T_4 synthesis and release from the thyroid. The effect of iodine may disappear after several weeks. The cardiovascular signs and symptoms of thyrotoxicosis are related to an increased adrenergic response. Thus, antiadrenergic agents, such as propranolol, may be used to alleviate symptoms. Digoxin may be needed to treat heart failure. These infants should also be observed for signs of respiratory compromise/tracheal obstruction by the large goiter. Surgery may be indicated in selected cases.

135. What is the definition of neonatal hypoglycemia?

Hypoglycemia is defined as a serum glucose less than 35 mg/dl in the term neonate and less than 25 mg/dl in the preterm or low birthweight neonate during the first 3 days of life. Beyond that time, a glucose of less than 45 mg/dl is considered abnormal.

136. When is hypoglycemia most likely to occur in a neonate?

During gestation, glucose is freely transferred across the placenta by the process of facilitated diffusion. However, after birth, the infant must adjust to the sudden withdrawal of this transplacental supply. In all infants, there is a nadir in blood sugar between 1 and 3 hours of life. This fall is accentuated in preterm infants, infants of diabetic mothers, infants with erythroblastosis fetalis, asphyxiated infants, and infants who are small or large for gestational age.

137. What are the clinical signs of hypoglycemia?

High-pitched cry, lethargy, apnea, seizures, cyanosis, tachypnea, and hypotonia.

138. How should infants with persistent hypoglycemia be evaluated?

   A. History with particular attention to:
      1. Maternal diabetes
      2. Blood group incompatibility
      3. Maternal toxemia and/or hypertension
      4. Maternal drugs
      5. Prior unexplained stillbirths and/or infant deaths
      6. Dextrose administered prior to delivery
   B. Physical Examination
      1. Size with respect to gestational age
      2. Features of erythroblastosis
      3. Features of infant of diabetic mother
      4. Features of Beckwith-Weidemann, i.e., omphalocele, macrosomia, macroglossia
      5. Hepatomegaly
      6. Cataracts
      7. Genital abnormalities
      8. Midline facial defects

C. Laboratory Evaluation
The optimal time to obtain the following studies is during an episode of hypoglycemia.
1. Glucose
2. Insulin
3. Human growth hormone
4. Cortisol
5. Lactate/pyruvate — if glycogen storage disease is suspected
6. Thyroid function — if hypopituitarism is suspected
7. Adrenal function

139. What disease states are associated with hypoglycemia?

Glucose Production Abnormalities
1. Premature infants
2. Small for gestational age infants
3. Stressed infants
   Hypothermia
   Asphyxia
   Sepsis or other serious infection
   Respiratory disease
4. Cardiac disease
   Cyanotic congenital disease
   Congestive heart failure
5. Inherited abnormalities
   Carbohydrate
      Type I glycogen storage disease
      Galactosemia
      Others
   Amino acid metabolism
      Tyrosinosis
      Methylmalonic aciduria
      Others
   Hormone deficiencies
      Growth hormone deficiency
      Hypopituitarism
      Others

Hyperinsulinemia
1. Infant of diabetic mother
2. Erythroblastosis fetalis caused by Rh incompatibility
3. Beckwith-Weidemann syndrome
4. Islet cell growth disturbances (such as adenoma and nesidioblastosis)
5. Tocolytic therapy with beta sympathomimetic drugs during labor

From Dransfield DA: Neonatal hypoglycemia and hypocalcemia. In Polin RA, Burg FD: Workbook in Practical Neonatology. Philadelphia, W.B. Saunders Co., 1983, p 55, with permission.

140. How should hypoglycemia be treated? How is refractory hypoglycemia treated?

Both symptomatic and asymptomatic hypoglycemia should be treated. The infant should first receive a bolus of intravenous glucose (200 mg/kg or 2 cc/kg of 10% dextrose) followed by a glucose infusion providing 6–8 mg/kg/min. Additional serum glucose concentrations should be determined to assure prompt correction and allow modification of the dose as needed. Certain infants may require more aggressive therapies such as higher concentration dextrose infusions, corticosteroids, or glucagon to attain euglycemia.

Refractory hypoglycemia is treated with corticosteroids (reduces peripheral glucose utilization and promotes gluconeogenesis), glucagon (releases glycogen from hepatic stores and promotes gluconeogenesis), or epinephrine (promotes glycogenolysis/gluconeogenesis, augments glucagon secretion, and inhibits insulin secretion). Diazoxide therapy should be used in only the most extreme cases after other therapies have failed.

141. What features are seen in Beckwith's syndrome?

Features include gigantism, macroglossia, visceromegaly, and omphalocele in association with severe hypoglycemia. Other reported anomalies include facial nevus flammeus, vertical earlobe grooves, microcephaly, renal medullary dysplasia, cytoplasia of the adrenal cortex, and hyperplasia of many other organs. Neonatal hypoglycemia, hypocalcemia, and polycythemia are frequently observed. Somatic overgrowth may be asymmetrical, resulting in hemihypertrophy. Patients are also at risk for the development of intraabdominal neoplasms, particularly nephroblastoma.

142. What abnormalities are associated with infants of diabetic mothers?

Metabolic Abnormalities
    Hypoglycemia
    Hypocalcemia
    Polycythemia
    Hyperbilirubinemia
Congenital Anomalies (multiple organ systems)
    Central nervous system
    Cardiovascular system
    Genitourinary system
    Limb defects

Functional Abnormalities
    Respiratory distress syndrome
    Renal vein thrombosis
    Asymmetric septal hypertrophy
    Birth trauma due to large size
    Neonatal small left colon syndrome

143. What is transient diabetes mellitus of infancy?

Transient neonatal diabetes is a syndrome described in growth-retarded neonates during the first 6 weeks of life. Symptoms include failure to thrive, dehydration, fever, hyperglycemia, and glycosuria. Minimal ketones are present. These infants are treated with insulin and complete recovery can be expected.

144. How should cardiomyopathy in infants of diabetic mothers be treated?

This cardiomyopathy is an asymmetrical septal hypertrophy with abnormal thickness of the right ventricular wall and intraventricular septum. Obstruction may or may not be present. Symptomatic infants should be treated with propranolol, whereas asymptomatic infants are simply observed following an echocardiogram. Digitalis therapy is contraindicated.

Respiratory System

145. How much pressure does it take to inflate the lungs of a normal infant at the moment of birth?

At the initiation of respiration shortly after birth, pressures of 40–70 cm H_2O are generated to inflate the neonatal lung.

146. Why do newborn infants breathe faster than adults?

The total work of breathing, which is the sum of elastic and resistance work, varies with ventilatory pattern (tidal volume and rate). The respiratory centers attempt to achieve a given minute ventilation with a pattern that minimizes work. This minimum energy expenditure is achieved at higher respiratory rates in infants than in adults (35–40 breaths/min vs. 16 breaths/min).

147. What causes pulmonary vascular resistance to decrease at the time of birth?

Pulmonary vascular resistance falls at birth with the onset of respiration and lung expansion. Both the rise in arterial oxygen tension and decrease in carbon dioxide tension directly affect the vessels by decreasing resistance. In addition, lung expansion itself permits increased flow to the pulmonary vasculature.

148. Who was Virginia Apgar?

Virginia Apgar was an anesthesiologist at Columbia Presbyterian Medical Center who introduced the Apgar scoring system to assess the newborn infant's response to the stress of labor and delivery.

149. How is an asphyxiated neonate identified?

It is not acceptable to label an infant as asphyxiated simply because of a low Apgar score. Asphyxiated neonates demonstrate abnormalities in multiple organ systems with CNS problems often most prominent. The cardinal features of hypoxic-ischemic encephalopathy include seizures, alterations of consciousness, and abnormalities of tone. Disorders of reflexes, respiratory pattern, oculovestibular response, and autonomic function are less significant components of this entity.

150. What organ systems are injured by perinatal asphyxia?

Virtually all organ systems are affected. Those most commonly involved are listed below.

CNS
  Hemorrhage
  Edema/necrosis
  Anoxic encephalopathy
Cardiovascular
  Dysrhythmia
  Myocardial dysfunction
  Right to left shunt
  Cardiogenic Shock
  DIC
Respiratory Tract
  Respiratory distress
  Pulmonary hemorrhage

Gastrointestinal Tract
  NEC
Urinary Tract
  ATN/renal failure
  Asphyxiated bladder syndrome
Endocrine
  SIADH
  Adrenal hemorrhage
  Pancreatic insult?
Integument

From Banagel and Donn: Fam Pract 22:539, 1986, with permission.

151. Which areas of the CNS are injured by hypoxia and ischemia?

In full-term infants, asphyxia produces injury in the peripheral and dorsal aspects of the cerebral cortex. Lesions involve gyri at the depths of the sulci as well as the neuronal nuclei of the basal ganglia. In preterm infants, injury is localized to the germinal matrix and the periventricular region while the cortex is spared. The major neuropathological varieties of neonatal hypoxic-ischemic encephalopathy are:

		Etiology
1.	Selective neuronal necrosis	Hypoxemia
2.	Status marmoratus	Hypoxemia
3.	Parasagittal cerebral injury	Ischemia
4.	Periventricular leukomalacia	Ischemia
5.	Focal and multifocal ischemic brain necrosis	Ischemia

152. When should epinephrine and sodium bicarbonate be given during a resuscitation in the delivery room?

In the severely asphyxiated newborn, the pediatrician should proceed immediately to ventilate with 100% oxygen. If the heart rate does not rise above 100 beats/min despite 2 minutes of adequate ventilation via endotracheal tube, epinephrine (0.1 cc/kg 1:10,000 dilution) should be administered via the endotracheal tube. If this measure is ineffective in establishing a normal heart rate, 1–2 mEq/kg of half-strength sodium bicarbonate should be given intravenously over several minutes.

153. What size endotracheal tubes should be used in neonates?

Gestational Age	ETT Size
<28 weeks	2.5 mm
29–32 weeks	3.0 mm
>32 weeks	3.5 mm

Another useful formula to bear in mind is that if ETT size (mm)/gestational age (weeks) is > 0.1, there is an increased risk for development of tracheal stenosis.

154. What is the best location for an endotracheal tube?

The endotracheal tube should be placed so that the tip is midway between the glottis and carina. Clinically, there should be equal breath sounds by auscultation bilaterally. As a guide to tube placement prior to chest x-ray confirmation, the following figure may be used. For orotracheal intubation, the lower line should be used for mouth to mid-trachea position.

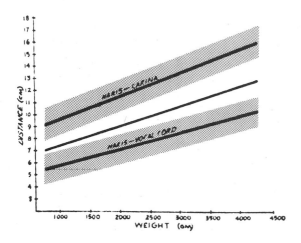

Endotracheal tube placement in neonates. (From Coldiron J: Pediatrics 41:823, 1968, with permission.)

155. What is the significance of "last gasp"?

During asphyxia, respiratory efforts initally increase in depth and frequency for up to 3 minutes, followed by approximately 1 minute of "primary apnea." Gasping then resumes for a variable period of time, terminating with the "last gasp," and is followed by "secondary apnea." A linear relationship exists between the duration of asphyxia and the recovery of respiratory function following resuscitation. Therefore, the longer artificial ventilation is delayed after the "last gasp," the longer it will take to resuscitate the infant.

156. What do hyperpnea and tachypnea signify in the neonate?

Hyperpnea refers to deep relatively unlabored respirations at mildly increased rates. This is typical of situations in which there is reduced pulmonary blood flow (e.g., pulmonary atresia) and results from ventilation of underperfused alveoli. Tachypnea refers to shallow, rapid, and somewhat labored respirations and is seen in the setting of low lung compliance (e.g., primary lung disease and pulmonary edema).

157. What is the difference between apnea and periodic breathing?

Apnea is defined as periods of cessation of respiration for > 10–15 seconds with or without cyanosis, pallor, hypotonia and/or bradycardia, or for < 10 seconds accompanied by bradycardia. Periodic breathing, which is commonly seen in preterm infants, is defined as recurrent sequences of respiratory pauses of 5–10 seconds followed by 10–15 seconds of rapid respirations. Periodic breathing is not associated with bradycardia. Both apnea and periodic breathing reflect lack of maturation of respiratory control centers in the preterm infant.

158. What is the differential diagnosis of apnea in the neonate and most likely etiology on day 1 and day 4 of life?

Apnea that presents on the first day of life is generally due to a known cause, as shown in the following figure, whereas that which presents on day 4 is more likely to be idiopathic and related to prematurity.

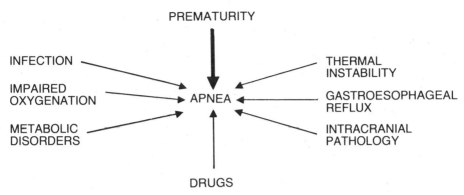

From Martin RJ, et al: J Pediatr 109:733, 1986, with permission.

159. When should apnea be treated?

In all cases of apnea, an underlying cause should be sought and treated if found. In idiopathic apnea, therapy should be initiated when episodes do not resolve with gentle tactile stimulation and require vigorous stimulation, or have a frequency of greater than two episodes per eight hour shift.

160. What methods are effective for treating apnea?

Several modalities are available for the treatment of apnea of prematurity: (1) use of oscillating water beds, (2) administration of continuous positive airway pressure (CPAP) (especially helpful in apnea with an obstructive component), (3) provision of supplemental oxygen (with or without CPAP), and (4) administration of respiratory stimulants (methyl-xanthines or doxapram). If supplemental oxygen is used, the PaO_2 must be carefully monitored either directly by arterial blood gases, or indirectly by non-invasive oxygen monitoring devices (e.g., pulse oximetry, transcutaneous oxygen monitor).

161. What are the indications for theophylline therapy in the neonate?

Theophylline is indicated in infants with apnea of prematurity who are experiencing greater than 1–2 episodes of apnea and bradycardia per eight hour shift. Theophylline is also given to provide bronchodilation in infants with bronchopulmonary dysplasia and to facilitate weaning of infants with RDS from ventilatory support.

162. What are the advantages of caffeine over theophylline for apnea of prematurity?

Caffeine demonstrates mostly central effects with less of an effect on smooth muscle. Theophylline, in contrast, is a cardiac stimulant and diuretic, and may cause gastrointestinal toxicity. Caffeine appears to have a wider therapeutic index, does not cause obvious toxicity even at plasma levels near 50 μg/ml, and has a longer half-life necessitating less frequent dosing schedules.

163. What are the indications for home monitoring in preterm infants with apnea?

The following are criteria for home monitoring as outlined by Spitzer and Fox:
1. History of severe apneic episodes
2. Thermistor documentation of apnea
3. Thermistor documentation of increased periodic breathing (> 5% sleep)
4. Sibling of victim of sudden infant death syndrome (SIDS)
5. Twin of SIDS victim
6. Severe feeding difficulties with apnea and bradycardia
7. ? Pulmonary, cardiac, and neurologic problems

164. What is the value of home monitoring?

At the Children's Hospital of Philadelphia, Spitzer and Fox have studied over 2000 infants presenting with apnea and, to date, no infant in whom cardiorespiratory monitoring has been used appropriately has died of SIDS. Also, families report that home monitoring is a positive and satisfying experience, alleviating the potential stress of living with an infant with apnea.

165. What perinatal factors are known to increase or decrease the incidence of respiratory distress syndrome (RDS)?

Increase Risk	Decrease Risk
Prematurity	Maternal toxemia
Maternal diabetes	Premature/prolonged rupture of mem-
History of RDS in siblings	branes
Male sex	Prenatally administered glucosteroids
Second-born twins	
Cesarean section	
Perinatal asphyxia	

166. What are the radiographic signs of RDS?

The radiographic signs of RDS are a diffuse reticulogranular pattern in both lungs with superimposition of air bronchograms. The x-ray is often described as showing a "ground glass" pattern.

167. What is the diuretic phase of RDS and what is its significance?

The diuretic phase of RDS is characterized by an 8–16 hour period of increased urine output occurring between 24 and 60 hours of life, during which urine output is at least 80% of fluid intake. This phase heralds a rapid improvement in lung function and recovery from RDS. Infants with a delayed diuresis are more likely to develop bronchopulmonary dysplasia.

168. What causes cyanosis in infants with RDS?

    1. Ventilation/perfusion mismatch due to atelectasis secondary to surfactant deficiency.

    2. Intrapulmonary shunting of blood due to pulmonary vasoconstriction secondary to hypoxemia and acidosis.

    3. Shunting across the foramen ovale and ductus arteriosus.

169. What is the Usher regimen?

The Usher regimen, a protocol developed for newborn infants with RDS, was designed to provide a protein-sparing amount of carbohydrate, prevent hyperkalemia, ensure adequate hydration, and correct metabolic acidosis. This approach, which preceded the availability of mechanical ventilation for newborn infants, called for the use of 10% glucose with up to 15 mEq of sodium bicarbonate per 100 ml of infusion depending on the patient's initial pH. Clinical trials conducted between 1957 and 1961 revealed that this regimen reduced mortality in patients with RDS by as much as two-thirds.

170. When should infants with RDS be mechanically ventilated?

Mechanical ventilation is initiated in infants with RDS when the diagnosis of respiratory failure is made.

    Laboratory criteria for respiratory failure
    1. respiratory acidosis with pH less than 7.20 and $PCO_2 > 60$.
    2. severe hypoxemia with PaO_2 less than 50–60 torr despite an FiO_2 of 0.7–1.0 and an adequate trial of continuous positive airway pressure.

    Clinical criteria for respiratory failure
    1. severe retractions
    2. cyanosis
    3. intractable apnea

171. What are the indications for paralysis in the neonate who is being mechanically ventilated?

The indications are controversial. Pancuronium is the drug most commonly used for this purpose, but also has some potentially serious side effects. Some authors recommend institution of this therapy when the patient (1) fights the ventilator breaths and is thus at risk for pneumothorax, or (2) requires greater than 75% oxygen and/or peak inspiratory pressures greater than 30 cm H_2O. Volpe has suggested that pancuronium be used to eliminate the fluctuating pattern of cerebral blood flow that results from a fluctuating blood pressure pattern. If left untreated, infants with that pattern of cerebral blood flow may have an increased risk for intraventricular hemorrhage.

172. What are the differences in blood oxygen content, oxygen saturation, and PO_2?

PO_2 is the partial pressure of oxygen in equilibrium with blood. The percentage of hemoglobin that is bound with oxygen at a given PO_2 is the *oxygen saturation*. The *oxygen content*, which is measured in volume %, is the total volume of oxygen bound to hemoglobin plus the volume dissolved in blood, the latter of which is generally negligible at normal values of PO_2. The oxygen content can be calculated as follows:

$$1.34 \text{ ml } O_2/\text{gm hemoglobin} \times \text{hemoglobin (gm/dl)} \times \text{oxygen saturation}$$

173. What are normal values for arterial pH, pCO_2, and base excess in healthy term infants?

pH	7.30–7.41
pCO_2	34–39 mm Hg
PO_2	60–90 mm Hg
Base excess	0–(23.3)
O_2 saturation	93–95%

174. In an infant receiving mechanical ventilation, what is an acceptable range for pH, PCO_2, and PO_2?

The goal of mechanical ventilation is to maintain the arterial PO_2 in the range of 50–80 mm Hg and arterial pH between 7.30 and 7.41. Earlier recommendations advocated maintenance of pCO_2 between 35 and 45 mm Hg. Some neonatologists now recommend that the pCO_2 be allowed to rise to levels as high as 55–60 mm Hg in order to minimize barotrauma. It is still controversial whether sustained hypercarbia has adverse side effects.

175. What mechanical ventilator settings are likely to affect PO_2 and PCO_2?

Since many ventilatory changes may affect both oxygenation and ventilation to some degree, the following table is an oversimplified but nevertheless useful guide:

Ventilator Setting	PO_2	PCO_2
PIP	↑	↓
PEEP	↑	↑ or NE
Frequency	↑ or NE*	↓
I:E	↑	NE†
FiO_2	↑	NE
Flow	↑	NE

NE = no consistent effect
* At very high respiratory rates, inspiratory time may be so short as to compromise oxygenation. Furthermore, at very high frequency there is an increase in inadvertent PEEP which can result in CO_2 accumulation.
† CO_2 elimination may be affected at extremely low expiratory times.

176. How do pressure limited-time cycled ventilators work?

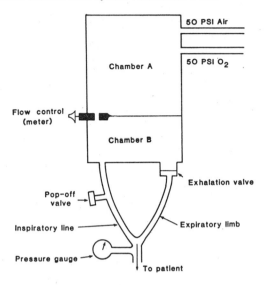

PSI=Pounds/square inch

Compressed air blended with oxygen is introduced into chamber A and regulated amounts are allowed to flow into chamber B, which is in contact with the patient. The actual pressure delivered to the infant is measured by a gauge in the inspiratory limb and the ventilator is cycled by the opening and closing of an exhalation valve. In a time-cycled ventilator this valve opens and closes when a preset time has been reached. While the valve is open, continuous flow is provided to avoid buildup of CO_2. (From Fox WW, Shutack JG: Positive pressure ventilation: pressure and time-cycled ventilators. In Goldsmith J, Karotkin E (eds): Assisted Ventilation in the Neonate. Philadelphia, W.B. Saunders, 1981, p 103, with permission.)

177. What is mean airway pressure? Which settings on the ventilator affect mean airway pressure?

Mean airway pressure (Pāw) is a measure of the average pressure to which the lungs are exposed during the respiratory cycle and can be calculated by dividing the area under the airway pressure curve by the duration of the cycle. Pāw is affected by changes in (1) inspiratory flow, (2) peak inspiratory pressure (PIP), (3) positive end-expiratory pressure (PEEP), and (4) ratio of inspiratory to expiratory time (I/E ratio).

178. What is "optimal PEEP" and how is it determined?

The "optimal PEEP" is the end-expiratory pressure at which oxygenation is maximal with minimum effect on cardiovascular function. The best way to determine optimal PEEP is controversial. In practice the PEEP setting is generally maintained at a level equal to 10% of the inspired oxygen concentration. For example if the inspired oxygen concentration is 60%, the PEEP should be kept in the 5–7 range; if 40%, the 4–5 range, etc.

179. What are the indications for continuous positive airway pressure (CPAP)?

CPAP should be initiated in infants with diffuse lung disease when an FiO_2 greater than 50% is required to maintain PaO_2 greater than 50 mm Hg. Many neonatologists maintain their patients in significantly higher inspired oxygen concentrations without CPAP and instead use clinical criteria such as significant grunting and retractions for intiation of CPAP.

180. What causes infants to grunt?

Infants with respiratory disease tend to expire through closed or partially closed vocal cords in order to elevate transpulmonary pressure and therefore increase lung volume. The latter effect results in an improved ventilation/perfusion ratio with better gas exchange. It is during the last part of expiration when gas is expelled through the partially closed vocal cords that the audible grunt is produced.

181. What is a hyperoxia test?

In patients with cyanosis, the hyperoxia test can be performed to distinguish among primary lung disease, cyanotic heart disease (CHD) and persistent pulmonary hypertension (PPHN). Briefly, the infant is placed in 100% oxygen and arterial oxygen tension is measured. A $PaO_2 > 100$ mm Hg is usually achieved in infants with primary lung disease, whereas a $PaO_2 < 100$ mm Hg is characteristic of CHD and PPHN. To distinguish the latter entities, 100% O_2 is administered while hyperventilating the patient. If the PaO_2 rises above 100 mm Hg, the diagnosis is presumed to be PPHN. If it does not, the most likely diagnosis is CHD.

182. What are the causes of bronchopulmonary dysplasia (BPD)?

Pathophysiologic events that contribute to the progressive development of chronic lung injury are oxygen toxicity, immaturity, barotrauma, air leaks, infection, congestive failure, and growth failure.

183. When should steroids be used in infants with BPD?

The use of steroids in BPD remains controversial. The proposed benefit is felt to be mediated by the following steroid actions: (1) stabilization of membranes and reduction of pulmonary edema, (2) enhancement of surfactant synthesis, (3) reduction of inflammation in injured small airways, and (4) reduction of bronchospasm. Serious side effects include: (1) hypertension, (2) hyperglycemia, (3) sepsis, (4) gastritis, and (5) adrenal suppression. Currently, corticosteroids have been used in infants approximately 2–6 weeks of age who have shown evidence of failure to wean from respiratory support with or without radiographic evidence of "exudative" BPD.

184. Is furosemide efficacious in treating infants with BPD?

Infants with BPD are at particular risk for the development of pulmonary edema due to abnormalities of lymphatic drainage as well as cardiac dysfunction secondary to cor pulmonale. Consequently, administration of diuretics to these patients results in improvements in both lung compliance and resistance as well as blood gases. These effects occur as a result of not only the diuretic-induced increase in sodium and water excretion, but also the increase in venous capacitance and reduction in venous return. It is controversial whether use of diuretics facilitates the weaning of infants from ventilatory support. Both furosemide and chlorthiazide therapy are associated with significant side effects.

185. What is surfactant?

Surfactant is a surface-active material comprised of a mixture rich in phosphatidylcholine (64%), phosphatidylglycerol (8%), and lesser amounts of proteins and other lipids. Surfactant acts as an anti-atelectasis factor in the alveolar lining by lowering surface tension at diminished lung volume and increasing it at high volumes. This allows for maintenance of functional residual capacity (FRC), which acts as a reservoir to prevent wide fluctuations in arterial oxygen and carbon dioxide tensions during respiration.

186. What tests can be done to estimate lung maturity prenatally?

Most prenatal tests for lung maturity are designed to detect the presence of surfactant. The following tests are those most commonly used:

1. *L/S ratio:* Since lecithin is a major component of surfactant, and sphingomyelin concentration is relatively constant during gestation, the L/S ratio can be used as a measure of lung maturity. An L/S of $\geq$ 2.0 carries a low risk of RDS and is generally attained at 34–35 weeks' gestation. While ratios of 1.5–2.0 carry a 40% risk of RDS, those values of $<$ 1.5 carry a risk of 75%. The L/S ratio is *not* reliable in pregancies with Rh disease or maternal diabetes. Furthermore, the test cannot be performed on fluid contaminated with blood or meconium.

2. *Phosphatidylglycerol (PG):* This surface-acting, stabilizing factor is present at greater than 35 weeks' gestation. Thus, its presence is indicative of lung maturity but its absence offers no definitive help in management. The measurement can be performed on blood- or meconium-contaminated fluid and is available as a standarized latex agglutination assay (Amniostat). Many clinicians quantitate both the L/S ratio and phosphatidylglycerol as part of a lung profile.

3. *Foam stability or shake test:* These tests depend on the ability of surfactant-rich fluid to form stable bubbles when mixed or shaken with ethanol. The foam stability index (FSI) has been developed as a standardized test using constant amounts of ethanol with different dilutions of amniotic fluid. Stable bubbles at $\geq$ 0.48 dilution are suggestive of mature lungs. The test is, however, limited by a high incidence of false-negative results.

4. *Fluorescence polarimetry:* This may be used to measure microviscosity of amniotic fluid which decreases as the lung matures. This method involves expensive equipment and is not routinely available.

5. *Optical density (OD) 650 nm:* The OD of phospholipids in amniotic fluid peaks at 650 nm. This test is rapid and routinely available; however, it may not be as reliable as other tests.

187. What are TTN, RDS type II, CPIP, and Wilson-Mikity syndrome?

Transient tachypnea of the newborn (TTN) is a syndrome characterized by respiratory distress in term or near-term non-asphyxiated newborn infants and is felt to be secondary to delayed resorption of fetal lung fluid. The characteristic x-ray findings are those of fluid in the interlobar fissures and central hypervascularity. This entity is sometime referred to as RDS type II because of many of the clinical similarities to RDS.

Chronic pulmonary insufficiency of prematurity (CPIP) is a syndrome characterized by the delayed onset of respiratory insufficiency in infants under 1250 gm. Other than poor lung volumes, the infants manifest minimal lung disease in the first 3 days of life followed by apnea, increased oxygen requirements, and atelectasis. Radiographically the lungs may be normal or exhibit mild abnormalities (microatelectasis, air bronchograms, small lung volumes, generalized haziness). The mechanisms proposed are abnormalities of surfactant turnover, respiratory muscle exhaustion and persistent secretion of fetal lung fluid.

Wilson-Mikity syndrome is seen in infants born at less than 36 weeks' gestation with no initial respiratory symptoms (or occasionally symptoms that have resolved) followed by the insidious onset of retractions and cyanosis. Radiographically the lungs range from normal in appearance to hyperinflated with large cysts. The prognosis is generally good.

188. What are the types of pulmonary interstitial emphysema (PIE)?

Pulmonary interstitial emphysema (PIE) presents as either diffuse (intrapulmonary) air collections or localized subpleural disease. The diffuse variety carries a high risk for mortality as well as for bronchopulmonary dysplasia in survivors. The severity of symptoms in localized disease is determined by the extent of the lobes involved.

189. What are the causes of PIE?

PIE is felt to be primarily a complication of mechanical ventilation causing rupture of air from the alveoli or small airways into the perivascular tissues of the lung.

190. How is PIE treated?

Since PIE is presumed to be a complication of mechanical ventilation, therapy for PIE is generally aimed at reduction of the peak inflating pressure and use of higher ventilator rates as necessary. In cases of localized PIE, dependent positioning of the involved lung as well as selective mainstem intubation and ventilation of the uninvolved lung have been shown to be beneficial. When medical management of localized PIE fails, surgical lobectomy may be considered.

191. What is insensible water loss?

Insensible water loss is the loss of water through the lungs during respiration and through evaporation from the skin. A rough guide to the amounts of insensible losses is given as follows:

Insensible Water Loss in Preterm Infants*

BIRTHWEIGHT (GM)	ML/KG/DAY
750–1,000	64
1,001–1,250	56
1,251–1,500	38
1,501–1,750	23
1,751–2,000	20
2,001–3,250	20

From Fanaroff AA, Martin RJ (eds): Neonatal-Perinatal Medicine: Diseases of the Fetus and Infant. St. Louis, C.V. Mosby, 1987, p 464, with permission.
*Nursed in humidified isolettes.

192. What factors are known to increase/decrease insensible water loss?

Factors Modifying Insensible Water Loss

FACTOR	DIRECTION OF CHANGE IN WATER LOSS
Prematurity	↑
Activity	↑
High humidity	↓
Fever	↑
Radiant warmer	↑
Phototherapy	↑
Mechanical ventilation	↓

From Fanaroff AA, Martin RJ (eds): Neonatal-Perinatal Medicine: Diseases of the Fetus and Infant. St. Louis, C.V. Mosby, 1987, p 464, with permission.

193. What are the clinical manifestations of pneumothorax?

Tachypnea, sudden deterioration in oxygen saturation, decreased breath sounds, signs of shock, shift of point of maximal impulse (PMI), hypertension with decreased pulse pressures, *or* hypotension.

194. What are the adverse consequences of hyperventilation and tolazoline?

Hyperventilation, a mainstay in the therapy of persistent pulmonary hypertension (PPHN), may cause chronic lung disease secondary to barotrauma. In addition, the hypocarbia caused by this modality may cause serious reductions in cerebral blood flow. However, it should be noted that developmental follow-up studies to date are encouraging. Finally, the resultant respiratory alkalosis may cause renal changes in the hydrogen ion/potassium exchange system, thereby impairing tubular function. Tolazoline, which is used as a pulmonary vasodilator in PPHN, also causes systemic vasodilation with hypotension. Additional toxicities include pulmonary hemorrhage, gastrointestinal hemorrhage, and thrombocytopenia.

Cardiovascular System

195. How does an EKG in the neonate differ from that in an older child or adult?

While the mass of the two ventricles is similar at mid-gestation, right ventricular growth is greater during the third trimester. The ECG during the newborn period normally reflects right ventricular dominance. As a consequence, the QRS complex shows a tall R wave in V_1, V_2 and a deep S wave on V_5, V_6. The leftward vectors are small. The normal newborn also has a rightward QRS axis of $+135°$ to $+180°$ (normal adult $0°$ to $+90°$), and a normal heart rate of 100–140 bpm.

196. How is right or left ventricular hypertrophy diagnosed in the neonate using the electrocardiogram?

Criteria for Right and Left Ventricular Hypertrophy in the Newborn

Right Ventricular Hypertrophy
    An R in lead aV_R of greater than 7 mm
    A qR pattern in V_1
    An RV_1 greater than 28 mm
    SV_6 greater than 13 mm
    A pure R wave (no q or S) in V_1 of 10 mm or greater
    Positive T in V_1 after day 5
Left Ventricular Hypertrophy
    R in V_1 greater than 9 mm
    R in V_6 greater than 17 mm in first week
    R in V_6 greater than 25 mm in first month
    Inverted TV_6 or T_1 with voltage changes
    Adult R/S progression; that is, SV_1 greater than RV_1 and RV_6 SV_6 (before day 3)

From Lees MH, King DH: The cardiovascular system. In Fanaroff AA, Martin RJ (eds): Neonatal-Perinatal Medicine: Diseases of the Fetus and Infant, 4th ed. St Louis, C.V. Mosby, 1987, p 648, with permission.

197. What prenatal factors may be associated with cardiac disease in the neonate?

Prenatal Historical Factor	Associated Cardiac Defect
1. Diabetes mellitus	1. Left ventricular outflow obstruction: asymmetric septal hypertrophy, aortic stenosis d-Transposition of the great arteries Ventricular septal defect
2. Lupus erythematosus	2. Congenital heart block
3. Rubella	3. Patent ductus arteriosus Pulmonic stenosis (peripheral)
4. Alcohol abuse	4. Pulmonic stenosis Ventricular septal defect
5. Trimethadione usage	5. Ventricular septal defect; tetralogy of Fallot
6. Lithium usage	6. Ebstein's anomaly
7. Aspirin abuse	7. Persistent pulmonary hypertension syndrome
8. Coxsackie B infection	8. Myocarditis
9. Beta blocker usage	9. Asymmetric septal hypertrophy

From Gewitz MH: Cardiac disease in the newborn infant. In Polin RA, Burg FD (eds): Workbook in Practical Neonatology. Philadelphia, W.B. Saunders Co., 1983, p 176, with permission.

198. What are the five "T"'s of congenital heart disease which present with cyanosis in the first days of life?

1. Tetralogy of Fallot
2. Transposition of the great arteries
3. Truncus arteriosus
4. Tricuspid atresia
5. Total anomalous pulmonary venous return

199. What is the differential diagnosis of cyanosis in the neonate?

Differential Diagnosis of Neonatal Cyanosis

CATEGORY	EXAMPLES	SIGNS	RESPONSE TO HYPEROXIA TEST	CHEST X-RAY	ARTERIAL BLOOD GASES
Heart disease with right to left shunt; *decreased* pulmonary blood flow	Tetralogy of Fallot Pulmonary atresia Tricuspid insufficiency	Hyperpnea Heart murmur Soft S_2	Minimal to nil	Variable heart size Diminished PVMs	pH normal or high pCO_2 low
Heart disease with right to left shunt; *increased* pulmonary blood flow	d-Transposition Anomalous pulmonary venous return	Tachypnea Loud S_2 Variable heart murmur	Minimal	Large heart (unless obstructed TAPVD) Increased PVMs	pH normal or low pCO_2 normal or high
Heart disease with heart failure; ventilation-perfusion mismatch	Coarctation syndrome Large left to right shunt Supraventricular tachycardia	Tachypnea Shock Heart murmur	Good response ($PaO_2 > 150$)	Large heart Pulmonary edema R/O pneumonia	pH low pCO_2 high
Primary pulmonary disease	RDS Group B Streptococcus Meconium aspiration Pneumothorax	Tachypnea Retractions Grunting, etc.	Good response (may need CPAP to prove)	Diagnostic appearance	pH low pCO_2 high
Metabolic disease	Hypoglycemia Methemoglobinemia	Variable: Tachypnea Flaccid Jittery, etc.	Minimal	Normal or large heart	pH normal or low pCO_2 normal
Polycythemia	Twin-Twin transfusion Intrauterine growth retardation	Plethora Signs of congestive heart failure	Minimal	Large heart Normal PVMs	Normal or low pH pGO_2 normal
Infection	Sepsis Myocarditis	Shock Marked peripheral cyanosis	Good	Large heart (unless hypoadrenal) Pulmonary edema	pH low pCO_2 high
Persistent fetal circulation	Meconium aspiration LGA baby Maternal salicylates	Hyperpnea Differential cyanosis	Variable—transiently good (with CPAP)	Normal heart size Decreased PVMs	pH low pCO_2 may be elevated
Neurologic disease	Intracranial bleed Seizure disorder	Tachypnea Focal signs Apnea	Good	Normal	pH low pCO_2 elevated

Modified from Lees MH: J Pediatr, 77:484, 1970. Abbreviations: PVMs, pulmonary vascular markings; CPAP, continuous positive airway pressure; TAPVD, total anomalous pulmonary venous drainage.

200. What causes congestive heart failure without a murmur in the neonate?
1. Myocarditis
2. Cardiomyopathy secondary to asphyxia, hypoglycemia, or hypocalcemia
3. Glycogen storage disease (Pompe's disease)
4. Cardiac arrhythmia
     paroxysmal supraventricular tachycardia
     congenital heart block
     atrial flutter and/or fibrillation
5. Arteriovenous malformations, e.g., CNS (vein of Galen)
6. Sepsis

201. How is paroxysmal atrial tachycardia (PAT) differentiated from other sinus tachycardias?
PAT may be distinguished from other sinus tachycardias as follows:
1. Persistent ventricular rate of over 180 bpm
2. A fixed or almost fixed "R-R" interval on EKG
3. Abnormal P-wave shape or axis or absent P-waves
4. Little change in heart rate with activity, crying or breathholding

202. What are the clinical manifestations of a patent ductus arteriosus in the neonate?
Tachypnea and tachycardia, bounding pulses, hyperdynamic precordium, systolic murmur or systolic and diastolic murmur, wide pulse pressures, labile oxygenation, and apnea.

203. Why does the ductus arterious remain patent in the preterm neonate?
Patency of the ductus arteriosus is maintained in the fetus by the combination of the relaxant effects of low oxygen tension and locally synthesized prostaglandin E. As term is approached, there is heightened sensitivity to oxygen tension as well as decreased responsiveness to the relaxant effects of prostaglandins. Thus, in preterm infants in whom these phenomena do not occur, the ductus tends to remain open.

204. Of what value is echocardiography for the diagnosis of a patent ductus arteriosus?
With the use of high-resolution, two-dimensional echocardiography, patent ductus arteriosus is detectable in 90% of cases. This sensitivity increases to 100% with the addition of pulsed Doppler to detect reversal of blood flow in the descending aorta during diastole. Nevertheless, the *clinical* assessment of a preterm infant with a PDA is generally adequate to guide therapeutic decisions. When the diagnosis of PDA is in doubt, the echocardiogram can help to confirm the diagnosis.

205. When should the ductus arteriosus be surgically ligated?
Surgical ligation of a patent ductus arteriosus is generally indicated in infants who have failed two courses of medical management including indomethacin. In infants where indomethacin is contraindicated (e.g., BUN > 30 mg/dl, creatinine > 1.8 mg/dl, platelet count < 60,000/mm^3, evidence of bleeding diathesis) and decompensation has occurred secondary to the PDA, surgical ligation should be performed.

206. What are the indications for indomethacin in the neonate?

Indomethacin is indicated in preterm infants with a *hemodynamically significant patent ductus arteriosus*. A clinically significant PDA is defined as one in which there is deteriorating respiratory status (e.g., tachypnea, apnea, carbon dioxide retention, increased ventilatory support, failure to wean ventilatory support) or evidence of congestive heart failure.

207. What are the indications for PGE$_1$ in the neonate?

Prostaglandin E$_1$ (PGE$_1$) is indicated in cardiac lesions with ductal dependent blood flow to either the pulmonary circulation (e.g., pulmonary atresia with intact ventricular septum, tricuspid atresia with intact ventricular septum, critical pulmonary stenosis) or the systemic circulation (e.g., critical coarctation of the aorta, interrupted aortic arch, hypoplastic left heart syndrome). *In infants with suspected congenital heart disease* in whom a specific diagnosis is not known (e.g., prior to transport to a tertiary care center), PGE$_1$ is clinically indicated in cases of profound cyanosis (PaO$_2$ < 25 mm Hg), poor perfusion and/or metabolic acidosis.

208. What are the major side effects of PGE$_1$?

Apnea, pyrexia, cutaneous flushing, seizures, hypotension, and bradycardia/tachycardia.

209. Where is the foramen ovale?

In fetal life the foramen ovale is the connection through which well-oxygenated blood from the placenta flows from the inferior vena cava to the left atrium.

210. What is the syndrome of persistent fetal circulation (PFC) and what are its clinical signs?

PFC refers to the combination of pulmonary hypertension and right-to-left shunting at the foramen ovale and/or ductus arteriosus in the absence of structural cardiac abnormalities. Patients are tachypneic and cyanotic. In addition, the pulmonary component of the second heart sound is loud. If ductal shunting is present, there may be differential cyanosis as confirmed by higher arterial oxygen tension in the right arm than in the descending aorta and legs.

Blood

211. What is the definition of anemia in a newborn infant (preterm/term)?

For the term infant, most authorities consider a venous blood hemoglobin of less than 13.0 g/dl or a capillary hemoglobin of less than 14.5 g/dl as consistent with anemia. In preterm infants beyond 32 weeks' gestation, hematologic values differ only minimally from full-term infants and therefore the same values may be used. In infants born prior to 32 weeks, mean hemoglobin values are lower as shown below:

Age (weeks)	Hb (g/dl)
12	8.0–10.0
16	10.0
20	11.0
24	14.0
28	14.5
34	15.0

212. What is the diagnostic approach to neonatal anemia?

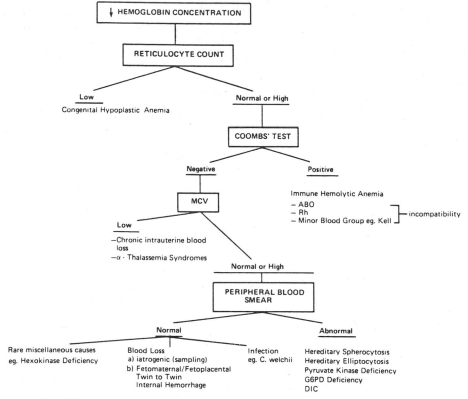

From Blanchette VS, Zipursky A: Assessment of anemia in newborn infants. Clin Perinatol 11:505, 1984, with permission.

213. What is the significance of P_{50}?

P_{50} is the arterial PO_2 value at which hemoglobin is 50% saturated. Therefore, this value reflects the position of the oxygen-hemoglobin dissociation curve and the relative tendency for oxygen to be delivered to the tissues. Differences in the proportions of fetal and adult hemoglobin, the concentration of DPG, and acid-base status will alter P_{50} values. The postnatal changes in P_{50} and hemoglobin-oxygen dissociation curves are shown below.

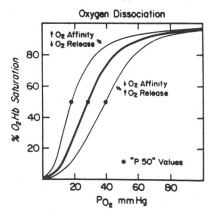

A typical hemoglobin-oxygen dissociation curve. The curve on the left represents that of a newborn. The middle curve is that of a normal older child or adult. The curve to the right is a "rightward shifted" curve seen as a compensatory phenomenon in many forms of anemia, hypoxia, and certain "low affinity" hemoglobinopathies, and in acidotic conditions. (From Stockman JA: Anemia of prematurity. Pediatr Clin North Am 33:115, 1986, with permission.)

214. What are the causes of physiologic anemia?

The fall in hemoglobin concentration that occurs in all infants during the first weeks of life is primarily the result of decreasing red blood cell mass, although hemodilution secondary to an expanding blood volume is a contributing factor. As is true in later life, the biochemical stimulus for hemoglobin synthesis is erythropoietin. Plasma erythropoietin levels decrease postnatally as tissue oxygen delivery improves (rightward shift of the hemoglobin-oxygen dissociation curve and increased cardiac output). A gradual rise in erythropoietin occurs as the hemoglobin concentration falls below 11 gm/dl.

215. When does the nadir of physiologic anemia occur in the term and preterm infant?

The nadir for physiologic anemia occurs at 8–12 weeks in term infants and earlier in preterm infants, depending on gestational age.

The mean and range of normal values for hemoglobin concentration and reticulocyte count of preterm and term infants. (From Dallman PR: Anemia of prematurity. Ann Rev Med 32:143, 1981, with permission.)

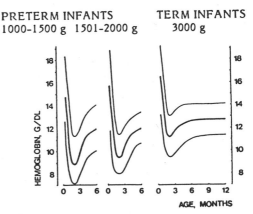

216. When should iron supplementation be started following birth?

In order to prevent iron-deficiency anemia, the following recommendations have been made by the American Academy of Pediatrics. In term infants, supplementation should be given no later than 4 months of age (versus 2 months of age in preterm infants). The recommended doses for term and preterm infants are 1 and 2 mg/kg/day, respectively. Recently, however, doses of 3 and 4 mg/kg/day have been recommended for infants with birthweights of 1000–1500 gm and < 1000 gm, respectively.

217. When does the switchover from fetal to adult hemoglobin synthesis occur in the neonate?

The switchover from production of hemoglobin F to hemoglobin A occurs in a very programmed fashion in the fetus and neonate (approximately 32 weeks' gestation). In fact, at birth, approximately 50–65% of hemoglobin is type F.

218. How low does the hemoglobin concentration fall physiologically in the newborn infant?

In the term infant, the hemoglobin concentration reaches a nadir of 11.4 ± 0.9 gm/dl (mean ± S.D.). In preterm infants, values 2 to 3 gm/dl lower are considered normal.

219. What are Bart's hemoglobin and Gower hemoglobin? What is their significance?

Bart's hemoglobin is a tetramer of the gamma globin chains and is normally present in trace amounts in the newborn. However, when present in higher percentage, it generally reflects a genetic defect of alpha globin chain production. Bart's hemoglobin is elevated in the following thalassemic syndromes: (1) silent carrier α-thalassemia trait: 1–2% Bart's hemoglobin, (2) α-thalassemia trait: 3–10% Bart's hemoglobin, (3) hemoglobin H disease: 20–40% Bart's hemoglobin, and (4) homozygous α-thalassemia: 80% Bart's hemoglobin (these infants are affected *in utero* and are always hydropic).

Hemoglobin Gower is an embryonic hemoglobin present normally between 10 and 12 weeks' gestation. There are two types: Gower 1 with $\zeta_2\epsilon_2$ structure and Gower 2 with $\alpha_2\epsilon_2$ structure. Embryonic hemoglobins are normally absent at birth but their presence in trace amounts (especially Gower 2) is associated with chromosomal anomalies (trisomy 13).

220. How is methemoglobinemia in the neonate diagnosed and treated?

Diagnosis. Clinically, newborns with methemoglobinemia present with generalized cyanosis in the absence of respiratory distress. A simple and rapid bedside test consists of collecting capillary blood from the infant's heel as well as from an adult control on white filter paper. The paper is waved in the air for 30 seconds to allow for oxygenation. If the infant's blood remains chocolate brown relative to the red adult blood, a methemoglobin level of greater than 10% is present. While mean methemoglobin values in preterm and term infants are 2.4% (range: 0.8–4.4) and 1.5% (range: 0.0–2.8), respectively, infants with methemoglobinemia generally have values greater than 10%. Hemoglobin electrophoresis may also be necessary to make the diagnosis of hemoglobin M disease (congenital methemoglobinemia).

Treatment. Infants with methemoglobinemia should be treated with a single IV dose of 1–2 mg/kg of methylene blue. Cyanosis should disappear and methemoglobin values should drop to normal within 60 minutes. In infants with acquired methemoglobinemia this single dose should suffice, provided the offending agent has been removed. However, in children with congenital cytochrome B_5 reductase deficiency, continued therapy with methylene blue or high-dose ascorbic acid (which directly reduces methemoglobin Fe^{+++} to oxy-hemoglobin Fe^{++}) is required.

221. What is the definition of polycythemia in the neonate?

Polycythemia is defined by a *venous* hematocrit of greater than 65%, since this exceeds the mean hematocrit found in normal newborns by two standard deviations.

222. What are the clinical manifestations of polycythemia?

Symptoms and Signs	Complications
Lethargy	Respiratory distress
Hypotonia	Congestive heart failure
Weak suck	Convulsions
Difficult to arouse	Peripheral gangrene
Irritable when aroused	Priapism
Plethora	Necrotizing enterocolitis
Cyanosis while active	Ileus
Vomiting	Acute renal failure
Tremulousness	
Easily startled	
Myoclonic jerks	
Hepatomegaly	
Jaundice	

From by Oski F, Naiman J (eds): Hematologic Problems in the Newborn. Philadelphia, W. B. Saunders Co., 1982, p 92, with permission.

223. What conditions or circumstances place an infant at risk for polycythemia and hyperviscosity?

Infants of diabetic mothers, intrauterine growth retardation, perinatal asphyxia, twin-to-twin transfusion (recipient), large placental transfusion (delayed cord clamping), and Beckwith's syndrome.

224. How should infants with polycythemia be managed?

Treatment of polycythemia with partial exchange transfusion is universally recommended for symptomatic infants (i.e., those with jitteriness, lethargy, seizures, respiratory distress, feeding intolerance, congestive heart failure, etc.). However, in asymptomatic infants, controversy exists regarding the need for treatment. In general, asymptomatic infants with a *venous* hematocrit of 65 to 70% may be closely observed, whereas those with values greater than 70% should also be treated because of the greater likelihood of co-existing hyperviscosity. Postnatal age should also be considered, because the hematocrit generally rises between 6 and 12 hours of life due to fluid shifts from the intravascular compartments. The amount of blood volume to be exchanged with crystalloid or colloid may be calculated using the following formula:

$$\text{Blood volume to be exchanged} = \frac{\text{Observed Hct} - \text{Desired Hct (55\%)}}{\text{Observed Hct}} \times \frac{\text{Blood Volume} \times \text{Body Wt.(kg)}}{(85-100\text{ml/kg})}$$

225. What is the definition of thrombocytopenia in the neonate?

Platelet counts below 100,000 should be considered abnormal in term or preterm neonates, whereas counts in the 100,000–150,000 range may be seen in some healthy newborns. Consequently, patients with counts in this latter category should have repeat counts as well as further studies if illness is suspected.

226. Contrast neonatal isoimmune and autoimmune thrombocytopenia.

Immune thrombocytopenias are caused by the transplacental passage of antibody from mother to infant, causing platelet destruction, and can be divided into two broad groups, which are compared below.

Thrombocytopenia Due to Maternal Antibody

	MATERNAL IDIOPATHIC THROMBOCYTOPENIC PURPURA ITP	ISOIMMUNE NEONATAL THROMBOCYTOPENIA
Estimated incidence	Uncertain ? 1 in 3000 births	1 in 5000 births
Offending antigen	Probably part of platelet membrane glycoprotein IIb-IIIa complex: on *all* platelets	PLA[1] (Zw[a]) or HLA: on father's and neonate's platelets but *not* mother's
Type of antibody	Maternal autoantibody	Maternal alloantibody (isoantibody) directed against foreign platelet antigen
Maternal platelet count	Reduced (unless splenectomy has been performed previously)	Always normal
Recurrence risk	Cannot be reliably estimated from maternal platelet count	50–85% (depending upon offending antigen and zygosity of father)

From Buchanan GR: Coagulation disorders in the neonate. Pediatr Clin North Am 33:212, 1986, with permission.

Similarities between babies with thrombocytopenia due to maternal ITP and to isoimmune thrombocytopenia include "well" appearance, lack of hepatosplenomegaly, risk of serious hemorrhage, general approach to management, and duration of thrombocytopenia postnatally (3–12 weeks).

227. What is the TAR syndrome?

Congenital amegakaryocytic thrombocytopenia with bilateral absence of the radii. This syndrome is believed to result from developmental defects early in embryogenesis and is inherited in an autosomal recessive manner. The bony abnormalities result in shortened forearms, flexion at the elbows and radial deviation of the wrist. Those who survive beyond the first year of life usually show gradual improvement in hematologic status.

228. What are the common causes of neonatal thrombocytopenia and how may they be differentiated?

Causes of Increased Platelet Destruction
    Maternal ITP
    Isoimmune thrombocytopenia
    Infection
    DIC
    Drugs
    Extensive localized thrombosis
    Critically Ill infants
    Giant hemangiomas
    Maternal lupus

Causes of Decreased Platelet Production
    Congenital amegakaryocytic
      hypoplasia (e.g., TAR)
    Bone marrow replacement
    Pancytopenias (e.g., Fanconi's
      anemia, trisomy 13 and 18)

Undetermined Mechanism
    Inborn errors of metabolism
    Congenital thyrotoxicosis

Etiologic Classification of Neonatal Thrombocytopenia

LABORATORY PARAMETER	INCREASED PLATELET DESTRUCTION	DECREASED PLATELET PRODUCTION
Platelet size	Increased	Normal
Platelet survival	Decreased	Normal
Platelet associated IgG	Often very increased	Usually normal, or slightly increased
Bleeding time	Usually prolonged	Prolonged
Other cell lines	Usually normal	Often abnormal
Megakaryocytes	Normal or increased	Decreased
Other bone marrow cell lines	Normal	Often decreased or abnormal

From Andrew M, Kolton J: Neonatal thrombocytopenia. Clin Perinatol 11:363, 1984, with permission.

229. When should thrombocytopenic infants receive a platelet transfusion?
Infants with platelet counts of less than 20,000 or those with clinical signs of bleeding regardless of the actual count should receive platelet transfusions.

230. How long should transfused platelets survive?
In cases where thrombocytopenia is not the result of increased platelet destruction, the platelet count will fall approximately 10% each day and reach pretransfusion levels in approximately 1 week.

231. When do the prothrombin time and partial thromboplastin time "normalize" to adult values?
The prothrombin time reaches adult values at approximately 1 week of age, while the partial thromboplastin time does not attain adult values until 2–9 months.

232. What are the normal values for prothrombin time (PT), partial thromboplastin time (PTT), and thrombin time (TT) in the neonate?

Normal Values for PT, PTT, and TT

ASSAYS OF COAGULATION FACTORS	NORMAL ADULT VALUES	PRETERM INFANT	TERM INFANT
Prothrombin time (sec)	10–14	12–14	11–15
Partial thromboplastin time (sec)	25–35	30–80	30–40
Thrombin time (sec)	15–25	17–25	15–20

From Buchanan GR: Coagulation disorders in the neonate. Pediatr Clin North Am 33:207, 1986, with permission.

233. How is disseminated intravascular coagulation (DIC) diagnosed in the neonate?
The laboratory findings in DIC include evidence of red cell fragmentation on peripheral smear, elevation of prothrombin time, partial thromboplastin time and thrombin time, thrombocytopenia, decreased levels of factors V, VIII, and fibrinogen, and in some cases the presence of fibrin split products.

234. How should newborn infants with DIC be managed?

Treatment of DIC should be directed primarily at the underlying disease rather than just at the coagulation defects. In many cases, treatment of the former will make specific treatment of the latter unnecessary. However, in cases where stabilization of coagulopathy is not imminent, treatment with fresh frozen plasma and platelets is recommended. In cases where fluid overload is a major concern, exchange transfusion with fresh whole blood may be used. However, this second approach is not superior to the first with respect to resolution of DIC. The use of heparin in DIC is currently reserved for cases of thrombosis of major vessels of purpura fulminans.

235. What is hemorrhagic disease of the newborn?

A hemorrhagic disorder of the first days of life caused by a deficiency of vitamin K–dependent factors (II, VII, IX, and X).

236. How can hemorrhagic disease of the newborn be prevented/treated?

Treatment or prophylaxis consists of intramuscular administration of 0.5–1 mg of vitamin K1 shortly after birth.

237. What is the Apt test?

The Apt test distinguishes fetal blood from swallowed maternal blood by relying on the differential sensitivity to alkali of adult and fetal hemoglobin.

The test is carried out as follows:

Method

Mix specimen (stool, vomitus, etc.) with an equal quantity of tap water. Centrifuge or filter. Supernatant must have pink color to proceed. To 5 parts of supernatant, add 1 part of 0.25 N (1%) NaOH.

Interpretation

A pink color persisting over 2 minutes indicates fetal hemoglobin. Adult hemoglobin gives a pink color that becomes yellow in 2 minutes or less, indicating denaturation of hemoglobin.

Reference: Apt L, Downey WS: J Pediatr 47:6, 1955.

238. What is the Kleihauer-Betke test?

In cases of suspected fetomaternal hemorrhage, the Kleihauer-Betke screen is used to detect the presence of fetal cells in the maternal circulation. This acid elution technique is based on the property of fetal hemoglobin to resist elution in an acid medium. In a stained maternal blood smear, the fetal cells stain darkly and the percentage of fetal red cells can be determined.

239. What is the D^u antigen?

D^u refers to a "D" antigen of very little reactivity. Individuals with the D^u antigen are frequently typed as Rh negative. D^u positive infants can suffer from hemolytic disease.

240. Which antigens make up the Rh complex?

The Rh antigen complex is made up of six possible antigens: C, c, D, d, E, e. The vast majority of isoimmunizations causing serious neonatal disease are the result of incompatibility to the D antigen. The non-D Rh antigens (E, C, c) have been shown to cause hemolytic disease and may be associated with mild to severe hydrops fetalis.

241. Why is the direct Coombs' test frequently negative or weakly positive in infants with ABO incompatibility?

There are fewer A or B antigenic sites on the newborn red cell, and there is also a greater distance between antigenic sites when compared to adults. There is also absorption of serum antibody by naturally occurring A and B substances scattered throughout body tissues, in foods, and gram-negative bacteria.

242. Contrast the features of DIC, hemorrhagic disease of the newborn, and liver disease.

Differentiating Features of Vitamin K Deficiency, Disseminated Intravascular Coagulation, and Liver Disease

FEATURES	VITAMIN K DEFICIENCY	DIC	LIVER DISEASE
History	No vitamin K given. Mother receiving barbiturates or anticonvulsants.	Vitamin K given.	Vitamin K given.
Associated disease	Infant usually not sick. Trauma may be precipitating factor.	Infant sick. Complications include sepsis, hypoxia, acidosis, hypothermia or obstetric accidents.	Infant sick. Hepatitis, metabolic disturbances such as hereditary fructose intolerance, galactosemia.
Site of hemorrhage	Usually gastrointestinal. Rarely skin or internal organs.	Generalized oozing into skin or internal organs, especially intracranial. Thromboses with gangrene rarely seen.	Mucosal and subcutaneous bleeding and bleeding into internal organs.
Time of onset	2nd or 3rd day after birth or later.	Usually immediate	Early or late
Capillary fragility	Normal	Usually abnormal	Usually abnormal
Bleeding time	Normal	Usually prolonged	Often prolonged
Prothrombin time	Very prolonged (5% or less)	Moderately prolonged	Very prolonged
Partial thromboplastin time	Prolonged	Prolonged	Prolonged
Thrombin time	Normal for age	Prolonged	Prolonged
Fibrin degradation products	Normal	Increased	Normal or increased
Fibrinogen	Normal	Often decreased	Decreased
Factor V	Normal	Decreased	Decreased
Factor VIII	Normal	Usually decreased	Normal
Factor XIII	Normal	Decreased	Normal
Platelet count	Normal	Decreased	Normal or occasionally decreased
Microangiopathic changes on peripheral smear	Absent	Present	Spur cells and/or target cells may be seen
Other associated physical findings	Nil	Depends on etiologic factors	Jaundice, hepatomegaly
Response to vitamin K	Dramatic*	Absent or minimal	Markedly diminished or absent

From Gross SJ, Stuart MJ: Hemostasis in the premature infant. Clin Perinatol 4:272–273, 1977, with permission.
Note: The differentiation between disseminated intravascular coagulation and liver disease (especially in fulminant hepatic failure) may be impossible since the entities may coexist. *Suboptimal response in the small premature infant.

243. What are the causes of hydrops fetalis?

Causes of Hydrops Fetalis

Severe chronic anemia *in utero*
    Erythroblastosis fetalis
    Homozygous alpha-thalassemia
    Chronic fetomaternal transfusion or twin-to-twin transfusion*
Cardiac failure
    Severe congenital heart disease
    Intrauterine arrhythmias
Hypoproteinemia
    Renal disease
    Congenital hepatitis
Infections (intrauterine)
    Syphilis
    Toxoplasmosis
    Cytomegalovirus

Modified from Blanchette V, Zipursky A: Neonatal hematology. In Avery GB (ed): Neonatology: Pathophysiology and Management of the Newborn. Philadelphia, J.B. Lippincott, 1987, p 651, with permission.
*Most important causes of nonimmune hydrops fetalis.

244. What is the significance of a single umbilical artery?

In the Collaborative Perinatal Study a single umbilical artery was found in 0.9% of deliveries. In the 14% of infants with this anomaly who died perinatally, 53% had additional abnormalities. Among the survivors, only 4% had additional abnormalities. Contrary to previously held views, urogenital anomalies are not more common than other developmental defects.

245. What are the best locations for umbilical venous and arterial catheters?

Insertion Distance for Umbilical Catheters (cm)

SHOULDER (LATERAL END OF CLAVICLE) TO UMBILICUS	AORTIC CATHETER TO DIAPHRAGM	AORTIC CATHETER TO AORTIC BIFURCATION	VENOUS CATHETER TO RIGHT ATRIUM
9	11	5	6
10	12	5	6–7
11	13	6	7
12	14	7	8
13	15	8	8–9
14	16	9	9
15	17	10	10
16	18	10–11	11
17	20	11–12	11–12

From Dunn PM: Localization of umbilical catheters by post mortem measurement. Arch Dis Child 41:69, 1966, with permission.

Neonatal Sepsis

246. What are the most common pathogens responsible for sepsis in the neonate?

Gram-negative bacteria (particularly *E. coli*) and group B streptococcus. Of note is the recent emergence of coagulase-negative staphylococci as the most common organisms responsible for nosocomial infections in most newborn intensive care units. As can be seen in the table (next page), the organisms most commonly responsible for neonatal sepsis vary significantly throughout the world.

Most Frequently Isolated Organisms in Neonatal Sepsis by Geographic Location

	BERLIN 1965–1978	NEW HAVEN 1966–1978	STOCKHOLM 1969–1978	MADRID 1971–1974	DALLAS 1973–1976	LONDON 1976–1979
Group B streptococci	27 (23%)	97 (25%)	33 (16%)	—	75 (39%)	7 (6%)
Escherichia coli	42 (36%)	122 (32%)	40 (19%)	39 (17%)	32 (17%)	6 (5%)
Klebsiella–Enterobacter	3 (3%)	56 (15%)	22 (10%)	99 (43%)	14 (7%)	5 (4%)
S. aureus	23 (19%)	24 (6%)	57 (27%)	62 (27%)	9 (5%)	5 (4%)
H. influenzae	—	11 (3%)	—	—	4 (2%)	—
S. epidermidis	—	2 (0.5%)	26 (12%)	—	—	55 (49%)
Enterococcus	1 (1%)	13 (3%)	(84%)	—	38 (20%)	—
P. aeruginosa	7 (6%)	9 (2%)	—	7 (%)	6 (3%)	8 (7%)
TOTAL	118	384	210	230	191	113

From Philip AGS: Neonatal Sepsis and Meningitis. Boston, G.K. Hall, 1985, with permission.

247. What pathogens are responsible for catheter-related sepsis in the neonate?
The pathogens emerging as the most common cause for catheter-related sepsis in the newborn in the United States are the coagulase-negative staphylococci. Additional organisms cultured from infants with intravascular catheters include *Staphylococcus aureus,* Candida species, Klebsiella and Enterobacter.

248. What is the pathogenesis of early-onset bacterial infections?
Blanc has designated the sequence of events responsible for early-onset bacterial infection the *"ascending amniotic infection syndrome."* Infection begins with colonization of the maternal genital tract. Pathogenic bacteria then spread upward through the cervix into the amniotic cavity, resulting in chorioamnionitis. Susceptible infants either inhale or swallow infected amniotic fluid and develop generalized sepsis. Although chorioamnionitis increases the risk of both fetal and neonatal infection, less than 5% of mothers with this condition deliver infected infants.

249. What perinatal factors are associated with an increased risk of sepsis?
Maternal fever and chorioamnionitis, premature and prolonged rupture of membranes, colonization with pathogens such as group B streptococcus, and prematurity. Other factors such as maternal septicemia or viremia, excessive manipulation of the fetus, and fetal monitoring are also important in the pathogenesis of neonatal infection. Of all the above factors, prematurity is the one most significantly associated with an increased risk of infection.

250. Can sepsis be distinguished from other causes of respiratory distress in the neonate?
Bacterial sepsis cannot be reliably distinguished from other causes of respiratory distress in the neonate. The earliest signs of bacterial sepsis are characteristically nonspecific. Although a history of perinatal risk factors and a physical examination noting tachycardia and poor perfusion are suggestive of infection, a specific diagnosis is confirmed only by the presence of a positive blood culture.

251. Of what value are prophylactic antibiotics in neonates?
They are of limited value in the prevention of bacterial sepsis during the newborn period, unless they are directed against specific illnesses for which the infant is at risk. Examples include silver nitrate or tetracycline prophylaxis to prevent ophthalmia neonatorum, or the use of BCG vaccination or isoniazid to prevent tuberculosis in infants at risk.

252. What are the common clinical presentations of neonatal infections?
It is important to note that initially, signs of sepsis may be minimal and nonspecific, often similar to those observed in many noninfectious processes.

**Clinical Signs of Bacterial Sepsis in 455 Newborn Infants
Studied at Four Medical Centers**

CLINICAL SIGN	PERCENTAGE OF INFANTS WITH SIGN
Hyperthermia	51
Hypothermia	15
Respiratory distress	33
Apnea	22
Cyanosis	24
Jaundice	35
Hepatomegaly	33
Lethargy	25
Irritability	16
Anorexia	28
Vomiting	25
Abdominal distention	17
Diarrhea	11

From Klein JO, Marcy SM: Bacterial sepsis and meningitis. In Klein JO, Remington JS (eds): Infectious Diseases of the Fetus and Newborn Infant. Philadelphia, W.B. Saunders Co., 1983, p 697, with permission.

253. What should a sepsis workup include for the neonate?
A complete blood count, blood cultures (preferably more than one set), CSF cell count, protein and glucose, and cultures. If respiratory distress is prominent, a chest film should be obtained. A urine culture should be included beyond the first few days of life. Urine cultures are infrequently positive in infants less than 72 hours of age except when associated with renal anomalies.

254. Of what value is the white blood count for identifying the infected or noninfected infant?
White blood cell counts are of limited value in the diagnosis of bacterial sepsis in the newborn period. In one-third of infants with proven bacterial disease, total WBC counts are normal, particularly early in the course of infection. On the other hand, less than 50% of infants with low ($<5000/mm^3$) or high ($>20,000/mm^3$) white counts demonstrate bacterial disease.

255. When should a lumbar puncture be part of the sepsis workup?
Always, unless the infant has cardiovascular instability or significant thrombocytopenia. A significant number (15–30%) of infants may have meningitis without bacteremia!

256. Which neutrophil indices are of value for identifying infection in newborn infants?
The most sensitive neutrophil index for identifying septic infants is the immature to total neutrophil ratio. Neutropenia is the most specific indicator. Overall abnormal neutrophil indices have not proven to be helpful for identifying infection in infants (low positive predictive value). When all neutrophil indices are normal, however, the likelihood of infection is extremely low (high negative predictive accuracy). (See table on next page.)

Neutrophil Values Predictive of Neonatal Bacterial Infection

	DIAGNOSTIC VALUE	POSTNATAL AGE
I. Neutropenia	<1800	birth
	<7800	12 hours
	<7200	24 hours
	<4200	48 hours
	<1800	72 hours & beyond
II. Increase in the	>.16	birth
ratio of immature	>.13	60 hours
to total	>.12	5 days & beyond
neutrophils		
III. Increased number	>5400	birth
of total	>14400	12 hours
neutrophils	>12600	24 hours
	>9000	48 hours
	>5400	72 hours & beyond
IV. Increased number	>1120	birth
of immature	>1440	12 hours
neutrophils	>1280	24 hours
	> 800	48 hours
	> 500	5 days & beyond

Adapted from Manroe, et al: J Pediatr 95:89, 1979.

257. Why do infected neonates display neutropenia more frequently than adults?

Neutropenia, which may be an ominous sign in septic infants, occurs more frequently in this group for several reasons: (1) there are smaller numbers of neutrophilic stem cells (colony-forming units) per unit body weight, (2) since stem cell proliferation in the neonate is maximal in the non-infected state, it cannot increase during infection, (3) release of marrow neutrophils is accelerated following the onset of infection in the neonate; therefore the neutrophil storage pool is rapidly depleted during the course of infection, and (4) the neutrophil storage pool and marrow proliferative pool are smaller in the neonate than in the adult.

258. Of what value is the gastric aspirate in the neonate?

Examination of gastric aspirates for leukocytes and bacteria was previously thought to be useful in identifying infants at risk for sepsis. However, the leukocytes are of maternal origin and the bacteria represent organisms colonizing or infecting the amniotic cavity. They do not necessarily indicate fetal or neonatal infection. Thus, results of gastric aspirate cultures are probably of minimal usefulness and may also be misleading.

259. Are the sedimentation rate and acute phase reactant determinations useful in the diagnosis of neonatal sepsis?

Several authors have advocated the use of sedimentation rates and acute phase reactants (C-reactive protein, fibrinogen, haptoglobin, and orosomucoid) to aid in the identification of neonates with bacterial sepsis. The greatest potential of the sepsis screen is to exclude infection when uncertainty exists about the clinical condition of a neonate in the first week of life. In most studies, sepsis screens have provided little data beyond white counts, neutrophil counts, and ratio of immature to total neutrophils, and currently are not widely used.

260. What are normal CSF values for healthy neonates? How do they change with meningitis?

Normal CSF values for healthy neonates are shown in the table. Frequently, there is a CSF pleocytosis with bacterial meningitis; however, its absence does not rule out meningitis. Protein levels may be elevated or normal, and glucose levels are often less than half of simultaneous blood sugar values.

CSF Examination in High-Risk Neonates without Meningitis

	TERM	PRETERM
WBC count (cells/mm^3)		
No. of infants	87	30
Mean	8.2	9.0
Median	5	6
SD	7.1	8.2
Range	0–32	0–29
+ 2 SD	0–22.4	0–25.4
Polymorphonuclear cells	61.3%	57.2%
Protein (mg/dl)		
No. of infants	35	17
Mean	90	115
Range	20–170	65–150
Glucose (mg/dl)		
No. of infants	51	23
Mean	52	50
Range	34–119	24–63
CSF/blood glucose (%)		
No. of infants	51	23
Mean	81	74
Range	44–248	55–105

From Sarf et al: J Pediatr 88:473, 1976, with permission.

261. What is the treatment for gram-negative meningitis in the neonate?

When treating gram-negative meningitis, drugs and dosages must be selected to achieve bactericidal cerebrospinal fluid (CSF) concentrations. Rapid sterilization of CSF may be difficult because the concentration of most antibiotics in CSF is below the minimum bactericidal concentrations for these organisms. In a four-year collaborative study, Mc-Cracken compared the efficacy of parenteral ampicillin and gentamicin with a regimen using parenteral antibiotics plus intrathecal gentamicin. There was no significant difference in morbidity and mortality between the two treatment groups. In a second collaborative study, the efficacy of systemic ampicillin and gentamicin was compared to a regimen employing systemic antibiotics plus intraventricular gentamicin. There was a significantly higher mortality in the group of infants who received systemic antibiotics plus intraventricular therapy (42.9% vs. 12.5%), and the study was terminated prematurely. In a subsequent study, McCracken demonstrated a similar outcome for infants with gram-negative meningitis receiving the combination of moxalactam and ampicillin as compared to ampicillin and amikacin. Cefotaxime is currently the preferred third-generation cephalosporin for the treatment of neonatal meningitis, and regimens employing cefotaxime, or ampicillin plus an aminoglycoside are thought to be equally efficacious.

262. What is the long-term neurologic prognosis for infants with meningitis?

Approximately 20–50% of infants who survive bacterial meningitis develop sequelae including hearing loss, communicating or noncommunicating hydrocephalus, abnormal speech, seizures, and mental and motor losses. Many infants appear relatively well at discharge, only to present later with perceptual difficulties or minimal brain damage.

263. Differentiate early- from late-onset group B streptococcal (GBS) sepsis.

Early-onset disease typically presents as shock with apnea and cardiovascular instability; late-onset disease is most commonly a focal infection. The GBS strains have been divided into serotypes based on the structure of their capsular polysaccharide antigens. Isolates from neonates without CNS involvement are evenly divided among serotypes I, II, and III; however, 90% of isolates from infants with meningitis (early or late onset disease) belong to serotype III.

Comparison of Early- and Late-onset GBS Disease

	EARLY ONSET	LATE ONSET
Age	≤5 days	≥10 days
Maternal complications	Frequent	Not frequent
Onset of disease	Fulminant	Insidious
Signs/symptoms	Cardiovascular instability or respiratory distress	Fever, lethargy, bulging fontanelle
CNS involvement	30%	80–90%
Mode of acquisition	Vertical	? Community/siblings
Serotypes	All	III (90%)
Mortality	30–50%	15–20%

264. How do the features of osteomyelitis in the neonate differ from those in the older child and adult?

1. Neonatal osteomyelitis almost invariably follows hematogenous dissemination.

2. Multiple foci of infection are frequently seen.

3. Septic arthritis is a frequent association, probably reflecting the spread of infection via blood vessels penetrating the epiphyseal plates.

4. Chronic osteomyelitis is infrequent.

5. The pathogens causing neonatal osteomyelitis are the same as those responsible for sepsis neonatorum.

265. What does the acronym TORCH mean?

Toxoplasma, other viruses, rubella, cytomegalovirus, and herpes virus.

266. What tests comprise a TORCH workup?

Diagnostic tests of value for identification of infants with congenital infection are shown below. Congenital infection may be confirmed or ruled out according to the criteria listed in the second table.

Diagnostic Approach to the Newborn Suspected of Being Congenitally Infected

NONSPECIFIC TESTS	SPECIFIC TESTS
Complete blood and platelet counts	Viral culture*:
Lumbar puncture	Oropharynx, urine, rectum;
Roentgenogram, long bones	Optional: CSF, conjunctiva
CT scan of head	Smears-skin lesions:
Ophthalmologic evaluation	FA stain
Audiologic evaluation	Dark-field examination
	Tzanck smear
	Serology†:
	Rubella: HAI, PHA, LA or ELISA screen for IgG antibody
	Toxoplasma: SF or IFA for IgG antibody
	Syphilis: VDRL or RPR
	Hepatitis B: HBsAg

From Plotkin SA, Alpert G: Pediatr Clin North Am 33:465, 1986, with permission.
*African green monkey kidney cell line must be inoculated. *HAI* = hemagglutination inhibition; *PHA* = passive hemagglutination; *LA* = latex agglutination; *SF* = Sabin-Feldman dye test; *IFA* = immunofluorescence test; *FA* = fluorescent antibody.
†Initial tests

How to Confirm or Rule Out Specific Congenital Infections

	CULTURE		SCREENING FOR SPECIFIC IgG ANTIBODY	
	Positive	Negative	Positive	Negative
Cytomegalovirus	Confirmed	Eliminated	Not indicated	Not indicated
Herpes simplex	Confirmed	Eliminated	Not indicated	Not indicated
Rubella	Confirmed	Not eliminated	Test-specific IgM antibody	Eliminated

```
                    +  /  \ −
                      /    \
                     ↓      ↓
              Confirmed   Ruled out*
```

Toxoplasma	Confirmed	Not eliminated	Test-specific IgM antibody	Eliminated

```
                    +  /  \ −
                      /    \
                     ↓      ↓
              Confirmed  Not ruled
                           out†
```

Syphilis			Specific treponemal test	Not eliminated

```
                    +  /  \ ↘ −
                      ↓   ↓
                 Possible‡ Ruled out
```

Hepatitis B			Confirmed§	Eliminated

From Plotkin SA, Alpert G: Pediatr Clin North Am 33:465, 1986, with permission.
*If culture is negative.
†Test mother, perform clinical and laboratory follow-up.
‡Test mother, compare titers, search for clinical evidence of infection, follow infant serologically.
§Screening in this case is for hepatitis antigen.

267. Why should the TORCH eponym be changed to CROTCHS?

It has recently been suggested, perhaps facetiously, that the TORCH eponym be changed to CROTCHS to emphasize the importance of cytomegalovirus infections. This more comprehensive acronym signifies the following: cytomegalovirus, rubella, (other), toxoplasma, coxsackievirus, herpes simplex, and syphilis. However, I doubt that this acronym will immediately suggest congenital infection, even to the most academic-minded physician.

268. Of what value is the quantitation of serum IgM for the identification of congenitally infected infants?

IgM levels in serum or cord blood have been used as screening tests for congenitally infected infants. Approximately 75% of infants who subsequently were diagnosed with a TORCH infection had elevated IgM levels. Conversely, there is a high incidence of false-positive IgM results. Rheumatoid factor is a convenient, although nonspecific, method of screening infants for congenital CMV infections. While 35–45% of infected infants have positive screens, false-positive results are infrequently noted. Rheumatoid factor may also be positive in the serum and CSF of newborns with toxoplasmosis.

269. What are the most common findings in congenitally infected infants? Which of them are most specific?

The figure (next page) summarizes common manifestations of symptomatic congenital rubella, cytomegalovirus, and toxoplasmosis. Those clinical findings which are considered relatively specific are listed in the table. Viruses other than those commonly associated with congenital infection can cause fetal wastage and perinatal disease. These include vaccinia and smallpox virus, varicella zoster virus, human immunodeficiency virus, and enteroviruses.

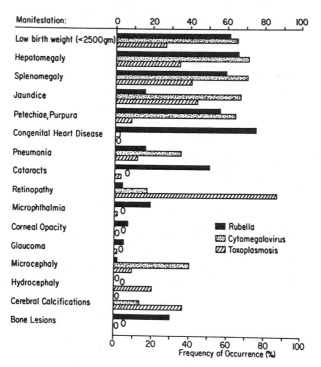

Manifestations of symptomatic congenital rubella and CMV infections and toxoplasmosis in the neonate. (From Overall JC Jr: Viral infections of the fetus and neonate. In Feigin RD, Cherry JD (eds): Textbook of Pediatric Infectious Diseases. Philadelphia, W.B. Saunders Co, 1981, p 690, with permission.

Relatively Specific Findings with Chronic Perinatal Infections

Congenital Rubella:	Eye: cataracts, cloudy cornea, pigmented retina
	Skin: blueberry muffin syndrome (erythrogenic arrest)
	Bone: vertical striation
	Heart: malformation (ductus, pulmonary artery stenosis)
CMV:	Microcephaly with periventricular calcifications
	Inguinal hernias in males
	Petechiae with thrombocytopenia
Toxoplasma:	Hydrocephalus with generalized calcifications
	Chorioretinitis
	Disproportionate elevation of CSF protein
Syphilis:	Osteochondritis and periostitis, eczematoid skin rash, mucocutaneous lesions (snuffles)
Natal Herpes:	Skin vesicles, keratoconjunctivitis
	Acute CNS findings
Hepatitis B:	Onset of jaundice and hepatosplenomegaly between one and six months of age
CMV:	Afebrile, protracted pneumonitis
Enterovirus:	Acute CNS findings, CSF pleocytosis

From Stagno S, Pass RF, Alford CA: Perinatal infections and maldevelopment. In Bloom AD, James LS (eds): The Fetus and the Newborn, Vol. 17, Series 1. New York, Alan R. Liss, Inc., 1981, with permission.

270. What are the late sequelae of congenital infections?

The late sequelae of chronic intrauterine infections are relatively common and occur in infants who are asymptomatic at birth. Most of these sequelae present later in childhood rather than infancy.

Late Sequelae of Chronic Intrauterine Infection

Cytomegalovirus	Hearing loss,* minimal* to severe brain dysfunction (motor, learning, language, and behavioral disorders)
Rubella	Hearing loss,* minimal* to severe brain dysfunction (motor, learning, language and behavioral disorders), autism,* juvenile diabetes, thyroid dysfunction, precocious puberty, progressive degenerative brain disorder*
Toxoplasmosis	Chorioretinitis,* minimal* to severe brain dysfunction, hearing loss, precocious puberty
Neonatal herpes	Recurrent eye and skin infection, minimal* to severe* brain dysfunction
Hepatitis B virus	Chronic subclinical hepatitis, rarely fulminant hepatitis

From Plotkin SA, Alpert G: Pediatr Clin North Am 33:465, 1986, with permission.
*Seen with infections that are subclinical in early infancy.

271. What is the preferred therapy for type II herpes simplex infection in the neonate?

The collaborative multicenter trial of acyclovir versus vidarabine in the treatment of neonatal type II herpes simplex is still in progress. Preliminary results indicate that both drugs decrease progression of disease from localized skin lesions to invasive CNS infection. However, the mortality rate in disseminated disease appears similar to that found in other studies. When vidarabine and acyclovir are compared, clinical responses to therapy appear equivalent, without apparent differences in toxicity.

272. What are the manifestations of congenital varicella?

Infants with congenital varicella may demonstrate either mild disease or severe systemic infection. Systemic symptoms include fever, poor feeding, pneumonia, vomiting, and respiratory distress with a mortality as high as 30%. In other cases, only a few vesicles are present without systemic abnormalities. Varicella zoster virus is also thought to cause a "congenital varicella syndrome," the principal features of which are summarized below.

Summary of Details in 18 Cases of Congenital Varicella Zoster

ILLNESS OR DEFECT	NO.
Maternal varicella in pregnancy	14
Maternal zoster in pregnancy	3
Maternal zoster varicellosus in pregnancy	1
Gestational age at maternal illness	8–20 weeks
Infants born "small for gestational age"	8
Cutaneous scars	13
Hypoplasia of a limb	10
Muscular atrophy	9
Rudimentary digits	5
Psychomotor retardation	7
Seizures	3
Muscular paralysis	4
Other CNS signs or symptoms Cortical atrophy Microcephaly Horner's syndrome	7

Table continued on next page.

Summary of Details in 18 Cases of Congenital Varicella Zoster *(Continued)*

ILLNESS OR DEFECT	NO.
Microphthalmus	8
Chorioretinitis	4
Cataracts and nystagmus	8
Facial asymmetry	3
Recurrent chest infections	4
Delayed development in infancy	7
Deaths	7
Survivors	11

From Hanshaw JB, Dudgeon JA, Marshall WC: In Viral Diseases of the Fetus and Newborn, 2nd ed. Philadelphia, W.B. Saunders Co., 1985, p 170, with permission.

273. How is hepatitis B virus transmitted to the neonate?

Hepatitis B virus is most commonly transmitted to the neonate either during the third trimester or near the time of delivery, although earlier transplacental infection may occur. Infants are also infected by fecal-oral transmission during the neonatal period, and by transmission through breast milk.

274. What are the clinical manifestations of congenital HTLV III infections?

The major clinical signs are listed in the table. Of note are several symptoms unique to the pediatric age group: pulmonary lymphoid hyperplasia, salivary gland enlargement, developmental delay, and dysmorphic craniofacial features.

Pediatric HTLV-III Infection—Major Findings (in Order of Frequency)*

Chronic pneumonitis (PLH;LIP)
Recurrent bacterial infections/sepsis
Oral thrush—persistent or recurrent
Diarrhea—chronic or recurrent
Lymphadenopathy (two or more sites)
Hepatosplenomegaly
Failure to thrive
Developmental delay
Encephalopathy
Small for gestational age
Thrombocytopenia
Salivary gland enlargement
Opportunistic infections
Kaposi's sarcoma
B-cell lymphoma

From Current Problems in Pediatrics, 1986, p 373, with permission.
*Based on study of 92 HTLV-III serologically positive infants.

275. How should infants born to PPD positive women be managed?

All infants born to mothers with a positive PPD should be separated from their mothers following delivery and treated with either BCG vaccination or INH prophylaxis. Infants born to mothers with suspected disease but not proven tuberculosis may be temporarily separated at birth until the mother is shown to be noninfectious. Other studies have advocated prophylactic INH administration to children at risk, although there must be guaranteed compliance with this regimen. BCG administration, a one-time immunization, has also been used, particularly when compliance cannot be ensured.

276. How does the treatment of syphilitic meningoencephalitis differ from congenital syphilis without CNS involvement?

Treatment for Congenital Syphilis

CONGENITAL SYPHILIS	DRUG	DOSE/KG
With neurosyphilis	Aqueous penicillin G	25,000 units IM or IV twice daily × 10 days
	Procaine penicillin G	50,000 units IM daily × 10 days
Without neurosyphilis	Benzathine penicillin G	50,000 units IM single dose

Modified from CDC MMWR 25:101, 1976. From Ingall D, Musher D: Syphilis. In Klein JO, Remington JS (eds): Infectious Diseases of the Fetus and Newborn Infant. Philadelphia, W.B. Saunders Co., 1983, p 367, with permission.

277. How is syphilitic meningoencephalitis diagnosed?
By examination of the CSF for pleocytosis (up to 200 mononuclear cells/mm^3), elevated protein (50–200 mg/dl), and a positive serologic test for syphilis (usually the VDRL).

278. What is the significance of hepatitis e antigen in the blood of a pregnant woman?
The hepatitis e antigen has been found in the sera of some HBsAg-positive women, and its presence is correlated with a high probability of transmission of the hepatitis virus to the neonate. However, babies born to mothers whose sera contain antibodies to the e antigen usually do not become infected. The presence of hepatitis e antigen in the serum of an asymptomatic carrier mother should alert physicians to the possibility of an infant at significant risk for neonatal hepatitis B virus infection.

279. What is the pseudoparalysis of Parrot?
Parrot's paralysis is the painful pseudoparalysis associated with the bony changes of syphilitic osteochondritis and periostitis. The presentation may be one of an irritable infant who does not want to move one or more limbs. The upper extremities are affected more commonly than the lower.

280. Which congenital infections cause cerebral calcifications?
Cerebral calcifications are most frequently observed in congenital toxoplasmosis and cytomegalovirus infections. Toxoplasmosis often produces dense round calcifications scattered diffusely throughout the white matter of the brain, although it may also present as curvilinear streaks in the basal ganglia. Infants with cytomegalovirus infections present with periventricular calcifications, but there is considerable overlap between the presentations of these two diseases. Herpes simplex has also been reported to cause massive bilateral calcifications of the cerebral hemispheres, as has congenital rubella infection. In rubella, radiographic documentation of intracranial calcifications is not a common finding.

281. How is systemic candidiasis diagnosed in the neonate?
Systemic candidiasis is best diagnosed by cultures of blood, urine, and CSF, or other body fluids that are generally sterile. Since cultures are only intermittently positive, multiple systemic cultures should be obtained. A urinalysis demonstrating budding yeasts or hyphae should raise suspicion of systemic infection. Gram stains of buffy coat smears may also demonstrate organisms. An ophthalmologic exam may indicate the presence of candidal endophthalmitis.

282. What is the preferred treatment of candidal sepsis and meningitis?
Systemic candidiasis is treated with amphotericin B intravenously for 4 weeks. Treatment is started at 0.1 mg/kg in a single daily dose infused over 4–6 hours. The dose is gradually increased over several days until a maximum daily dosage of 0.5–1.0 mg/kg is achieved. 5-Flucytosine (50–150 mg/kg/day) should be used to supplement amphotericin B if the infection is severe, the organism is resistant to amphotericin, or the central nervous system is involved.

283. What are the clinical presentations of listeriosis in the newborn?

Infection caused by *Listeria monocytogenes* may occur during the first few days of life (early-onset disease) or present beyond the first week (late-onset disease). Infants present with variable symptoms including vomiting, lethargy, jaundice, seizures, respiratory distress, and myocarditis. Skin and pharyngeal lesions (roseoles or focal cutaneous granulomas) may also be present. Meningitis occurs but is more common with late-onset disease. Neonatal listeriosis should be suspected in the following circumstances: (1) maternal history of prior stillbirth or repeated abortions; (2) placental pathology including funisitis, chorioamnionitis, or placental villous granulomas; and (3) neonatal hepatosplenomegaly and granulomas of the skin and posterior pharynx.

284. How frequent is gonococcal conjunctivitis in babies who have had silver nitrate or erythromycin drops?

The rate of occurrence of gonococcal conjunctivitis is less than 0.03% following eye prophylaxis with silver nitrate or erythromycin.

285. What is the value of granulocyte transfusion for the infected neonate?

Neutropenia is frequently observed in septic neonates, and has been correlated with a poor outcome. As a consequence, granulocyte transfusion has been suggested as an adjunctive immunologic therapy. Unfortunately, there are few randomized controlled studies in human neonates. Most studies to date report an improved survival following white cell transfusion with few or no side effects. Data from adults also suggest that the transfused white cells retain functional properties. Because there is a paucity of data from controlled trials demonstrating efficacy, granulocyte transfusions in newborn infants should be reserved for the most critically ill infants after conventional therapies have failed.

Granulocyte Transfusions in the Newborn Infant

AUTHOR	SOURCE	N	OUTCOME	COMMENTS
Laurenti et al	J. Pediatr. 98:118, 1981	38	Improved survival in treatment group	Mostly gram-negative infections with onset beyond age 2 days. Nonrandomized study.
Christensen et al	Pediatrics 70:1, 1982	16	Improved survival in treatment group	Randomized study of infants with severe NSP depletion.
Wheeler et al	Ped. Inf. Dis. 3:407, 1982	3	Study group too small to assess outcome	—
	Pediatrics 79:422, 1987	20	Study group too small to assess outcome	—
Cairo et al	Pediatrics 74:887, 1984	23	Improved survival in treatment group	Randomized study. Only 3 infants had NSP depletion. Mixture of septic and "R/O sepsis" infants.
	J. Pediatr. 110:935, 1987	35	Improved survival in treatment group	Randomized study. Infants receiving WBC had less fulminant disease.
Addo-Yobo et al	Pediatr. Res. 19:330A, 1985	4	All treated infants survived	Buffy coat transfusions. No control group with severe NSP depletion.
Baley et al	Pediatrics 80:712, 1987	25	No benefit to granulocyte transfusions in infants with or without NSP depletion	Randomized trial. Noted fall in P_aO_2 with 3 PMN transfusions

286. What is the value of exchange transfusion for the infected neonate?
As with granulocyte transfusion, there is little controlled data supporting the role of exchange transfusion in neonatal septicemia. Although the mechanism responsible for improved survival is unknown, likely possibilities include the administration of opsonins or functional granulocytes. Because of potential serious side effects, this therapy should also be used with caution.

Urinary System

287. What percentage of kidneys are palpable in the newborn period?
Nearly all kidneys are palpable if they're there!

288. What is the differential diagnosis of an enlarged kidney in the neonate?
The differential diagnosis of kidney enlargement includes tumor, renal vein thrombosis, hydronephrosis, polycystic kidney and multicystic renal disease.

289. What are the classic manifestations of renal vein thrombosis?
The classic manifestations of renal vein thrombosis are renal enlargement, hematuria, and thrombocytopenia, with or without evidence of disseminated intravascular coagulation.

290. What are the major causes of renal failure in the neonate? Which laboratory studies are useful for differentiating pre-renal from intrinsic renal failure?

Major Causes of Renal Failure in the Neonate

PRERENAL	POSTRENAL OBSTRUCTION	INTRINSIC RENAL FAILURE
Hypotension caused by:	Urethral obstruction	Congenital abormalities
Septic shock	Posterior urethral valves	Cystic dysplasia
Maternal antepartum	Imperforate prepuce	Hypoplasia
hemorrhage	Urethral stricture	Agenesis
Twin-to-twin	Urethral diverticulum	Polycystic kidneys
hemorrhage	Megaurethra	Inflammatory
Neonatal hemorrhage	Ureterocele	Congenital syphilis or
Cardiac surgery	Ureteropelvic or	toxoplasmosis
Congestive heart failure	ureterovesical	Pyelonephritis
Asphyxia neonatorum	obstruction	Vascular
Dehydration	Extrinsic tumors	Venous thrombosis
	compressing bladder	Cortical necrosis
	outlet	Arterial thrombosis
	Neurogenic bladder	Disseminated intravascular
		coagulation
		Acute tubular necrosis
		Perinatal asphyxia
		Dehydration
		Shock
		Nephrotoxins

From Rahman N et al. Clin Perinatol 8:242, 1981, with permission.

$$Fe_{Na} = \frac{Urine\ Na}{Serum\ Na} \times \frac{Serum\ Cr}{Urine\ Cr} \times 100$$

Summary of Diagnostic Indices in Neonates with Oliguria

DIAGNOSTIC INDICES	RENAL FAILURE	PRERENAL OLIGURIA	P VALUE
U_{Na} (mEq/L)	63.41 ± 34.7	31.41 ± 19.5	<.01
U/S sodium	0.45 ± 0.22	0.23 ± 0.14	<.01
U/S urea	5.78 ± 2.89	29.64 ± 17.90	<.01
U/S creatinine	9.67 ± 3.57	29.24 ± 15.60	<.05
RFI	11.62 ± 9.61	1.29 ± 0.82	<.01
FE_{Na} urea	12.11 ± 11.50	1.01 ± 0.63	<.01
FE_{Na} creatinine	4.25 ± 2.18	0.95 ± 0.55	<.01

From Mathew OP, et al. Pediatrics 65:57, 1980, with permission.

291. What are the associated findings of renal agenesis?
Oligohydramnios, Potter's facies (low-set ears, micrognathia, hypertelorism, epicanthal folds, and mongoloid slant to the eyes), and pulmonary hypoplasia. Other associated abnormalities are vernix nodules (amnion nodosum), single umbilical artery, esophageal, duodenal or anal atresia, colonic agenesis, and Meckel's diverticulum. The internal genitalia are often abnormal and sirenomelia has been observed. Unilateral renal agenesis is infrequently associated with other anomalies.

292. What is prune belly syndrome?
Prune belly syndrome consists of absent abdominal musculature, redundancy and wrinkling of the abdominal wall skin, protrusion of the abdominal organs, bilateral cryptorchidism, and urinary tract dilatation. The kidneys may be hypoplastic but there is frequently adequate renal parenchyma on one side. The bladder is usually large and the ureters dilated and tortuous.

293. What are the adverse effects of furosemide in the neonate?
(1) Electrolyte disturbances, including hyponatremia, hypokalemia, hypochloremia, and dehydration, (2) calciuresis with nephrolithiasis and osteopenia, and (3) ototoxicity in the presence of renal failure.

294. What is acceptable urine output and how is the value derived?
The minimum and maximum volumes of urine output are determined by the amount of solute to be excreted and the maximal renal diluting and concentrating ability (which are 30–50 mOsm/L and 700–800 mOsm/L, respectively). Most clinicians find a urine output of at least 2 cc/kg/hr acceptable. This value, however, is a calculated one based on an average solute intake, and knowledge about the concentrating and diluting capacities of the neonatal kidney. Infants with high solute intakes may need more urine output, and those with low intakes may need less.

295. What are the presenting signs of neonatal urinary tract infection?
Signs and symptoms are nonspecific and rarely are referable to the urinary tract, except in neonates with renal anomalies. More common symptoms include anorexia, hyperbilirubinemia, vomiting, diarrhea, and weight loss.

Nervous System

296. What behavioral states may be confused with seizures?
A variety of "seizure-like" behaviors, which show no evidence of simultaneous EEG discharges consistent with seizures, are believed to originate in the brainstem and spinal cord without superimposed inhibitory cortical influences. These include jitteriness, movements during REM sleep, "rowing" and "bicycling" movements (which may in some situations represent seizures), decorticate and decerebrate posturing, and autonomic dysfunctions.

297. How are seizures differentiated from tremors in the neonate?
Jitteriness is a movement disorder of neonates characterized primarily by tremulousness and is frequently confused with seizures.

Jitteriness Versus Seizures

CLINICAL FEATURES	JITTERINESS	SEIZURE
Abnormality of gaze or eye movement	0	+
Movements exquisitely stimulus-sensitive	+	0
Predominant movement	Tremor	Clonic jerking
Movements cease with passive flexion	+	0

298. What are the most common etiologies for seizures in infants <24 hours, 24–72 hours, and >72 hours of age?

Etiology of Neonatal Seizures in Relation to Time of Seizure Onset

	TIME OF ONSET		
ETIOLOGY	0–24 hours	24–72 hours	>3 days
Hypoxic-ischemic encephalopathy	+	+	−
Intracranial hemorrhage	+	+	−
Hypoglycemia	−	+	−
Hypocalcemia	−	+	+
Intracranial infection	−	−	+
Developmental defects	+	+	+
Drug withdrawal	+	+	+

299. What is an acceptable workup in a newborn infant with seizures?

The workup should include a careful prenatal and natal history as well as a complete physical examination. Laboratory studies should include blood for glucose, electrolytes, calcium, phosphorus and magnesium. A lumbar puncture should be performed to rule out meningitis, and an ultrasound or CT scan should be obtained when intracranial hemorrhage or a developmental defect is suspected. Additional studies, where warranted, include a blood ammonia level, and blood and urine for organic and amino acid analysis.

300. How should an infant with seizures be treated?

Due to the potential deleterious effects of seizures on the central nervous system, initiation of therapy is urgent. The following therapies should be administered only *after* ventilation and perfusion are adequately established:

Acute Therapy of Neonatal Seizures

With hypoglycemia
    Glucose, 10% solution: 2 ml/kg, IV followed by an infusion supplying 4–8 mg/kg/min
Without hypoglycemia
    Phenobarbital: 20 mg/kg, IV
    If necessary, additional phenobarbital: 5–20 mg/kg, IV
    Phenytoin: 20 mg/kg, IV
    Calcium gluconate, 5% solution: 4 ml/kg IV (monitor EKG during infusion)
    Magnesium sulfate, 50% solution: 0.2 ml/kg, IM
    Pyridoxine: 50–100mg, IV

From Volpe J (ed): Neurology of the Newborn. Philadelphia, W.B. Saunders Co., 1987, p 149, with permission.

301. What is the treatment for refractory seizures in the neonate?

Frequent and recurrent seizures are not uncommon in newborns and are especially common in the setting of asphyxia. If seizures are refractory to a full 40 mg/kg initial dose of phenobarbital, phenytoin up to 20 mg/kg is administered. If seizures still persist, addition of drugs in the benzodiazepine family (e.g., diazepam, lorazepam) or paraldehyde is generally effective. It is important to make sure that no underlying biochemical disturbance is present before the serum levels of anticonvulsants are raised to maximal concentrations. Although pyridoxine-dependent seizures are rare, a trial dose of pyridoxine should be administered intravenously to infants with recurrent seizures of uncertain etiology. If possible, simultaneous EEG recording should be performed to document the cessation of seizure activity and the normalization of the EEG within minutes.

302. Of what prognostic value is the interictal EEG in a neonate with seizures?

It may be helpful in providing prognostic information regarding neurologic outcome. The following table is a composite of two of the largest series including both term and preterm infants.

Prognosis of Neonatal Seizures — Relation to EEG*

EEG BACKGROUND	NEUROLOGIC SEQUELAE (%)
Normal	10
Severe abnormalities[†]	90
Moderate abnormalities[‡]	50

From Volpe J (ed): Neurology of the Newborn. Philadelphia, W. B. Saunders Co., 1987, p 145, with permission.
*Based primarily on data reported by Rowe et al (Electroencephalogr Clin Neurophysiol 51:219, 1981) and Lombroso (In Wasterlain CG et al (eds): Advances in Neurology. New York, Raven Press, 1983, p 101) and includes both full term and premature infants.
[†]Burst-suppression pattern, marked voltage suppression, and electrocerebral silence.
[‡]Voltage asymmetries and "immaturity".

303. Are seizures without concurrent hypoxia or acidosis harmful in a neonate?

Although the hypoxemia and hypercarbia that accompany seizures may result in brain injury, CNS damage can be produced by other associated events as well: (1) increased cerebral blood flow accompanying seizures may result in hemorrhagic infarction of vulnerable vascular beds (e.g., the germinal matrix in premature infants), (2) changes in the concentrations of critical high energy phosphate compounds (e.g., ATP, phosphocreatine) may lead to irreparable injury, (3) depletion of brain substrates such as glucose despite increased cerebral blood flow, and (4) excessive release of synaptic excitatory amino acids such as glutamate which exert a toxic effect at sites where they would otherwise serve as neurotransmitters (experimental animal data).

304. Should all seizures be treated?

Seizures in the neonatal period often signal life-threatening illness or a disorder that may lead to irreversible brain injury. Therefore, they should be promptly treated if clinical suspicion is high. After the results of diagnostic studies are available, and anticonvulsant therapy has been optimized, seizures of very brief duration are occasionally left untreated.

305. What perinatal events increase the likelihood of a subdural bleed?

Subdural hemorrhages in the neonate are thought to represent traumatic lesions. Therefore they occur in clinical settings in which the head is excessively molded: (1) a relatively large infant passing through a relatively small birth canal, (2) unusually rigid pelvic structures, (3) a very brief labor not allowing time for the pelvis to expand, or very long labor causing prolonged head compression, and (4) use of difficult technical maneuvers at delivery.

Pathogenesis of Neonatal Subdural Hemorrhage

AT RISK	PREDISPOSING FACTORS
Mother	Primiparous
	Older multiparous
	Small birth canal
Infant	Large full term > premature
Labor	Precipitous
	Prolonged
Delivery	Breech extraction
	Foot, face, brow presentation
	Difficult forceps extraction
	Difficult rotation

From Volpe J (ed): Neurology of the Newborn. Philadelphia, W.B. Saunders Co., 1987, p 287, with permission.

306. What are the indications for a subdural tap?

A subdural tap is useful in the diagnosis of subdural hematomas located along the cerebral convexities. However, CT is probably safer and therefore a preferable alternative. From a therapeutic standpoint, a subdural tap is indicated to reduce signs of increased intracranial pressure and to prevent the development of craniocerebral disproportion, which is characterized by a rapid increase in head size resulting in perpetuation of subdural bleeding.

307. How is a subdural effusion distinguished from normal CSF?

Subdural effusions are believed to result from transudation of fluid high in albumin through abnormally permeable channels in the subdural membrane. As a result, subdural effusions are higher (by approximately 40 mg/dl) in total protein than simultaneously drained CSF from the lumbar-subarachnoid space. In addition, the protein in subdural effusions is comprised of 62–72% albumin versus that in CSF which is 35–45% albumin.

308. What is the prognosis for infants with acute subdural hematomas?

Prognosis with acute subdural hemorrhage depends on the particular type. Patients with lacerations of the tentorium and falx as well as occipital diastasis have a uniformly poor prognosis with nearly 100% mortality. In the rare survivor of lacerations of the tentorium and/ or falx, hydrocephalus secondary to obstruction of CSF flow at the tentorial notch is common. The outcome in smaller posterior fossa hematomas is better, but depends on the rapidity of diagnosis and intervention. In one series of patients who underwent surgical evacuation, 72% were normal or minimally abnormal on follow up, 17% were left with major sequelae, and 11% died. Those who did not undergo evacuation had a favorable outcome in 44%, major sequelae in 12%, and death in 44% of cases. Favorable outcome can be expected in 50–80% of infants with a convexity subdural hemorrhage. The remainder are left with focal cerebral signs and occasionally hydrocephalus.

309. What causes subarachnoid hemorrhage (SAH)?

SAH in the neonate is believed to result from traumatic or hypoxic events that increase either traction on, or flow through, small fragile vascular channels which are the remnants of anastomoses present during brain development between the leptomeningeal arteries.

310. What are the clinical manifestations of SAH in the neonate?

1. Asymptomatic. In most cases, only small amounts of hemorrhage have occurred and minimal or no clinical signs are present.

2. "Well baby with seizures." In patients without significant hypoxic-ischemic encephalopathy, seizures secondary to SAH have their onset on the second day of life. In the interictal period, these babies appear well.

3. Catastrophic deterioration. In rare instances, newborn infants with large subarachnoid hemorrhages follow a rapidly fatal course characterized by coma, respiratory disturbance, seizures, loss of brainstem reflexes, and flaccidity.

311. What is the value of a lumbar puncture for the diagnosis of intracranial hemorrhage?

The finding of blood in CSF is a frequent correlate of intracranial hemorrhage in the newborn. Although "traumatic" lumbar punctures are often cited as the cause of "bloody taps," one series showed that 92% of infants with bloody spinal fluid had blood demonstrable by CT scan in their ventricles or subarachnoid space. (Other authors have suggested that up to 50% of CSF samples with red cells may represent traumatic "taps".) Additional CSF findings consistent with hemorrhage are xanthochromia, elevated protein and hypoglycorrhachia.

312. What is the frequency of subependymal–intraventricular hemorrhage (SEH-IVH) in the neonate?

Multiple series addressing this question have used CT scans and ultrasonography to define an incidence of between 34 and 43% for periventricular-intraventricular hemorrhages in premature infants. These figures include hemorrhages of all grades of severity (i.e., grades I–IV).

313. What are the clinical presentations of IVH?

1. A catastrophic deterioration characterized by an inexorable evolution in minutes to hours. Major features include stupor or coma, respiratory disturbances including apnea, generalized tonic seizures, "decerebrate" posturing, fixed pupils, flaccid quadriparesis, and absent "doll's eyes". Associated features include falling hematocrit, bulging anterior fontanelle, hypotension, bradycardia, temperature instability, metabolic acidosis and abnormal water homeostasis (inappropriate secretion of antidiuretic hormone or diabetes insipidus).

2. A saltatory deterioration that follows a stuttering evolution over hours to days. Important features include altered level of consciousness, decreased motility, decreased tone, abnormal eye movements (e.g., downward vertical drift, skew deviation) and an abnormally tight popliteal angle (<130° for premature infants and <110° for term infants).

3. A clinically silent syndrome that is often associated with an unexplained fall in hematocrit or failure of hematocrit to rise after transfusion.

314. How are SEH and IVH classified?

Most systems of classification include a grading system according to increasing severity as follows:

Grade I	germinal matrix hemorrhage only
Grade II	intraventricular hemorrhage *without* ventricular dilatation
Grade III	intraventricular hemorrhage *with* ventricular dilatation
Grade IV	grade III hemorrhage *with* intraparenchymal involvement

Volpe has abandoned the grade IV classification in favor of "intraventricular hemorrhage with intracerebral involvement" in order to emphasize the importance of the extent of parenchymal involvement rather than the grade of hemorrhage in determining prognosis.

315. How is SEH-IVH diagnosed?

When CT or ultrasound is not routinely available, lumbar puncture may aid in the diagnosis of IVH. The classic CSF findings are: presence of red blood cells, elevated protein, xanthochromia, and decreased glucose. However, a significant proportion of infants with IVH will not have blood in the lumbar subarachnoid space at the time of puncture. The mainstays of diagnosis therefore are CT and cranial ultrasound, with the latter offering the advantages of availability at the bedside, lack of ionizing radiation, and decreased expense. CT remains particularly useful in detecting complicating subdural hemorrhage, posterior fossa lesions, and cerebral parenchymal involvement.

316. Should all preterm infants be examined by cranial ultrasound?

Because of the relative noninvasiveness of ultrasound, most neonatologists recommend that a single cranial ultrasonogram be obtained in the first week of life in infants born at less than 35 weeks' gestational age.

317. What are the best times to perform an ultrasound examination of a neonate?

In series of infants studied by ultrasonography, approximately 50% had the onset of hemorrhage in the first day of life, an additional 25% on the second day, and another 15% on the third day. Thus, a single scan on the fourth day of life would be expected to detect greater than 90% of hemorrhages. However, it is important to note that approximately 20–40% of hemorrhages show evidence of extension within 3–5 days after initial diagnosis. Thus a second scan is indicated after about five days after the first to determine the maximal extent of hemorrhage.

318. What is the pathophysiology of IVH in the preterm neonate versus the term infant?

Although IVH is predominantly a lesion of premature infants, many cases have been documented in term infants. Although factors related to cerebral blood flow, venous pressure, and vascular integrity are applicable in both settings, the term infant is unique; 50% of cases involve trauma related to difficult deliveries (e.g., breech extraction and forceps rotation) and 25% have *no* definable pathogenic factors.

319. What is the difference between ventriculomegaly and posthemorrhagic hydrocephalus?

Both ventriculomegaly and hydrocephalus may follow IVH. While ventriculomegaly is the result of periventricular cerebral atrophy secondary to white matter hypoxic injury, hydrocephalus results from ventricular dilatation caused by disturbances in CSF dynamics.

320. Of what prognostic value are technetium brain scans and CT scans in the evaluation of asphyxiated neonates?

In addition to providing information concerning the site and extent of brain injury, the technetium brain scan can provide prognostic data based on the presence and persistence of findings. On short-term followup, 72% of asphyxiated infants with normal scans were normal, whereas 76% of those infants with abnormal scans either died or had significant neurologic sequelae. Furthermore, 100% of infants whose scans remained abnormal at 3–9 weeks of age displayed neurologic abnormalities. CT has also been used to delineate the prognosis of asphyxiated newborns. While asphyxiated term infants with normal CT scans rarely display significant neurologic sequelae, those with diffuse hypodensity or significant intraparenchymal hemorrhage are rarely normal on followup. However, in one-third of cases where there is limited hypodensity and no intracerebral hemorrhage, the outcome cannot be readily predicted. In preterm infants ultrasound is as effective as, and more convenient than, CT for determining prognosis.

321. What is the mechanism of pyridoxine-dependent seizures in the neonate?

The probable molecular defect in pyridoxine-dependent seizures is a disturbance in the binding of pyridoxal-5-phosphate (the active form of pyridoxine) to the apoprotein of glutamic acid decarboxylase, which is necessary for the synthesis of the inhibitory neurotransmitter, gamma-amino butyric acid (GABA).

322. What is the prognosis for infants with neonatal seizures?

The most important determinant of neurologic prognosis is the nature of the neuropathologic process underlying the seizures. Although much of the data does not extend to school age, the following table represents the experience of multiple authors.

Prognosis of Neonatal Seizures — Relation to Neurologic Disease

NEUROLOGIC DISEASE*	NORMAL DEVELOPMENT (%)
Hypoxic-ischemic encephalopathy	50
Intraventricular hemorrhage	<10
Primary subarachnoid hemorrhage	90
Hypocalcemia	
Early onset	50
Late onset	100
Hypoglycemia	50
Bacterial meningitis	50
Developmental defect	0

From Volpe J (ed): Neurology of the Newborn. Philadelphia, W.B. Saunders, 1987, p 145, with permission.
*Prognosis is for those cases with the stated neurologic disease when seizures are a manifestation (this value usually will differ from *overall* prognosis for the disease).

323. How effective are serial lumbar punctures for preventing posthemorrhagic hydrocephalus?

Although lumbar punctures are useful in lowering increased intracranial pressure and for treatment of posthemorrhagic hydrocephalus, they are of *no* benefit for the *prevention* of hydrocephalus.

324. Following an IVH, is ventriculomegaly without increased intracranial pressure a benign condition?

Ventriculomegaly without increased intracranial pressure usually is secondary to cerebral atrophy and evolves to a state of stable ventricular size, neither decreasing as in transient hydrocephalus, nor increasing as in persistently progressive hydrocephalus.

325. What are the adverse effects of compressive head wrapping?

The rationale for compressive head wrapping for neonatal hydrocephalus is derived from animal experiments that showed the degree of hydrocephalus was markedly greater when the skull was expansile rather than fixed because of the absence of sufficient pressure to drive CSF reabsorption. However, apnea, bradycardia, and extreme irritability have been seen in babies treated with this modality. These complications are felt to be the result of abrupt rises in intracranial pressure, which in one clinical series rose from baseline levels of 200–250 to 500–700 mmHg.

326. Why does perinatal asphyxia increase the likelihood of development of IVH?

Asphyxia, probably through associated myocardial failure, results in increased cerebral venous pressure and resultant hemorrhage. Furthermore, hypoxia may acutely increase cerebral blood flow and lead to hemorrhage from the fragile endothelial-lined capillaries in the germinal matrix.

327. What are the major causes of arthrogryposis multiplex congenita?

The development of fixed joints with decreased movement results from impaired intrauterine mobility usually secondary to muscle weakness. The basis for this weakness has been localized to every major level of the motor system as follows:

Causes of Arthrogryposis Multiplex Congenita

SITE OF MAJOR PATHOLOGIC FINDINGS	EXAMPLES
Cerebrum	Developmental anomalies Hydrocephalus
Anterior horn cell	Werdnig-Hoffmann disease Lumbosacral meningomyelocele
Peripheral nerve or root	Polyneuropathy
Neuromuscular junction	Myasthenia gravis
Muscle	Congenital muscular dystrophy
Primary disorder of joint and/or connective tissue	Marfan's syndrome
Intrauterine mechanical restriction	Uterine abnormality and oligohydramnios

Adapted from Volpe J (ed): Neurology of the Newborn. Philadelphia, W. B. Saunders Co., 1987, p 473.

328. Why shouldn't a cephalhematoma be aspirated?
Aspiration may introduce infection.

329. What percentage of infants with a cephalhematoma have an underlying skull fracture?
Between 5 and 25% (two series). Most often these are linear fractures that do not require therapy except for radiologic followup to assure healing.

330. How are the following abnormalities distinguished by physical examination: cephalhematoma? caput succedaneum? subgaleal hematoma?
These three major forms of extracranial hemorrhage occur in distinct tissue planes as illustrated by the following figure and can thus be distinguished as outlined in the table:

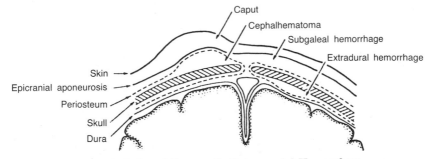

Major Varieties of Traumatic Extracranial Hemorrhage

LESION	FEATURES OF EXTERNAL SWELLING	INCREASES AFTER BIRTH	CROSSES SUTURE LINES	MARKED ACUTE BLOOD LOSS
Caput succedaneum	Soft, pitting	No	Yes	No
Subgaleal hematoma	Firm, fluctuant	Yes	Yes	Yes
Cephalhematoma	Firm, tense	Yes	No	No

From Volpe J (ed): Neurology of the Newborn. Philadelphia, W.B. Saunders Co., 1987, pp 639–640, with permission.

331. What is Erb's paralysis?
Erb's palsy, the more common form of neonatal brachial plexus injury, involves cervical nerve roots 5 and 6 and in 50% of cases cervical root 7 as well. Clinically, the patient displays

weakness of shoulder abduction and external rotation, elbow flexion and supination, wrist extension, and finger extension. Consequently, the upper extremity is held adducted, internally rotated, and pronated. The affected wrist and fingers are held in the "waiter's tip" position. Examination of the reflexes in these patients reveals absence of the biceps reflex, a Moro's reflex characterized by hand movement but no shoulder abduction, and the presence of the palmar grasp. Approximately 5% of patients with Erb's palsy also have ipsilateral diaphragmatic involvement.

332. What is Klumpke's palsy?
Weakness of the distal upper extremity. The vast majority of patients display proximal as well as distal weakness, with the latter attributable to injury to the lower spinal nerve roots (i.e., C8 and T1). The hand in affected infants is held extended at the fingers and wrist. Approximately one-third of cases are associated with Horner's syndrome.

333. What is the outcome of neonatal brachial plexus palsy?
Approximately 90% of patients have normal examinations by 12 months of age. Onset of recovery within 2 weeks and involvement of only the proximal upper extremity are both favorable prognostic signs.

334. What is the "Statue of Liberty" splint?
The Statue of Liberty splint was used to place the limb affected by a brachial plexus injury in a position at the shoulder, elbow, and wrist that was opposite from that assumed by the unsupported limb. This splint is no longer recommended because of the risk of contractures in the newly assumed extremity position.

335. Which nerve roots are affected with a brachial plexus injury?
Brachial plexus injury results from trauma to cervical nerve roots 5 to 8 (C5 to C8) and thoracic root 1 (T1).

336. How should brachial plexus injury be treated?
Therapy of brachial plexus injury must be aimed at preventing contractures. For the first 7–10 days the arm should be gently immobilized against the abdomen to minimize further hemorrhage and/or swelling. Following this initial period, passive range of motion exercises at the shoulder, elbow, wrist, and hand should be performed. In addition, wrist splints to stabilize the fingers and avoid contractures should be used.

337. When should myelomeningocele be surgically repaired?
Surgical closure of myelomeningocele should be performed "early" to prevent infection and loss of motor function. Prevailing opinion had been that closure should be performed in the first 24–48 hours of life. However, recent series have demonstrated no increase in infection rate when surgery was performed even after 7 days of life, especially when prophylactic antibiotics were administered. Therefore, the defect should be repaired relatively promptly, but families should be given enough time to make a rational decision.

338. Which infants with myelomeningocele are poor candidates for surgical closure?
Infants with myelomeningocele who are most likely to die despite treatment, or who are likely to be severely handicapped if they survive are those with (1) absence of lower limb function other than hip flexors, adductors, and quadriceps, (2) gross enlargement of the head, (3) kyphosis, (4) associated gross congenital anomalies, and (5) major birth injuries.

339. What are the advantages of a "selective approach" in infants with neural tube defects?
Advocates of a selective approach emphasize the reduction in the number of severely handicapped children who require vast amounts of medical supervision and hospitalizations, and whose families require large amounts of social support.

340. How should the parents of an infant with neural tube defect be counselled regarding future pregnancies?
At the present time, neural tube defects are felt to be the result of an interplay of genetic and environmental influences. While the overall incidence of myelomeningocele varies from 1–5/1000 live births in various series, there is an increased incidence in families with prior children with this defect.

341. What is the risk of alkali administration in the newborn infant?
Alkali administration, in particular sodium bicarbonate, must be used judiciously in the newborn because of the risks of (1) IVH associated with administration of hyperosmolar solutions, (2) hypernatremia, and (3) hypercarbia in patients with respiratory insufficiency.

342. What is the prognosis in traumatic facial nerve injury in the newborn infant?
The prognosis for recovery in traumatic facial nerve injury is excellent, with the majority demonstrating return of normal function in 1 to 3 weeks and the rare patient with residual deficit after several months.

343. What is the Möbius syndrome?
It is a congenital condition characterized by facial diplegia and bilateral abducens palsies. Tongue weakness and talipes equinovarus are also seen in one-third of cases. This syndrome is believed to result from both developmental aberrations as well as destructive processes (e.g., *in utero* hypoxia).

344. What are the clinical manifestations of phrenic nerve paralysis?
Phrenic nerve paralysis generally occurs in clinical settings predisposing to traction injury such as abnormal presentations, dysfunctional labor, augmented labor, large fetal size and fetal distress. In the first hours after birth, the infant manifests signs of respiratory distress with accompanying hypoxemia and hypercapnia. Over the next several days the infant may show improvement or at least stabilize. Only in the most severe cases does frank respiratory failure occur secondary to atelectasis and/or pulmonary infection. Approximately 80–90% of cases are associated with brachial plexus injury.

345. When should infants with phrenic nerve paralysis be treated surgically?
Surgical plication of the diaphragm is recommended in cases where intermittent positive pressure ventilation has been required for longer than 2 months.

346. What is the prognosis for infants with diaphragmatic paralysis?
Despite improvements in management, the mortality associated with unilateral diaphragmatic paralysis ranges from 10–15%, and for bilateral lesions (where prolonged ventilatory support is required) approaches 50%. Recovery in patients with unilateral disease can be expected to occur in approximately 6–12 months.

Bibliography

1. Creasy RK, Resnik R: Maternal Fetal Medicine: Principles and Practice. Philadelphia, W.B. Saunders Co., 1984.
2. Fanaroff AA, Martin RJ (eds): Neonatal-Perinatal Medicine Diseases of the Fetus and Infant, 4th ed. St. Louis, C.V. Mosby Co., 1987.
3. Nathan DG, Oski FA (eds): Hematology of Infancy and Childhood, 3rd ed. Philadelphia, W.B. Saunders Co., 1987.
4. Remington JS, Klein JO (eds): Infectious Diseases of the Fetus and Newborn Infant, 2nd ed. Philadelphia, W.B. Saunders Co., 1983.
5. Smith CA, Nelson NM: The Physiology of the Newborn Infant, 4th ed. Springfield, IL, Charles C Thomas, 1976.
6. Thibeault DW, Gregory GA (eds): Neonatal Pulmonary Care, 2nd ed. Norwalk, CT, Appleton-Century-Crofts, 1986.
7. Volpe J (ed): Neurology of the Newborn, 2nd ed. Philadelphia, W.B. Saunders Co., 1987.

NEPHROLOGY

John W. Foreman, M.D.

1. What is diurnal enuresis?

Daytime wetting (diurnal enuresis) is defined as a lack of bladder control during waking hours in a child old enough to maintain control. In otherwise normal children diurnal enuresis is not considered a problem until 2½–3 years of age. A study in Swiss children showed that daytime bladder control was present in 40% of 2-year-olds, 78% of 3-year-olds, and 98% of 4-year-olds. During the first several years after being toilet trained, many children wet themselves when they postpone voiding because they are so engrossed in their current activities. This is probably normal if it occurs less than twice a week.

2. What are the causes of diurnal enuresis?

1. *Organic causes* for diurnal enuresis account for less than 5% of affected children. Of these, urinary tract infections are probably the most common cause. An ectopic ureter should be suspected if dampness is constantly present; most children with diurnal enuresis have intermittent wetness. Rarely a neurogenic bladder can be a cause of this problem. Severe lower urinary tract obstruction can lead to bladder distention with overflow incontinence. Finally, pelvic masses such as presacral teratoma, hydrocolpos, or fecal impaction, which press on the bladder, can lead to stress incontinence with running, coughing, or lifting.

2. *Physiologic types* of daytime wetting include vaginal reflux of urine, giggle incontinence, and urgency incontinence. Reflux of urine into the vagina during micturition occurs frequently; after normal voiding, when such a girl stands up and walks, the urine seeps out of the vagina and wets the underpants. Treatment consists of simply advising the child to spread her labia and spend a few extra minutes sitting on the toilet after voiding. Giggle incontinence is a sudden, involuntary, uncontrollable and complete emptying of the bladder when giggling or laughing. Tickling or excitement may also lead to this problem. Urgency incontinence can be defined as an attack of intense bladder spasms that leads to abrupt voiding and wetting.

3. *Psychogenic causes* of daytime wetting are stress-related. Wetting can occur in any child who is significantly frightened. Chronic stress, such as the loss of a close relative, marital discord, or hospitalization, can also lead to this kind of daytime wetting. The resistant child is one who is about 2½ years of age, and refuses to be toilet trained. These are usually males who are predominantly or totally wet. Often this situation has occurred because of high-pressured attempts at toilet training. Most children with daytime wetness and nighttime dryness have a behavioral basis for the problem.

Recommended Workup for Organic Causes Daytime Wetting

History
    Dysuria, frequency, hematuria
    Continuous dampness vs. intermittent wetness
    Previous urinary tract infection
Physical Examination
    Abdominal examination for distended bladder or impaction
    Genital examination
    Perianal sensation, anal tone, rectal examination
    Lower back examination for lipoma or birthmark
    Stress incontinence assessment
    Urine stream assessment
Laboratory Studies
    Urinalysis
    Urine culture (females)

From Schmitt BD: Daytime wetting (diurnal enuresis). Pediatr Clin North Am 29:9–20, 1982, with permission.

Differential Diagnosis of Nonorganic Daytime Wetting

CHARACTERISTICS	URGENCY INCONTINENCE	STRESS RELATED	RESISTIVE CHILD
Sex	Females > 90%	Equal	Males 70%
Time of onset	Primary (unless UTI-induced)	Acquired	Primary (never toilet trained)
Frequency of wetting (% of voidings)	<10%	Variable	90%
Frequency and urgency	Yes	Yes	No
Associated nocturnal enuresis	Many	Some	*
Precipitating event	No	Yes	No
Parents punish or lecture	No	No	Yes
Only uses toilet if reminded	No	No	Yes
Associated encopresis	No	Few	Many

From Schmitt BD: Daytime wetting (diurnal enuresis). Pediatr Clin North Am 29:9–20, 1982, with permission.

*Same as general population for that age group.

3. What are the indications for radiographic evaluation of the urinary tract in a child who develops a urinary tract infection (UTI)?

Radiographic studies of the urinary tract should be performed in every male child following the first UTI. There is some controversy, however, as to whether one should wait for the second UTI in females. Between 50 and 80% of girls with one UTI will in fact have a second UTI. Therefore, the majority of female children will eventually undergo an anatomic evaluation. Since there still is a reasonably high incidence of anatomic abnormalities in females (especially those who present at a younger age), it would be prudent to schedule radiographic studies after the first infection. In older female children and teenagers with symptoms strictly referable to cystitis, it is reasonable to wait until the second infection before performing an evaluation. The incidence of anatomic abnormalities in older female children is much smaller than in younger individuals. One of the anatomic concerns is whether ureteric reflux is present. This necessitates a voiding cystourethrogram. Both an IVP (or renal ultrasound) and a voiding cystourethrogram should be obtained in children with UTIs.

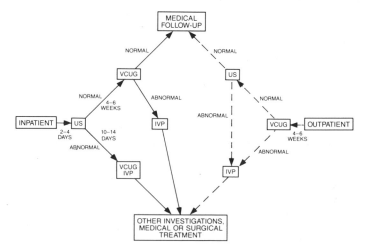

Algorithm for initial radiologic evaluation of children with urinary tract infection. Protocol for inpatients is described by solid arrows and protocol for outpatients by dashed arrows. IVP, intravenous pyelography; US, renal ultrasonography; VCUG, voiding cystourethrography. (From Alon U, Pery M, Davidai G, Berant M: Ultrasonography in the radiologic evaluation of children with urinary tract infection. Pediatrics 78:58–64, 1986, with permission.)

4. What are the indications for prophylactic antibiotics in a child with a history of UTIs?

There are no clear indications. They are often used in children with multiple recurrences (and grade I or no reflux) to minimize stress within a family. Prophylactic antibiotics are also useful in minimizing the number of days missed at school in children with recurrent infections. Children who have grade II or higher reflux should be given prophylactic antibiotics in an attempt to prevent further UTIs and subsequent renal injury until the reflux resolves. Children with various forms of obstructive uropathy who are prone to UTIs (such as the child with posterior urethral valves) should also receive prophylactic antibiotics.

5. What are the types of reflux seen in voiding cystourethrograms? What other common abnormalities can be seen on a voiding cystourethrogram?

International Grading Classification

Grade I	ureter only
Grade II	ureter, pelvis and calyces; no dilatation, normal calyceal fornices
Grade III	*mild dilatation* and/or tortuosity of the ureter and *mild* dilatation of the renal pelvis; *minor* blunting of the fornices
Grade IV	*moderate dilatation* and/or tortuosity of the ureter and moderate dilatation of the renal pelvis and calyces; *maintenance* of the papillary impressions in the *majority* of calyces
Grade V	*significant blunting* of the majority of the fornices; the papillary impressions are no longer visible in the majority of the calyces; *gross* dilatation and tortuosity of the ureter; *gross* dilatation of the renal pelvis and calyces

From Duckett JD, Bellinger MF: A plea for standardized grading of vesicoureteral reflux. Eur Urol 8:74–77, 1982, with permission.

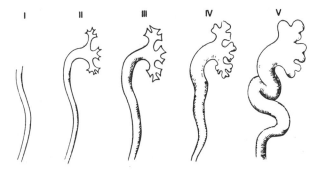

Besides demonstrating reflux, a number of other bladder abnormalities may be observed. A diverticulum may be seen, especially in the presence of outflow obstruction. A posterior urethral valve or a urethral stricture can be detected during the voiding phase of the study. A ureterocele may be seen and appears as a filling defect in the bladder. Other features to note are the capacity of the bladder and whether the wall is thickened from muscular hypertrophy or is smooth.

6. How should urinary reflux be managed?

Grade I reflux does not extend into the kidney and has not been associated with renal injury; therefore, nothing should be done. Approximately 75% of children with grades II or III reflux will improve with time, usually at a rate of 10%/year. Nightly administration of nitrofurantoin or trimethoprim/sulfamethoxazole is usually effective in preventing further infections. Urine cultures should be obtained every 3 months and whenever symptoms of an infection are present. Reevaluation of the child for presence of reflux, the renal size, and the extent of scarring should be done every 2 years until the reflux resolves. Radionuclide voiding cystourethrograms and renal ultrasound or radionuclide renograms may substitute for the traditional IVP and voiding cystourethrogram, since these procedures expose the child to less irradiation. Grade V reflux should be surgically corrected since the risk of renal damage is high, especially in the infant, and the chance of resolving spontaneously is low. It is presently unclear whether Grade IV reflux should be corrected surgically or followed as outlined above for Grades II and III. This decision should be individualized in consultation with a pediatric urologist or nephrologist.

7. How is cystitis distinguished from pyelonephritis?

With difficulty. Many nephrologists avoid the issue and simply refer to the infection as a UTI. Pyelonephritis tends to have more constitutional symptoms such as fever, rigors, and flank and back pain, while cystitis has more bladder symptoms such as wetting, dysuria, frequency, and urgency. Some studies have suggested that an elevation in the sedimentation rate or C-reactive protein can distinguish between them. Pyelonephritis tends to be associated with a rise in these indices, but there is enough overlap between cystitis and pyelonephritis to make the distinction difficult in the individual patient. Detection of antibody-coated bacteria (a sign of upper tract disease in the adult) is not helpful in the pediatric age group. The "gold standard" for differentiating between these two sites is to culture bladder urine, then sterilize the bladder by washing it with an antiseptic solution, and culture the subsequent urine (bladder washout technique). This, obviously, is not designed for the average patient in the office. The presence of white cell casts, impaired urinary concentrating ability, or enlarged kidneys on x-ray or ultrasound indicates pyelonephritis. In most situations the best guess is based on the history and physical examination.

8. What indices are used to distinguish prerenal azotemia from established renal failure?

Prerenal Azotemia vs. Renal Failure

PARAMETERS	PRERENAL	RENAL
Urine osmolality	> 500	< 350
Urine/plasma osmolality	> 1.3	< 1.1
Urine/plasma urea	> 8	< 3
Urine/plasma creatinine	> 40	< 20
FeNa*	$< 1\%$	$> 2\%$
RFI†	$< 1\%$	$> 2\%$

*FeNa
(Fractional excretion of Na) $= \dfrac{U_{Na} \cdot P_{creatinine}}{P_{Na} \cdot U_{creatinine}} \times 100$

†RFI
(Renal Failure Index) $= \dfrac{U_{Na} \cdot P_{creatinine}}{U_{creatinine}}$

The FeNA and RFI can be done on an untimed "spot" urine. These tests are useful only in patients with hypovolemia in whom one is trying to distinguish prerenal oliguria from established acute tubular necrosis (ATN). Patients with postrenal causes (obstruction) tend to have values similar to ATN patients, while patients with acute glomerulonephritis have values similar to prerenal patients. Diuretics, especially potent loop diuretics, invalidate all of these indices.

9. What is the Schwartz formula for estimating creatinine clearance?

$$\text{Creatinine clearance in ml/min/1.73m}^2 = \frac{\text{height(cm)} \times (.55)}{\text{Serum creatinine (mg/dl)}}$$

This formula was derived from children with ages ranging from 6 months to 20 years. It is best applied to children over 2 years when glomerular filtration rate (GFR) bears a constant relationship to surface area.

Reference: Schwartz GJ, Haycock GB, Edelmann CM Jr, Spitzer A: Pediatrics 58:259–263, 1976.

For full-term infants from 1–52 weeks of age, Schwartz and colleagues also derived an estimate of glomerular filtration rate using the formula:

$$\text{Creatinine clearance (ml/min/1.73m}^2) = \frac{0.45 \times \text{length (cm)}}{\text{Serum creatinine (mg/dl)}}$$

Reference: Schwartz GJ, Feld LG, Langford DJ: J Pediatr 104:849–854, 1984.

10. What is the mechanism of action of loop diuretics and what are the associated side effects and consequences?

Furosemide acts principally in the medullary diluting segment of the ascending limb of the loop of Henle where it inhibits chloride reabsorption and secondarily inhibits sodium and potassium reabsorption. The onset of action is within 1 hour of oral administration and 5 minutes of IV administration with a peak effect by 2 hours. The duration is 6–8 hours. Furosemide also inhibits calcium and magnesium reabsorption in the loop such that up to 30–35% of the filtered load can be lost. The usual side effects of furosemide are the consequence of its diuretic action, namely volume contraction, hyponatremia, hypokalemia, and metabolic alkalosis. Because of the hypercalciuric effect, it has been linked to renal stone formation in neonates after prolonged administration. Ototoxicity has been observed after large intravenous doses, especially in patients with reduced renal function. Furosemide is a sulfonamide and patients with sulfonamide sensitivity may have an allergic reaction.

11. What is the mechanism of action of thiazide diuretics and what are the associated side effects and consequences?

Thiazide diuretics, hydrochlorothiazide and chlorothiazide, act by directly inhibiting sodium reabsorption in the early portion of the distal tubule. There is also an effect on sodium and chloride reabsorption by the proximal tubule. This effect is not usually observed clinically because increases in sodium and chloride delivery out of the proximal tubule are compensated for by increased reabsorption by the uninhibited loop of Henle. Onset of action ranges from 1–2 hours with a peak at 4–6 hours and duration of 12–24 hours. Thiazide diuretics are useful in treating edema, although they are less potent than furosemide. They are useful as antihypertensives and are more potent than furosemide in this regard. They are also useful in the treatment of hypercalciuria, nephrogenic diabetes insipidus, and proximal renal tubular acidosis. The side effects of these agents are volume contraction, hypokalemia, hyperuricemia and rarely hyperglycemia.

12. What is the normal anion gap from infancy to adulthood?

The anion gap or delta is the difference between the serum sodium and the sum of the serum chloride plus serum bicarbonate usually measured as total CO_2. This difference represents the unmeasured anions such as organic acids, sulfate, and phosphate. The mean anion gap in children from age 9 months to 19 years is 8 ± 2 mEq/L if the blood is assayed immediately; however, if the blood is analyzed 4 hours later, the mean is closer to 11 mEq/L, which is similar to that of adults (12 ± 2 mEq/L). An elevated anion gap, in practice, occurs when this difference is greater than 15–16 mEq/L.

References: Flanagan CM, Drott HR, Norman ME: Pediatr Res 17:349A, 1983.
Emmett M, Narins RG: Medicine 56:38, 1977.

13. What are the causes of an elevated anion gap acidosis?
Shock
Diabetes mellitus
Renal failure
Diarrhea of infancy
Inborn errors of metabolism
     (e.g., maple syrup urine disease)
Poisonings
    Salicylates
    Ethanol
    Methanol
    Ethylene glycol

14. How limited is the respiratory response to metabolic alkalosis?
Metabolic alkalosis occurs when there is a net gain of alkali or loss of acid. This leads to a rise in the serum bicarbonate concentration and pH. In metabolic alkalosis, as in metabolic acidosis, there is a measure of respiratory compensation in response to the change in pH. This is accomplished by alveolar hypoventilation, but this response is limited, owing to the overriding need to maintain an adequate blood oxygen concentration. Usually the pCO_2 will not rise above 50–55 torr in spite of severe alkalosis.

15. What are the differential diagnosis and pathophysiology for a child presenting with primary metabolic alkalosis?
Metabolic alkalosis can be divided into two major categories based on the urinary chloride concentration. In the first category, the urine chloride concentration is less than 10 mEq/L, and the metabolic alkalosis is responsive to volume expansion with a saline infusion. The classic example is pyloric stenosis, in which persistent vomiting with loss of hydrochloric acid and fluid generates a rise in plasma bicarbonate concentration and extracellular volume contraction. This extracellular volume contraction stimulates aldosterone production and proximal tubular bicarbonate reabsorption, maintaining the raised plasma bicarbonate concentration despite an increased filtered load. Hypokalemia develops because of an increased exchange of sodium for potassium in the distal nephron under the influence of the elevated serum aldosterone concentration. The development of hypokalemia exacerbates the alkalosis by promoting the exchange of intracellular potassium for extracellular hydrogen ion and also hydrogen ion for sodium in the distal nephron. This gives rise to the "paradoxical aciduria" in the face of systemic alkalosis. Treatment of this form of metabolic alkalosis is aimed at correcting the volume contraction with an infusion of saline. The restoration of intravascular volume promotes the excretion of the excess bicarbonate, normalizing the plasma pH. Excessive diuretic use will lead to metabolic alkalosis through the development of volume contraction from sodium chloride losses and hypokalemia from potassium chloride losses. The urine chloride in this situation will be high while the diuretic is present and then will fall when the drug is stopped. The alkalosis will persist in spite of stopping the diuretic until the extracellular volume and potassium losses are restored.

The second type of metabolic alkalosis is unresponsive to saline and is associated with a high urine chloride concentration and often hypertension. Mineralocorticoid excess plays a central role in the generation of the acid-base disturbances in most cases. Primary aldosteronism is the classic example in which persistently elevated aldosterone secretion leads to increased sodium and chloride reabsorption and volume expansion. With the onset of volume expansion, other mechanisms, such as "third factor," act to inhibit sodium reabsorption in the proximal tubule, flooding the distal tubule with sodium salts. Here, the exchange of luminal sodium for potassium and hydrogen ions generates a metabolic alkalosis, especially when potassium intake is limited. The resulting hypokalemia enhances sodium bicarbonate reabsorption. Most of the saline-unresponsive forms of metabolic alkalosis are quite uncommon in pediatrics, except that caused by the exogenous administration of steroids.

Causes of Saline-responsive Metabolic Alkalosis	Causes of Saline-resistant Metabolic Alkalosis
Pyloric stenosis	Primary hyperaldosteronism
Vomiting	(extremely rare in pediatrics)
Upper GI suction	Hyperreninemic hypertension
Congenital chloride diarrhea	Renal artery stenosis
Laxative abuse	Heritable block in steroid hormone synthesis
Diuretic abuse	17α-OH deficiency
Cystic fibrosis	11β-OH deficiency
Chloride-deficient formulas in infants	Licorice
Posthypercapnia syndrome	Liddle's syndrome
Poorly reabsorbable anion	Bartter's syndrome
administration	Severe potassium deficiency
Post-treatment of organic acidemias	

16. What is Bartter's syndrome?

Bartter's syndrome is probably the result of a primary disturbance in sodium or chloride transport leading to volume contraction and increased aldosterone secretion. This, in turn, results in hypokalemia and alkalosis in the manner previously described for primary aldosteronism. These children are characterized by failure to thrive, metabolic alkalosis, resistance to the hypertensive effects of an angiotensin II infusion, polyuria, and profound hypokalemia. The urinary chloride in this illness is quite high, as are the plasma renin and aldosterone concentrations. However, these children are usually in a state of volume contraction in contrast to the volume-expanded state found with other causes of metabolic alkalosis and high urinary chloride.

17. What are the common causes of hyperkalemia in the pediatric age group?

Factitious—*in vitro* hemolysis
Renal failure
Acidosis
Tumor lysis
Severe trauma—crush injuries, burns
Rhabdomyolysis
Excessive administration—usually IV
Adrenal causes
    Complete block of 21-hydroxylase (adrenogenital syndrome)
    Adrenal insufficiency
Drugs
    Potassium-sparing agents—spironolactone, triampterene, amiloride
    Prostaglandin inhibitors
    Angiotensin-converting enzyme inhibitors—captopril, enalapril
    Arginine HCl—growth hormone stimulation test
Prematurity—aldosterone unresponsiveness
Type 4 renal tubular acidosis
Familial periodic paralysis

18. What are the common causes of hypokalemia?

Diuretics, occasionally laxatives
Metabolic alkalosis—especially secondary to pyloric stenosis
Diabetic ketoacidosis
Diarrhea
Renal tubular acidosis, types 1 and 2
Fanconi syndrome
Bartter's syndrome
Hyperreninemic hypertension—renal artery stenosis
Hyperaldosteronism—usually secondary to cirrhosis or congestive heart failure

19. What are the clinical presentations of hyperkalemia and hypokalemia?
Symptoms of hyperkalemia and hypokalemia are vague and overlap. Both conditions lead to an alteration in the electrical potential of the cell membrane, impairing electrical conduction. Hyperkalemia often causes muscle weakness and occasionally cramping and paralysis. Rarely, seizures may occur. Hypokalemia also causes muscle weakness. Paralysis is more common with hypokalemia and can cause apnea, which is the usual cause of death. Mental confusion may be present. Both disturbances of potassium cause cardiac abnormalities. Hypokalemia can cause premature contractions, especially junctional contractions, and paroxysmal tachycardias. These arrhythmias are worsened by digitalis.

20. What is the definition of "significant" proteinuria?
Protein excretion of more than 6 mg/m^2/hr on a timed urine collection. Children with nephrosis excrete more than 40 mg/m^2/hr. The upper limit of protein excretion in adults is 150 mg/day. The urine protein/urine creatinine ratio has been used to estimate protein excretion. A value less than 0.2 (mg protein/mg creatinine) is considered normal in a child older than 2 years.

21. Is a urine dipstick accurate for quantitating proteinuria?
The urine dipstick gives an estimate of the protein concentration in a sample of urine. Unless the total volume of urine is known, however, an estimate of the amount of protein lost cannot be made. The dipstick reacts principally with albumin and may read negative when the major urinary protein is something other than albumin. In practice, a urine dipstick reading greater than "trace" requires repeating and some explanation, although it may be due to such non-renal causes as exercise, fever, and contamination of the urine specimen with the benzalkonium chloride used to clean the patient for a urine culture. As to accuracy, the dipstick is accurate enough for monitoring patients with proteinuria and it is cost effective for detecting proteinuria ($0.15–.25 by dipstick versus $30 by hospital laboratory). One can be misled in patients with large urinary outputs since the dipstick may show only trace amounts of protein when in fact substantial proteinuria exists. Here, precise quantitation may be necessary.

22. What constellation of clinical findings defines nephrotic syndrome?
The nephrotic syndrome consists of heavy proteinuria (>40 mg/hr/m^2), hypoalbuminemia, edema, and hyperlipidemia. The most common cause, especially in toddlers and pre-schoolers, is minimal change disease.

23. What is the mechanism of hyperlipidemia associated with severe proteinuria?
Elevations in the plasma concentrations of cholesterol and triglycerides are characteristically seen in children with nephrotic syndrome. Low density lipoproteins (LDL) and very low density lipoproteins (VLDL) are also increased, but high density lipoproteins (HDL) may be high, normal, or low. The mechanisms underlying these lipid alterations include both enhanced hepatic production of VLDL and decreased peripheral catabolism/utilization of VLDL. With very low plasma oncotic pressure, conversion of VLDL to LDL may be impaired. HDL may be lost in the urine in severely proteinuric states. Although total cholesterol rises in most nephrotics, the ratio of LDL to HDL cholesterol may actually be low. It is this ratio which is more predictive of the risk of atherosclerosis and it varies from patient to patient. Lowering of plasma lipids with an infusion of albumin suggests that the oncotic pressure or possibly the plasma viscosity is an important determinant of these abnormalities. Normalization of the plasma lipids, however, is usually the last feature of the nephrotic syndrome to resolve.

24. What are the indiations for furosemide and albumin therapy in nephrotic syndrome?

Intravenous albumin followed by a potent diuretic such as furosemide is used to induce a diuresis in a child with nephrotic syndrome. This measure is only temporary, since the rise in albumin will lead to increased protein excretion, returning the serum level to the previous steady-state value. However, it is useful in a child with incapacitating anasarca in conjunction with other measures such as sodium restriction and steroids. Furosemide and albumin are also used in children with cellulitis and skin breakdown due to edema, and in those with respiratory embarrassment from pleural effusions. In more acute situations the pleural space should be drained with a needle. Albumin alone is useful in the child with a rising BUN secondary to decreased renal perfusion. This is most often seen after vigorous diuretic therapy. Albumin alone is also indicated in the nephrotic child with shock from hypovolemia to promote transfer of interstitial water into the intravascular compartment. The usual course of action is to give 0.5–1 gm/kg of 25% albumin intravenously over 1–2 hours followed by 1–4 mg/kg of furosemide (euphemistically called the "albumin-Lasix sandwich"). Respiratory rate and blood pressure should be monitored during the treatment, and the diuretic administered earlier if the blood pressure rises significantly or if there is difficulty with respiration.

25. What are the recommended primary and secondary therapies for idiopathic nephrosis?

The primary treatment of idiopathic nephrotic syndrome is steroids, usually prednisone. Various doses have been recommended ranging from 2 mg/kg/day to 60 mg/m^2/day with a maximum dose of 80 mg. Alternate-day steroids are not particularly effective in inducing a remission. Multiple doses throughout the day are more effective than a single daily dose. Daily steroids are continued until the urine is free of protein or for a complete month regardless of protein excretion. The daily prednisone is then followed by a course of alternate-day therapy for 1–3 months. A mistake often made is to stop the steroids too quickly. Our approach is to treat the initial episode of nephrosis with 2 mg/kg/day of prednisone for 1 month, then give that same dose every other morning as a single dose and begin tapering the steroids over the next 2 months. Relapses are treated similarly except the switch to alternate-day steroids is done when the urine dipstick shows a negative or trace reaction for protein for several days.

Secondary therapies for idiopathic nephrotic syndrome include cytotoxic drugs (cyclophosphamide and chlorambucil), prostaglandin inhibitors, and diuretics. Cytotoxic drugs are considered in the child in whom the steroids have become more harmful than helpful. Indications for cytotoxic agents include significant growth failure, aseptic necrosis of bone, severe hypertension, gross obesity, and cataracts. Some children who were initially responsive to steroids but later become resistant may again become responsive after a course of cytotoxic drugs. Cyclophosphamide is given as a single daily dose of 2.5 mg/kg and chlorambucil as 0.2 mg/kg for 2–4 months usually in association with low-dose prednisone. The immediate risk of both of these medications is infection, especially with leukopenia. The white blood count should be monitored weekly with cessation of therapy if the total white count is less than 4,000 cells/mm^3 or the neutrophil count is less than 1500 cells/mm^3. Cystitis can be seen with both agents, although it is more common with cyclophosphamide and can be hemorrhagic. This risk can be reduced by giving cyclophosphamide in the morning and maintaining a good fluid intake throughout the day. Both agents can cause infertility and malignancy, although these risks are difficult to quantitate and are probably low in the doses previously mentioned.

Patients resistant to prednisone and cytotoxic drugs may be helped with prostaglandin inhibitors, such as indomethacin, although there is a risk of acute renal failure. Finally, in such patients, diuretics in various combinations are useful.

26. When should renal biopsy be performed in a child with nephrosis?

A renal biopsy is not necessary in the majority of children with nephrosis. It is reasonable to consider a biopsy in children with idiopathic nephrotic syndrome under the age of 1 year or over age 10–12 years since the incidence of minimal change disease in such children is much less. Children with hypocomplementemia, azotemia not responsive to volume and albumin, gross hematuria, and red cell casts on urinalysis should also have a biopsy to aid in the decision whether to treat with steroids. A number of studies have pointed out that the response to prednisone is nearly as good as a biopsy in predicting whether the pathology is minimal change or not. Complete remission of the proteinuria indicates a high (80–90%) likelihood of minimal change disease, and no response about a 95% chance that it is not. Gamblers and weathermen would love those odds. Children who have no response or only some reduction in their proteinuria after a month of therapy should be biopsied. A more difficult issue is when to biopsy children with frequent relapses, and this usually is a matter of nephrologic style. One approach is to biopsy them when the consideration of adding cytotoxic agent is raised or when they become steroid resistant.

27. What is the mechanism of hypercoagulability associated with nephrotic syndrome?
The mechanism is multifactorial. The hyperviscosity of the blood in many nephrotics plays a role. Elevations in fibrinogen and other clotting factors have been described, as well as a decrease in fibrinolysis. Low levels of antithrombin III are often observed in children with nephrosis.

28. What organisms are responsible for peritonitis in children with nephrotic syndrome?
Pneumococcus remains an important cause of spontaneous peritonitis in children with nephrosis, although gram-negative organisms, especially *E. coli,* account for 25–50% of cases.

29. What chronic infections are associated with membranous glomerulonephritis?
The most common infectious agent associated with membranous nephropathy is hepatitis B. In most children, the liver function studies are entirely normal. The HB_S antigen should be looked for in otherwise normal patients with membranous nephropathy. This lesion has also been observed in congenital and secondary syphilis and malaria.

30. Which diseases present with nephritis and nephrosis in the pediatric age group?

Diseases That Present with Nephritis and Nephrosis

HEMATURIA (Gross or Microscopic)	ACUTE GLOMERULONEPHRITIS	NEPHROTIC SYNDROME
IgA nephropathy (Berger's disease)	Acute proliferative	Minimal change disease
Benign recurrent hematuria	Poststreptococcal	Focal glomerulosclerosis
Alport syndrome	SBE	Membranous nephropathy
Henoch-Schonlein purpura	IgA nephropathy (Berger's disease)	Membranoproliferative glomerulonephritis
	Rapidly progressive	Mesangial proliferative
	Membranoproliferative	SLE
	Hemolytic-uremic syndrome	Congenital nephrotic syndrome
	Henoch-Schonlein purpura	
	SLE	

31. How is renal tubular acidosis (RTA) classified and how does each variety present during childhood?
There are four main types of RTA. In type 1 RTA there is an impairment in distal acidification; in type 2 there is an impairment in bicarbonate reclamation; type 3 is a combination of types 1 and 2; and type 4 is secondary to a lack of, or an insensitivity to aldosterone. All four types are associated with a hyperchloremic, normal anion gap acidosis.

Types 1, 2, and 3 are associated with hypokalemia, whereas type 4 RTA is characterized by hyperkalemia in addition to hyperchloremic acidosis. Hypercalciuria is typical of type 1 RTA which in conjunction with hypocitraturia often leads to nephrocalcinosis and renal calculi. Type 2 is often part of a more global defect of proximal tubule function, the *Fanconi syndrome,* characterized by aminoaciduria, hypophosphatemia, glycosuria, and rickets. Type 4 RTA is most commonly observed in patients with obstructive uropathy, congenital adrenal hyperplasia and adrenal insufficiency. Other symptoms and signs which are common with all forms of renal tubular acidosis are growth failure, polyuria, polydipsia, recurrent dehydration, and vomiting.

Clinical and Laboratory Characteristics of Renal Tubular Acidosis in Children

	TYPE 1 (classic, distal)	TYPE 2 (Proximal)	TYPE 3 (Hybrid)	TYPE 4 Aldosterone deficiency)
Growth failure	+++	++	++	+++
Hypokalemic muscle weakness	++	+	+	Hyperkalemia
Nephrocalcinosis	Frequent	Rare	±	Rare
Low citrate excretion	+++	±	±	±
Fractional excretion of filtered HCO$_3$ at normal serum bicarbonate levels (%)	<5	>15	5–15	<15
Daily alkali treatment (mEq/kg body weight)	2 to 4	2 to 14	2 to 14	2 to 3
Daily potassium requirement	Decreases with correction	Increases with correction	±	

From Chan JCM: J Pediatr 103:327, 1983, with permission
+, Present, ++, common, +++, very common; −, not present; ±, variable.

32. What are the causes of proximal renal tubular acidosis?

Transient
Idiopathic or genetically transmitted
Hyperparathyroidism
Acetazolamide
Sulfanilamide
Leigh's encephalopathy
Metachromatic leukodystrophy
Fanconi syndrome
    Idiopathic
    Hereditary
    Cystinosis
    Tyrosinemia

Fanconi syndrome (cont'd)
    Galactosemia
    Glycogen storage disease
    Hereditary fructose intolerance
    Lowe's syndrome
    Wilson's disease
    Outdated tetracycline
    Heavy metal poisoning
    Multiple myeloma
    Renal transplantation
    Vitamin D deficiency
    Cytochrome c oxidase deficiency

33. What are the causes of distal renal tubular acidosis?

Sporadic
Hereditary
Sickle cell anemia
Ehlers-Danlos syndrome
Medullary cystic disease
Carbonic anhydrase B defect
Sjogren's syndrome
Systemic lupus erythematosus
Hypergammaglobulinemia
Amphotericin B
Chronic pyelonephritis

Hydronephrosis
Secondary to nephrocalcinosis
    Idiopathic
    Hyperthyroidism
    Hyperparathyroidism
    Vitamin D intoxication
    Hereditary fructose intolerance
    Wilson's disease
    Fabry's disease
    Medullary sponge kidney

34. How is the diagnosis of proximal or distal renal tubular acidosis (RTA) confirmed?

The first step in the evaluation of a child with suspected RTA is to demonstrate a "normal" anion gap acidosis by measuring the serum electrolytes and pH. Next, one needs to document whether the child can acidify his or her urine by lowering the pH to less than 5.5. At that time, a measure of hydrogen ion secretion should be obtained by measuring the titratable acidity (normal >70 μEq/min/1.73m²). This should be done at a time of systemic acidosis (serum bicarbonate <18 mEq/L). Many children with RTA spontaneously achieve this degree of acidosis, so maneuvers to further acidify them are unnecessary and risky. If acidosis is not spontaneously present and the question remains as to whether the child can develop a normal urinary hydorgen ion gradient (lower the urine pH to <5.5), then acidifying agents such as ammonium chloride (75–150 mEq/m²) or arginine hydrochloride (100–150 ml of a 10% solution IV) can be used. Furosemide (1 mg/kg IV) will also stimulate the distal tubule to secrete hydrogen ion, often obviating the need to use ammonium chloride. During an infusion of ammonium chloride, the urine pH and hydrogen ion excretion should be monitored hourly along with the serum bicarbonate and potassium concentrations. Hydrogen ion secretion by the distal tubule can also be assessed by raising the urine pH to 7.0 or greater with exogenous bicarbonate and then measuring both the urine and blood pCO_2 anaerobically (requires bladder catheter). Normal children will develop a urine pCO_2 that is at least 30 torr greater than the blood pCO_2.

To evaluate the proximal nephron's ability to reabsorb bicarbonate, sodium bicarbonate ($NaHCO_3$) can be infused intravenously until the urine pH (which previously was less than 6.0) reaches 6.0. The serum bicarbonate concentration when this occurs is defined as the bicarbonate threshold, and is normally >21 mEq/L in infants and $>22-23$ mEq/L in older children. This method, however, is quite cumbersome and measuring the fractional bicarbonate excretion at a time when the serum bicarbonate concentration is normal yields comparable information on the proximal tubule's ability to reclaim filtered bicarbonate. The normal value is $<5\%$; children with proximal defects excrete $>15\%$.

$$\text{Fractional excretion of bicarbonate} = \frac{(U_{HCO_3} \times \text{plasma creatinine}) \times 100}{\text{Plasma } HCO_3 \times U \text{ creatinine}}$$

Diagnostic Procedures in Children with Renal Tubular Acidosis

SPECIAL TESTS	CLINICAL ASSOCIATION
Ammonium chloride (75 mEq/M²) acid loading test	Type 1 RTA: urine pH >6 and net acid excretion <70 μEq/min/1.73 m²
Urine PCO₂-blood PCO₂ after alkali load to increase urine PCO₂ (at urine pH >7.0)	Type 1 RTA: urine PCO₂-blood PCO₂ is <30 torr
Bicarbonate loading to return carbon dioxide value to normal; fractional excretion of bicarbonate: (urine HCO₃ × plasma creatinine)	Type 2 RTA: fractional excretion of bicarbonate $>15\%$
(Plasma HCO₃ × urine creatinine)	
Plasma renin activity, etc.	Type 4 RTA (see table below)

Differential Diagnosis of Type 4 Renal Tubular Acidosis Characterized by Hyperkalemia, Hyponatremia, and Metabolic Acidosis

	SERUM CORTISOL	URINE 17-OHS	URINE 17-KS	PLASMA RENIN ACTIVITY	SERUM ALDOSTERONE	RESPONSE TO MINERALO-CORTICOID
Addison disease	↓	↓	↓	↑	↓	Yes
21-hydroxylase deficiency	↓	↓	↑↑	↑	↓	Yes
Hypoaldosteronism	N	N/↑	N/↑	N/↑	↓	Yes
Pseudohypoaldosteronism	N	N	N	↑↑↑	↑↑↑	No
Chronic renal failure	N	N	N	↓	↑	No
Spitzer syndrome	N	—	N	–	N	No

From Blachus Y, Kaplan BS, Griffel B, et al: Clin Nephrol 11:281, 1979, with permission.
17-OHS, 17-hydroxycorticosteroid; 17-KS, 17-ketosteroid; N, Normal concentration.

35. What is the classic triad of clinical findings in hemolytic-uremic syndrome (HUS)?
Microangiopathic hemolytic anemia (blood smear showing RBC fragments and schistocytes), azotemia, and thrombocytopenia. Of the three, thrombocytopenia may not always be present.

36. What other diseases should be considered in the differential diagnosis of HUS?
HUS in a young child is not generally confused with other disorders. Acute autoimmune hemolytic anemia can occasionally be confused with HUS, especially if hemoglobinuria has caused renal injury. The blood smear in this disorder is quite different from HUS, and the Coombs' test is positive in the former and negative in the latter. In the older child and teenager, distinguishing thrombotic thrombocytopenia purpura (TTP) from HUS can be difficult. However, TTP is quite rare in children and tends to have marked CNS involvement and less renal disease. Systemic vasculitis, such as lupus erythematosus, can cause microangiopathic hemolytic anemia, thrombocytopenia, and azotemia. These disorders, however, usually involve many organs and are associated with a number of abnormal laboratory tests, such as hypocomplementemia, anti-nuclear antibody positivity, and positive tests for circulating immune complexes, which easily distinguish them from HUS. Shock, especially with septicemia, can lead to disseminated intravascular coagulopathy, which causes thrombocytopenia and a microangiopathic anemia. Many such children also develop acute renal failure. Shock is the dominant problem in these children, which is not typically a part of HUS. Further, these children have marked abnormalities of the clotting system in addition to thrombocytopenia, which is not typical for children with HUS.

37. What other disorders should be considered in the differential diagnosis of renal vein thrombosis?
Renal vein thrombosis usually occurs in the sick infant, especially in the first month of life. Dehydration, shock, septicemia, asphyxia, and cyanotic congenital heart disease (especially following angiography) are predisposing factors. The usual presenting features are a sudden change in the infant's clinical condition associated with hematuria, oliguria, proteinuria, and a flank mass. Thrombocytopenia is common but hypertension is not. An IVP is often not helpful, since the kidney with the thrombosis usually does not visualize. An ultrasound study, demonstrating the renal vein clot and an enlarged kidney, or a radionuclide study is usually more useful. The differential diagnosis includes acute tubular or cortical necrosis, multicystic dysplasia, renal arterial thrombosis, adrenal hemorrhage, renal trauma, hydronephrosis, neuroblastoma, nephroblastomatosis, and Wilms' tumor.

38. What biomedical data suggest myoglobinuria as the etiology of acute renal failure?
Myoglobinuria or hemoglobinuria should be considered whenever the urine dipstick indicates significant blood but few or no red blood cells are observed in the sediment from fresh urine. One should remember, however, that red blood cells will lyse if allowed to stand at room temperature for a long time. This is especially true if the urine is alkaline or dilute. Adding ammonium sulfate (2.8 gm to 5 ml of urine) will precipitate hemoglobin and clear the urine of the brown or red color secondary to this pigment. The dipstick test should also become negative. Since ammonium sulfate does not precipitate myoglobin, no effect will be seen. In children with myoglobinuria there is often evidence of rhabdomyolysis, myalgia, and weakness, and muscle enzymes are elevated. If renal failure occurs, the creatinine rises very quickly secondary to the loss of creatine from muscle. The ratio of BUN/serum creatinine will often be less than 10. (Normally, in renal failure it is 20 to 1 or greater.) Hemoglobinuria is caused by massive hemolysis, which can be suspected by a pink to red discoloration of the serum.

39. What is the three glass test?
The three glass test involves having the subject void initially into one glass, then into the second glass, and then at the end into a third glass. Hematuria found only in the first glass suggests a lesion in the urethra. Blood in the third glass supposedly indicates bladder neck and trigone pathology. Blood in all three glasses suggests that the bleeding is from the bladder, ureter, or kidney. Usually, getting a child to void in one cup is a major

accomplishment let alone three different ones. Needless to say, the three glass test has not been particularly useful in pediatrics. Three glasses are probably more useful at the local pub.

40. What organism should be suspected when a patient presents with symptoms of UTI and a very alkaline urine?

Proteus. This enzyme cleaves urea, liberating ammonia and raising the pH to 8 or higher. At this pH, triple phosphate crystals that resemble coffin lids may be present in the urine. Pseudomonas and occasionally *E. coli* may also produce urease.

41. How do glucosuria and proteinuria affect urine specific gravity?

The specific gravity is the ratio of the weight of a volume of urine to a similar volume of water. It is affected by the number and weight of the particles in the urine. Because of their weight, glucose and protein can affect the specific gravity. For each 1 gm/dl of protein, the specific gravity is increased by 0.003, and for each 1 gm/dl of glucose by 0.004. In practice this usually does not affect the clinical interpretation as to whether the urine is concentrated or not.

42. Which substances give a positive urine "Clinitest"?

Glucose, fructose, galactose, pentose, lactose, cephalosporins, and large amounts of ascorbic acid.

43. What is the cause of Tamm-Horsfall protein?

Tamm-Horsfall protein is a large mucoprotein secreted into the urine by cells of the thick ascending limb of the loop of Henle. It is the matrix of a cast.

44. What causes black urine?

Black or dark brown urine is observed in children with alkaptonuria due to the excretion of homogentisic acid. The urine does not turn black immediately, but only after exposure to air. Black urine can also be seen in melanotic sarcoma from melanin excretion. Brown urine is often observed in glomerulonephritis.

45. What are the indications for peritoneal dialysis or hemodialysis in the child with acute renal failure?

Peritoneal dialysis or hemodialysis should be instituted when other more conservative medical interventions have failed to control the problems associated with renal failure. Specific indications for dialysis include hyperkalemia unresponsive to potassium restriction and Kayexalate administration; hypertension, congestive failure, or edema secondary to volume overload that is unresponsive to volume restriction and diuretics; significant acidosis that cannot be treated with sodium bicarbonate because of volume overload; and signs of uremia such as stupor or coma, seizures, gastrointestinal bleeding, and pericarditis. The least clear indication is an elevated BUN concentration. Dialysis is usually instituted when the BUN concentration reaches 100 mg/dl, although it may be started sooner or later in individual patients depending on whether they are recovering from or just developing renal failure. A final indication for dialysis is drug overdose or intoxication.

46. What is the inheritance pattern of adult and childhood polycystic kidney disease?

Adult polycystic kidney disease is inherited in an autosomal dominant pattern and infantile or childhood polycystic kidney is inherited in an autosomal recessive pattern. Indeed, a better nomenclature is to refer to these two disorders by the inheritance pattern, rather than as adult and childhood polycystic disease, since autosomal dominant polycystic disease can present anytime during childhood.

47. Which renal calculi are acid- or alkali-insoluble and how should each kind of calculi be treated?

Calcium oxalate stones, the most common type of renal calculi, are unaffected by the urine pH. These stones can be treated with thiazide diuretics, which increase renal calcium reabsorption. Calcium phosphate stones, which occur in distal renal tubular acidosis, respond to treatment with alkali. Uric acid stones form in acid urine and also respond to alkalinization. Additional therapy for these stones includes a reduction in purine intake and allopurinol to block the formation of uric acid. Urine alkalinization, in addition to penicillamine and a large fluid intake, helps to prevent formation of cystine stones. Struvite or infection stones form in extremely alkaline urine. Urine acidification along with antibiotics are the cornerstones of treatment for these stones.

48. Which entities are known to cause renal papillary necrosis?
Diabetes, analgesic abuse, sickle cell trait and disease, pyelonephritis, urinary tract obstruction, and hypotension (usually in neonates).

49. What is the mechanism of acidosis in chronic renal failure?
The most common mechanism of acidosis in chronic renal failure is the retention of nonvolatile acids produced from the catabolism of protein. This acidosis is associated with an elevated anion gap and usually appears when the glomerular filtration rate drops below 30% of normal. Interestingly, it tends to be nonprogressive. The serum bicarbonate concentration is maintained in the 12–18 mEq/L range because bone salts are used to buffer the acid at the expense of further renal osteodystrophy. Hyperchloremic, "non-delta" acidosis can also be seen in chronic renal failure. This usually occurs with diabetic nephropathy and obstructive uropathy. The mechanism of this acidosis presumably is from decreased aldosterone production or decreased tubular sensitivity to aldosterone, which results in diminished distal tubular acidification.

50. What is the significance of red cell casts in the urine?
Finding red cell casts on urinalysis almost always indicates the presence of glomerulonephritis. They have, however, been observed after strenous exercise and renal trauma (including renal biopsy).

51. What are the causes of chronic glomerulonephritis?
    Membranoproliferative glomerulonephritis
    Membranous glomerulopathy
    Alport's syndrome
    Systemic lupus erythematosus
    Focal glomerulosclerosis
    Diffuse proliferative glomerulonephritis
    Henoch-Schonlein purpura
    Crescentic glomerulonephritis (rapidly progressive GN)
    Berger's disease (IgA nephropathy)
These are the main causes of chronic glomerulonephritis. Strictly speaking, membranous glomerulopathy and focal glomerulosclerosis are not inflammatory diseases so they are not glomerulonephritides. Hemolytic-uremic syndrome is another important cause of chronic renal failure but is not a chronic glomerulonephritis.

52. What is the significance of white cell casts in the urine?
White cell casts are found in a variety of renal disorders. They are noted in patients with acute glomerulonephritis (especially poststreptococcal glomerulonephritis), although red blood cell casts are more common. White blood cell casts are the typical casts in interstitial nephritis and pyelonephritis. Indeed, the presence of white cell casts in a child with a urinary tract infection indicates pyelonephritis.

53. Which glomerulonephritides are associated with hypocomplementemia?
    Poststreptococcal
    Other post-infectious causes (may have normal complement)
    Subacute bacterial endocarditis
    Shunt nephritis
    Systemic lupus erythematosus
    Membranoproliferative

54. What serum and urine findings characterize total body potassium depletion?

The only serum finding that characterizes total body potassium depletion is a low serum potassium concentration with a normal or low blood pH. With an alkaline blood pH, a low serum potassium concentration may only indicate a shift of this ion from extracellular to intracellular space without total body depletion. The urine findings reflect the underlying cause rather than a low body potassium level. If the total body potassium depletion has resulted from renal tubular acidosis, then the urine will have a relatively high potassium concentration with an alkaline pH. If the cause of the potassium depletion is secondary to poor intake (a very unusual circumstance), then the urine will contain little potassium. With severe vomiting from pyloric stenosis, the urine may be acid and contain a large amount of potassium in spite of the hypokalemic metabolic acidosis.

55. What causes green or blue urine?

Methylene blue and indigo blue can make the urine blue. Vegetable dyes and paint from toys can be ingested by young children and turn their urine blue, green, red, or any other color. Often changing the pH of the urine will alter the color.

56. What causes milky urine?

The precipitation of calcium phosphate or urates can turn the urine milky, especially when stored in the refrigerator. Warming the urine to body temperature causes these precipitated salts to return to solution, removing the milky appearance. Purulent material associated with infections of the bladder and urethra may also cause the urine to appear milky. Lymph can also cause a milky urine as a result from lymphatic obstruction (rare cause of milky urine).

57. What causes red urine?

Red urine can be caused by blood, porphyrins, beets, blackberries, vegetable dyes, drugs such as phenolphthalein which is used in laxatives, and urates (especially in neonates). Hemoglobinuria and myoglobinuria usually cause a brown color. *Serratia marcescens* can produce a red pigment, making the diaper red.

58. What causes pneumaturia?

Pneumaturia is the passage of gas bubbles in the urine. It can occur as a result of a fistula between the bladder and the bowel or vagina. Fistulae can be congenital abnormalities or result from infection, neoplasms, inflammatory bowel disease, or instrumentation of the bladder. Rarely, urinary tract infections with gas-producing bacteria can lead to pneumaturia. This condition is most often observed in diabetics.

59. Describe the grading scheme for hypospadias and the implications of each grade?

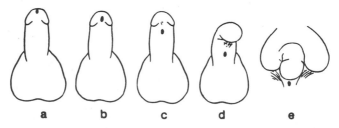

Degree of hypospadias. (a) normal meatus, (b) coronal or glandular, (c) distal shaft, (d) proximal shaft, (e) perineal with bifid scrotum and penoscrotal transposition. (Penoscrotal hypospadias not depicted). (From Perlmutter AD: Hypospadias. In Edelmann CM Jr (ed): Pediatric Kidney Disease. Boston, Little, Brown and Co., Boston, 1978, p 1235, with permission.)

Hypospadias occurs in 1–2/1000 live births and is the result of failure or delay in midline fusion of the urethral folds. It is often associated with a ventral band of fibrous tissue (chordee) which causes ventral curvature of the penis, especially with an erection, making intercourse difficult or impossible. In assessing hypospadias, it is useful to describe where the urethral meatus appears—glandular, distal shaft, proximal shaft, or perineal—and also the degree and location of chordee. A number of associated genitourinary abnormalities have been described with hypospadias including meatal stenosis, inguinal hernias, undescended testes, and an enlarged utricle masculinus (vestigial vagina). The incidence of these abnormalities rises sharply with the more severe degrees of hypospadias. In the mild forms of hypospadias, which account for the majority of cases, radiography or endoscopy of the urinary tract is unnecessary. The treatment of hypospadias is surgical repair usually as a one-step procedure. With the advent of microsurgical techniques, the optimal time for repair appears to be 9–18 months of age.

60. How common is renal trauma?
About 5% of childhood trauma involves the kidney, making it a relatively uncommon event. About 10% of the kidneys injured have underlying abnormalities such as hydronephrosis, a horseshoe kidney, or ectopy, making them more vulnerable to injury.

61. What physical findings suggest genitourinary trauma?
Fractured lower ribs
Flank mass, contusion, or wound
Lower abdominal mass or tenderness
Pelvic fracture
Genital swelling or discoloration
Inability to void
Blood at urethral meatus
High-riding prostate
Hematuria

62. What are the steps in the evaluation of suspected renal trauma?
The workup must evaluate the overall condition of the child; the type, location and extent of injury; and the status of the contralateral kidney. Minor contusions and lacerations of the kidney are best managed conservatively. These decisions are best left to a pediatric urologist or surgeon. Two caveats are in order: (1) The degree of hematuria bears no relationship to the degree of injury. (2) The absence of hematuria does not exclude severe renal injury, although 80–90% will have hematuria. With the general availability of computerized tomography (CT), many centers advocate its use over conventional IVP because of its ability to detect trauma to abdominal structures other than the urinary tract. If trauma to the urethra is suspected, such as with pelvic fractures, catheterization of the urethra should not be attempted until the integrity of the urethra is established with a urethrogram.

63. What are the pros and cons of routine circumcision for all infants?
Wallerstein recently reviewed this issue and stated that there is little or no medical evidence to recommend routine circumcision of male newborns. Indeed, the American Academy of Pediatrics in 1971 and in 1975 stated that there is no valid medical indication for circumcision in the neonatal period. This position was reaffirmed in 1978 and 1983. The practice has been largely abandoned in Great Britain and Western Europe. The arguments marshalled for routine circumcision are prevention of penile cancer, reduction in the transmission of venereal disease, promotion of good hygiene, and prevention of phimosis. There is virtually no evidence supporting any of the goals. There is no difference in the incidence of penile carcinoma in countries that routinely circumcise and those that do not. No good evidence is available supporting the concept that circumcision inhibits the transmission of venereal disease. The last two arguments are largely a matter of ignorance. Pediatricians have advised mothers that proper penile hygiene from birth requires full retraction of foreskin to clean smegma from the glans, a task virtually impossible because the foreskin is firmly attached to the glans in almost all newborns. Separation occurs normally in several months to several

years. The foreskin can be forcibly retracted, but this involves tearing the two tissues apart which is painful and may result in bleeding. The proper care of the foreskin in infancy is to simply leave it alone. Because it is the norm to have a non-retractile foreskin in infancy, it is extremely difficult to make the diagnosis of phimosis at this age. However, the majority of uncircumcised males will not develop this, so circumcising all male infants for a small minority does not make sense.

The arguments against circumcision are that (1) it is painful; (2) there is a risk of infection, and meatal stenosis is not uncommon, and (3) there is a risk of mutilating or amputating the penis or glans as a result of the circumcision. On balance, there are no valid *medical* reasons for routinely circumcising all male infants.

Recently, Wiswell and Roscelli reported an increased incidence of urinary tract infection in uncircumcised male infants. Their data suggest a 1% incidence of urinary tract infection in the first year of life of uncircumcised males versus a 0.1% incidence in circumcised males. This risk does not appear to be great enough to recommend routine circumcision, but does point out the need to look for urinary tract infection in a febrile, uncircumcised male infant.

References: Wallerstein E: Circumcision: The uniquely American enigma. Urol Clin North Am 12:123–132, 1985.

Wiswell TE, Roscelli JD: Corroborative evidence for the decreased incidence of urinary tract infections in circumcised male infants. Pediatrics 78:96–99, 1986.

64. In what percentage of UTIs will there be no white blood cells in the urine?
In up to 30% of UTIs there are no or few white blood cells in the urine. Most of these, however, are in children with recurrent infections.

65. Are urine Gram stains helpful?
Yes, Gram stains can help to determine whether the infection is due to a gram-positive organism, such as enterococcus, or a more common gram-negative organism. A Gram stain is probably not necessary in the evaluation of a nontoxic child with dysuria, but is especially useful in the toxic youngster with clinical evidence of pyelonephritis. The trick, of course, is not Gram staining your hands or shirt.

66. What are the indications and contraindications for a suprapubic bladder aspiration?
A suprapubic bladder aspiration is indicated in any child under the age of 2 in whom an uncontaminated specimen of urine is desired for culture. In the infant, the bladder tends to be an anterior abdominal organ, especially when full, making puncture relatively easy. The difficulty lies in timing, just as it is in asking for a date. You can't get blood out of stone or urine out of an empty bladder. It is best to perform the bladder tap 1/2 to 1 hour after a feeding. Commonly, children will void just as you start to insert the needle. Compressing the penis in males or putting upward pressure on the urethra by placing a finger in the rectum on females can obviate this problem to some extent. You know you have inserted the needle too far if you stick your finger. The procedure is illustrated below.

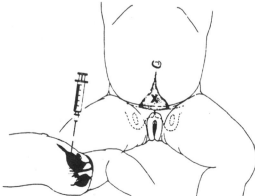

Suprapubic aspiration of the bladder (X indicates needle entry site). (From Hughes WT, Buescher ES: Pediatric Procedures, 2nd ed. Philadelphia, W.B. Saunders Co., 1980, p 288, with permission.)

There are no strict contraindications to a bladder tap. The incidence of complications arising from it are remarkably low. They include abdominal wall abscess, bladder hematoma, bleeding, anaerobic septicemia (presumably from bowel penetration), and intestinal perforation. It would be prudent to avoid a bladder tap in a child with a marked bleeding diathesis, or marked ileus with significant bowel distention. Catheterization of the bladder in these circumstances would be safer.

67. When are undescended testicles best repaired?

The optimal time for surgery on an undescended testes is between 18 months and 2 years of age. Cryptorchidism usually resolves without intervention. Seventy-five percent of full-term and 90% of premature cryptorchid newborns will have full testicular descent by age 9 months. In the second year of life ultrastructural changes in the seminiferous tubules of the undescended testes begin to appear, which may be halted by orchipexy. Eighteen to twenty-four months is also considered an optimal time psychologically to operate.

68. What physical findings should prompt a search for an underlying renal abnormality?

Abdominal mass	Neonatal ascites
High imperforate anus	Oligohydramnios
Perineal hypospadias	Anuria-oliguria (especially in the neonate)
Exstrophy of the bladder	Aniridia, hemihypertrophy (Wilms' tumor)
Ambiguous genitalia	Poor urinary stream
Prune belly abdomen	Persistent wetness

Bibliography

1. Alon U, Pery M, Davidai G, Beraut M: Ultrasonography in the radiologic evaluation of children with urinary tract infection. Pediatrics 78:58, 1986.
2. Churchill BN, Sheldon CA: Common urinary tract problems in children. Pediatr Clin North Am 1987.
3. Edelman CM Jr (ed): Pediatric Kidney Disease. Boston, Little, Brown & Co., 1978.
4. Fine RN, Nissenson AR: Dialysis Therapy. Philadelphia, Hanley & Belfus, 1986.
5. Foreman JW, Chan JCM: Chronic renal failure in children. J Pediatr 113:793, 1988.
6. Holliday MA, Barratt TM, Vernier RL: Pediatric Nephrology. Baltimore, Williams & Wilkins, 1987.
7. Ingelfinger JR: Pediatric Hypertension. Philadelphia, W.B. Saunders, 1982.
8. Kelalis PP, King LR, Belman AB: Clinical Pediatric Urology, 2nd ed. Philadelphia, W.B. Saunders Co., 1985.
9. Kolvin I, MacKeith RC, Meadow SR: Bladder Control and Enuresis. London, W. Heinemann Medical Books Ltd., 1973.
10. Kunin CM: Detection, Prevention and Treatment of Urinary Tract Infections, 3rd ed. Philadelphia, Lea & Febiger, 1987.
11. Retik AB, Cukier J: Pediatric Urology. In Libertino JA (series ed): International Perspectives in Urology. Baltimore, Williams & Wilkins, 1987.
12. Schrier RW (ed): Renal and Electrolyte Disorders, 3rd ed. Boston, Little, Brown & Co., 1986.
13. Stamey TA: Pathogenesis and Treatment of Urinary Tract Infections, 2nd ed. Baltimore, Williams & Wilkins, 1980.
14. Williams DI, Johnston JH (eds): Paediatric Urology, 2nd ed. London, Butterworth, 1982.

NEUROLOGY

Robert Clancy, M.D.

1. What are the cardinal symptoms of urea cycle defects and organic acidurias?

The mitochondrion is the cell's powerhouse. Body tissues such as brain and muscle that demand a major expenditure of energy are especially vulnerable to an interruption of their energy supply secondary to disturbed mitochondrial function. As such, brain, muscle, heart, liver, and the GI and renal transport systems fail predominantly due to clinical disorders of the mitochondrion. A variety of conditions can abruptly embarrass mitochondrial function and result in a multisystem crisis. In the newborn period, urea cycle defects and organic acidemia may produce an acute form of encephalopathy manifested initially as feeding intolerance, vomiting, and lethargy, which progress rapidly to cerebral edema, coma, seizures, flaccid paralysis, respiratory depression, reduced gag reflex, and ultimately death. These signs are not specific for mitochondrial failure but suggest overwhelming, widespread CNS dysfunction. Their differential diagnosis includes sepsis, meningitis, intracranial hemorrhage, stroke, or any catastrophic neurologic illness.

Modes of Presentation of Urea Cycle Defects

1. Neonatal catastrophe—masquerading as sepsis neonatorum
   a. Seizures, hypertonicity, vomiting, coma, death
   b. Extreme elevations of NH_3: over 1000 $\mu g/dl$
2. Subacute presentation in infancy
   a. Recurrent vomiting and growth failure
   b. Intermittent ataxia
   c. Seizures, mental retardation, developmental regression
3. Presentation later in childhood
   a. Psychomotor retardation
   b. Intermittent ataxia
   c. Vomiting, protein intolerance—history of poor feeding during infancy
   d. Overt symptoms after mild illness
4. Asymptomatic variant
   a. Usually shows amino acid abnormality without hyperammonemia

From Cohn RM, Roth KS (eds): Metabolic Disease: A Guide to Early Recognition. Philadelphia, W.B. Saunders Co., 1983, p 138, with permission.

Modes of Presentation of Organic Acidemias

Neonatal Catastrophe
   Acidosis (anion gap)
   Ketosis and ketonuria
   Tachypnea
   Neurologic findings
   Neutropenia, anemia, and thrombocytopenia
Failure to Thrive and Vomiting During the First Year of Life
   Deterioration with infection or diarrhea
   Vomiting
   Progressive delay in psychomotor development
   Acidosis—usually seen with exacerbations but is occasionally persistent
   May be history of protein intolerance leading to symptoms
   Neurological symptoms with exacerbations
Onset After the First Year of Life
   Episodes of ketoacidosis following a minor infection
   May be lethargy, seizures, or coma with such attacks

From Cohn RM, Roth KS (eds): Metabolic Disease: A Guide to Early Recognition. Philadelphia, W.B. Saunders Co., 1983, p 360.

2. What are the acceptable criteria for pronouncing a patient brain dead?

Criteria for the determination of brain death in infants and children have recently been proposed. Brain death is said to have occurred when all brain functions are irreversibly lost. Spinal cord, peripheral nerve, or reflex muscular activity may persist despite brain death. The clinical hallmark of brain death is deep, unremitting, unresponsive coma. Consciousness requires the presence of (1) an intact brainstem, which contains the "on and off" switch of vigilance—the ascending reticular activating system; and (2) the cerebral hemispheres, which house the content of consciousness such as memories, thoughts and skillful motor control. Patients with suspected brain death should be observed over a period of 12–24 hours for:

1. Unresponsive coma and the absence of eye opening, extraocular movements, vocalizations, or other cerebral-generated activity.

2. Absent brainstem reflexes such as the pupillary light reflex, reflex extraocular movements (elicited by irrigation of the ears with cold water or doll's eyes reflex), eye blink generated by hand clap, spontaneous respirations, gag reflex, coughing, or sucking.

3. Absent cerebral cortical activity as evidenced by a properly recorded "flat," "isoelectric" or "ECS" (electrocerebral silence) EEG, the absence of blood flow to the hemispheres by cerebral arteriography, or the presence of intracranial pressure that exceeds mean blood pressure for several hours.

The most difficult patients in whom to diagnose brain death are the neonate and infants under 2 months. For this age group, more stringent criteria are recommended: (1) The diagnosis of brain death should be deferred until the infant is at least 1 week old. (2) The patient should be observed in the "brain dead state" for at least 48 hours before the declaration of brain death and the termination of life support.

Reference: Volpe J: Brain death determination in the newborn. Pediatrics 80:293–297, 1987.

3. Which anticonvulsants are teratogenic?

About one-third of women with epilepsy experience an increase in their usual seizure frequency during pregnancy or have seizures confined to pregnancy (gestational epilepsy). Convulsive maternal seizures may be harmful or fatal to the fetus. Therefore it is prudent to recommend anticonvulsant treatment during pregnancy, usually with a single effective drug. Only the anticonvulsant trimethadione is unequivocally teratogenic and absolutely contraindicated during pregnancy. Epileptic mothers have a two- to three-fold increased risk of having offspring with congenital malformations. The suspicion of drug-related mutagenesis or teratogenesis is complicated by evidence that epilepsy per se in the mother or father is associated with a higher risk of fetal malformation. Many believe that phenytoin produces a relatively common and distinctive "fetal phenytoin syndrome," and valproate may be associated with an enhanced risk of neural tube defects. Carbamazepine seems to be the "safest" choice from the perspective of fetal malformations. Primidone and phenobarbital are also considered relatively safe.

References: Goyle Shobha, Maurya AK, Kailash S, Maheswari MC: Mutagenic risk in epileptic patients before and after anticonvulsant therapy. Epilepsia 28:81–86, 1987.

Janz D: The teratogenic risk of antiepileptic drugs. Epilepsia 16:165, 1975.

4. What features make febrile seizures atypical?

A simple febrile seizure occurs as a (1) generalized convulsion; (2) relatively brief attack (less than 15 minutes) and (3) a solitary event (one attack per 24 hours). Simple febrile seizures usually occur early in the course of the febrile illness. This observation relates more to the cause of the fever and seizure. For example, in meningitis or encephalitis the fever may appear for a considerable period of time before the seizure occurs. The purpose of defining the atypical or complex febrile seizure is to alert the physician to possible complicating factors: (1) A focal seizure raises the concern of a localized or lateralized functional disturbance of the central nervous system. (2) An unusually long seizure (over 15 minutes) also raises the suspicion that something more than fever may be present and that neurologic sequelae can result. (3) Repeated seizures within a 24-hour period likewise imply a potentially more serious disorder or the possibility of impending status epilepticus.

5. How common are febrile seizures?
Febrile seizures affect 2–5% of children under 6 years of age.

6. What is the purpose of treating febrile seizures?
To prevent the recurrence of more febrile seizures.

7. When and how should a child with febrile seizures be treated with anticonvulsants?
Despite the ubiquity of febrile seizures, no consensus of management has been adopted. For most children, simple febrile seizures are an unwanted but transient and innocent disruption of their health and treatment is not mandatory. Treatment may be considered in the very young child if febrile seizures recur and in those with preexisting neurologic abnormalities or with complex febrile seizures. The available approaches to febrile seizures include:

1. The continuous daily prophylactic administration of phenobarbital to produce a minimum serum level of 15 μg/ml. Comparable protection against febrile seizures may be achieved with valproate, but children in this age group are in the highest risk group for hepatotoxicity so its use is not recommended under age 2 years. The daily use of primidone (15–20 mg/kg/day) is effective but probably has little advantage over phenobarbital.

2. The intermittent use of diazepam suppositories at the first sign of febrile illness. Suppositories are not available in the United States but the intravenous solution can be administered as a retention enema. It is well established that the *intermittent use* of phenobarbital plays no effective role in febrile seizure prophylaxis.

Neither carbamazepine nor phenytoin appear effective in preventing the recurrence of febrile seizures.

References: Knudsen FU, Vestermark S: Prophylactic diazepam or phenobarbitone in febrile convulsions: A prospective controlled study. Arch Dis Child 53:660–663, 1978.

Nelson KB, Ellenberg JH: Prognosis in children with febrile seizure. Pediatrics 61:720–727, 1978.

8. How likely are febrile seizures to recur?
About 30% of affected children will have a recurrence after the first febrile seizure. The risk of recurrence is modified by the patient's age: 50% will recur at least once if the patient's first seizure occurred before the first birthday. In this age group, there is also a 30% chance of *multiple* recurrences compared to an 11% risk of multiple recurrences if the first seizure occurred after age 1 year. Thus, many physicians do not recommend prophylactic treatment unless the first febrile seizure occurred under age 1 year.

9. How dangerous are febrile seizures?
The exact risk of death or permanent neurologic disability following a febrile seizure is uncertain. A well-studied group of children was furnished by the Collaborative Perinatal Project in which there were no deaths or persistent neurologic deficit in the majority of affected children. Only 4.3% of that group had a seizure longer than 30 minutes. There was not an enhanced risk of intellectual impairment if the child was developmentally and neurologically normal before the first febrile seizure.

10. What is the risk of epilepsy following febrile seizure?
The risk of later epilepsy depends on several variables. In otherwise normal children with simple febrile seizures, the risk of epilepsy is only 1%. The risk of epilepsy is higher if: (1) there is a close family history of nonfebrile seizures; (2) prior neurologic or developmental abnormalities existed; or (3) the patient had an atypical or complex febrile seizure defined as focal seizures, seizures lasting longer than 15 minutes and multiple attacks within 24 hours.

11. Should an EEG or other study be obtained in an atypical febrile seizure?
The decision to perform ancillary diagnostic testing on a patient with an atypical febrile seizure requires experience and careful clinical judgment. Most children with their first

atypical febrile seizure should undergo an examination of cerebrospinal fluid to rule out intracranial infection. Children with focal motor seizures or postictal lateralized deficits (motor paresis, unilateral sensory or visual loss, sustained eye deviation, or aphasia) require a CT scan, for they may harbor a structural abnormality. The immediate performance of an EEG offers limited insight into the patient's disease. Prominent generalized postictal slowing is not unexpected. Definite focal slowing suggests a possible structural abnormality. The interictal EEG should return to normal within 1 week after a simple febrile seizure. A definite *epileptiform abnormality* in the setting of febrile seizure may represent:

1. An inherited EEG trait if a close relative has genuine epilepsy (children may inherit an "abnormal EEG" from an epileptic parent without actually inheriting clinical epilepsy).

2. A sporadic, unrelated, epileptic EEG abnormality (about 2–3% of healthy children with no family history of epilepsy have an incidental unexpected epileptiform EEG abnormality but do not develop clinical seizures).

3. A "lowered seizure threshold" with the implication that the febrile seizure may have been an early expression of genuine epilepsy precipitated by the stress of fever and threatens to recur without the provocation of fever.

12. Differentiate epileptic from nonepileptic neonatal seizures.
In the most general sense of the term, a neonatal "seizure" is an abnormal unexpected "attack" of altered nervous function which interrupts the natural flow of infantile behavior. Epileptic neonatal seizures are those abnormal clinical events ("seizures") that occur simultaneously with electrographic seizures. Nonepileptic neonatal seizures are those abnormal clinical events that occur in the absence of electrographic seizure patterns. Clinical and electrographic seizures may coincide or dissociate, even in the same child.

13. What are the most common types of seizures in the neonatal period?
The most common clinical neonatal seizure is the so-called "subtle" seizure. Rather than arising as an abrupt dramatic "convulsion" with obvious forceful twitching or posturing of the muscles, the subtle seizure appears as an unnatural, repetitive, stereotyped choreography featuring oral-buccal-lingual movements, eye blinking, nystagmus, lip smacking, or complex integrated limb movements (swimming, pedaling, or rowing) and other fragments of activity drawn from the limited repertoire of normal infant activity.

14. What is the anticonvulsant of choice for petit mal epilepsy? Why?
Ethosuximide (trade name Zarontin). Most patients with petit mal epilepsy have only absence attacks during which there is some disturbance of consciousness, alertness, or reactivity while the EEG shows the classic pattern of generalized 3 per second spike and slow-wave discharges. Ethosuximide is currently the drug of choice for several reasons:

1. It works well for many patients. It not only stops the clinical attacks of absence but it often normalizes the EEG by "erasing" the 3 per second spike-wave discharges.

2. It is well tolerated by most patients. Although rare cases of serious bone marrow, liver, or dermatologic disorders have occurred, routine or frequent blood test are not considered obligatory by most physicians.

3. It has a relatively long serum half-life (40 hours). Thus once or twice a day dosing is appropriate and represents a real convenience to the patient.

4. It is relatively inexpensive.

15. What percentage of patients with petit mal seizures also have occasional grand mal seizures?
About 30%.

16. What is the drug of choice for coexisting petit mal and grand mal seizures? Why?
Valproate. Its broad spectrum of activity provides excellent coverage for both seizure types. In fact, many physicians consider valproate the drug of choice for absence seizures alone. Most patients with absence seizures are older than 2 years, at which time there is little risk of hepatotoxicity from valproate. Despite the relatively short elimination half-life (6–16 hours), twice a day dosing with divalproex (trade name: Depakote) may be used. Valproate is considered to have a very low risk of unwanted cognitive side effects.

17. What is the anticonvulsant of choice for idiopathic grand mal epilepsy?
The "traditional" anticonvulsants (phenobarbital, primidone, phenytoin) are no longer considered the drugs of choice for grand mal seizures for many age groups. (Phenobarbital remains the drug of choice for neonatal seizures.) Recent studies have shown that most of the major anticonvulsants do a comparably good job at reducing or eliminating seizure recurrences. Since many children with seizures will require treatment for years, some even for a lifetime, the question is rightly raised about the impact of the chronic use of anticonvulsant drugs on the body and brain. For example, the long-term consumption of phenytoin may be associated with coarsened facial features, hirsutism, and gingival hyperplasia. Perhaps more importantly there is a growing awareness of mental side effects affecting behavior, mood, cognitive processing, memory, and attention provoked by phenobarbital and phenytoin. For these reasons carbamazepine and valproate have emerged as the current drugs of choice for grand mal seizures.
    Reference: Mattson RH, Cramer JA, Collins JF, et al: Comparison of carbamazepine, phenobarbital, phenytoin and primidone in partial and secondarily generalized tonic-clonic seizures. N Engl J Med 313:145–151, 1985.

18. How quickly can anticonvulsants be discontinued?
In practice, all anticonvulsants are gradually tapered rather than abruptly discontinued even though there is no actual *withdrawal state* produced by a "cold turkey" reduction of most anticonvulsants. For example, the abrupt discontinuation of phenytoin, carbamazepine, valproate, and ethosuximide characteristically produces no withdrawal symptoms that feature seizures. In contrast, there is the occasional appearance of a withdrawal syndrome of agitation, signs of autonomic overactivity, and seizures which follows the precipitous elimination of habitually consumed diazepam or short-acting barbiturates (such as secobarbital). The long elimination half-life of phenobarbital lessens the risk of withdrawal symptoms following abrupt discontinuation. Most neurologists gradually taper and discontinue anticonvulsants so as not to invite the return of seizures following the loss of necessary drug therapy. The duration of tapering is highly variable and seems to reflect personal preference. Some physicians employ the following rule of thumb for tapering anticonvulsants: 25% of the total daily dose is withdrawn for a period of five elimination half-lives ($5 \times T\frac{1}{2}$).

19. If you suspect that a child has petit mal seizures, what can you do to induce a seizure?
Hyperventilation for at least 3 minutes is a useful provocative maneuver to precipitate an absence seizure in a child with petit mal epilepsy. Young patients may be coaxed into overbreathing if the doctor makes a game of it. Hold a tissue paper in front of the child's mouth. Instruct the patient to keep breathing fast enough to keep the tissue aloft. The time of day is another consideration bearing on the appearance of petit mal seizures. Some children have attacks only at certain times such as in the early morning or immediately after awakening. Many families now have available the use of electronic video recording equipment. Ask the family to make a home movie of the spell which you can then observe by replaying the tape.

20. Which anticonvulsants cannot be given intramuscularly?

Routes of Administration of Anticonvulsants

ANTICONVULSANT	ACCEPTABLE ADMINISTRATION ROUTES			
	Oral	Rectal*	Intravenous	Intramuscular†
Phenobarbital	X		X	X
Phenytoin	X		X	
Diazepam	X	X	X	X
Valproate	X	X		
Carbamazepine	X	X		

*Graves Nina M, Kriel Robert L: Rectal administration of antiepileptic drugs in children. Pediatr Neurol 3:321–326, 1987.
†IM injections are not recommended to treat serious acute seizure disorders. The speed and completeness of IM absorption may be unacceptably variable, especially with benzodiazepines.

21. What are the common disorders that mimic epilepsy?

There are many conditions which are characterized by the sudden onset of abnormal consciousness, awareness, reactivity, behavior, posture, tone, sensation, or autonomic function. Syncope, breath-holding spells, migraine, hypoglycemia, narcolepsy, cataplexy, gastroesophageal reflux, parasomnias (night terrors, sleep walking, sleep talking, nocturnal enuresis) feature an abrupt or "paroxysmal" alteration of brain function and suggest the possibility of epilepsy. Perhaps one of the most difficult attacks to distinguish is the "pseudoseizure," also called a pseudoepileptic seizure or hysterical seizure. These abnormal attacks are outwardly modeled after the patient's subconscious or conscious perception of what a seizure should look like and occur without any abnormal electrical discharges of neurons in the central nervous system.

22. What are the common side effects of phenytoin?

Phenytoin (Dilantin) promotes connective tissue growth that is ultimately manifest as gum hyperplasia, coarsening of the facial features, hypertrophic (keloid) scar formation, and sometimes Dupuytren's contractures. Facial and body hair growth is also stimulated. Lowered serum folate levels may eventually produce a megaloblastic anemia or mild peripheral neuropathy. The consumption of phenytoin may accelerate the hepatic elimination of vitamin D, resulting in rickets. The neurologic side effects include subtle mood, behavioral, or cognitive effects, even within the normal therapeutic range. Signals of overmedication include nystagmus (blood level > 20 μg/ml), ataxia (> 30 μg/ml), and somnolence (> 40 μg/ml). Irreversible ataxia and cerebellar atrophy from Purkinje cell depletion may follow chronic phenytoin overmedication.

23. How does valproate affect serum levels of other drugs?

Caution should be exercised when administering valproate stimultaneously with other anticonvulsants. Valproate has significant effects on the serum levels of other anticonvulsants.

Effects of Adding Valproate to Preexisting Anticonvulsants
Elevated Serum Levels
  Phenobarbital
  Primidone
  Ethosuximide
  Carbamazepine
Reduced Serum Levels
  Phenytoin (the free or unbound fraction may be increased despite a reduction of total serum phenytoin concentration)

Effects of Adding Other Drugs to Existing Valproate Regimen
No Change in Serum Levels
  Ethosuximide
  Clonazepam
Reduced Serum Levels
  Phenobarbital
  Primidone
  Carbamazepine

24. How are seizures differentiated from breath-holding?

Loss of consciousness is not an infrequent complaint and may arise from many (benign or pathological) neurologic or systemic conditions. First be aware that a "convulsion" (forceful involuntary contractions of the skeletal musculature) may follow even a simple faint. "Convulsive syncope" refers to the presence of mild brief stiffening, eye rolling, clonic or myoclonic limb twitches in the moments following loss of consciousness and postural tone due to a faint. Syncope (loss of consciousness secondary to transient cerebral hypoperfusion) is preceded by a prodrome of feeling faint, graying-out of vision, muffled hearing, sweating, and nausea. Loss of consciousness due to a grand mal seizure is abrupt, as though a switch was suddenly thrown, turning off consciousness.

Breath-holding spells feature loss of consciousness secondary to syncope. Two mechanisms may operate. (1) A child may deliberately hold his breath, Valsalva, and turn blue. These are called cyanotic breath-holding attacks and occur after a suitable triggering stimulus. (2) A child may reflexly develop bradycardia or transient asystole with or without true apnea, precipitated by a painful or unpleasant surprise such as a trivial blow to the occiput following a stumble or fall. This second type of breath-holding is called "pallid infantile syncope," "reflex anoxic seizures," or "white breath-holding attack."

The loss of consciousness with a generalized seizure may arise any time and is not triggered by a specific stimulus. The attacks can occur while awake or asleep and usually have more prominent motor signs with frank tonic stiffening and sustained clonic jerking.

25. What is rolandic epilepsy? How is it diagnosed?

Rolandic epilepsy (benign focal epilepsy of childhood) is a common epilepsy syndrome that has received little recognition in the United States. The following criteria establish the diagnosis:

1. It begins during school age in otherwise healthy and neurologically normal children.

2. The seizures are "idiopathic" or familial (rolandic epilepsy may be inherited in an autosomal dominant fashion).

3. The clinical seizures may be simple or complex, partial or generalized seizures. The simple partial seizure may begin during the daytime as a sensory disturbance on the tongue or focal clonic facial twitching. During sleep generalized seizures seem to predominate.

4. The EEG shows a distinctive type of sharp-slow wave discharges localized to the rolandic (central, midtemporal, central-temporal, or sylvian) regions.

5. Ancillary neurodiagnostic tests are normal.

Rolandic epilepsy is often referred to as a benign syndrome because: (1) the individual is otherwise normal; (2) the seizures are usually easily controlled with low doses of a single anticonvulsant; and (3) the seizures virtually always abate after puberty.

Reference: Loiseau P, Pestre M, Dartigues JF, et al: Long-term progression in two forms of childhood epilepsy: Typical absence seizure and epilepsy with rolandic (centrotemporal) EEG foci. Ann Neurol 13: 642–648, 1983.

26. What is the risk of epilepsy following an isolated seizure?

The risk of recurrence after a single epileptic seizure is uncertain but may be as low as 25 to 50%. The exact risk probably depends on the seizure type, the patient's age, concurrent neurologic problems such as mental retardation or cerebral palsy, family history, and the results of the EEG examination. All patients with a solitary seizure deserve a careful and thoughtful medical and neurologic evaluation to exclude important and treatable etiologies. However, anticonvulsant treatment is not mandatory in all cases. The decision to treat should be made after discussing all the pros and cons of therapy with the patient and family. Many physicians prefer to await the appearance of a second seizure before committing the patient to long-term anticonvulsant therapy.

Reference: Annergers JF, Shirts SB, Houser WA, Kurland LT: Risk of recurrence after an initial unprovoked seizure. Epilepsia 27:43–50, 1986.

27. What causes pinpoint pupils?

Pupillary size represents a dynamic balance between the constricting influence of the third nerve (representing the parasympathetic autonomic nervous system) and the dilating influence of the ciliary nerve, which conducts fibers of the sympathetic nervous system. Pinpoint pupils imply that the constricting influence of the third cranial nerve is not balanced by opposing sympathetic dilatation. This could result from a *structural lesion in the pons* through which descend the sympathetic pathways. Small, reactive pupils also accompany some metabolic disorders. Opiates such as heroin or morphine produce pinpoint pupils that resemble those seen in pontine lesions. A variety of other agents also produce constriction of the pupils including propoxyphene, organophosphates, carbamate insecticides, barbiturates, clonidine, meprobamate, and pilocarpine eye drops, as well as mushroom or nutmeg poisoning.

28. When are "doll's eyes" movements considered normal or abnormal?

The oculovestibular reflex (also called oculocephalic, proprioceptive head-turning reflex, or doll's eyes reflex) is an ocular movement reflex that produces conjugate movements of the eyeballs within the bony orbits in response to stimulation of the organs of balance. This reflex is named after the "expensive" toy dolls with mechanically movable eyes that roll up and down when the doll's head is tilted. (Contrast that with the "inexpensive" toy dolls whose eyes are painted on their faces and are thus immobile.) The input or afferent signal of the doll's eyes reflex originates in the semicircular canals and proprioceptors of the cervical musculature and spinal joint position sensors. The efferent limb of the reflex is mediated through the "movers" of the eye (the third and sixth cranial nerves) joined by the medial longitudinal fasciculus.

1. In healthy awake newborn infants (who cannot inhibit or override the reflex with willful eye movements), the reflex is easy to elicit and is a normal finding.

2. In healthy, awake, *mature* individuals, normal vision overrides the reflex, which is thus normally absent.

3. In coma with preserved brainstem function, the depressed cortex does not override the reflex and doll's eyes movements will occur in response to rapid head rotation. Indeed, the purpose of eliciting this reflex in the comatose patient is to demonstrate that the brainstem still functions normally.

4. In coma with brainstem damage, the neural circuits that carry out the reflex are impaired and the reflex is abolished.

Be sure to elicit the reflex correctly before concluding that it is absent: the eyelids are held open while the head is briskly rotated from side to side. Be careful that there is no cervical spine instability! A positive response is contraversive conjugate eye deviation (head rotates to the right and both eyes deviate to the left). Next the head is rapidly flexed and extended. During flexion the eyelids may open reflexly (doll's eyelid phenomenon), allowing one also to test levator palpebral function.

29. What is spasmus nutans?

Spasmus nutans is a rare, acquired movement disorder of unknown etiology beginning between ages 4 months and 14 months. The full triad consists of head tilt (torticollis), head nodding, and nystagmus. The condition often presents first with the head nodding, which is out of synchrony with the speed, direction and tempo of the nystagmus. The condition lasts several months to years and usually fades by age 5 years. The nystagmus is present in the primary position (with the patient looking straight ahead) but is characteristically unilateral or markedly asymmetrical. The nystagmus has a pendular quality. (A pendulum arm sweeps arcs of *equal* magnitude and velocity). The direction of the nystagmus can be horizontal, vertical, or rotatory and may vary with the direction of gaze. Spasmus nutans has occasionally been associated with developmental abnormalities or optic chiasmal gliomas. Therefore a CT scan should be obtained before reassuring the parents of the benign nature and favorable outcome of the disorder.

30. Is the cherry-red spot characteristic of Tay-Sachs disease?

A cherry-red spot is due to the abnormally pale appearance of the ganglion nerve cells that surround the relatively normal fovea. It is not pathognomonic for Tay-Sachs disease. Occlusion of the central retinal artery results in pale coagulation necrosis of the retina. The fovea lacks an inner cell layer and receives its vascular supply from the choroidal vessels. Hence, in occlusion of the central retinal artery, the normally perfused fovea stands out as a cherry-red spot in contrast to the rest of the white ischemic retina. A variety of inborn errors of metabolism also result in cherry-red spots: Farber's disease, Niemann-Pick (Groups A and C) disease, infantile Gaucher's, metachromatic leukodystrophy, generalized GM1 gangliosidosis, Sandhoff's disease, and mucolipidosis Type 1.

31. What is the differential diagnosis of ptosis?

Ptosis is the downward displacement of the upper eyelid due to dysfunction of the muscles that elevate the eyelid. A drooping eyelid may represent "pseudoptosis" from swelling of the eyelid caused by local edema or active blephorospasm. True ptosis results from weakness of the eyelid muscles or interruption of its nerve supply. Primary muscular etiologies of ptosis include congenital ptosis, which may occur alone or in the setting of Turner's or Smith-Lemli-Opitz syndrome. Ptosis may also occur in myasthenia gravis, botulism, and some muscular dystrophies. Neurologic causes of ptosis include the Horner's syndrome, which results from the interruption of the sympathetic supply to Muller's smooth eyelid muscle, and third nerve palsy, which innervates the levator palpebral muscle.

32. What is a Marcus-Gunn pupil and in what disease is it noted?

The pupils are normally equal in size due to the consensual light reflex: light entering either eye produces the same strength "signal" for constriction of both the stimulated and nonstimulated pupil. Some diseases of the maculae or optic nerves affect one side more than the other. For example, a meningioma may develop on one optic nerve sheath. As a result of unilateral or asymmetrical optic nerve dysfunction, a Marcus-Gunn pupil (afferent pupillary defect) may result.

33. How is a Marcus-Gunn pupil detected?

By the "swinging flashlight test," which is conducted as follows:

1. The patient is examined in a dim room and fixation is directed to a distant target (this permits maximal pupillary dilation due to lack of direct light and accommodation reflexes).

2. Light presented to the "good" eye produces equal constriction of both pupils. The flashlight is swung briskly over the bridge of the nose to the eye with the "defective" optic nerve. The abnormal pupil remains momentarily constricted from the lingering effects of the consensual light response. However, the impaired eye with its reduced pupillomotor signal soon escapes the consensual reflex and actually dilates despite being directly stimulated with light. The pupil that paradoxically dilates to direct light stimulation displays the "afferent defect."

34. What is the Marcus-Gunn reflex?

The Marcus-Gunn reflex, also known as the jaw-winking phenomenon, presumably arises from a congenital "miswiring" of the oculomotor and trigeminal nerves. In this anomaly ptosis follows jaw closure and eyelid elevation follows jaw opening.

35. What is the proper workup for a child with opsoclonus-myoclonus?

Opsoclonus-myoclonus (also called infantile polymyoclonus syndrome or acute myoclonic encephalopathy of infants) is a rare but distinctive movement disorder that presents as "dancing eyes and dancing feet." Opsoclonus is characterized by wild, chaotic, fluttering, irregular, rapid, conjugate bursts of eye movements (saccadomania). Myoclonus is sudden shock-like muscular twitches of the face, limbs, or trunk. The anatomic site of pathology is the cerebellar outflow tracts, including the dentato-rubro-thalamo-cortical networks. The etiology of the clinical syndrome may be direct viral invasion, postinfectious encephalopathy, or neuroblastoma. Neuroblastoma is a malignant tumor of early childhood which arises from neural crest ectoderm. The adrenal medulla and sympathetic chain in the abdomen or chest are common sites of origin. Determination of urinary excretion or catacholamine metabolites (VMA test) is a useful screening test. CT scan or ultrasonic examination of the abdomen may also detect the presence of a malignant mass. If there is a strong clinical suspicion of pheochromocytoma, complete workup would include VMA spot test, complete blood count, intravenous pyelogram, chest x-ray, skeletal survey, bone marrow examination, and bone scan.

36. How can the cause of eye deviation be localized in a child with nystagmus?

Nystagmus is defined as relatively rhythmic oscillatory eye movements. Many adjectives are used to describe the clinical characteristics of nystagmus which are useful in localizing the site of the pathology.

Vestibular nystagmus. The vestibular system plays a major role in the conscious and unconscious coordination of posture, tone, and balance. Sustained changes of posture are modulated by the otoliths (utricles and saccules) and movements from acceleration are mediated by the semicircular canals. Artificial stimulation of the vestibular apparatus can create an illusion of movement (vertigo) and the generation of jerk nystagmus. Jerk nystagmus has two parts and is named for the direction of the normal corrective fast phase. The slow movement is the pathological component. For example, left beating jerk nystagmus implies that the fast phase is directed to the left and the abnormal slow phase is directed to the right. Everyone recalls the medical school mnemonic "cows" which describes the resulting jerk nystagmus due to irrigation of a normal ear with cold or hot water: cold water irrigation produces a nystagmus with the fast phase opposite the irrigated side; warm water irrigation produces a nystagmus whose fast phase is on the same side as the irrigated ear. Most vestibular abnormalities behave as a destructive lesion and mimic the effects of cold water irrigation. Consider the example of a patient with an acute destructive lesion of the *right* vestibular apparatus. The patient's symptoms (identical to those caused by cold water irrigation of the right ear) include:

1. Jerk nystagmus with beating of the fast phase opposite to the stimulated ear (in this case, a *left* jerk nystagmus).

2. An illusion of movement with the subjective sensation of spinning to the right and a tendency to fall to the right, past pointing to the left and the experience that the external environment is moving to the left.

Lesions of the peripheral vestibular system (the semi-circular canals) classically produce complaints of brief but intense vertigo and sometimes deafness or tinnitus. The nystagmus tends to beat in only one direction regardless of the direction of gaze.

Lesions of the central neurologic connections of the vestibular system (the vestibular nuclei and pathways) rarely cause tinnitus or hearing loss and typically produce complaints of mild sustained vertigo. The direction of jerk nystagmus may reverse as the direction of gaze changes.

Ataxia is the neurologic sign *par excellence* of cerebellar disease. Loss of the smooth, orderly execution of muscular coordination can produce an unsteady gait (as opposed to the conscious nauseating experience of perceived movement, swaying, or spinning called vertigo). Additional clinical neurologic signs of cerebellar disease are hypotonia, intention tremor, dysdiadochokinesia, scanning speech, dysmetria, and nystagmus. Because there are numerous intimate anatomical and functional connections between the vestibular system and the cerebellum, nystagmus in some patients with cerebellar disorders may behave similarly to vestibular disorders. However, there are several varieties of nystagmus or abnormal eye movements which are more or less specific for cerebellar disorders. An acute cerebellar hemispheric lesion may induce an ipsilateral horizontal gaze paresis with deviation of the eyes to the opposite side. This may be followed by gaze paretic nystagmus with the fast component ipsilateral to the side of the injury. Periodic alternating nystagmus, vertical upbeat nystagmus, rebound nystagmus, ocular dysmetria or flutter, and opsoclonus all indicate the presence of a cerebellar disorder rather than a vestibular one.

37. What forces mediate pupillary constriction and dilation?

Pupil size represents a balance between the opposing forces of constriction and dilation. Pupillary constriction is mediated by the parasympathetic arm of the autonomic nervous system via the Edinger-Westphal nucleus whose efferent fibers run within the third cranial nerve (the oculomotor nerve — the "mover" of the eye) and activate a ring of constricter muscle fibers in the iris. Pupillary dilation is mediated by sympathetic fibers that originate in the hypothalamus, descend through the brainstem, exit the spinal cord at T1, ascend in the cervical sympathetic chain, and ultimately innervate a ring of radially oriented dilation fibers via the long ciliary nerve.

38. How are pupillary size, equality, and reactivity to light evaluated in premature infants?

A well-developed "dazzle reflex" ensures that the infant forcefully grimaces and tightly closes the eyes in response to a strong light stimulus. It is difficult to see the pupils through tightly closed eyelids! (Tip: if the infant is lying supine, turn off the overhead lights and illuminate the pupils obliquely.) Second, the pupil may be difficult to see through the incompletely transparent cornea of the very small premature infant or in heavily pigmented irises. Consistent reactivity to light is present by a conceptional age of 31 weeks. It may, however, be noticeable as early as 29 weeks. Prior to that time the examiner may note that the pupils are relatively equal and of changing diameter, fluctuating from time to time depending on sleep, alertness, activity, or stress. However, an immediate brisk direct light response may not be evident.

> References: Meltzoff AN, Moore MK: Imitation of facial and manual gestures by human neonates. Science 198:75, 1977.
>
> Robinson RJ: Assessment of gestational age by neurological examination. Arch Dis Child 41: 437–447, 1966.

39. What is the significance of abnormal pupillary size or abnormal reactions to light?

Such abnormalities are highly important neurologic signs that may indicate the presence of primary ocular disease, optic nerve dysfunction, oculomotor palsies, brainstem herniation, or Horner's syndrome (meiosis, ptosis, anhidrosis).

40. What is the Babinski response?

Cutaneous stimulation of the lateral outer sole produces reflex movement of the great toe. Most healthy children and adults have a flexor plantar response. The Babinski reflex is the presence of extension of the great toe in response to stroking the plantar surface of the foot and may indicate immaturity or abnormality of the pyramidal tracts.

41. How is the Babinski response elicited?

Ideally the response should be elicited with the patient awake and the head midline. The lateral sole is smartly stroked with a sharp object. Beware that midline stimulation of the foot produces a plantar grasp and excessively painful stimulation provokes bulk foot and limb withdrawal reflex.

42. Why is interpretation of the Babinski response controversial?

When the traditional or classic neurologic examination is conducted on a neonate, the interpretation of the physical findings is fraught with hazards. Even simple plantar stimulation has a conflicting literature associated with it. Richmond Paine's classic study of neurologic signs in infants describes the presence of an *extensor* toe sign up to the age of 1 year in 75% of normal babies. Other experienced clinicians insist that plantar stimulation causes *flexion* of the great toe. These discrepancies are presumably related to differences in examination technique rather than biological differences in the patients studied. The results of plantar stimulation must be integrated with the entire motor examination, including symmetry of the reflex, presence of abnormal tone or posture, sustained clonus, and motor development.

Reference: Paine RS, Brazelton TB, Donovan DE, et al: Evolution of postural reflexes in normal infants and in the presence of chronic brain syndromes. Neurology 14:1036–1048, 1964.

43. At what age does handedness develop?

Normal infants show a hand preference (cerebral dominance or handedness) by 17 to 18 months.

44. How is hand preference demonstrated?

The preferred hand is stronger than the nondominant side, more likely to reach for desired objects and more capable of skillful execution and delicate manipulation such as grasping eating utensils, pencils or small objects. The abnormally premature development of a strong hand preference may be an indicator of motor dysfunction in the opposite hand from hemiplegia or Erb's palsy. Persistent fisting of the "nondominant" hand, asymmetrical lateral protective reflexes, or parachute response and asymmetric tone or deep tendon reflexes are additional clues to suggest a lateralized motor abnormality.

45. Which extremities are affected in spastic quadriplegia, paraplegia, hemiplegia, and monoplegia?

1. Spastic quadriplegia (tetraplegia) denotes weakness of all four extremities with the legs more abnormal than the arms.

2. Diplegia or paraplegia connotes an abnormality affecting both legs.

3. Hemiplegia implies that the arms and legs on the same side are involved, usually with the arm worse than the leg. Double hemiplegia implies the presence of bilateral brain injury affecting all four limbs, with each arm worse than the corresponding leg.

4. Monoplegia is the involvement of any one extremity.

46. If a lumbar puncture (LP) is traumatic, is the cell count still useful as a diagnostic test?

The CSF cell count and differential can still be useful after a "traumatic" LP caused by the local entry of blood from the procedure itself. Take the following steps to maximize information yield:

1. Immediately spin down one tube of CSF. Recent blood does not have time to discolor the normal, crystalline, colorless CSF. The presence of xanthochromia implies preexisting blood at least 12 hours old.

2. The traumatic introduction of red blood cells guarantees the presence of serum proteins as well. CSF protein is artificially elevated by 1 mg % for each 1,000 red blood cells per cubic millimeter. Example: a traumatic lumbar puncture yielded 20,000 red blood cells per cubic millimeter and a CSF protein of 85 mg %. The "corrected" CSF protein is 65 mg % (85 mg % − 20 mg %), which is abnormally high.

3. The CSF cell count must be compared to the peripheral white and red blood cell count. Example: a traumatic lumbar puncture yielded 20,000 RBC/mm³ and 90 WBC/mm³. If the patient has a peripheral white blood count of 10,000 WBC/mm³ and a red blood cell count of 5,000,000 RBC/mm³, the ratio of "WBC/RBC" is 10,000/5,000,000 or 2 WBC/1,000 RBC. In our example, the peripheral blood count has traumatically contaminated the CSF and introduced 20,000 RBC/mm³ × 2 WBC/1,000 RBC or 40 WBC/mm³. The "corrected" CSF white cell count is 50 WBC/mm³ (90−40), which is also excessively high.

47. What are the common causes of elevated CSF protein?

Elevated CSF protein is a nonspecific finding encountered in a variety of neurologic disorders. Several common etiologies should be considered:

1. Infection: tuberculous meningitis, acute bacterial meningitis (pneumococcus, meningococcus, *H. influenzae*), syphilitic or viral meningitis, or encephalitis.

2. Inflammation such as Guillain-Barré syndrome, multiple sclerosis, peripheral neuropathy, or postinfectious encephalopathy.

3. Tumor of the cerebral hemispheres or spinal cord.

4. Vascular accidents such as cerebral hemorrhage (including subarachnoid hemorrhage, subdural hemorrhage, intracerebral hemorrhages) or stroke due to cranial arteritis, diabetes mellitus, or hypertension.

5. Degenerative disorders involving white matter disease (such as Krabbe's disease).

6. Metabolic disorders such as uremia.

7. Toxins such as lead.

48. What predisposing factor should be considered in patients with recurring meningitis?

Some infections are inherently recurrent. Mollaret's meningitis by its nature features recurrences of infection. Chronic relapsing encephalomyelitis may also produce repetitive bouts of inflammation of the cord or hemispheres. Multiple bouts of meningitis may also be seen in individuals with congenital or acquired immunodeficiency. There are a variety of anatomical causes of recurring meningitis. Predisposing congenital defects include myelomeningocele, neurenteric cysts, and midline or spinal dermal sinuses. Occult encephaloceles may leak and introduce microorganisms into the spinal fluid. Acquired anatomical causes of recurrent infection include CSF leaks from a skull fracture at the base of the brain which extend into the sinuses or petrous pyramid. Basilar skull fractures are recognized by bleeding from the middle ear or CSF otorrhea. Fractures of the base of the anterior fossa produce CSF rhinorrhea through a damaged cribiform plate.

49. What is meningismus?

The term "meningismus" has various meanings. It is most commonly used to refer to the signs and symptoms of meningeal irritation associated with meningitis (abnormal CSF profile) including headache, nuchal rigidity, Kernig's and Brudzinski's signs. Some physicians also use "meningismus" to describe headache or stiff neck seen without meningitis such as in the setting of a cerebellar hemisphere infarction.

50. What are the physical signs of meningeal irritation in the neonate?

In neonates the physical signs of meningeal irritation may be overshadowed by systemic dysfunction such as poor feeding, respiratory distress, or jaundice. Perhaps this is because meningitis commonly follows seeding of the meninges by systemic sepsis. Only a few patients present predominantly with frank neurologic signs such as coma, seizures, or abnormal posture. Pure nuchal rigidity can occur but is rare in the newborn. More commonly, there is widespread increase of extensor tone in the neck, trunk, and limb musculature. Meningismus is not seen in every patient of any age even with advanced purulent meningitis, and should not be considered a *sine qua non* for the diagnosis.

51. What is the meaning of "meningism"?

"Meningism" was commonly used in the older medical literature to denote the sudden onset of headache and mild meningeal signs without meningitis in the setting of an acute febrile illness. These symptoms follow acute systemic viral or bacterial infections such as streptococcal pharyngitis or roseola infantum. The CSF profile is normal except for mildly increased CSF pressure.

52. Which congenital infections cause cerebral calcifications and how do the patterns help with diagnosis?

1. CMV is a congenital viral infection that produces a calcified mold of the ventricles.

2. Herpes simplex virus is related to CMV and may also cause intracranial calcifications that are not typically periventricular. A relatively rare form of neonatal herpes infection is the result of transplacental transmission of the virus early in pregnancy, leading to abortion or congenital anomalies featuring intracranial calcifications, microcephaly, choreoretinitis, and

intrauterine growth retardation. More commonly, previously well infants acquire the virus at birth from the maternal birth canal and later develop an acute, fulminant, disseminated viral sepsis or a more restricted viral encephalitis.

3. Toxoplasmosis produces the classic triad of congenital hydrocephalus, diffuse intracranial calcification, and bilateral chorioretinitis. Multiple calcifications are scattered homogeneously and indiscriminately in both cerebral hemispheres. Less frequently only two or three discrete foci of calcifications may be seen.

4. Rubella acquired by the mother and transmitted to the fetus in the first trimester behaves as a teratogen with resulting prematurity, low birth weight, cataracts, deafness, cardiac defects, "salt and pepper" retinitis, and microcephaly. Calcification is not usually seen.

53. What noninfectious diseases cause cerebral calcifications?

Injured nerve cells often become "leaky" and permit the excessive intracellular entry of calcium, which behaves as a mitochondrial toxin. Indeed the calcium ion plays a key role in effecting neuronal death and hence has promoted conspicuous interest in the pharmacologic use of calcium entry blocking agents, which may divert this pathologic process. Calcium salts may be microscopically visible within individual "mineralized neurons" or may precipitate in macroscopic abundance visible by skull x-ray or CT scan. The presence of grossly visible intracerebral calcification implies subacute or chronic disease. Acute brain injury does not lead to immediate CNS calcification.

Classification of Pathologic Intracranial Calcifications in Infants and Children

	INCIDENCE	
ENTITY	Among all calcifications	Within entity
Developmental		
Tuberous sclerosis	Common	47%
Sturge-Weber syndrome	Common	50%
Neurofibromatosis	Rare	<1%
Cockayne syndrome	Rare	Common
Fahr syndrome	Rare	100%
Lipoid proteinosis	Rare	Common
Miscellaneous familial types	Rare	Common
Basal cell nevus syndrome	Rare	Common
Lissencephaly	Rare	Rare
Wilson Disease	Rare	Rare
Inflammatory		
Cytomegalic inclusion disease	Common	40%
Other viral diseases		
Herpes simplex	Rare	Occasional
Congenital rubella	Rare	Rare
Polioencephalitis	Rare	Rare
Congenital toxoplasmosis	Common	60%
Bacterial infections		
Pyogenic meningitis	Rare	Rare
Tuberculous meningitis	Rare	50%
Tuberculoma	Rare	1% to 8%
Other parasitic infections		
Cysticercosis	Rare	Occasional
Paragonimiasis	Rare	40%
Echinococcosis	Rare	Rare
Trichinosis	Rare	Rare
Coccidioidomycosis	Rare	Rare

Table continued on next page.

Classification of Pathologic Intracranial Calcifications
in Infants and Children *(Continued)*

	INCIDENCE	
ENTITY	Among all calcifications	Within entity
Neoplastic		
Craniopharyngioma	Common	70%
Astrocytoma	Occasional	7%
Ependymoma	Occasional	6%
Teratodermoid	Occasional	Common
Other neoplasms		
Meningioma	Rare	Common
Oligodendroglioma	Rare	Common
Choroid plexus neoplasm	Rare	Occasional
Medulloblastoma	Rare	Rare
Corpus callosum lipoma	Rare	Common
Secondary retinoblastoma	Rare	Occasional
Pituitary adenoma	Rare	Rare
Chordoma	Rare	Rare
Meningeal leukemia	Rare	Rare
Meningeal neuroblastoma	Rare	Rare
Undifferentiated neuroec-todermal neoplasm	Rare	Occasional
Postradiation calcification	Occasional	Occasional
Vascular		
Subdural hematoma	Common	10%
Extradural hematoma	Rare	Rare
Intracranial hematoma	Rare	Rare
Arteriovenous malformation	Occasional	20%
Vein of Galen anomaly	Rare	Rare
Aneurysm	Rare	Rare
Vascular hamartoma	Rare	Rare
Anoxia	Rare	Rare
Vessel wall	Rare	Rare
Therapeutic radiation	Rare	Rare
Unknown	Rare	Rare
Endocrine		
Hyperparathyroidism	Rare	Occasional
Hypoparathyroidism	Rare	53%
Pseudohypoparathyroidism	Rare	45%
Pseudopseudohypoparathyroidism	Rare	Rare
Toxic		
Carbon monoxide	Rare	Occasional
Lead poisoning	Rare	Occasional
Vitamin D intoxication	Rare	Rare
Hypercalcemia	Rare	Occasional
Methotrexate (intrathecal)	Rare	Unknown

From Swaiman KF, Wright FS (eds): The Practice of Pediatric Neurology. St. Louis, C.V. Mosby Co., 1982, p 119, with permission.
Modified from Harwood-Nash DC, Fitz CR: Neuroradiology in Infants and Children, vol. I. St. Louis, C.V. Mosby Co., 1976, pp 147 and 148.

54. What is the normal pattern of head growth in premature infants?

There is no single criterion for "normal" head growth of the premature baby. Many important factors bear on the growth rate: the presence of an intraventricular hemorrhage, nutritional status, and the general physical well-being of the infant as reflected in the presence of respiratory distress syndrome, sepsis, or congenital heart defect. The average rate of head growth for sick premature infants during the first four months of life is 0.25 cm per week. In healthy, growing, feeding, premature babies the average rate of head growth is 1.1 cm per week for the first 2 months of life and decreases to about 0.5 cm per week for the next 2 months.

References: Marks KH, Maisels MJ, Moore E, et al: Head growth in sick premature infants — a longitudinal study. J Pediatr 94:282–285, 1979.

Sher PK, Brown ST: A longitudinal study of head growth in pre-term infants. 1: Normal rates of head growth. Dev Med Child Neurol 17:705–710, 1975.

55. What is Rett syndrome?

Rett syndrome is a newly described neurodegenerative condition that exclusively affects girls. After a normal birth and early infancy, developmental arrest begins around 7 to 18 months of age followed by severe decline of cognitive skills and loss of purposeful hand movements. Once the condition enters a prolonged quiescent stage over decades of life, the individual has profound dementia, microcephaly, ataxia, spastic paraparesis, seizures, and characteristic hand wringing and respiratory stereotypies. The diagnosis is established on clinical grounds and the fundamental cause is unknown.

Reference: Hagberg B, Aicardi J, Dias K, Ramos O: A progressive syndrome of autism, dementia, ataxia and loss of purposeful hand use in girls: Rett's syndrome: Report of 35 cases. Ann Neurol 14: 471–479, 1983.

56. What is the differential diagnosis of acquired torticollis?

One of the early signs of normal motor development is the acquisition of head control. Head position is the result of multiple somatic and neurologic influences which ordinarily result in a properly aligned head carriage. Consequently, many disorders can result in an abnormal head position and produce torticollis:

CNS Causes
    Cerebellar hemisphere tumor
    Herniation of cerebellar tonsils
    Basal ganglia disorders — dystonia
        musculorum deformans, spasmotic
        torticollis, Wilson's disease, etc.
Vestibular Causes
    Benign paraoxysmal torticollis of infancy
    Acute labyrinthitis
Ocular Causes
    Spasmus nutans
    Trochlear nerve palsy

Local Musculature Causes
    Chronic scarring from trauma
    Spasm from local adenopathy or acute
        trauma
    Local tetanus
Cervical Spine Causes
    Bony torticollis (congenital spinal
        abnormalities such as Klippel-Feil
        syndrome)
Systemic Causes
    Retropharyngeal abscess
    Gastroesophageal reflux

57. What is the significance of a burst suppression pattern in an EEG?

The term "burst suppression" refers to a very abnormal EEG pattern observed in a variety of serious diffuse acute encephalopathies such as meningitis, encephalitis, head injury, or hypoxic-ischemic injury. The ongoing EEG activity is no longer uninterrupted and continuous but rather appears as a sudden "burst" of abnormal electrical patterns followed by an abnormal "suppression" of brain waves. This EEG pattern originates from the cerebral cortex, which is no longer operating under the influence or guidance of the midbrain and thalami due to disruption of their connecting fibers. Burst suppression is not specific from an etiologic viewpoint. Many neurologic illnesses can produce it if they are diffuse and sufficiently severe. The significance of a burst suppression EEG is that it indicates an important acute, severe disturbance of brain functioning. Burst suppression is often considered an ominous EEG prognostic sign because many with this abnormality will die and survivors are at high risk for permanent neurologic sequelae. Burst suppression can sometimes appear briefly as an immediate postictal finding that quickly evolves into a less abnormal state. This does not necessarily indicate an unfavorable outcome. The intravenous administration of benzodiazepines to stop status epilepticus can also result in a transient burst suppression background. Similarly, large doses of barbiturates or general anesthesia may cause a reversible burst suppression EEG with an expected return to normalcy after the drug is discontinued. Finally, some children with infantile spasms and a hypsarrhythmic EEG will display a "burst suppression" EEG pattern only during sleep.

58. What is Cushing's law?
Cushing's law dictates that an elevation of intracranial pressure will result in an increase of blood pressure to a point slightly above the pressure exerted on the medulla oblongata.

59. What are the components of Cushing's triad and what is their significance?
Cushing's triad consists of the development of slow or irregular respirations, slow pulse, and elevated blood pressure resulting from an increase of intracranial pressure. Cushing's triad may be observed in children with increased intracranial pressure or compression of the posterior fossa, which houses the medullary circulatory control center.

60. What are the common features of myelomeningocele?
Children with "myelomeningocele" have a complex, multifaceted, congenital disorder of structure which represents a dysraphic state—a defective closure of the embryonic neural groove. In its full expression it is typified anatomically by:
1. The presence of unfused or excessively separated vertebral arches of the bony spine (spina bifida).
2. Cystic dilation of the meninges which surround the spinal cord (meningocele).
3. Cystic dilation of the spinal cord itself (myelocele).
4. A spectrum of congenital *cerebral* abnormalities.

61. Which congenital cerebral disorders are associated with myelomeningocele?
1. A type II Arnold-Chiari malformation may occur in which the hindbrain is abnormal and enclosed in a small posterior fossa. The medulla oblongata and the "tonsils" of the cerebellum are displaced or herniated downward to occupy the normal position of the upper cervical cord. The impaired egress of CSF caused by aqueductal stenosis commonly results in hydrocephalus. Arnold-Chiari malformations sometimes coexist with other abnormalities of the cerebral cortex.
2. More severe cerebral malformations may occur in the maximal expression of the "dysraphic state." Incomplete closure of the cranial bones results in cranium bifidum. Protrusion of abnormal brain tissue through the defective skull bone results in an encephalocele. Gross failure of neural groove fusion results in craniorachischisis, or in its maximal form, anencephaly.
3. Hydrocephalus: 95% of children with thoracic or high lumbar myelomeningocele have associated hydrocephalus. The incidence decreases progressively with more caudal spinal defects to a minimum of 60% if the myelomeningocele is located in the sacrum. Hydrocephalus per se does not cause the mental retardation associated with this syndrome. (Recall that children with appropriately treated congenital hydrocephalus due to simple aqueductal stenosis usually have normal psychomotor development). Mental retardation is usually attributed to acquired secondary CNS infection or subtle microscopic anomalies of neuronal migration and differentiation which may coexist with the macroscopically visible malformation of the hindbrain.

62. What is the prognosis for motor and sensory function of the lower limbs in children with myelomeningocele?
The prognosis depends directly on the level of the spinal lesion. Those with sacral defects will functionally walk with minimal assistive devices. Those with thoracic lesions have extensive motor disability and may possibly learn to walk but only with the use of assistive devices. Regardless of the level of the lesion, most (90%) will lack bowel and bladder control.

63. Can myelomeningocele be diagnosed prenatally?

The fundamental cause of myelomeningocele is unknown. Genetic influences appear to materially modify the risk of affected offspring. Prenatal diagnosis is available in the form of determination of the amniotic fluid level of alpha-fetoprotein. The bony spinal defect can sometime be visualized by prenatal ultrasonography.

Reference: Leonard CO: Counseling parents of a child with meningomyelocele. Pediat Rev 4: 317–322, 1983.

64. What is the differential diagnosis of stridor in a child with meningomyelocele?

Stridor in an infant with meningomyelocele is usually due to dysfunction of the vagus nerve, which innervates the muscles of the vocal cords. In their *resting* position, the edges of the vocal cords meet in the midline. Hence, in bilateral vagal nerve palsies, the free edges of the vocal cords are closely opposed and obstruct air flow, resulting in stridor. In symptomatic patients the motor nucleus of the vagus nerve may be congenitally hypoplastic or aplastic. More commonly, the vagal dysfunction is believed to arise from a mechanical traction injury secondary to hydrocephalus, which produces progressive herniation and inferior displacement of the abnormal hindbrain. Shunting the hydrocephalus may alleviate the traction and improve the stridor. Sometimes the later recurrence of stridor indicates reaccumulation of hydrocephalus due to ventriculo-peritoneal shunt failure.

65. What are the "early" signs of spinal cord compression?

Early spinal cord compression may be easily overlooked before flagrant motor or sensory signs are prominent. Some early clinical clues that may be helpful in detecting spinal cord compression promptly include:

1. Scoliosis producing sustained poor posture.

2. Back pain or abdominal pain that begins abruptly or paroxysmally during *sleep*.

3. Increased sensitivity of the spinal column to local pressure or percussion.

4. In extramedullary tumors that compress the cord, prodromal pains of *radicular* distribution are common because such tumors often arise from the posterior nerve roots themselves.

5. Bowel or bladder dysfunction may be a presenting feature of *sacral* or *conus medullaris* compression.

6. Since the somatotopic organization of sensory fibers places the sacral and lumbar dermatomes nearest to the cord surface, extrinsic compression commonly results first in diminished sensation in the anogenital region and lower limbs.

66. What is the origin of the word "migraine"?

Ancient Greek physicians recognized a specific type of recurring head pain that was unilateral and affected half of the head. The modern word "migraine" is a modification of the archaic term hemicranium.

67. At what age can children begin to have migraine headaches?

About 20% of migraineurs suffer their first headache before the age of 10 years.

68. What are the clinical features of a migraine headache?

1. The attacks of headache are discrete. There is a distinct beginning, middle, and end of the headache. Sleep usually ameliorates the head pain. The patient is entirely well between headaches. Migraine does not usually begin explosively. Explosive-onset headaches should raise the concern of intracranial hemorrhage or pheochromocytoma.

2. In children who are predisposed, a precipitant may trigger the individual headache attack. Lack of sleep, glaring lights, motion, smoke, or specific foods can bring about an attack. For some, migraine is a psychosomatic illness in the sense that stress, worry, or anxiety (the psyche) can bring on a disorder of the body (the soma) in the form of headache.

In contrast, the diagnosis "tension headache" does not connote emotional tension but rather tension of the scalp musculature whose prolonged contraction is the source of the head pain.

3. The pain of migraine is classically unilateral but may be bilateral or diffuse. Most children localize the center of their pain as temporal, frontal, or retro-orbital. The quality of the pain is often described as throbbing, pounding, or hammering, occasionally synchronous with the beating of the heart. Some migraineurs apply pressure to the superficial temporal artery (they hold their heads) to temporarily reduce the pain.

4. Migraine is a systemic disorder. Temporary gastroparesis causes dilatation of the stomach with resulting nausea and vomiting. The appetite is reduced and many become irritable. There may be increased urine output or diarrhea. Edema may cause puffy eyes or bloated fingers. Migraineurs may complain of cold hands or feet, mild fever, tachycardia, or sweating.

69. How common are classic migraines in children?

Some children cannot articulate their symptoms adequately to justify the unequivocal diagnosis of "migraine." Instead, their headaches are labelled "undifferentiated." With the passage of time the diagnosis may be clarified. Most migraineurs have common migraine. A distinct minority have classic migraine with the characteristic visual auras of scintillating scotomas (colorful, shimmering, fluorescent blind spots), fortification phenomena (zigzag, angular, visual hallucinations), or visual obscuration.

70. How should children with migraine be managed?

The first step in successful management is to make a correct diagnosis. If the description of the headache is compatible with migraine, the physical and neurologic examination should be normal. Specifically check the following:

1. Height and weight should be normal for age. Pituitary tumor, craniopharyngioma, or partial ornithine transcarbamylase deficiency may all result in growth failure and yet mimic migraine headache. The head circumference should be normal, thus ruling out hydrocephalus.

2. The skin should be checked for abnormalities. Throbbing headaches are common in individuals with neurofibromatosis or systemic lupus erythematosus. Both of these disorders have easily recognizable skin manifestations.

3. The blood pressure should be normal.

4. No sinus tenderness or pain with head movement (implying cervical spine disease) should be detected. The patient should be examined for the presence of carious teeth, misaligned bite, or disordered chewing and jaw opening, implying the presence of temporomandibular joint dysfunction.

5. The neurologic examination should be normal.

If the physician is comfortable that "migraine" is the basis of the headache, the next question to be considered is how frequent, severe, or disabling the condition is.

1. If the headaches are infrequent and do not materially disrupt the lifestyle or school attendance of the patient, the migraineur should be treated symptomatically with simple analgesics. Sleep is very helpful. If appropriate, specific migraine remedies such as ergotamine tartrate (Cafergot) can be used.

2. If the headaches are frequent or severe enough to functionally disrupt the patient's lifestyle, the physician may consider these options for *prophylactic* treatment:
- Migraine elimination diet (chocolate, nuts, monosodium glutamate, nitrites in processed meats, aged cheese, etc.).
- Biofeedback.
- The most practical treatment is pharmacotherapy available as: ergonovine maleate, propranolol, amitriptyline, calcium channel blockers (verapamil), cyproheptadine (Periactin), clonidine (Catapres), or methysergide.
- Metoclopramide (Reglan) can be used to promote gastric motility and increase speed of absorption of antimigraine medications.

71. What are the clinical findings in cavernous sinus thrombosis?

Within the confined space of the cavernous sinus lie all three cranial nerves which move the eye (oculomotor, trochlear, and abducent nerves) and the upper two divisions of the trigeminal nerve (ophthalmic V_1 and maxillary V_2). The venous drainage of the orbit exits via the cavernous sinus. Orbital infections thus quickly spread to these contiguous venous structures and result in an acute thrombophlebitis. Thrombosis of the venous channels of the cavernous sinus results in desperate systemic illness with fulminant constitutional signs such as fever, headache, prostration, and local signs of proptosis, prominent redness, swelling, and edema of the eyelid and bulbar conjunctiva (chemosis), visual loss, papilledema, ophthalmoplegia (due to dysfunction of cranial nerves III, IV and VI) and paraesthesias, numbness, or local pain in the distribution of V1.

72. What are the clinical findings in lateral sinus thrombosis?

The venous drainage of the deep and superficial structures of the brain is channeled through a series of connecting vascular pathways including the superior sagittal sinus, the inferior sagittal sinus, the occipital sinus, and straight sinus. These major venous drainage pathways meet at the confluence of sinuses (torcular herophili). The *lateral* or *transverse* sinuses connect the torcular herophili to the jugular vein and thus are a major channel for venous exit. Thrombosis of the lateral sinus can result from traumatic skull fracture, thrombophlebitis from suppurative otitis media, mastoiditis, or carcinoma. Slowed venous flow and coagulation may be seen in the context of congenital heart disease, dehydration, hypotension, polycythemia, leukemia, hypernatremia, or obstruction of the superior vena cava or jugular veins. As a result of obstructed venous outflow, the reabsorption of CSF in the subarachnoid villi of the superior sagittal sinus is impeded and intracranial pressure increases. The subsequent clinical picture features the usual signs and symptoms of intracranial hypertension and commonly ear pain on the side of the thrombosed lateral sinus. If there is retrograde propagation of the venous clot, progressive focal neurologic signs and seizures may also develop, reflecting sequential necrosis of brain tissue.

73. What are the characteristic features of pseudotumor cerebri?

The condition pseudotumor cerebri (PTC) produces an increase of ICP in the absence of a demonstrable mass lesion. The characteristic features include:
1. Headache, fatigue, vomiting, anorexia, stiff neck, and diplopia from increased ICP.
2. A normal neurologic examination except for papilledema or a sixth nerve palsy.
3. A normal CT scan except sometimes for small ventricles.
4. Normal CSF profile with the exception of an elevated opening pressure.

74. What causes pseudotumor cerebri?

Although there are multiple possible causes, over 90% of cases are "idiopathic." Among the reported causes are:
1. Drugs: tetracycline, nalidixic acid, nitrofurantoin, corticosteroids, and excess vitamin A.
2. Endocrinologic disorders: many affected patients are obese women with irregular menstrual periods. Hypoparathyroidism and Turner's syndrome are rare causes.
3. Thrombosis of the dural venous sinuses due to head trauma, otitis media, mastoiditis, or obstruction of the jugular veins in the superior vena cava syndrome.

75. What morbidity is associated with pseudotumor cerebri?

Visual loss. Patients with well-developed papilledema may complain of fleeting visual loss (obscurations) that may be accentuated by the Valsalva maneuver or by standing up. This sign is believed to represent reduction of optic nerve blood flow due to arterial compression. Visual obscurations do not necessarily imply imminent "stroke" of the optic nerves.

76. What treatment is recommended for severe cases of pseudotumor cerebri?

Patients with sustained visual field loss or severe refractory headache are candidates for treatment. Specific treatment depends on the presence of an identifiable etiology which should be removed when possible. For example, the cessation of the offending medication such as tetracycline or weight reduction in obese patients is recommended. Nonspecific treatment includes the administration of acetazolamide, furosemide, or hydrochlorothiazide and sometimes corticosteroids. In severe cases surgical intervention is available in the form of the installation of a lumboperitoneal shunt or optic nerve sheath decompression.

77. What are the tubers of tuberous sclerosis?

Tuberous sclerosis is a classic member of a family of disorders called phakomatoses, whose distinctive malformations of the nervous system are associated with small tumors (phakomas or lentil-like neoplasia of skin, eye, and brain). The brain may be dysplastic. The neurons themselves may appear microscopically abnormal, giant, or bizarre. The macroscopic disorganization of the brain may result in circumscribed, nodular *cortical* malformations which are firm to the touch. The tuber ("potato") is a nest of bizarre monstrous neurons or giant glial cells on the cortical surface. CT scans in tuberous sclerosis often reveal rounded, calcified deposits that lie along the wall of the ventricle. These are due to small, subependymal, calcified nodules of astrocytes called "candle gutterings."

78. What is a shagreen patch and what is its significance?

The diagnosis of tuberous sclerosis is usually entertained in the triad of mental retardation, epilepsy, and characteristic skin lesions. The cutaneous signs include adenoma sebaceum, hypopigmented macules (also called ashleaf spots or nevi anemici), and the shagreen patch ("peau de chagrin"). This cutaneous lesion is usually found in the lumbosacral area, is raised, pigmented, and irregular, and resembles coarsely grained leather.

79. Name the three forms of the disease complex of von Recklinghausen's neurofibromatosis and describe the features of each.

1. A *peripheral* form with multiple peripheral nerve sheath tumors is associated with café-au-lait spots, axillary freckling, lisch iris nodules and other physical stigmata. The peripheral form is the most common, and is frequently associated with nontumorous neurologic complications including macrocephaly, headaches, mental retardation, learning disabilities, attention deficit disorder, and seizures. Gliomas of the optic nerve, chiasm, hemispheres, or brainstem are the most common types of associated tumors.

2. A *central* form features multiple intracranial and intraspinal tumors. There is a rare form of neurofibromatosis described in a limited number of kindreds. In the central form of neurofibromatosis, schwannomas, also called neurinomas or neurilemmomas, envelop the axons of the peripheral nerve roots as they leave the central nervous system. Within the cranial cavity the acoustic nerve, particularly its vestibular branch, is most commonly involved. A typical feature is bilateral acoustic schwannomas. Multiple tumors may be present. In the spinal cord, Schwann cell tumors may develop on the spinal nerve roots and multiple meningiomas may be present.

3. A *visceral* form in which ganglioneuromas and nerve sheath tumors involve the viscera and autonomic nerve system may be associated with peripheral neuroblastomas, adrenal ganglioneuromas, and pheochromocytomas.

80. What endocrine abnormalities are seen in patients with craniopharyngioma prior to treatment?

Craniopharyngiomas are relatively common tumors which are believed to develop from nests of squamous cells which embryologically originate near the junction of the infundibular stalk and the adenohypophysis. Many believe these collections of epidermal cells represent the vestigial remnants of Rathke's pouch. Craniopharyngiomas are among the most common supratentorial tumors in childhood. Due to their sensitive location deep at the brain's base, the clinical presentation features:

1. Growth failure from a primary reduction of growth hormone output due to compression of the pituitary gland or hypothalamus. Subclinical hypothyroidism from inadequate production of TSH may also be seen.

2. Visual disturbances are common and include optic atrophy, papilledema, or visual field cut due to compression of the optic tracts and chiasm.

3. Headaches are attributed to increased intracranial pressure with or without hydrocephalus.

4. Enuresis, polydipsia, or polyuria from diabetes inspidus.

81. Which spinal segments do each of the common reflexes test?

Localizations of Reflexes

DEEP TENDON REFLEX	SUPERFICIAL REFLEX	PERIPHERAL NERVE	SEGMENTAL ORGANIZATION
	Pupillary	Optic/oculomotor	CN II-III
Jaw jerk		Trigeminal	CN-V
	Corneal	Trigeminal/facial	CN V-VII
	Gag	Glossopharyngeal/ vagal	CN IX-X
Biceps		Musculocutaneous	C5-C6
Brachioradialis		Radial	C5-C6
Triceps		Radial	C6-C7-C8
Finger flexion		Median/ulnar	C7-T1
Abdominal reflex		Thoracic	T8-T12
	Umbilical	Thoracic	T8-T12
	Cremasteric	Genitofemoral	L1-L2
Adductor		Femoral/obturator	L2-L4
Quadriceps		Femoral	L2-L3-L4
Gastrocsoleus		Sciatic	L5-S2
	Plantar reflex	Sciatic	S1-S2
	Anal wink	Pudendal	S3-S4-S5

82. What is the difference between a muscle fibrillation and fasciculation?

The anatomical unit of histological organization of striated skeletal muscle is the *fiber*, microscopically visible as a long cylindrical cell with numerous nuclei dispersed along its length. Numerous parallel fibers are grouped together into *fascicles*, visible to the naked eye. The functional unit of organization of skeletal muscle is the *motor unit* which includes (1) the anterior horn cell or alpha motor neuron, whose cell body lies in the ventral gray mass of the spinal cord; (2) its axon, which leaves the cord in the ventral root and courses in the peripheral nerve wrapped in its myelin sheath; and (3) several target muscle fibers within the same fascicle. Thus, the smallest natural amount of muscle activity is the firing of one motor neuron, producing contraction of its multiple target fibers.

Some neuromuscular diseases affect the nerve cell body, axon, or muscle fibers to generate small, local, spontaneous muscular twitches or contractions called fibrillations or fasciculations. A fibrillation is the spontaneous contraction of an *individual muscle fiber*. It produces no shortening of the muscle and cannot be observed through the skin but may rarely be visible in the tongue. Fibrillations are detected by an electromyographic (EMG) examination and recognized as irregular, asynchronous, brief (1–5 milliseconds), low voltage (20–300 microvolts), electrical discharges of the muscle fiber that recur with a frequency of 1 to 30 per second. They usually arise in the setting of denervation from injury to the cell body or axon but may also occur in primary disorders such as myopathy.

A fasciculation is the spontaneous, relatively synchronous contraction of *numerous fibers within a fascicle* which belong to the same motor unit. The contraction may produce a visible movement of the muscle and can be seen through the skin. On EMG examination the electrical discharge of the fasciculation is distinctly longer (8–20 msec) and has a higher voltage (2–6 mV) than the fibrillation potential. Fasciculations recur at irregular intervals with a frequency of 1 to 50 per minute. Benign fasciculations in the calf and small muscles of the hands or feet can be seen in some healthy people. Fasciculations are not characteristic of primary muscle diseases. They are usually associated with denervation of any cause but are especially prominent in disorders of anterior horn cells such as Werdnig-Hoffmann disease.

83. What are the symptoms and signs of neonatal myasthenia gravis? How is persistence of symptoms treated?

Passively acquired neonatal myasthenia. Infants born to myasthenic mothers may be the recipients of an immunoglobulin that crosses the placenta and binds to the acetylcholine receptor protein (AchRP) of striated muscle. Signs and symptoms of weakness occur in about 12% of affected offspring and typically arise within the first hours or days of life. Pathologic muscle fatigability commonly causes feeding difficulty, generalized weakness, hypotonia, and respiratory depression. Ptosis and impaired eye movements occur in only 15% of cases. The weakness virtually always resolves as the body burden of anti-AchRP immunoglobulin diminishes. Symptoms typically persist about 2 weeks but may require several months to disappear entirely. General supportive treatment is usually adequate, but oral or IM neostigmine may help to diminish symptoms.

Congenital myasthenia presents primarily with extraocular muscle and facial weakness and commonly persists through childhood. Generalized weakness does not occur until later in infancy. Although the mother is not myasthenic, other siblings may be similarly affected, and an autosomal recessive inheritance is suspected. The daily use of neostigmine may be symptomatically helpful.

Familial infantile myasthenia also occurs in siblings, although the mother is not myasthenic. The clinical presentation is severe, congenital, generalized weakness and flaccidity with preserved extraocular movements. The weakness responds to neostigmine and usually subsides within a few weeks only to resurface during a myasthenic crisis in later infancy.

84. How can neonatal myasthenia gravis be differentiated from infant botulism?

Very few cases of botulism have been reported in neonates. Symptoms have always occurred after discharge from the neonatal nursery. Botulism is usually heralded by constipation followed by early facial and pharyngeal weakness, ptosis, and *dilated, sluggishly reactive* pupils with diminished deep tendon reflexes. The injection of Tensilon does not improve muscle strength. EMG examination demonstrates distinctive abnormalities such as brief small amplitude polyphasic potentials (BSAPs) and an incremental response in the amplitude of evoked muscle potentials to repetitive nerve stimulation. Stool cultures may be positive for the toxin or clostridia organism in the feces.

Myasthenia gravis usually presents at birth or within the first few days of life. There may be a family history of myasthenia in the mother or siblings. The distribution of weakness depends on the specific subtype of myasthenia but pupils and deep tendon reflexes are spared. The EMG examination shows a distinctive progressive decline in the amplitude of compound motor action potentials with repetitive stimulation of the nerve. Tensilon temporarily improves the patient's clinical strength and also abolishes the pathologic EMG response to repetitive stimulation.

85. How does infant botulism differ from botulism in adults?

Adult botulism usually results from the ingestion of preformed toxin produced in contaminated foods by the microorganism *Clostridium botulinum*. Adult botulism usually produces a *descending* paralysis with the following evolution of weakness: blurred vision (due to paralysis of the muscles of accommodation), ptosis, diplopia, dysphagia, dysphonia, dyspnea, and limb weakness. This contrasts with the classic evolution of weakness in Guillain-Barré syndrome, which usually produces an *ascending* paralysis and sometimes sensory disturbances such as painful dysesthesias.

Infantile botulism presents as a gradual, progressive, hypotonic areflexic weakness due to colonization of the GI tract by the Clostridium microorganism, which then elaborates the paralyzing toxin *in situ*. Constipation and poor feeding are the harbingers of ptosis, faulty head control, and eventual weakness of the bulbar and somatic musculature.

86. What are some of the common systemic causes of hypotonia?

Hypotonia is a common but nonspecific sign in neonates and young infants.

1. It may represent a nonspecific sign in any acute serious medical illness such as sepsis, shock, dehydration, or hypoglycemia.

2. It may be encountered in the context of chromosomal abnormalities such as Down's syndrome.

3. It may represent a disturbance of connective tissue, producing excessive joint laxity.

4. It is commonly encountered in metabolic encephalopathies such as hypothyroidism, Lowe's syndrome, or Canavan's disease.

5. It may indicate the presence of a CNS disorder such as cerebellar dysfunction, acute spinal cord disease, neuromuscular disorder, hypotonic cerebral palsy, or benign congenital hypotonia.

In the absence of an acute encephalopathy the differential diagnosis of hypotonia is best approached by asking the question: Does the patient have normal strength despite the hypotonia or is the patient weak and hypotonic? The combination of weakness and hypotonia usually points to an abnormality of the anterior horn cell or the peripheral neuromuscular apparatus.

87. How should a patient with newly diagnosed Landry-Guillain-Barré (LGB) syndrome be monitored?

LGB (acute idiopathic polyradiculoneuritis) is the most common acute or subacute polyneuropathy encountered in clinical practice. The fundamental neuropathology is the presence of multifocal areas of inflammatory demyelination of nerve roots and peripheral nerves. As a result of the loss of the healthy myelin covering that embraces the axon of the peripheral nerve, the conduction of nerve impulses (action potentials) may be blocked or dispersed. The resulting clinical effects are predominantly motor — the evolution of flaccid, areflexic paralysis. There is a variable degree of motor weakness. Some have mild brief weakness, whereas fulminant paralysis occurs in others. Sensory symptoms such as painful dysesthesias are not uncommon but are overshadowed by the motor signs.

Early clinical monitoring is focused on the development of bulbar or respiratory insufficiency. Bulbar weakness features unilateral or bilateral facial weakness, diplopia, hoarseness, drooling, depressed gag reflex, or dysphagia. Frank respiratory insufficiency may be preceded by air hunger, dyspnea, or a soft muffled voice (hypophonia). The autonomic nervous system is occasionally involved as signified by the presence of labile blood pressure and body temperature. The contemporary management of LGB includes the following:

1. Observation in an intensive care unit with frequent monitoring of vital signs.

2. The early institution of plasmapheresis where available.

3. In the presence of bulbar signs, the patient is placed NPO and the mouth is suctioned frequently. Hydration is maintained intravenously and nutritional support provided by NG feedings.

4. The vital capacity is measured frequently. In children, the normal vital capacity (VC) may be calculated as: $VC = 200 \text{ cc} \times \text{age (in years)}$. If the vital capacity falls below 25% of normal, endotracheal intubation is carried out. Careful pulmonary toilet is conducted in an attempt to minimize atelectasis, aspiration, and pneumonia.

5. Meticulous nursing care includes careful positioning of the patient to prevent pressure sores, compression of peripheral nerves, and venous thrombosis.

6. Physical therapy is conducted to prevent the development of contractures by passive range of movement exercises and splinting to maintain physiologic hand and limb postures until muscle strength returns.

88. What CSF findings are characteristic of LGB?

The classic CSF finding is LGB is the "albuminocytologic dissociation." Most common infections or inflammatory processes generate an elevation of white blood cell count *and* protein. The CSF profile in LGB includes a normal cell count with elevated protein, usually in the range of 50 to 100 mg %. At the onset of disease, however, the CSF protein may be normal until protein elevation evolves during the early weeks of the illness.

89. What is the differential diagnosis of a polyneuropathy?

Acute polyneuropathy is usually caused by the Guillain-Barré syndrome. However, acute intermittent porphyria, diphtheritic neuropathy, and arsenic or thallium poisoning may also produce an acute polyneuropathy. Chronic polyneuropathy may be subdivided into those conditions that produce pure sensory disturbances, or a mixture of sensory and motor signs as described in the tables below.

Chronic Sensory Neuropathies

CLINICAL PRESENTATION	POTENTIAL ETIOLOGIES
Sensory Loss Only	
All sensory modalities	Toxins* (drugs, metals, industrial solvents)
(+/− ataxia)	Hereditary sensory neuropathy type II
	Carcinoma
	Vitamin E deficiency
	Tabes dorsalis
Limited sensory modalities	Hereditary sensory neuropathy type I
(pain and temperature only)	Congenital sensory neuropathy
	Diabetes mellitus
	Decrease in alpha lipoprotein
	Leprosy
Autonomic nervous system	Riley-Day syndrome
(dysautonomia and reduced pain and	Diabetes mellitus
temperature sensation)	Fabry's disease
	Amyloidosis
Mixed Sensory and Motor Chronic Polyneuropathy	
Primary axonal damage	Nutritional
(slightly reduced nerve conduction	Drugs
velocities; reduced amplitude of	Toxins*
compound action potentials and reduced	Hereditary motor and sensory neuropathy
amplitude of sensory action potentials	type III
with denervation of muscles)	Vasculitis
	Diabetes mellitus
	Uremia
	Carcinoma
Primary demyelination	Hereditary motor and sensory neuropathy
(markedly slow nerve conduction	type I or II
velocities with reduced or dispersed	Multiple myeloma
action potential without evidence of	Refsum's disease
muscle denervation)	Metachromatic leukodystrophy
	Krabbe's disease
	Nieman-Pick disease

*Examples of toxins that may produce neuropathy:

Isoniazid	Hydralazine	Nitrofurantoin	Kanamycin
Vincristine	Insecticides	Arsenic	Lead
Mercury	Phenytoin	Acrylamide	Dapsone
Nitrous oxide	Metronidazole	Chlorambucil	

90. What are hereditary neuropathies?

Some disorders of the peripheral nerve are not the result of acquired disorders such as diabetes or acute inflammation but rather result from an inherited molecular or biochemical disturbance. Although relatively uncommon, they collectively account for a substantial percentage of neuropathies that are supposedly "idiopathic." They present as a chronic, slowly progressive, noninflammatory degeneration of the nerve cell body, peripheral axon or Schwann cells (myelin). The neurologic consequences may be predominantly sensory (e.g., congenital insensitivity to pain), predominantly motor (e.g., spinal muscular atrophy or Werdnig-Hoffmann disease), or mixed motor and sensory abnormalities (e.g., Charcot-Marie-Tooth).

91. What are the clinical signs of Werdnig-Hoffmann disease?

The hallmark of Werdnig-Hoffmann disease is gradual progressive muscle weakness, hypotonia, and areflexia. As the anterior horn cells of the spinal cord wither and die, the voluntary somatic musculature weakens and atrophies. The resulting clinical picture features an awake baby (the third cranial nerve is not affected so the eyes remain open and eye movements are preserved) with a facial diplegia (cranial nerve VII), open jaw (weakness of cranial nerve V), drooling (dysfunction of cranial nerves VII, IX, and X), and a small, weak, fasciculating tongue (denervation of cranial nerve XII). There are a few feeble movements of the distal extremities, and the legs are habitually positioned in a resting "frog-leg" posture. The anal sphincter and anal wink reflex remain operational. Early in the disease the cry weakens to a muffle, respirations become "paradoxical," and death follows aspiration or chronic respiratory insufficiency.

92. What are the common causes of peripheral seventh nerve palsy?

Facial weakness due to a lesion of the facial nerve (cranial nerve VII) is common. The facial weakness involves both the upper and lower face and affects both emotional and volitional facial movements. Any part of the nerve can be disturbed: the nucleus itself, the axon as it passes through the substance of the pons, or the peripheral portion of the nerve. Common etiologies include:

1. Trauma
2. Developmental hypoplasia or aplasia including the Möbius anomalad.
3. Bell's palsy (usually idiopathic but may follow nonspecific viral infections).
4. Infections including the Ramsey-Hunt syndrome (herpes zoster invasion of the geniculate ganglion producing herpetic vesicles behind the ear and painful paralysis of facial nerve); Lyme disease; local invasion from suppurative mastoiditis or otitis media; mumps, varicella or enterovirus neuritis; sequelae of bacterial meningitis; and parotid gland infection, inflammation, or tumor.
5. Guillain-Barré syndrome.
6. Tumor of the brainstem or cerebellar pontine angle tumors.
7. Inflammatory disorders such as sarcoidosis.

Bibliography

1. Barlow C: Headaches and Migraine in Childhood. Philadelphia, J.B. Lippincott Co., 1985.
2. Bell WF, McCormick F: Increased Intracranial Pressure in Children, 2nd ed. Philadelphia, W.B. Saunders, 1978.
3. Bell WF, McCormick F: Neurologic Infections in Children, 2nd ed. Philadelphia, W.B. Saunders, 1981.
4. Fenichel G: Neonatal Neurology, 2nd ed. New York, Churchill Livingstone, 1985.
5. Holmes GL: Diagnosis and Management of Seizures in Children. Philadelphia, W.B. Saunders, 1987.
6. Menkes JH: Textbook of Child Neurology, 3rd ed. Philadelphia, Lea and Febiger, 1985.
7. Swaiman KF: Pediatric Neurology: Principles and Practice. St. Louis, C.V. Mosby, 1989.
8. Volpe J: Neurology of the Newborn, 2nd ed. Philadelphia, W.B. Saunders, 1987.
9. Weiner HL, Levitt LP: Pediatric Neurology for the House Officer, 3rd ed. Baltimore, Williams and Wilkins, 1988.

ONCOLOGY

Beverly Lange, M.D.

1. What are favorable and unfavorable prognostic indicators in childhood leukemia?

Prognostic Factors in Acute Lymphoblastic Leukemia

FACTOR	FAVORABLE	UNFAVORABLE
WBC	$<10,000/mm^3$	$>10,000/mm^3$
Age	2–10 years	<1 yr, >10 yrs
Immunophenotype	CALLA+, non-T cell	CALLA−, SIG+, Cyμ+, T cell
Morphology	L1	L2, L3
Chromosomes	Normal	Translocations: t9;22, t4;11, t8;14, t2;8, t8;22, t1;19
DNA content	Normal or hyperdiploid	Hypodiploid, haploid
Bulky disease	Absent	Present
Sex	Female	Male

Reference: Bleyer WA, et al: The staging of childhood acute lymphoblastic leukemia: strategies of the Children's Cancer Study Group and a three-dimensional technic of multivariate analysis. Med Pediatr Oncol 14:271–280, 1986.

Prognostic Factors in Acute Nonlymphoblastic Leukemia

FACTOR	FAVORABLE	UNFAVORABLE
WBC	$<100,000$	$>100,000$
Age	<17 years	>60 years
Morphology	Myelocytic	Monocytic
Chromosomes	Normal, t8;21, 47 + 8	$-x, -y, -7, -5$
Onset	Abrupt	Preleukemia, myelodysplasia, secondary leukemia

Reference: Grier HE et al: Prognostic factors in childhood acute myelogenous leukemia. J Clin Oncol 5:1026–1032, 1987.

2. Why do infants with acute leukemia under 1 year of age have a worse prognosis than older children?

Infants tend to have leukemias that are biologically different from the usual common acute lymphoblastic leukemia. They may have unfavorable translocations, i.e., t4;11 or t9;11, or lack CALLA surface antigen. Both these features are found in mixed lineage or biphenotypic leukemias. They often have high white counts and bulky extramedullary disease at diagnosis; CNS relapse is quite frequent. The younger the infant, the worse the outlook.

Reference: Reamon G et al: Acute lymphoblastic leukemia in infants less than one year of age. J Clin Oncol 3:1513–21, 1985.

3. What is the most common malignant neoplasm of childhood?

Acute lymphoblastic leukemia.

4. What is the most common solid malignancy of childhood?

As a group, brain tumors. Astrocytomas are the most common brain tumors. Primitive neuroectodermal tumors (PNET), such as medulloblastoma and ependymoma, are next most frequent.

5. Which neoplasms are associated with hemihypertrophy?

Wilms' tumor, hepatoblastoma, and adrenal cortical carcinoma are associated with hemihypertrophy either as part of Beckwith-Wiedemann syndrome or in isolation. One to 3% of Wilms' tumor patients have hemihypertrophy.

Reference: Breslow NE, Beckwith JB: Epidemiological features of Wilms tumor: results of the National Wilms Tumor Study. J Natl Cancer Inst 68:429–436, 1982.

6. What cancers are associated with Down's syndrome? Klinefelter's syndrome? Fanconi's anemia? 13q− syndrome?

Down's syndrome. Children with Down's syndrome have a 1 in 95 chance or 30-fold increased risk of developing acute leukemia. They have an extraordinary risk of developing acute megakaryoblastic leukemia, especially in the neonatal period or early infancy. They are at slightly increased risk of developing retinoblastoma and testicular germ cell tumors.

References: Wilson MG, Ebbin AJ, et al: Chromosomal anomalies in patients with retinoblastoma. Clin Genet 12:1, 1977.

Saka Shita C, Koyanagi T, et al: Congenital anomalies in children with testicular germ cell tumors. J Urol 124:889–891, 1980.

Klinefelter's syndrome. Patients with Klinefelter's are also at risk for developing germ cell tumors of the testes and mediastinum and possibly acute nonlymphocytic leukemia.

Reference: Nuits-Homsma SHM, Muller H, Pad Geraedst JPM: Klinefelter's syndrome and acute non-lymphocytic leukemia. Blut 44:15–20, 1981.

Fanconi's anemia. Patients with Fanconi's anemia are at increased risk for acute nonlymphocytic leukemia, hepatoma (following androgen therapy), and squamous cell carcinoma of the mucosal surfaces.

Reference: Ortonne J, et al.: Squamous cell carcinomas in Fanconi anemia. Arch Dermatol 117:443–444, 1981.

13q− syndrome. Patients with 13q14 deletion are at risk for retinoblastoma, pinealblastoma, and osteogenic sarcoma.

Reference: Kitchin FD, Ellsworth RM: Pleiotrophic effects of the gene for retinoblastoma. J Med Genet 11:244–246, 1974.

7. How is neuroblastoma classified and what is the prognosis for each clinical stage?

International Classification of Neuroblastoma

Stage I:	Localized tumor grossly excised with or without microscopic residual disease; lymph nodes negative microscopically.
Stage IIA:	Unilateral tumor incompletely excised with lymph nodes negative microscopically.
Stage IIB:	Unilateral tumor completely or incompletely excised with positive ipsilateral regional lymph nodes; identifiable contralateral lymph nodes negative microscopically.
Stage III:	Tumor infiltrating across the midline incompletely excised with or without lymph node involvement; or unilateral tumor with contralateral regional lymph node involvement.
Stage IV:	Dissemination of tumor to distant lymph nodes, bone marrow, bone, liver and/or other organs.
Stage IVS:	Localized primary tumor as defined for Stage I or IIA with dissemination limited to liver, skin, or bone marrow in an infant ≤12 months of age.

Patients with Stage I or II disease have nearly a 90% chance of cure with surgery alone. Children whose disease is not controlled with surgery frequently have unfavorable biologic features such as unfavorable histology (i.e., many mitotic figures and/or karyorrhexis), an elevated serum ferritin and/or an amplified N-myc cellular oncogene.

Patients with Stage III disease have a 50% chance of cure with surgery, radiation, and chemotherapy. Their prognosis is also determined by biologic features at diagnosis.

Patients with Stage IV disease have about a 20% chance of long-term survival. Age is an especially important prognostic variable in that those under 1 year have a considerably better outlook.

Patients with Stage IVS disease have greater than an 80% chance of long-term survival with supportive care alone. Infants under age 6 weeks may die of liver failure or mechanical problems related to a big liver. Few patients with stage IVS disease actually progress to typical Stage IV disease with bone and extensive marrow involvement.

Reference: Brodeur GM, Seeger RC, et al: International criteria for diagnosis, staging and response to treatment in patients with neuroblastoma. In Advances in Neuroblastoma Research. New York, Alan Liss, in preparation.

8. What are the indications for granulocyte transfusions in the infected granulocytopenic cancer patient?

The only established indication for granulocyte transfusion in the febrile neutropenic cancer patient is a blood culture persistently positive for gram-negative bacteria in a patient receiving appropriate antibiotics. The use of granulocytes in typhlitis, abscesses, pneumonitis, fungemia, or persistent fever is not established.

Reference: Alavi JB, et al: Leukocyte transfusions in acute leukemia. N Engl J Med 296:706–711, 1977.

9. What is the best way to monitor the cardiac toxicity associated with chemotherapy?

Cardiac toxicity is usually associated with the anthracyclines, adriamycin, and daunomycin. It is most important not to exceed doses known to be associated with cardiomyopathy, and to estimate a one-third increase in "effective cardiotoxic dose" if the heart has been irradiated. Reduction in shortening fraction in face of an adequate preload suggests early damage. It is generally recommended to perform an echocardiogram before anthracycline is begun, at 200 mg/m^2, 300 mg/m^2, 400 mg/m^2 and at each 50 mg/m^2 thereafter and 1 year after therapy stops. There is no formula for predicting when heart failure will occur in a given individual. The risk of clinical myocardiopathy is about 5% at 450-500 mg/m^2. Infusion therapy rather than bolus therapy may increase the tolerance to high doses.

10. What childhood solid tumors are capable of completely replacing the marrow?

Neuroblastoma, non-Hodgkin's lymphoma, and less commonly rhabdomyosarcoma, Ewing's tumor, and medulloblastoma can replace the marrow. Hodgkin's disease affects the marrow in a patchy distribution. Carcinomas are rare in children but may replace the marrow when they occur.

11. What are leukemic lines and how can they be differentiated from growth arrest lines?

Leukemic lines are transverse bands of diminished density at the end of the metaphyses of long bones. These lines are a nonspecific finding and may occur in major illnesses as a manifestation of poor health and suboptimal bone metabolism.

Reference: Wilson JKV: The bone lesions of childhood leukemia: A survey of 140 cases. Radiology 72:672, 1959.

12. Which children with acute lymphoblastic leukemia (ALL) should receive cranial irradiation? Why?

In the 1970s virtually all children with ALL were treated with prophylactic cranial irradiation to prevent CNS leukemia. However, irradiation causes learning problems in young children. More recently it has been shown that many children can be treated with repetitive instillations of intrathecal methotrexate and/or cytosine arabinoside. High doses of intravenous methotrexate and Ara-C may also have a protective effect on the CNS. Any child who has overt leukemic meningitis probably needs craniospinal irradiation or extraordinary doses of chemotherapeutic agents that penetrate into the meninges. Some children with very high white counts or rare lymphomatous parenchymal brain disease require radiation therapy. Chemotherapy alone is effective prophylaxis for most patients, but it has not yet been demonstrated to eradicate established disease.

References: Meadows AT, Massari DJ, et al: Declines in IQ scores and cognitive dysfunctions in children with acute lymphocytic leukaemia treated with cranial irradiation. Lancet 1015-1018, 1981.

Sullivan MP, Chen T, et al: Equivalence of intrathecal chemotherapy and radiotherapy as central nervous system prophylaxis in children with acute lymphatic leukemia: A pediatric oncology group study. Blood 60:948–958, 1982.

13. What percentage of children with ALL can successfully achieve a first remission?

Almost all (98%) children with ALL achieve remission with combination chemotherapy. Some require only vincristine, prednisone, and L-asparaginase; others with unfavorable features may require additional therapy such as daunomycin.

Reference: Bleyer WA, et al: The staging of childhood acute lymphoblastic leukemia: strategies of the Children's Cancer Study Group and a three-dimensional technic of multivariate analysis. Med Pediatr Oncol 14:271–280, 1986.

14. What is the duration of the first remission in ALL and acute myelogenous leukemia? How does the prognosis change in children who relapse?

The majority of children with ALL survive relapse-free, so the median duration of first remission has not been reached. If relapse occurs in the CNS or testes, many children can still be cured with irradiation and additional chemotherapy. If relapse occurs in the marrow within 18 months of diagnosis, the chance of cure with either chemotherapy or marrow transplant is less than 10%. If marrow relapse occurs later than 18 months from diagnosis, and especially if it occurs after treatment has been stopped, intense chemotherapy or marrow transplant may offer prolonged second remission and possibly cure to over 25% of patients.

Between 70 and 75% of children with acute myeloid leukemia achieve remission; median remission duration is about 14 months. About 10% of the patients die from infectious or hemorrhagic complications during induction and another 10–20% fail to respond to the initial therapy. Of the children who achieve remission, between 40–50% survive 5 years. If disease recurs, it is usually fatal. Transplant may cure some patients who relapse.

References: Creutzig U, Ritter J, et al.: Improved treatment results in childhood acute myelogenous leukemia: A report of the German cooperative study. AML-BFM. Blood 78:298–304, 1985.

Steuber CP: Therapy in childhood acute nonlymphocytic leukemia (ANLL). Am J Pediatr Hematol Oncol 3:379–388, 1981.

15. Following initiation of treatment, what special risk does promyelocytic leukemia carry?

Patients with acute promyelocytic leukemia are prone to hemorrhagic or thrombotic diathesis. This results from release of procoagulant activity from the promyelocytic granules. When disseminated intravascular coagulation (DIC) has started prior to therapy, hemorrhagic problems are the usual presenting chief complaint. These problems are aggravated by treatment. In addition, patients with promyelocytic leukemia are even more prone to fatal infectious complications than other patients with different subtypes of myeloid leukemia. In the past heparin has been used to prevent or treat DIC but is of unproven efficacy. Our current approach is to use blood products such as platelets and plasma to control the intravascular coagulation.

References: Goldberg MA, Ginsburg D, et al: Is heparin administration necessary during induction chemotherapy for patients with acute promyelocytic leukemia? Blood 79:187–191, 1987.

Kantarjian HM, Keating MJ, et al: Acute promyelocytic leukemia. Am J Med 80:789–797, 1986.

Chan KW, Steinherz PG, Miller DR: Acute promyelocytic leukemia in children. Med Pediatr Oncol 9:5–15, 1981.

16. What is the difference between the adult and juvenile types of chronic myelogenous leukemia?

Adult Versus Juvenile Chronic Myelogenous Leukemia

	ADULT CML	JUVENILE CML
General health	Well	Ill
Splenomegaly	Marked	Moderate
Hepatomegaly	Usually absent	Usually present
WBC	>100,000/μm^3	<100,000/μm^3
Differential	Mostly granulocytes	Monocytosis
Platelets	>400,000	<150,000

Table continued on next page.

Adult Versus Juvenile Chronic Myelogenous Leukemia *(Continued)*

	ADULT CML	JUVENILE CML
LAP[A]	Decreased or absent	Normal
Chromosomes	Ph[1]	Normal or −7
Growth *in vitro*	Granulocytic colonies	Monocytic colonies or increased clusters
Median Survival	3 yr	9 mo–1 yr, but variable
Therapy	Bone marrow transplant	Bone marrow transplant

LAP[A] = leukocyte alkaline phosphastase; Ph[1] = Philadelphia chromosome (t9;22)

Cao A: Juvenile chronic myelogenous leukemia. Lancet 1:1002, 1970.
Chessells JM, et al: The Ph chromosome in childhood leukemia. Br J Haematol 41:25–41, 1979.
Nix WL, Ferbach DJ: Myeloproliferative diseases of childhood. Am J Pediatr Hematol Oncol 3:397–407, 1981.

17. Which childhood cancers can be successfully treated with bone marrow transplantation?

1. Chronic myeloid leukemia in chronic phase
2. Preleukemic syndromes
3. Acute myeloid leukemia in first or second remission
4. Acute lymphoblastic leukemia failing induction, or in second or possibly third remission
5. Non-Hodgkin's lymphoma in second remission
6. Neuroblastoma in first or second remission
7. Multiply relapsed Hodgkin's disease

Transplantation for all diseases except acute leukemia and chronic myeloid leukemia is still investigational.

Reference: Report of an International Cooperative Study: Bone-Marrow Autotransplantation in Man. Lancet 960–962, 1986.

18. What is the age distribution of children with Hodgkin's lymphoma?

Hodgkin's disease is uncommon before 5 years of age, but there are rare cases under 3 years. In North America the peak incidence occurs in the second decade of life with a slight male predominance. It continues into young adulthood and then decreases in frequency until the sixth decade. The sex ratio changes from male predominance to female predominance after 12 years of age.

References: Fraumani JF Jr, Li FP: Hodgkin's disease in childhood: An epidemiologic study. J Natl Cancer Inst 42:681–691, 1969.

Young JL, Miller RW: Incidence of malignant tumors in U.S. children. J Pediatr 86:254-258, 1975.

19. What are the non-Hodgkin's lymphomas?

Non-Hodgkin's lymphomas include a heterogeneous group of malignant solid tumors that are of lymphoid origin. The classification of non-Hodgkin's lymphoma is still disputed. In general, it is divided according to the extent of spread in the body and histology. The disease is either localized or disseminated. Localized tumors are limited to either a node or an area such as the appendix or a tonsil, and may include some regional surrounding nodes. It can also originate in bone. The tumor cells may spread to the bone marrow or spinal fluid much like leukemia, or disseminate throughout the abdomen and pleural space.

Histology is divided into lymphoblastic and nonlymphoblastic types. The most common type of lymphoblastic lymphoma occurs in the mediastinum and probably originates in the thymus. Disease is virtually always disseminated at diagnosis. Nonlymphoblastic lymphomas include Burkitt's lymphoma or peripheral T-cell lymphomas. Burkitt's lymphoma often occurs in the retroperitonium and is usually disseminated. The classification of lymphomas of childhood is very different from that of adults.

20. Which is the most common leukemia in the neonate?

Leukemia in the neonate is always acute and is about equally divided between lymphoid and nonlymphoid leukemia. Those with a non-lymphoid leukemia may undergo spontaneous regression, especially in patients with Down's syndrome.

21. Which tumor has the quickest doubling time?

Burkitt's lymphoma. The generation time of the Burkitt cell is between 24 and 36 hours. However, the actual doubling time is less than that because there is a very high spontaneous cell death rate. Some T-lymphoblastic leukemia/lymphomas have a doubling time similar to that of Burkitt cells.

Reference: Iverion U, Iverion OH, Ziegler JL, et al: Cell kinetics of African cases of Burkitt's lymphoma. Eur J Cancer 8:305–308, 1972.

22. How is Hodgkin's lymphoma classified and what is the prognosis for each category?

Hodgkin's lymphoma, like non-Hodgkin's lymphoma, is classified according to stage of disease and histology.

Ann Arbor Staging

Stage I: A single lymph node region (I) or a single extralymphatic organ or site (I_E).
Stage II: Two or more lymph node regions on the same side of the diaphragm (II).
Stage III: Involvement of lymph node regions on both sides of the diaphragm (III), which may also be accompanied by localized involvement of extralymphatic organ or site (III_E) or by involvement of the spleen (III_S).
Stage IV: Diffuse or disseminated involvement of 1 or more extralymphatic organs or tissues with or without associated lymph node enlargement.

Hodgkin's disease is also staged according to whether or not there are symptoms. Those with no symptoms are referred to as A. Patients with documented fever, involuntary weight loss greater than 10%, and/or night sweats are considered to have B disease. Intractable pruritus may also be a symptom of Hodgkin's disease but is not among the B symptoms used for staging.

Stage is determined both clinically and pathologically. Clinical staging refers to staging that is done without histologic proof. Pathologic staging refers to biopsy proven disease in a given region and usually refers to patients who have had a staging laparotomy and splenectomy to determine the extent of disease. For example, a patient who is symptom-free and who has a positive node in his neck and a mass in the mediastinum but nothing else detectable on physical examination or radiologic studies is said to have *clinical* stage IIA disease. If the patient goes on to have a staging laparotomy and splenectomy, and no disease is found, he would then be considered to have *pathologic* stage IIA disease.

The Rye, New York Histologic Classification*

	LYMPHOCYTES	R/S CELLS	OTHER	INCIDENCE
Lymphocyte predominant	Many	Few	Histiocytes	5%
Nodular sclerosing	Many	Few or many	Bands of refractile fibrosis	70%
Mixed cellularity	Many	Few or many	Eosinophils Histiocytes	20–30%
Lymphocyte depletion	Few	Many	No refractile fibrosis	<5%

*This classification is based on the relative number of lymphocytes and of Reed-Sternberg cells.

The prognosis for children with Hodgkin's disease is excellent in that the majority are cured. For stages I and IIA, the 5-year relapse-free survival is in excess of 80% for patients treated with radiation only and may be in excess of 90% for patients given radiation and chemotherapy. For stage IIB prognosis is less good, especially if there is a massive mediastinal tumor, but 5-year survival is still in excess of 80%. The same survival figures also pertain to stage IIIA disease but treatment generally is more extensive than that for a patient with limited stage II disease. For stage IV disease, 5-year relapse-free survival is in excess of 60–70%.

Reference: Carbone PP, Kaplan HS, et al: Report of the committee on Hodgkin's disease staging classification. Cancer Res 31:1860–1861, 1971.

23. Which tumor carries the greatest risk for tumor lysis syndrome? When is the syndrome most likely to present?

The tumor that carries the greatest risk for tumor lysis syndrome is Burkitt's lymphoma with disseminated intraabdominal and retroperitoneal disease. Tumor lysis syndrome consists of hyperuricemia, hypokalemia, hyperphosphatemia, and hypocalcemia. Rarely, the tumor lysis syndrome occurs before the patient begins treatment, but most often it starts within 24 hours of beginning chemotherapy and may persist for 4 to 5 days. Tumor lysis syndrome can be fatal because of hyperkalemia or hypocalcemia; it can be lessened in severity or prevented by allopurinol, alkalinization, and aggressive hydration at 2–4 times maintenance rates.

Reference: Cohen LF, Bar JE, MaGrath IT, et al: Acute tumor lysis syndrome: A review of 37 patients with Burkitt's lymphoma. Am J Med 68:486–490, 1980.

24. What laboratory monitoring should be done for patients at risk for tumor lysis syndrome?

Laboratory monitoring should include serum sodium, potassium, calcium, phosphorus, BUN, creatinine, uric acid, and urine pH, specific gravity, and volume prior to initiating treatment. Blood pressure and sensorium should be followed. Chemotherapy should not be instituted until there is a urine specific gravity ≤ 1.010 and a pH of ≥ 7.0. These laboratory studies should be repeated 4–6 hours later and then every 4–12 hours, depending on the severity of the abnormalities that follow initiation of treatment. If metabolic abnormalities occur, an echocardiogram and/or EEG may be necessary.

Reference: Cohen LF, Bar JE, MaGrath IT, et al: Acute tumor lysis syndrome: A review of 37 patients with Burkitt's lymphoma. Am J Med 68:486–490, 1980.

25. What are the most common presentations of neuroblastoma?

The most common presentation of neuroblastoma is that of generalized disease in a child less than 5 years of age (88%). Fifty-five percent of children with generalized disease are under age 2. Most children with neuroblastoma are irritable and ill, and they often have exquisite bone pain, proptosis, and periorbital ecchymoses. Seventy percent of neuroblastomas arise in the abdomen; half of these arise in the adrenal and the other half in the parasympathetic ganglia distributed throughout the retroperitonium and the paravertebral area in the chest and neck. The tumor produces and excretes catecholamines, which can cause systemic symptoms such as sweating, hypertension, diarrhea, and irritability. Most neuroblastomas are disseminated. Children with localized neuroblastoma may have symptoms referable to a mass such as Horner's syndrome. Some may have no symptoms but the condition may be detected on a routine newborn examination when an adrenal mass is felt, or on a chest radiograph taken for other reasons where an incidental posterior mediastinal mass is seen.

26. What percentage of patients with neuroblastoma have elevated catecholamines? Which catecholamines are elevated?

About 70% of the neuroblastomas excrete vanillylmandelic acid (VMA) in the urine. If all catecholamine metabolites (VMA, homovanillic acid [HVA], dopamine, epinephrine, norepinephrine or their metabolites) are measured, 95% of patients will have elevated values. A high ratio of HVA to VMA and the absence of any "catecholamine" excretion are considered unfavorable prognostic factors.

Reference: Siegel SE, Laug WE, Harlow PJ, et al: Patterns of urinary catecholamine metabolite excretion. In Neuroblastoma Research. New York, Raven Press, 1980.

27. Which childhood cancers can be congenital?

In a 30-year period at the M.D. Anderson Hospital, there were 423 infant neoplasms, of which 24 (5%) occurred in neonates and could be considered congenital. These were distributed as follows: fibrosarcoma, 8; neuroblastoma, 6; CNS tumors, 3; leukemia, 3; retinoblastoma, 2; histiocytosis X, 1; and malignant melanoma, 1.

Reference: Cangir A, Shallenberger RC, Choroszy M: Malignant neoplasms in neonatal period. Proc Am Soc Clin Oncol 6:A847, 1987.

28. Which childhood cancers are associated with an increased alpha-fetoprotein?

Increased alpha-fetoprotein is associated with germ cell tumors, including endodermal sinus tumors of the ovary and testicular yolk sac carcinoma, hepatocellular tumors, and retinoblastoma. Normally, alpha-fetoprotein is synthesized in the liver, yolk sac, and the GI tract of the fetus. Synthesis usually stops at birth; it disappears with a half-life of 3.5 days. Elevated serum levels are most commonly seen with nonmalignant liver disease. Levels remain elevated for 5–7 weeks after resection of the tumor but persistence beyond that time is suggestive of residual disease.

References: Alpert ME, Uriel J, Nechaud B: Alpha fetoglobulin in the diagnosis of human hepatoma. N Engl J Med 278:984, 1968.

Masopust J, Kithier K, Radl J, et al: Occurrence of fetoprotein in patients with neoplasm and non-neoplastic diseases. Int J Cancer 3:364, 1968.

29. Which congenital anomalies are associated with Wilms' tumor?

Congenital abnormalities associated with Wilms' tumor include genitourinary anomalies (4.4%), hemihypertrophy (2.9%), and aniridia (1.1%). The genitourinary anomalies include hypoplasia of the kidney, fusion or ectopia of the kidney, duplication of the collecting system, and hypospadias. Multiple pigmented nevi and hemangiomas are also associated with hemihypertrophy and Wilms' tumor. Patients with aniridia may have associated eye lesions, mental retardation, or deformities of the skull or the face. Wilms' tumor has also been described in patients with neurofibromatosis.

References: Miller RW, Fraumeni JF, Manning MD: Association of Wilms tumor with aniridia, hemihypertrophy, and other congenital malformations. N Engl J Med 270:922, 1964.

Pendergrass TW: Congenital anomalies in children with Wilms' tumor. Cancer 37:403, 1976.

30. What are the common causes of congestive heart failure in patients with Wilms' tumor?

Heart failure is uncommon in this disease. Heart failure in patients with Wilms' tumor is usually iatrogenic and is most commonly caused by a combination of irradiation and radiomimetic antitumor antibiotics such as adriamycin and actinomycin-D. Radiation alone is unlikely to cause heart failure, but the addition of the cardiac toxic antibiotic adriamycin may add to damage. Actinomycin-D is not cardiotoxic but can contribute to heart damage by its radiomimetic affect. Heart failure can also be caused by the upward spread of a renal vein tumor thrombus to the heart, causing tamponade.

31. What percentage of patients with Wilms' tumor have hematuria?

About 15%.

32. What are favorable prognostic indicators in Wilms' tumor?

The most important prognostic factors include the presence of metastases and tumor histology. In the National Wilms' Tumor Study, patients with no metastatic disease had an actuarial survival of 83%, whereas 31% of those with liver metastases and 5% of children with pulmonary metastases survived. Anaplastic, sarcomatous, or clear cell histology are all unfavorable prognostic factors. Additional unfavorable factors include age over 2 years (especially patients with Wilms' who are not children), positive regional lymph nodes, operative spillage of tumor, large size of the tumor, direct extension within the abdomen, and invasion of extrarenal vessels.

Reference: Breslow NE, Palmer NF, Hill LR, et al: Wilms' tumor prognostic factors for patients without metastases at diagnosis—results of the National Wilms' Tumor Study. Cancer 41:1577, 1978.

33. What are the common bony tumors of childhood and when do they present?

The two common primary tumors of bone in children are osteogenic sarcoma and Ewing's sarcoma. Osteogenic sarcoma most commonly occurs during the adolescent growth spurt. It rarely occurs in young children. Ewing's tumor has a peak incidence in adolescents but may be seen in patients as young as 2–4 years of age. Its incidence increases progressively in the first two decades of life.

34. What is the prognosis for children with osteosarcoma?

In 1989, between 40 and 70% of children with osteosarcoma will be alive without evidence of metastatic disease 2 years after diagnosis if they are treated with amputation or limb-salvage procedure plus multi-agent chemotherapy. Some of these children will develop pulmonary metastasis at a later time, and a proportion of these can be saved with thoracotomy and more chemotherapy. Without the use of chemotherapy, only 20% of the children will be free of metastatic disease 1 year after diagnosis.

Reference: Link M, et al: The effect of adjuvant chemotherapy on relapse-free survival in patients with osteosarcoma of the extremity. N Engl J Med 314:1600–1606, 1986.

35. Osteosarcoma is generally located in which part of the bone?

The metaphyses of long bones of the extremities. Sixty percent of the tumors are located in the metaphyses of the knee, that is, the proximal tibia or distal femur.

36. What are the most frequent sites of origin of rhabdomyosarcomas? What sites of origin have a favorable or unfavorable prognosis?

Head and neck (28%), genitourinary region (21%), extremities (18%), and the orbit (10%). The survival of patients with head and neck tumors ranges from nearly 100% of those with orbital disease to 14% of those with metastatic disease. Virtually all patients with orbital rhabdomyosarcoma are cured of their disease. Most head and neck tumors cannot be resected completely, and there is frequently gross residual tumor left behind after surgery (Group III). Survival in this group is roughly 50%. Most children with genitourinary rhabdomyosarcoma in whom the disease is completely excised surgically will survive. If, however, there is residual disease at surgery (as most commonly occurs), 72% will survive. Those with metastatic disease have a 37% survival. The survival rate has improved somewhat over the past few years.

Reference: Maurer HM, Donaldson M, Gehan EA, et al: The Intergroup Rhabdomyosarcoma Study: Update, November 1978. Natl Cancer Inst Monogr 56:61, 1981.

37. What is the most common secondary tumor in patients with bilateral retinoblastoma?

Osteogenic sarcoma. In the past when the primary tumor was treated with radiation therapy in high doses, the incidence of osteosarcoma was as high as 33% and the tumors were often in the orbit. Without any radiation therapy, only 5% of children with bilateral retinoblastoma develop osteosarcoma, and the osteosarcoma usually occurs in the femur.

Reference: Sagerman RH, Cassady JR, Tretter P, Ellsworth RM: Radiation induced neoplasia following external beam therapy for children with retinoblastoma. Am J Roentgenol Radium Ther Nucl Med 105:529, 1969.

38. What is the mechanism of secondary tumors in children with retinoblastoma?

It is believed to be a genetic linkage on chromosome 13 between a gene that predisposes to osteosarcoma and one that predisposes to retinoblastoma. Alternatively, the gene for the two diseases could be the same. Development of primary tumors is presumed to be a result of deletion of a regulatory gene. This gene has been cloned and sequenced, and the hypothesis can be tested. There is also a dose-response effect of radiation therapy, producing secondary osteosarcoma in the orbit.

Reference: Friend SH, et al: A human DNA segment with properties of the gene that predisposes to retinoblastoma and osteosarcoma. Nature 323:643–646, 1986.

39. Which cancers are most commonly associated with a secondary neoplasm?

Cancers Commonly Associated with a Secondary Neoplasm

PRIMARY TUMORS	SECONDARY TUMORS
Retinoblastoma	Osteosarcoma
	Pinealblastoma
Hodgkin's disease	Acute nonlymphoblastic leukemia
	Non-Hodgkin's lymphoma
	Sarcoma in radiation field
	Thyroid carcinoma
Acute lymphoblastic leukemia	Brain tumors
	Non-Hodgkin's lymphoma
Sarcomas	Sarcomas

40. What role does genetic evaluation have in patients with retinoblastoma?

Patients with retinoblastoma and their families should have genetic counseling. Patients or parents who are suspected to be gene carriers include those with bilateral disease or multiple tumors in one eye, those with a family history of retinoblastoma, and those with one or more affected offspring. With familial retinoblastoma, the risk of disease in subsequent offsprings is 30–50%. Among these offspring, half will have bilateral tumors. In counseling parents of a child with familial retinoblastoma, it is important to discuss the risk of other tumors in patients who are gene carriers. Cure rates for retinoblastoma are excellent; however, osteosarcoma is a more sinister and less curable disease. The risk to the offspring of the patient with unilateral sporadic retinoblastoma or to subsequent offspring of unaffected parents with a negative family history and one affected offspring is relatively low.

Reference: Vogel F: Genetics of retinoblastoma. Hum Genet 52:1, 1979.

41. What diseases can present with leukocoria?

Retinoblastoma
Toxocara canis
Persistent hyperplastic primary vitreous
Coats' disease
Large chorioretinal coloboma
Retinopathy of prematurity (retroenteral fibroplasia)

Congenital cataract
Retinal dysplasia
Medulloepithelioma (diktyoma)
Congenital retinal fold

Reference: French-Howard GL, Ellsworth RM: Differential diagnosis of retinoblastoma: A statistical survey of 500 children. I. Relative frequency of lesions which simulate retinoblastoma. Am J Ophthalmol 610, 1965.

42. Virilization may be associated with which childhood cancer?

The tumors that cause virilism are most commonly those which produce large quantities of dihydroepiandrosterone (DHA), a 17-ketosteroid. Tumors producing testosterone may also cause virilization. Most commonly these are benign tumors of the adrenal; rarely they are malignant. However, the distinction between carcinoma and benign adenoma is frequently difficult. Occasionally males with primary hepatic neoplasms may become virilized because of production of androgens by the tumor.

Reference: Burr IM, Graham T, Sulliven J, et al: A testosterone-secreting tumor of the adrenal producing virilization in a female infant. Lancet 2:643, 1973.

43. Which common germ cell tumors occur in children?

Germ cell tumors are benign or malignant neoplasms that are derived from the primordial germ cells. Teratomas that are mature are benign. The most common germ cell tumor is a histologically benign mature cystic teratoma occurring in the sacrococcygeal area. Germ cell tumors can occur outside the gonads in brain, kidneys, mediastinum, lung, liver, or stomach. Malignant germ cell tumors include embryocarcinomas, choriocarcinomas, teratocarcinomas, endodermal sinus tumors (yolk sac tumor), dysgerminomas, seminomas, and mixed germ cell tumors.

44. What is the most common ovarian tumor of childhood?

Germ cell tumors in girls (in contrast, women develop stromal tumors most commonly). The most frequent ovarian germ cell tumors are dysgerminomas followed by endodermal sinus tumors, teratomas, and mixed germ cell tumors. Stromal tumors are rare.

Reference: Norris HJ, Jensen RD: Relative frequency of ovarian neoplasms in children and adolescents. Cancer 30:713, 1972.

45. Which cancers have a significantly higher incidence in black children? White children?

Wilms' tumor has a higher incidence in black female infants. Ewing's tumor is about 30 times more common in whites than in blacks. Hodgkin's disease is rare in Orientals.

Reference: Cutler SJ, Young JL Jr (eds): Third national cancer survey: incidence data, NCI Mongr. 41, DHEW Pub No. (NIH) 75-787, Washington, D.C., U.S. Government Printing Office, 1975.

46. Are there any known transplacental carcinogens?

Diethylstilbestrol, which was used to prevent spontaneous abortion, has been associated with an increased risk of vaginal cancer in the female offspring. Recently, it has been reported that there is a tenfold increased risk of monoblastic leukemia in the infants of mothers who smoke marijuana. It has been suggested that sedatives and a number of nonhormonal drugs are transplacental carcinogens, but this is not proven. It has also not been proved that cigarette smoke or the use of oral contraceptives are transplacental carcinogens.

47. What is the differential diagnosis of generalized lymphadenopathy?

Infectious Diseases
  Viral
    Infectious mononucleosis
    Cytomegalovirus infection
    Human immunodeficiency virus
    Hepatitis
  Bacterial
    Disseminated streptococcus
    Subacute bacterial endocarditis
    Salmonella
  Parasitic
    Toxoplasmosis
    Malaria
  Fungal
    Brucellosis
    Coccidioidomycosis
    Histoplasmosis
    Mycobacteria infection
    Tuberculosis
  Unknown
    Kawasaki disease

Collagen Vascular
  Juvenile rheumatoid arthritis
  Systemic lupus erythematosus
  Sjogren's syndrome
Drug Reaction
  Phenytoin
  Allopurinol
  Hydralazine
Immunologic
  Chronic granulomatous disease
  Mucocutaneous lymph node syndrome
Other
  Sarcoid
  Generalized reactive hyperplasia
  Sinus histiocytosis
  Benign giant lymphoid hyperplasia
  Castleman's disease
Malignant
  Hodgkin's disease
  Non-Hodgkin's lymphoma
  Neuroblastoma leukemia
  Metastatic tumors

Reference: Zuelzer, Caplan: The child with lymphadenopathy. Semin Hematol 12, 1975, p 12.

48. Which cancers are often associated with splenomegaly?

Acute leukemia, chronic myeloid leukemia, chronic myelomonocytic leukemia, Hodgkin's disease, and non-Hodgkin's lymphoma. It is debatable whether histiocytosis X is a malignancy, but when disseminated it is usually associated with splenomegaly. Solid tumors rarely metastasize to the spleen to the point of causing splenomegaly.

49. What is the etiology of the diabetes mellitus noted in patients receiving chemotherapy for acute lymphoblastic leukemia?

Patients receiving chemotherapy for acute lymphoblastic leukemia may develop diabetes mellitus as a result of the prednisone therapy. Patients who develop steroid-induced diabetes often have some family history of diabetes. Steroid-induced diabetes is almost always self-limited. Patients can also develop diabetes as a sequela of hemorrhagic pancreatitis caused by L-asparaginase. The pancreatitis may completely destroy the islet cells; this form of diabetes requires lifelong insulin therapy.

50. Should children receiving chemotherapy be given routine immunizations?

Children who are receiving chemotherapy can be given routine diphtheria/tetanus/pertussis immunization when they have discontinued the intensive part of treatment. They should not be given live virus vaccines (measles, mumps, rubella, and polio). They can receive the Salk vaccine for polio protection but the response may be suboptimal. Patients with severe pulmonary disease secondary to the malignancy or cancer treatment should receive influenza immunization. They can receive Pneumovax and Prohibit (*H. influenzae* diphtheria conjugate) if otherwise clinically indicated. The response to these immunizations of children receiving chemotherapy is likely to be suboptimal, particularly if their treatment includes steroid, cyclophosphamide, or radiation therapy. However, there is no evidence that tolerance is induced with immunization.

51. Which tumors most commonly cause superior vena cava (SVC) syndrome? What are the symptoms of SVC syndrome?

The tumors associated with superior vena cava obstruction in childhood are most commonly non-Hodgkin's lymphoma, Hodgkin's disease, and, rarely, neuroblastoma or sarcomas. Nonmalignant causes include infections such as histoplasmosis or tuberculosis. Iatrogenic causes are most frequent in pediatrics and are usually a result of vascular thrombosis from cardiovascular surgery for congenital heart disease, shunting for hydrocephalus, or catheterization for venous access.

Symptoms of SVC syndrome or superior mediastinal syndrome are cough, hoarseness, dyspnea, orthopnea, and chest pain. Patients with substantial obstruction may also show anxiety, confusion, and lethargy, and have headaches, distorted vision, and a sense of fullness in the ears and head. Symptoms are aggravated by lying supine or flexing tightly. Signs of SVC syndrome include swelling of the face or neck, and/or upper extremities, plethora, cyanosis, suffusion, edema of the conjunctiva, diaphoresis, wheezing, and stridor.

Reference: Janin Y, Becker J, Weiss L, Schneider K: Superior vena cavae syndrome in childhood and adolescence: A review of the literature and report of three cases. J Pediatr Surg 17:219, 1982.

52. What are the indications for prophylactic penicillin in splenectomized children?

Children who have had splenectomy are at high risk for hyperacute infection with pneumococcus, *Hemophilus influenzae,* and other encapsulated bacteria. Ideally, all children should receive pneumococcal and *Hemophilus influenzae* immunization prior to splenectomy. This is possible only when splenectomy is elective. The high-risk period for infection is the first 2 years following splenectomy, especially the first month. Most physicians give prophylactic penicillin to all children for at least the first month after splenectomy. Many hematologists and oncologists recommend lifelong prophylactic penicillin. The strongest argument for prophylactic penicillin comes from the study of patients with sickle cell disease. These children have the same infectious problems as patients who have had surgical splenectomy for hematologic diseases or neoplasm. Patients with sickle cell disease who were randomized to receive prophylactic penicillin had significantly fewer deaths and life-threatening infections than patients who were not taking prophylaxis.

Reference: Gaskin M, Verter J, Wilbods G, Ed L, et al: Prophylaxis with penicillin in children with sickle cell anemia. N Engl J Med 314:1593, 1986.

53. What is the incidence of severe infection in patients who have been splenectomized?

The incidence depends on the age of the child and the underlying disorder. In initial studies of pediatric patients with Hodgkin's disease, the risk of hyperacute infection following splenectomy was estimated to be 10%. This has been reduced to 1–2% because of immunization, prophylactic penicillin, and patient and physician awareness. Patients with thalassemia are a relatively high-risk group for postsplenectomy sepsis, whereas the patients with hereditary spherocytosis over 5 years of age and patients who are splenectomized after trauma are at low risk (<1%).

References: Chilcote RR, Baehner RL, Hammond GD: Septicemia meningitis in children splenectomized for Hodgkin's disease. N Engl J Med 295:798, 1976.

Hayes DM, Terderg J, Cheng PT: Complications related to 234 staging laparotomies performed in the intergroup Hodgkin's disease in childhood study. Surgery 96:471, 1984.

54. Where are the most common central nervous system (CNS) tumors in childhood and where do they present?

In contrast to brain tumors in adults, most brain tumors in children are infratentorial. The most common histologic subtypes are medulloblastoma (primitive neuroectodermal tumor or PNET) and cerebellar astrocytoma, ependymoma and brain stem glioma. The supertentorial tumors that occur are mostly gliomas involving the cortical hemispheres or hypothalamus. Craniopharyngiomas are also common.

Reference: Ertel I: Brain tumors in children. Cancer 30:306–321, 1980.

55. Where do brain tumors metastasize?

Most brain tumors do not metastasize; they are fatal because of local invasion. Some may disseminate through the cerebrospinal fluid or "drop" metastases to the spinal cord or the cauda equina. Medulloblastoma may metastasize to bone or bone marrow. Rarely lymph nodes, liver, or pancreas may be involved.

Reference: Lewis MB, Nunes LB, Powell DE, Schneider BI: Extraaxial spread of medulloblastomas. Cancer 31:1287, 1973.

56. Which CNS tumors are associated with a favorable or unfavorable prognosis?

The prognosis in patients with CNS tumors depends on histology, location, extent of surgical resection, and to some extent the age of the child. Estimated 5-year survival rates are:

Five-Year Survival Rates in Patients with CNS Tumors

ANAPLASTIC	FIVE-YEAR SURVIVAL
Astrocytoma (Grade III)	45% RT and chemotherapy, 20% RT
Astrocytoma (Grade IV) (Glioblastoma multiforme)	40% RT and chemotherapy, 0% RT
Medulloblastoma	50% RT and chemotherapy, 20% RT
Pontine glioma	20% RT and chemotherapy

RT = radiation therapy.

57. Which posterior fossa tumor is commonly associated with erythrocytosis? Why?

Cerebellar hemagioblastoma. This tumor can secrete erythropoietin.

58. Spinal tumors can be extramedullary, extradural, or extramedullary-intradural. Which tumors are most commonly seen in each area?

Most pediatric tumors are epidural, including neuroblastoma, non-Hodgkin's lymphoma, and sarcomas.

59. What are the common presenting signs of spinal cord tumors?

Eighty percent of children with spinal cord compression have back pain, either local or radicular. Any child with cancer and back pain should be considered to have spinal cord compression until proven otherwise. A detailed physical examination with estimation of strength, reflexes, anal tone, and determination of a sensory level is mandatory.

References: Ch'ien LT, Kalwinsky DK, Peterson G, et al: Metastatic epidural tumors in children. Med Pediatr Oncol 10:455–462, 1982.

Portenoy RK, Lipton RB, Foley KM: Back pain in the cancer patient, an algorithm for evaluation and management. Neurology 37:134–138, 1987.

60. Which childhood cancers commonly metastasize to the lungs?

Wilms' tumor, osteosarcoma, Ewing's sarcoma, rhabdomyosarcoma, and low-grade, soft-tissue sarcomas such as fibrosarcoma and synovial sarcoma. Wilms' tumor and Hodgkin's disease can have lung metastases at diagnosis. Neuroblastoma and non-Hodgkin's lymphoma rarely cause pulmonary parenchymal disease.

61. What are the clinical manifestations of the histiocytosis "X" syndromes?

Eosinophilic Granuloma
　　Solitary lytic bone lesion
　　　(skull, long bones, ribs, pelvis, vertebral body)
Multiple Eosinophilic Granuloma (Hand-Schüller-Christian disease)
　　Lytic bony lesions
　　Proptosis
　　Diabetes insipidus
　　Hanging molars
　　Lymphadenopathy
Letterer-Siwe
　　Lytic bony lesions
　　Hepatosplenomegaly
　　Adenopathy
　　Draining ears
　　Cholesteatomas
　　Mastoid destruction
　　Diffuse skin lesions
　　Seborrhea
　　Failure to thrive
　　Pulmonary infiltration
　　Restrictive pulmonary disease

62. What is the proper treatment for hyperuricemia?

The treatment for hyperuricemia due to maligancy is allopurinol, alkalinization, and hydration.

References: Holland P, Holland NH: Prevention and management of acute hyperuricemia in childhood leukemia. J Pediatr 72:358–366, 1968.

Allegretta GJ, Weisman SJ, Altman AJ: Metabolic and space-occupying consequences of cancer and cancer treatment. Pediatr Clin North Am 32:601–611, 1985.

63. What are the common clinical manifestations of hypercalcemia?

Neuromuscular
　　Lethargy
　　Apathy
　　Depression
　　Fatigue
　　Hypotonia
　　Obtundation
　　Stupor
　　Coma
Cardiovascular
　　Bradycardia
　　Arrhythmia
　　Digitalis toxicity

Gastrointestinal
　　Anorexia
　　Nausea
　　Vomiting
　　Constipation
　　Ileus
Renal
　　Polyuria
　　Nocturia

Reference: Harguindey S, Decastro L, et al: Hypercalcemia complicating childhood malignancies. Cancer 44:2280–2290, 1979.

64. Which cancers and chemotherapeutic agents are associated with the syndrome of inappropriate secretion of antidiuretic hormone (SIADH)?

SIADH occurs with CNS tumors, lung tumors (especially small cell carcinoma in adults), lymphoma, or gastrointestinal carcinoma. It is also associated with vincristine or cyclophosphamide therapy.

Bibliography

1. Altman AJ, Schwartz AD: Malignant Diseases of Infancy, Childhood and Adolescence, 2nd ed. Philadelphia, W.B. Saunders, 1983.
2. DeVita VT Jr, Hellman S, Rosenberg SA (eds): Cancer: Principles and Practice of Oncology, 2nd ed. Philadelphia, J.B. Lippincott, 1985.
3. Holland JF, Frei E III (eds): Cancer Medicine, 2nd ed. Philadelphia, Lea and Febiger, 1982.
4. Nathan DG, Oski FA (eds): Hematology of Infancy and Childhood, 3rd ed. Philadelphia, W.B. Saunders, 1987.
5. Pizzo PA, Poplack DG: Principles and Practice of Pediatric Oncology. Philadelphia, J.B. Lippincott, 1988.
6. Poplack DG (ed): The Leukemias. Pediatric Clinics of North America, vol. 35, August 1988.

ORTHOPEDICS

Douglas A. Boenning, M.D.
Nancy R. Freedman, M.S.N.

1. What are the signs and symptoms of congenital hip dislocation (CHD)?

Early signs of CHD in a newborn infant include a positive Ortolani's sign (palpable "clunk" with reduction of the dislocation), a positive Barlow's test (pressure applied over the lesser trochanter causes hip dislocation), asymmetric thigh or gluteal folds, and apparent shortening of one leg on the side of the dislocation. Ortolani's sign disappears after the age of 1–2 months, when the head of the femur can no longer be reduced. Later signs of CHD include a limping gait and Galeazzi's sign (femoral shortening on the side of the dislocation).

2. What factors are associated with an increased risk of CHD?

Breech presentation, positive family history, first pregnancy, female gender, amniotic fluid abnormalities (especially oligohydramnios), premature rupture of membranes, and large birth weight.

3. What is the incidence of CHD?

2.5 to 6.5 per 1000 live births. Over 50% of these cases are not detected on neonatal screening examinations, and repeated testing of infants' hips beyond the newborn period is vitally important.

4. What is the recommended therapy for CHD?

The recommended treatment is to keep the legs abducted and the hips and knees flexed, so the developing head of the femur is kept within the acetabulum. Two commonly used devices are the Pavlik harness and the Frejka splint. Use of two or three diapers to keep the hip abducted generally is not recommended for CHD, as this method does not provide reliable stabilization.

5. Why is CHD so uncommon in preterm infants?

Unlike term infants, smaller infants born prematurely rarely have CHD because they are not subject to intrauterine compression during the later stages of pregnancy.

6. What is the characteristic presentation of slipped femoral epiphysis?

A slipped capital femoral epiphysis generally occurs in an obese preadolescent or adolescent boy who presents with a limp and hip pain (sometimes referred to the knee). The child's hip is maintained in a position of external rotation and adduction. Although less common, slipped capital femoral epiphysis can also occur in girls and in children who are tall and thin.

7. What is the most common cause of a painful hip in a child less than 10?

Toxic synovitis—a usually self-limited, mild inflammation of the hip joint of unclear etiology. It is also called "transient synovitis," "irritable hip," and "coxitis fugax."

8. How can toxic synovitis be differentiated from septic arthritis?

Toxic Synovitis Versus Septic Arthritis

TOXIC SYNOVITIS	SEPTIC ARTHRITIS
History	
Preceding URI with or without low-grade fever	Fever
Hip or referred knee pain	Usually large joint involvement (hip, ankle, knee, shoulder, elbow)
Limp	
Physical	
Refusal to bear weight	Exquisite pain, swelling, warmth
Can delicately elicit range of motion in affected hip joint	Marked resistance to mobility
Laboratory	
ESR normal or mildly elevated	ESR markedly elevated
Mild peripheral leukocytosis	Leukocytosis with "left shift"
Negative blood culture	Often positive blood culture
Joint fluid cloudy	Joint fluid purulent
Negative Gram stain	Often positive Gram stain
Radiographs	
Occasionally demonstrate fluid in the joint space	Widening of joint space
	Possible associated bony findings (early osteomyelitis)

9. What entities are associated with absent radii?

VATER syndrome (anomalies of vertebrae, anus (imperforate), tracheoesophageal region and radii), Fanconi's anemia, congenital thrombocytopenia (TAR syndrome), and Holt-Oram syndrome (associated with a secundum ASD).

10. What is Sprengel's deformity?

Sprengel's deformity (congenital elevation of the scapula) is a failure of scapular descent during fetal life, resulting in an elevated, hypoplastic scapula. The affected side of the neck is shorter and fuller and gives the appearance of torticollis. A fibrocartilaginous band or omovertebral bone may bridge the space between the medial upper scapula to the spinous process of a cervical vertebrae. Abduction of the ipsilateral arm is limited to 90°. Sprengel's deformity is associated with congenital scoliosis and renal anomalies.

11. What is the differential diagnosis for scoliosis?

Scoliosis is a lateral curvature of the spine; kyphosis and lordosis are posterior and anterior curvatures, respectively. Together they are referred to as spinal deformities. About 1–2% of the pediatric population have a spinal deformity but very few are severe enough to require treatment: 85%—idiopathic; 5%—congenital (including hemivertebrae and vertebral fusions); 5%—neuromuscular (cerebral palsy, polio, spinal muscular atrophy, muscular dystrophy); and 5%—miscellaneous (Marfan's, Ehlers-Danlos, tumors).

12. Are males or females more likely to have scoliosis?

Females are 5 times more likely than males.

13. How is screening for scoliosis performed?

The child should be dressed only in underwear or as minimal clothing as possible. From the back and side, the child is examined sitting and bending forward. The following signs suggest scoliosis:

1. Uneven shoulders.
2. Waist crease asymmetry that does not disappear on sitting. Most waist crease asymmetries are due to minor leg-length discrepancies.
3. Prominent scapula.

4. Asymmetry of paraspinal muscles or rib cage in the thoracic spine while bending (>0.5 cm in lumbar region and >1.0 cm in thoracic region).

5. Excessive thoracic kyphosis in forward bending position when viewed from the side. If significant spinal deformity is suggested, an orthopedic consultation should be obtained.

Reference: Bunnell W: Spinal deformities. Pediatr Clin North Am 33:1475–1487, 1986.

14. What are the indications for surgical correction of scoliosis?

(1) Curvature greater than 40–50°; (2) progressive worsening of scoliosis between 25 and 40° despite brace therapy; (3) and curvatures producing an unacceptable cosmetic appearance. Various surgical options are available, including Harrington rod insertion and spinal fusion.

15. Distinguish postural from structural scoliosis.

Postural Versus Structural Scoliosis

	POSTURAL	STRUCTURAL
No. of curves	One	Usually more than one
Convexity of curve	Right or left	85% to the right
Rotation of vertebrae	Absent	Present
Flexibility	Voluntarily corrected	Cannot be completely corrected voluntarily
	Disappears with recumbency or suspension	Part of curvature is fixed
Radiographs	No structural changes	Late structural changes

16. In which vertebra is spondylolisthesis most likely to occur?

L5. This condition of forward slipping of the vertebra is due to a developmental defect in the vertebral arch (pars interarticularis), which can separate the vertebra into two parts. It should be considered in the differential diagnosis of acute or chronic pediatric low back pain.

17. What is the differential diagnosis for torticollis?

Infection: cervical adenitis, retropharyngeal abscess, meningitis.

Trauma: atlanto-axial dislocation (especially in Down's syndrome), rotatory subluxation, soft tissue trauma, birth trauma with hematoma of sternocleidomastoid muscle.

Congenital conditions: congenital muscular torticollis, Klippel-Feil syndrome (fusion of cervical vertebrae), strabismus, vascular ring, abnormal skin webs (pterygium colli).

Miscellaneous: oculogyric crisis, tumor, Sandifer's syndrome (severe gastroesophageal reflux and esophagitis).

18. When does the mass of congenital muscular torticollis disappear?

The mass is usually soft, nontender, mobile and contained within or attached to the sternocleidomastoid muscle. Histologically, it consists of dense fibrous tissue. It reaches its maximal size at 1 month and disappears by 4–6 months.

19. What are the most common bacterial agents in osteomyelitis?

In order of frequency:

Neonates: (1) *Staphylococcus aureus;* (2) group B streptococcus; (3) Enterobacteriaceae (Salmonella, *E. coli,* Pseudomonas, Klebsiella).

Children: (1) *Staphylococcus aureus* (80%); (2) group A streptococcus; (3) *Hemophilus influenzae.*

20. Is it safe to treat children with osteomyelitis with oral antimicrobial agents?

Oral antimicrobial therapy may be considered under the following conditions: (1) an identified organism; (2) adequate surgical debridement; (3) improving clinical course on IV antibiotics; (4) patient does not vomit or have diarrhea; (5) adequate serum levels obtained on oral therapy; (6) reliable parents and/or patient.

Reference: Morrissey RT, Shore SL: Bone and joint sepsis. Pediatr Clin North Am 33:1551–1564, 1986.

21. What is the pathophysiology of Osgood-Schlatter disease?

This entity consists of painful swelling of one or both tibial tubercles at the insertion of the patellar tendon. The disease is very common in adolescents, usually beginning between the ages of 11 and 15. Vigorous exercise results in stressful pulling of the patellar tendon. Although the tubercles do enlarge from this repetitive strain, the primary problem appears to be a low-grade tendinitis and subsequent new heterotopic bone formation in the distal tendon itself. Ossicles have been found in the tendon separate from the tubercle and their removal provides relief. Fortunately, this entity rarely requires surgery. Restriction of activity for two to three weeks and gradual resumption of activity usually diminishes the symptoms. The year 1903 was a banner one for the tibial tubercle, as Osgood and Schlatter, working independently, both described the phenomenon.

22. What are the osteochondroses?

They are a group of disorders in which degeneration and aseptic necrosis of unclear cause involve the ossification or growth centers. Recalcification then occurs. The patient usually presents with pain at the affected site. The commonly affected sites and eponyms (generally named after the first describer) include:

Tarsonavicular bone	Kohler's disease
Capitellum of the elbow	Panner's disease
Carpal lunate	Kienböck's disease
Distal ulnar epiphysis	Burn's disease
Head of the femur	Legg-Calvé-Perthes disease
Head of the second metatarsal	Freiberg's disease

23. What are some inborn errors of metabolism that cause rickets?

Any condition that causes a phosphaturic state, such as: (1) cystinosis, (2) galactosemia, (3) Wilson's disease, (4) hereditary fructose intolerance, or (5) hereditary tyrosinemia.

24. What are some inborn errors of metabolism that cause rickets?

The pathologic abnormalities of rickets result primarily from osteoid overgrowth due to poor mineralization. The bones become weak and distorted. Among the signs of rickets are:

Craniotabes	"Pigeon breast," or sternal protrusion
Delayed suture and fontanelle closure	secondary to the use of accessory muscles
Frontal thickening and bossing	Harrison's groove, a rim of rib indentation
Defective tooth enamel	at the insertion of the diaphragm
Palpably widened spongy epiphyses	"Rachitic rosary," or enlarged costochondral
at wrists and ankles	junctions
Femoral and tibial bowing	

25. What causes osteoporosis in children?

Insufficient calcified bone with osteoid overgrowth is osteomalacia (also called rickets in a young child); insufficient bone mass with osteoid overgrowth is osteopenia. The structural consequences of both of these entities, particularly fracture susceptibility, constitute the syndrome of osteoporosis. In children this condition is usually secondary to other problems such as immobilization, chronic renal or liver failure, renal tubular acidosis, steroids, malabsorption, or heparin therapy. Osteoporosis is associated with Turner's syndrome, osteogenesis imperfecta, homocystinuria, and may also be seen in a primary juvenile idiopathic form. The vertebrae and ends of long bones are usually affected. More commonly, the term osteoporosis is used in association with osteopenia.

26. What is the inheritance pattern of osteogenesis imperfecta (OI)?

There are several types of OI. The most common, type I (1:30,000 live births), is autosomal dominant. OI congenita, type II, is a lethal form of the disease and is autosomal recessive.

27. What skeletal abnormality is associated with the McCune-Albright syndrome?

Polyostotic fibrous dysplasia (i.e., fibrous tissue replacing bones). The fibrous dysplasia occurs most commonly in long bones and the pelvis, and may result in deformity and/or increased thickness of bone.

28. What is craniosynostosis?

Craniosynostosis, or the premature fusion of sutures, leads to abnormal skull growth and shape. Referral to a pediatric neurosurgeon is indicated at the time of diagnosis.

29. What are the varieties of craniosynostosis?

Craniosynostosis

DIAGNOSIS	SUTURE	SHAPE
Plagiocephaly	Unilateral coronal synostosis	Facial asymmetry
Trigonocephaly	Metopic synostosis	Triangular configuration
Acrocephaly, oxycephaly	Coronal and lambdoidal	High, peaked, conical skull
Brachycephaly	Coronal	Short, broad cranium
Scaphocephaly	Sagittal synostosis	Long, narrow cranium

From Curry T: Problems/issues of newborn care. In Schwartz MW (ed): Principles and Practice of Clinical Pediatrics. Chicago, Year Book Medical Publishers, Inc., 1987, p 217, with permission.

30. How is craniosynostosis distinguished from overlapping sutures in a neonate?

Overlapping sutures in the newborn result from compression of the skull during the birth process. If the sutures are not fused, they will quickly separate as the brain undergoes rapid growth in the first weeks of life. A persistent ridge is indication for a roentgenogram to assess whether the suture is prematurely fused.

31. What is nursemaid's elbow and how is it treated?

Subluxation of the radial head caused by a sudden pull or jerk on the forearm in toddlers and pre-schoolers. The injury occurs when the child is suddenly lifted by one arm, commonly yanked over a curb or up onto his feet after a fall. The annular ligament surrounding the radial head is torn. Radiographs are normal. The child presents with a flexed, painful elbow with forearm pronated and clamped to the side. Treatment involves medial rotation of the forearm and replacement of the radial head. A trick is to ask the child for permission to look at the hand without disturbing the elbow. With the examiner's other hand placed over the radial head, traction is applied at the same time the forearm is medially rotated. The child will usually cry or protect the arm afterwards, but within 15 minutes the child will start to move the arm spontaneously.

32. What are the pathologic stages in Legg-Calvé-Perthes (LCP) disease?

LCP is a condition of aseptic necrosis of the femoral head involving children primarily ages 4–10. The first phase is the incipient or synovitis stage. Lasting 1–3 weeks, this stage is characterized by an increase in hip-joint fluid and a swollen synovium associated with reduced movement. The second stage is avascular necrosis. Lasting 6 months to 1 year, the blood supply stops to part (or all) of the head of the femur. That portion of the bone essentially dies, but the contour of the femoral head remains unchanged. The third and longest pathologic stage of LCP is fragmentation or regeneration and revascularization. Lasting 1–3 years, the blood supply returns and causes both resorption of necrotic bone and laying down of new immature bone. Permanent hip deformity can occur in this last stage. It is important to note that plain radiographs may lag behind the progression of the disorder by as much as 3–6 months. Radionuclide bone scans are much better because early ischemia and avascular necrosis are depicted as decreased localizations of isotope.

33. What is osteochondritis dissecans?

It is another aseptic necrosis syndrome. It occurs when a section of articular cartilage and underlying bone undergoes necrosis secondary to trauma or ischemia. The necrotic section of cartilage and bone detaches completely or partially and lodges in the contiguous joint. Males are more commonly affected and complain of pain on strenuous physical activity with associated findings of stiffness, swelling, clicking, and occasional locking. The knee, elbows, ankle, and hip are commonly affected joints. The diagnosis of osteochondritis dissecans is usually made on the basis of a plain radiograph. The primary long-term concern is degenerative arthritis, particularly if substantial areas of large joints are involved.

34. What are the characteristic x-ray changes, clinical findings, and history in a child with an osteoid osteoma?

Osteoid osteoma is typically seen in older children and adolescents and exhibits a male predominance (M/F 2 to 1). Most children complain of localized pain usually in the femur and tibia; however, arms and vertebrae may also be involved. Radiographs and CT scans demonstrate an osteolytic area surrounded by densely sclerotic reactive bone. Bone scans reveal "hot spots." The site is usually less than 1 cm in diameter and arises at the junction of old and new cortex. Pathologically the lesion is highly vascularized fibrous tissue with an osteoid matrix and poorly calcified bone spicules surrounded by a dense zone of sclerotic bone.

35. What are the three phases of a bone scan?

The phases are generally demarcated by the time elapsed since injection of the radionuclide dye. Phase I—the "angiographic phase." The dye passes in the first few seconds through the large blood vessels and provides early assessment of regional vascularity and perfusion. Phase II—the "blood pool phase." Usually obtained in the first minutes after an injection, this phase highlights the movement of the dye into extracellular spaces of soft tissue and bone. Phase III—obtained 1½ to 3 hours after injection. The dye localizes in the bone with minimal soft tissue imaging. The three-phase process is used to differentiate soft tissue from bony abnormalities. At times, a phase IV study may be done by rescanning for the same dye at 24 hours, which further minimizes soft tissue background activity.

36. What is the Salter-Harris fracture classification?

Devised in 1963, this is a classification of growth plate (physis) injuries for purposes of description, treatment and prognosis.

Type I: epiphysis and metaphysis separate; usually no displacement occurs due to the strong periosteum; radiograph may be normal; tenderness over the physis may be the only sign; normal growth after 2–3 week cast immobilization

Type II: fragment of metaphysis splits with epiphysis; usually closed reduction; casting is for 3–6 weeks (longer for lower extremity than upper extremity); growth usually not affected, except distal femur and tibia

Type III: a partial plate fracture involving a physeal and epiphyseal fracture to the joint surface; occurs when growth plate is partially fused; closed reduction more difficult to achieve

Type IV: extensive fracture involving epiphysis, physis, metaphysis, and joint surface; high risk for growth disruption unless proper reduction (usually done operatively) is obtained

Type V: crush injury to the physis; high risk for growth disruption

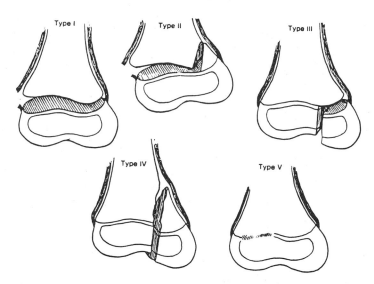

From Sherk H: Musculoskeletal injuries. In Fleisher G, Ludwig S (eds): Textbook of Pediatric Emergency Medicine. Baltimore, Williams & Wilkins, 1983, p 953, with permission.

37. What is the Thurston-Holland sign?
This sign is the small section of metaphyseal bone that remains attached to the epiphysis in a type II fracture. It is diagnostic of injury to the growth plate.

38. What are the most common fractures in children?
Growth plate fractures, those occurring at the ends of long bones, are most common in children. This site is where children's bones are weakest, and ossification is not yet complete. Buckle (compression) and greenstick (incomplete) fractures are also common.

39. What is the most common pathologic fracture in children?
Also called secondary fractures, these are fractures through a bone that is weakened by a pathologic process. The most common such fracture is through unicameral bone cysts (also called simple bone cysts). These cysts usually occur in the metaphysis of a long bone, most frequently the humerus. They occur predominantly in males, are usually asymptomatic (until a fracture occurs), are centrally located in the bone, and are often quite large.

40. What should be noted on physical examination in a child with a suspected fracture?
Assess "the five P's" in the affected extremity: Pain and point tenderness, Pulse (distal to the fracture), Pallor, Paresthesia (distal to the fracture), and Paralysis (distal to the fracture). The involved extremity should also be carefully examined for deformity, swelling, crepitus, discoloration, and open wounds. A primary concern in any evaluation is a distal neurovascular compromise, which may require immediate surgical intervention.

41. What are indications for open reduction of a fracture?
An open reduction is an operative reduction in which pins are fixed into the separate fragments to promote proximity for healing. Indications include (1) failed closed reduction (often in older children with displaced forearm, tibial, or femoral fractures); (2) displaced intra-articular fractures; (3) displaced Salter-Harris III and IV fractures (to prevent premature growth plate closure); and (4) patients with head trauma.

Reference: Conrad EU, Rang MC: Fractures and sprains. Pediatr Clin North Am 33:1523–1539, 1986.

42. What is the treatment for a clavicular fracture without neurovascular compromise?
Place a child with a clavicular fracture in a figure-of-eight (or clavicle) strap until healing is progressing and the child is comfortable. The figure-of-eight strap decreases the pain caused by motion, promotes healing, and reduces the chance of a prominent bump appearing at the fracture site. The strap needs to be worn snugly and not removed for bathing. Complete union occurs in 10–14 days in infants and in 4–5 weeks in toddlers and younger children, but the splint can be removed earlier. The resulting callus of healing takes about 2 years to disappear through bone remodeling.

43. What is a Colles' fracture?
Commonly, this refers to a group of complete fractures of the distal radius with varying displacement of the distal fragment. The fracture is classically due to a fall injury, as the outstretched hand, dorsiflexed wrist, and pronated forearm strike the ground in an effort to brace the fall.

44. What is a boxer's fracture?
A palmar, angulated fracture of the distal fifth metacarpal, often the result of a bad temper unleashed.

45. How long does a fractured femur take to heal?
In a newborn, 3 weeks. In a 20-year-old, 20 weeks.

46. What is the difference between subluxation and dislocation?
Subluxation is an incomplete or partial dislocation.

47. What is the value of casting for an ankle sprain?
There is disagreement whether casting is beneficial; however, casting may increase comfort, prevent reinjury during healing and improve overall rehabilitation.

48. Why are sprained ligaments uncommon in children?
Growth plates are weaker than ligaments and thus pathology will develop in the growth plate, such as a Salter-Harris epiphyseal fracture or a buckle fracture, before the ligaments tear or rupture.

49. What is bone remodeling? In which fractures will remodeling of bone _not_ occur?
Remodeling is the correction of bony deformities, usually fractures, which occurs spontaneously in a growing child. Fractures that will not remodel require closed or open reduction to realign the segments: intra-articular fractures; fractures with excessive shortening, angulation, or rotation; displaced epiphyseal plate fractures; and midshaft or diaphyseal fractures.

Reference: Conrad EU, Rang MC: Fractures and sprains. Pediatr Clin North Am 33:1523–1539, 1986.

50. What condition does this child have?

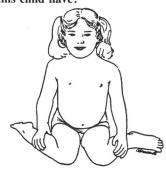

This is femoral anteversion (or medial femoral torsion), which is a common cause of in-toeing in younger children. This child is demonstrating the reverse tailor position, a sign of the internally rotated hip. Normally, with a child lying prone and knees flexed at 90°, the hip cannot be rotated internally more than 70°. Most cases resolve and only with a very severe deformity is correction warranted. (Figure reproduced from Staheli LT: Torsional deformity. Pediatr Clin North Am 33:1382, 1986, with permission.)

51. What are the causes of in-toeing gait (pigeon-toeing)?
The condition may be due to problems anywhere in the lower extremity.

Foot: metatarsus adductus
      talipes equinovarus (clubfoot)
      pes planus (flat feet)
Leg: tibial torsion, internal
      genu valgum (knock knees)
      tibia vara (Blount's disease)
      bow legs
Hip: femoral anteversion (also known as medial femoral torsion)
      paralysis (polio, myelomeningocele)
      spasticity (cerebral palsy)
      maldirected acetabulum

Reference: Tunnessen W: Signs and Symptoms in Pediatrics, 3rd ed. Philadelphia, J.B. Lippincott Co., 1987.

52. What are "shin splints"?
This term is used to describe the pain and cramping felt in the anterior compartment of the lower leg after strenuous exercise. It is rare in children but may be seen in teenagers who exercise (especially jogging and running in track) after an extended period of inactivity. The pain results from muscle strain, swelling and cramping, particularly of the flexor digitorum longus muscle, which flexes the lateral four toes and plantarflexes the foot at the ankle joint. The muscle swelling may contribute to ischemia. If you have never experienced shin splints, try snowshoeing for a few hours. It may be the ultimate test of the anterior tibial muscles.

53. What is the most common congenital foot abnormality?
Metatarsus adductus. The term metatarsus varus is also used, although they do describe slightly different forefoot positions.

54. What is metatarsus adductus?
A kidney-shaped foot with the front part of the foot (forefoot) turned inward. It is believed to result from intrauterine constriction. Most cases are mild and flexible, with the foot easily dorsiflexed and the lateral aspect easily straightened by passive stretching. Improvement usually occurs within 2 months with passive stretching exercises. Rigid, more fixed deformities may require casting.

55. What are the common causes of foot pain in the three age groups listed below?

Probable Causes of Foot Pain by Age

AGES 0 TO 6 YEARS	AGES 6 TO 12 YEARS	AGES 12 TO 19 YEARS
Ill-fitting shoes	Ill-fitting shoes	Ill-fitting shoes
Foreign body	Foreign body	Foreign body
Occult fracture	Accessory navicular bone	Ingrown toenail
Osteomyelitis	Occult fracture	Pes cavus

Table continued on next page.

Probable Causes of Foot Pain by Age *(Continued)*		
AGES 0 TO 6 YEARS	AGES 6 TO 12 YEARS	AGES 12 TO 19 YEARS
JRA (if other joints involved)	Tarsal coalition (peroneal spastic flat foot)	Hypermobile flat foot with tight Achilles tendon
Rheumatic fever	Ingrown toenail	Ankle sprains
(Hypermobile flat foot)	Ewing's sarcoma	Stress fracture
	(Hypermobile flat foot)	Ewing's sarcoma
		Synovial sarcoma

From Gross RH: Foot pain in children. Pediatr Clin North Am 33:1397, 1986, with permission.

56. What is the differential diagnosis for pes cavus?

Pes cavus, or high-arched feet, can result from disruption of the longitudinal arch of the foot due to contractures or disturbed muscle balance. A neurologic cause should be suspected. The differential diagnosis includes normal familial variant, spina bifida, cauda equina lesion, peroneal muscle atrophy, Friedreich's ataxia, and Hurler's syndrome.

57. What is a clubfoot?

There are actually different types of clubfoot, all variations of a foot twisted out of shape. The term is commonly used to refer to talipes equinovarus (TEV), which occurs in about 1 per 1000 live births and is the predominant type in 95% of clubfeet. The hindfoot remains rigidly inverted, the forefoot is adducted, and dorsiflexion is limited. The inability to dorsiflex the foot is a key distinguishing feature between TEV and metatarsus adductus. In TEV, there is subluxation or dislocation of the talocalcaneonavicular joints.

58. What generalized developmental syndromes are associated with clubfoot?

Arthrogryposis
Caudal regression syndrome
Cerebral palsy
Craniocarpotarsal dysplasia
Diastrophic dwarfism

Larsen's syndrome
Meningomyelocele
Progressive muscle atrophy (peroneal type)
Spinal cord tumor
Myotonic dystrophy

59. What is a Denis-Browne splint?

The splint consists of a metal bar connected to shoes or straps about the feet. The bar provides varying degrees of external rotation. The splint is used in children with tibial torsion where spontaneous correction is not occurring and infrequently in some children with clubfoot.

60. What is Blount's disease?

Tibia vara, or Blount's disease, is a medial angulation of the tibia in the metaphyseal region due to a growth disturbance in the medial aspect of the proximal tibial epiphysis. In the infantile type the child is usually obese, an early walker, and develops pronounced bow legs during the first year of life. In the adolescent variety, the onset occurs during late childhood or early adolescence. It is distinguished from the infantile type in being unilateral in 90% of cases, with resultant leg shortening.

61. Which long bone is most frequently absent congenitally?

The fibula. Absence of the fibula may be partial or complete and is usually unilateral. The involved leg is shortened and commonly demonstrates bowing of the tibia and slight shortening of the femur. The foot usually shows a severe deformity with equinus and valgus deformities with absence of or abnormal development of lateral phalanges.

62. What are the long-term effects of uncorrected leg-length discrepancy?

Equinus contracture of the ankle, scoliosis, low back problems, and late degenerative arthritis of the hip.

Reference: Moseley CF: Leg-length discrepancy. Pediatr Clin North Am 33:1585–1586, 1986.

63. What is the Trendelenburg test?

If a normal individual stands on one leg, ipsilateral hip abductors (primarily the gluteus medius) prevent the pelvis from tilting, and balance is maintained. Children over 4 years of age can usually stand this way for at least 30 seconds. If the opposite side of the pelvis does tilt or the trunk lurches to maintain balance, this is a positive Trendelenburg sign. It may be an indicator of muscle weakness (due to muscular or neurologic pathology) or of hip instability (such as acetabular dysplasia).

64. What is infantile cortical hyperostosis?

Caffey's disease (or syndrome), which usually occurs before 6 months of age, is a condition of unknown etiology that consists of tender, nonsuppurative, cortical swellings of the shafts of bone, most commonly the mandible and clavicle. It remits spontaneously, but exacerbations may persist for several years. In severe cases, corticosteroids may be helpful.

65. What is the difference between valgus and varus deformities?

There are some things that seem to be destined to be learned, forgotten, and relearned many times as a rite of passage. The Krebs cycle is one. This is another. The terms refer to angular deformities in the musculoskeletal system. If the distal part of the deformity points toward the midline, the term is varus. If the distal part points away from the midline, the term is valgus. For example, in knock-knees, the lower portion of the deformity points away, so the term is genu valgum.

66. Which four muscles constitute the rotator cuff?

Supraspinatus, infraspinatus, teres minor, subscapularis (most major league pitchers know them well).

67. What is craniotabes? What is its significance?

It is a condition in which abnormally soft, thin skull bones buckle under pressure and recoil like a ping-pong ball. It is best elicited on the parietal or frontal bones and is usually associated with rickets in infancy. It may also be seen in hypervitaminosis A, syphilis, and hydrocephalus. Craniotabes may be normal during the first 3 months of life.

68. What connective tissue disorder did Paganini supposedly have that accounted for his great dexterity?

Ehlers-Danlos syndrome.

69. What bony disorder did Toulouse-Lautrec have?

A rare form of dwarfism called pyknodysostosis, characterized by short stature, coarsening of the face, thickened and brittle bones, thickened lips, and drooling. His parents were cousins.
    Reference: Smithsonian, November 1985.

Bibliography

1. Bradford DS, Lonstein JE, Moe JH, et al: Moe's Textbook of Scoliosis and Allied Spinal Deformities, 2nd ed. Philadelphia, W.B. Saunders, 1987.
2. Chung SMK: Hip Disorders in Infants and Children. Philadelphia, Lea & Febiger, 1981.
3. Dickson JH (ed): Spinal deformities. In Spine: State of the Art Reviews, vol. 1, no. 2. Philadelphia, Hanley & Belfus, Inc., 1987.
4. Ferguson AB: Orthopaedic Surgery in Infancy and Childhood, 5th ed. Baltimore, Williams & Wilkins, 1982.
5. Fleisher G, Ludwig S: Textbook of Pediatric Emergency Care, 2nd ed. Baltimore, Williams & Wilkins, 1988.
6. Jones KL: Smith's Recognizable Patterns of Human Malformation, 4th ed. Philadelphia, W.B. Saunders, 1988.
7. Katz JF: Common Orthopedic Problems in Children. New York, Raven, 1981.

8. Lovell WW, Winter RB: Pediatric Orthopaedics, 2nd ed. Philadelphia, J.B Lippincott, 1986.
9. Lovinger RD: Rickets. Pediatrics 66:359-365, 1980.
10. Maroteaux P: Bone Diseases of Children. Philadelphia, J.B Lippincott, 1978.
11. Nelson JD, Bucholz RW, Kusmiesz H, et al: Benefits and risks of sequential parental-oral cephalosporin therapy in suppurative bone and joint infections. J Pediatr Orthop 2:255-262, 1982.
12. Rockwood CA Jr, Wilkins KE, King RD: Pediatric Fractures. Vol. 3 of Rockwood CA Jr., Green DP: Fractures, 2nd ed. Philadelphia. J.B., Lippincott, 1984.
13. Salter RB: Textbook of Disorders and Injuries of the Musculoskeletal Structure, 2nd ed. Baltimore, Williams & Wilkins, 1983.
14. Scoles PV: Pediatric Orthopedics in Clinical Practice. Chicago, Year Book Publishers, 1982.
15. Sharrard WJW: Paediatric Orthopaedics and Fractures, 2nd ed. Oxford, Blackwell Scientific Publications, 1979.
16. Silverman FN: Caffey's Pediatric X-ray Diagnosis, 8th ed. Chicago, Year Book, 1985.
17. Staheli LT (ed): Common Orthopedic Problems. Pediatr Clin North Am vol. 33, no. 6, December 1986.
18. Tachdjian MO: The Child's Foot. Philadelphia, W.B. Saunders, 1985.
19. Tachdjian MO: Pediatric Orthopedics. Philadelphia, W.B. Saunders, 1972.
20. Tunnessen W: Signs and Symptoms in Pediatrics, 3rd ed. Philadelphia, J.B. Lippincott, 1987.
21. Way LW (ed): Current Surgical Diagnosis and Treatment. Norwalk, CT: Appleton and Lange, 1988.

PULMONOLOGY

Robert W. Wilmott, M.D.

Asthma

1. What is the usual age of onset of symptoms in childhood asthma?

Approximately 50% of childhood asthma develops before 3 years of age and nearly 100% of children present by age 7 years. The more severely affected children usually present in infancy and the milder cases present later in childhood. The signs and symptoms of asthma may be evident early in life; however, the child displaying such signs may be erroneously diagnosed as having recurrent pneumonia or "wheezy bronchitis."

2. What proportion of childhood asthmatics will "outgrow" their symptoms?

Popular pediatric teaching has been that most children with asthma will "outgrow their symptoms." While many children will improve with time, not all studies support that contention. A careful study of patients with asthma who were followed longitudinally from infancy noted that two-thirds of the subjects were still symptomatic and that one-third of those with persistent asthma missed significant amounts of time from work or had to restrict athletic activities. However, it is safe to say that many children with asthma have milder symptoms as they grow older, and that the asthma is usually easier to manage by using metered dose inhalers (which are usually ineffective until a child is at least 8 years old).

References: Williams H, McNicol KN: Prevalence, natural history, and relationship of wheezy bronchitis and asthma in children. An epidemiological study. Br Med J 4:321-325, 1969.

Martin AJ, Landau LI, Phelan PD: Asthma from childhood to age 21: the patient and his disease. Br Med J 284:380–382, 1982.

3. Is asthma more common in males or females?

Asthma is two to three times more common in boys than in girls until the onset of puberty. It becomes more common in women after puberty.

4. What mechanisms lead to airway obstruction during an acute asthma attack?

The pathophysiology of airway obstruction in asthmatics and the sequence of events that leads to status asthmaticus are incompletely understood. It appears that an attack may be analogous to the late reaction noted after bronchial provocation with inhaled allergen. There are three main components to airway obstruction: bronchospasm, mucosal edema, and plugging of airways by thick secretions. These abnormalities are probably secondary to the release of mediators from mast cells and eosinophils. The mast cell mediators include histamine, leukotrienes, platelet activating factor, and neutrophil chemotactic factor. Major basic protein and eosinophil cationic protein are released from the eosinophil.

5. What clinical signs correlate best with severity of respiratory disease during an acute asthmatic attack?

Markedly increased respiratory rate

Pronounced retractions (especially sternocleidomastoid retractions)

Altered mental state (agitation, drowsiness)

Diminished breath sounds. Wheezing may be absent if flow rates are very low.

Increased pulsus paradoxus. This is performed by measuring the blood pressure and noting the difference in pressure between the point at which the systolic pressure is initially heard (intermittently) and the point at which the systolic pressure is heard with every heart beat. Normally, this is less than 10 mm Hg.

6. In children with chronic cough (especially nocturnal), but with little or no history of wheezing, what testing should be done?

The differential diagnosis should include asthma, chronic sinusitis, cystic fibrosis, inhaled foreign body, and immune deficiency. The choice of laboratory tests should be guided by the history and physical examination. The following tests should certainly be considered:

Chest radiograph
Pulmonary function tests before and after bronchodilation
Sweat test
Immunoglobulins
Exercise test to document exercise-induced bronchospasm
Sinus radiographs

7. What is the usefulness of the chest radiograph during an acute exacerbation of asthma?

The chest radiograph will usually show only hyperinflated lung fields and increased bronchial markings (you hope!). However, a chest radiograph may be taken at this time to exclude pneumothorax (rare), pneumomediastinum (5%), and pneumonia or atelectasis (approximately 20%).

8. How useful are pulmonary function tests in following children with asthma?

Pulmonary function tests (PFTs) are only moderately useful during an acute attack of asthma. It is often difficult to make any measurements at all in severe status asthmaticus because of dyspnea. By contrast, PFTs are very useful in the longitudinal evaluation of outpatients with asthma in demonstrating a satisfactory response to therapy, and for identifying the severely obstructed, hyperinflated asymptomatic patient who has a poor prognosis if unrecognized.

9. What are the usual findings on arterial blood gas sampling during acute asthma attacks?

The most common finding is hypocapnea because of hyperventilation. Hypoxemia is also usually present unless the child is being treated with oxygen. Hypercapnia is therefore a serious sign which suggests that the child is tiring or is becoming severely obstructed. This finding should prompt reevaluation and consideration of admission to an intensive care unit.

10. In a child hospitalized for asthma, at what rate should the fluids be run?

This is a controversial question! One conventional answer is that asthmatics should receive 150% of maintenance requirements because of large insensible pulmonary water losses in hyperventilating patients. However, severely obstructed patients are at risk of developing inappropriate ADH secretion, and I recommend giving less fluid in this situation, and monitoring the plasma and urine electrolytes and urine specific gravity at regular intervals.

11. What other entities should be considered in the differential diagnosis of the wheezing child?

Cystic fibrosis
Foreign body inhalation
Congestive heart failure
Immune deficiency

Viral infections
Tracheobronchomalacia
Gastroesophageal reflux with aspiration

12. Which asthmatics should be admitted to hospital?

Children with a history of sudden deterioration
Children who have not cleared in the emergency room after three subcutaneous doses of epinephrine or three treatments with adrenergic aerosols followed by a bolus of intravenous theophylline
Children with an adverse social history

13. When should mechanical ventilation be considered in the child with status asthmaticus?

Hypercapnia ($PaCO_2$ greater than 50 mm Hg)

Uncompensated respiratory acidosis

Altered mental status (lethargy, hypotonia, decreased response to pain)

14. What types of oral bronchodilators are available for home management of asthma? What are the advantages and disadvantages of each?

Oral Bronchodilators for Home Management of Asthma

TYPE	ADVANTAGES	DISADVANTAGES
β_2	Quick acting Do not need levels	Short duration Theoretical risk of tachyphylaxis Side effects: tremor, anxiety, hyperactivity
Short-acting theophylline	May be more effective than the β_2 drugs	Side effects: nausea hyperactivity, vomiting, seizures, nervousness, cardiac dysrhythmia Need therapeutic level monitoring Individual variations in clearance
Sustained-release theophylline	Steady levels	Side effects are the same as those seen with short-acting theophylline preparations Toxic patients may have continued absorption from GI tract

15. What are the appropriate doses of theophylline for children of various ages?

Dosages of Theophylline

AGE	TOTAL DAILY DOSE (mg/kg/24 hr)
Infants 6–51 wk	$0.2 \times$ (age in wks + 5)
Children 1–9 yr	24
Children 9–12 yr	20
Adolescents 12–16 yr	18
Adults	13 or 900 mg/day (whichever is less)

From Canny GJ, Levison H: The modern management of childhood asthma. Pediatr Rev Commun 1:123–162, 1987, with permission.

16. What role does cromolyn sodium have in the treatment of asthma?

Cromolyn can be very effective if administered correctly by inhalation on a regular basis. While its greatest value is in treating allergic (extrinsic) asthma, many children with asthma respond to cromolyn empirically and it is not necessary to document an allergic etiology before commencing a trial of therapy. Often a β_2 agonist is prescribed as well and used as needed for any breakthrough symptoms. Exercise-induced asthma can be treated effectively in many children by administration of cromolyn 15 minutes before activity. Cromolyn inhibits mast-cell degranulation (blocking mediator release) and also reduces airway hyperactivity by unknown mechanisms. It has no bronchodilator properties and is thus not useful in the acute setting. Children with known allergies to dogs, cats, or horses where exposure to the allergen is anticipated (!!!) can be treated with cromolyn beforehand. However, it may be necessary to use both the nasal and the ophthalmic preparations if oculonasal symptoms have been a problem. There is no way to provide complete protection if the allergen exposure is sufficiently heavy.

17. What is the treatment for exercise-induced asthma?

The most effective therapy is two puffs of a β_2 agonist such as albuterol by metered dose inhaler 10–15 minutes before exercise. Cromolyn is also useful, although it is not as potent as the β_2 drugs; it can be used in combination with them. Other approaches include several short warm-up sprints before exercising, and warming and humidifying the inhaled air (such as using a face mask for skiing).

18. What are the factors that affect theophylline clearance?

Increased Clearance	Decreased Clearance
Age (increased in children)	Age (decreased in infants)
Low carbohydrate, high protein diet	High carbohydrate, low protein diet
Charcoal broiled meat	Caffeine
Cigarette smoking	Macrolide antibiotics (e.g., erythromycin)
Marijuana smoking	Cimetidine
Chronic ethanol intake	Viral infections
Cystic fibrosis	Cor pulmonale
	Congestive cardiac failure
	Liver disease

From Canny GJ, Levison H: The modern management of childhood asthma. Pediatr Rev Commun 1:123–162, 1978, with permission.

Cystic Fibrosis

19. What is the incidence and inheritance pattern of cystic fibrosis (CF)?

Incidence

> Caucasians: 1:2,000
> Black population in U.S.A.: 1:17,000
> North American Indians: 1:80,000
> Orientals (Hawaii): 1:90,000

Inheritance Pattern

Cystic fibrosis is inherited as an autosomal recessive condition. There has been much speculation that there could be more than one gene for cystic fibrosis. This could account for the clinical diversity of CF, but there is no evidence to support the contention. Recent genetic studies all agree that there only is one locus for the gene in the center of the long arm of chromosome 7. However, the possibility that there are multiple alleles at this locus has not been excluded.

20. What are the causes of false-positive and false-negative sweat tests?

False-positive Sweat Tests*

Malnutrition†	Type I glycogen storage disease
Celiac disease	Hypoparathyroidism
Untreated adrenal insufficiency	Atopic dermatitis
Anorexia nervosa	Pupillotonia-areflexia and segmental
Renal diabetes insipidus	hypohidrosis
Ectodermal dysplasia	Mucopolysaccharidosis
Fucosidosis	Klinefelter's syndrome
Familial cholestasis	Hypogammaglobulinemia
Untreated hypothyroidism	

False-negative Sweat Tests

1. Peripheral edema
2. Administration of the antibiotic cloxacillin
   (this observation is not well substantiated)

---

*From Ruddy RM, Scanlin TF: Abnormal sweat electrolytes in a case of celiac disease and a case of psychosocial failure to thrive. Clin Pediatr 1987; 26:83–89, 1987, with permission.
†This is the most common cause of a clinical dilemma.

21. Which organisms are most frequently recovered from the tracheobronchial secretions of children with CF?

Children with CF have a typical chronological sequence of infection. This sequence is not invariable, but it is a useful guide:

	Common	Uncommon
Infant	S. aureus	E. coli
		Klebsiella sp.
Young child	H. influenzae	
Older child through adulthood	P. aeruginosa	P. cepacia

22. What is the clinical significance of mucoid pseudomonas or *E. coli?*

These mucoid gram-negative bacteria synthesize complex carbohydrates that give them a slimy, gelatinous colonial morphology. For example, the mucoid strains of *P. aeruginosa* elaborate a gel that is closely related to alginic acid. It is rare to isolate mucoid strains of these bacteria except in subjects with cystic fibrosis. Therefore the isolation of a mucoid strain should always suggest the possibility of that disease. It appears that the synthetic pathway for the production of alginate in *P. aeruginosa* is activated by the microenvironment of the lungs in patients with CF. Whether these observations apply to *E. coli* is less clear. Mucoid *P. aeruginosa* is rarely cultured from other chronically infected sites.

23. What is the pathophysiology of rectal prolapse in CF?

Rectal prolapse is a common complication of CF—approximately 23% of patients are affected. Possible explanations include:

Poor nutrition with defective connective tissue supporting structures.

Chronic coughing which raises intra-abdominal pressure.

Abnormal bowel movements (increased volume of stools with abnormal consistency).

24. What is the life expectancy of children with CF? What are the complications that influence life expectancy?

The median survival rate for all patients with cystic fibrosis in 1987 was approximately 29 years. Factors that appear to influence survival rates are:

1. Gender. Males have better survival rates than females.

2. Colonization with virulent bacteria. *Pseudomonas aeruginosa* and *Pseudomonas cepacia* are more serious pathogens which are difficult to clear once the patient is persistently infected. Patients who are chronically colonized with *P. aeruginosa* have significantly worse survival rates than other patients with CF.

3. Meconium ileus at birth used to be considered a negative prognostic indicator, but it does not appear to be a significant factor in the 1980s. Improved neonatal care and surgical techniques, and the increased use of parenteral nutrition in the neonatal period are thought to account for the improved outlook.

4. Nasal polyps appear to be a positive prognostic indicator. Patients with polyps appear to have milder pulmonary disease. This is a surprising observation, and there is no obvious explanation for this phenomenon.

References: Drake Lee AB, Pitcher-Wilmott RW: The clinical and laboratory correlates of nasal polyps in cystic fibrosis. Int J Pediatr Otorhinolaryngol 1982; 4:209–214, 1982.

Stern RC, Boat TF, Wood RE, et al: Treatment and prognosis of nasal polyps in cystic fibrosis. Am J Dis Child 1982; 136:1067–1070, 1982.

5. Cor pulmonale is one of the late complications of CF because progressive obstructive airway disease leads to the development of pulmonary hypertension and respiratory failure. The prognosis after developing cor pulmonale is very poor, with a 1-year survival rate of only 20%.

6. Pneumothorax is associated with moderate to advanced lung disease in patients with CF. Therefore air leak has traditionally been regarded as a poor prognostic sign. The prognosis has been improving now that pneumothoraces are being managed aggressively at major cystic fibrosis centers.

25. Are steroids beneficial in the treatment of CF?

The definitive answer to this question may not be available until the Cystic Fibrosis Foundation's Multi-center Study is completed in 1991. The reason for performing this study was a report of a randomized, double-blind, placebo-controlled trial of alternate-day prednisone therapy. After four years the treatment group was found to have improved pulmonary function, a reduced frequency of hospital admissions, and significantly greater heights and weights. This earlier study was not as comprehensive or as powerful as the current multi-center trial. Therefore, it would be wise to wait for the results of the new study before prescribing steroids routinely to "reduce the inflammatory component of cystic fibrosis lung disease." Therefore, the current indications for the use of corticosteroids in CF are: status asthmaticus, allergic bronchopulmonary aspergillosis, and hypersensitivity reactions.

Reference: Auerbach HS, Kirkpatrick JA, Williams M, Colten HR: Alternate-day prednisone reduces morbidity and improves pulmonary function in cystic fibrosis. Lancet 2:686–688, 1985.

26. How are recurrent pneumothoraces in CF managed?

Medical treatment includes chemical pleurodesis with intrapleural instillation of tetracycline or quinacrine. Surgical treatment includes parietal pleurectomy (also known as pleural stripping) or pleural abrasion with dry gauze/abrasive pads. The morbidity and the efficacy of medical and surgical therapy appear to be similar. It should be noted that an extensive pleurodesis may make a CF patient ineligible for treatment by heart-lung transplantation. The most appropriate therapy is therefore a limited surgical pleurodesis if it appears that the patient may become a candidate for a heart-lung transplant in the future.

27. How is hemoptysis managed in CF?

Minor Hemoptysis (< 1 oz blood)
> Examine the patient if hemoptysis represents a new problem.
> Check coagulation studies, hemoglobin, sputum culture.
> Start antibiotics if the patient has an infection.
> Stop irritating, inhaled medications (Mucomyst).
> Stop percussion for the time being and substitute vibration and postural drainage.

Moderate Hemoptysis (1–6 oz blood)
> All of the above.
> Type and cross-match blood.
> Consider hospital admission for observation.

Major Hemoptysis (> 6 oz blood)
> All of the above.
> Admit to hospital.
> Transfuse if indicated.
> Evaluate for Gelfoam embolization of the bleeding bronchial artery or for a partial pneumonectomy.

Infections of the Respiratory Tract

28. What is the pathophysiology of the pulmonary disease in bronchiolitis?

Viral infection with respiratory syncytial virus is the precipitating cause in 80% of infants. Influenza virus, para-influenza type 3, and rhinovirus can produce a similar clinical pattern. The infection causes inflammatory edema of the small airways with infiltration by lymphocytes and plasma cells. Bronchospasm may also be present, although the relative contribution of bronchospasm to wheezing is controversial. Changes in the diameter of small airways cause increased airway resistance with tachypnea and wheezing, and right to left shunting due to ventilation/perfusion inequalities. Increased secretion of mucus and desquamation of epithelial cells may lead to atelectasis of subsegments, segments, or even lobes because of airway occlusion. Late complications include an increased incidence of reactive airway disease, and minor abnormalities of pulmonary function.

29. What are the signs and symptoms of impending respiratory failure in bronchiolitis?
Beware of infants with lethargy, reduced breath sounds, and cyanosis. Such patients are in impending respiratory failure and should have an arterial blood gas determination.

30. A 5-month old infant has bronchiolitis due to respiratory syncytial virus (RSV). What should the parents be told about the risk of future wheezing?
The risk of developing asthma is increased in children with a history of RSV bronchiolitis. Estimates of risk range from 30% to greater than 50%.

31. When is ribavirin therapy indicated in bronchiolitis?
Ribavirin, an anti-viral agent, has been marketed aggressively for RSV bronchiolitis. However, it should be reserved for the treatment of patients with congenital heart disease, bronchopulmonary dysplasia, immune deficiency, or onset of respiratory failure. Ribavirin is not indicated for the treatment of mild cases of RSV bronchiolitis. The diagnosis of RSV infection should be confirmed by immunofluorescence, as it has not been substantiated that ribavirin has any place in the therapy of para-influenzal or adenoviral infections.

32. What are the most common pathogens responsible for retropharyngeal abscesses? What are the radiographic findings on the lateral neck film?
Mixed infections of anaerobes and aerobes (including streptococci, *Staphylococcus aureus* and Hemophilus) are the rule in this condition. The x-ray findings include airway narrowing and widening of the retropharyngeal space. Normally, the retropharyngeal space is approximately the width of one vertebral body.
  Reference: Brook I: Microbiology of retropharyngeal abscesses in children. Am J Dis Child 141:202–204, 1987.

33. Children of what age group are most susceptible to retropharyngeal abscess? Why?
This disease is most common between ages 1 and 6. There are several small lymph nodes in the retropharyngeal space which usually disappear by age 4 or 5. These lymph nodes drain the posterior nasal passages and the nasopharynx, and may become involved if those sites are infected.

34. What are the indications for tonsillectomy in a child with a peritonsillar abscess?
All children who have had a peritonsillar abscess should be referred for a tonsillectomy 4–5 weeks later to reduce the risk of recurrence.

35. Cold agglutinins are often present during illness with *Mycoplasma pneumoniae*. What are "cold agglutinins" and how specific are they for mycoplasmal infections?
Cold agglutinins are IgM antibodies that agglutinate red cells by reacting with the I antigen. A titer of 1:64 or greater supports the diagnosis of *Mycoplasma pneumoniae* infection. Other respiratory infections, especially viral infections, can also give a positive result. A single cold agglutinin titer of >1:64 is therefore not conclusive evidence of infection with *M. pneumoniae*. However, in combination with a high antimycoplasma antibody titer, a cold agglutinin titer of 1:64 is diagnostic.

36. What are the distinguishing features of croup and epiglottitis?

Distinguishing Features of Croup and Epiglottitis

CROUP	EPIGLOTTITIS
Symptoms	
Prodromal upper respiratory infection	Rapid onset
Harsh, brassy cough	Little coughing
Hoarseness	Muffled voice
Slightly sore throat	Pain in throat

Table continued on next page.

Distinguishing Features of Croup and Epiglottitis *(Continued)*

CROUP	EPIGLOTTITIS
Signs	
Mild fever	High fever ($>39°C$)
Not toxic	Toxic appearance
Variable distress	Severe distress; sits upright; may drool saliva
Harsh inspiratory stridor	Low-pitched inspiratory stridor
Expiratory sounds uncommon	May have a low-pitched expiratory sound
Tongue blade examination is normal	Tongue blade examination may precipitate complete airway obstruction and is therefore hazardous to the patient. It may reveal a swollen red epiglottis.
Radiology	
Subglottic narrowing	Edema of epiglottis and aryepiglottic folds (a positive "thumb" sign)

37. What are the common pulmonary diseases in children with AIDS?

Both infectious and noninfectious pulmonary diseases are common presenting complaints in children with AIDS: These include:

Pneumocystis carinii pneumonia

Cytomegalovirus pneumonia

Pulmonary lymphoid hyperplasia or lymphoid interstitial pneumonia

Pulmonary candidiasis

Legionella pneumophila pneumonia

Infection with *Mycobacterium avium intracellulare*

38. How often are blood cultures positive in children with pneumonia?

Blood cultures are positive in 20–30% of cases of bacterial pneumonia. Despite this low sensitivity, blood cultures should be sent when the diagnosis of pneumonia is being considered, as the specificity of a positive culture is high.

39. What is the value of a nasopharyngeal culture in a child with pneumonia?

The technique has very limited value. The correlation between organisms colonizing or infecting the upper respiratory tract and those that may be infecting the lower respiratory tract is poor. Normal children may be colonized with α-hemolytic streptococcus, *S. aureus*, or *H. influenzae*. The interpretation of results of such cultures is therefore only slightly more reliable than reading tea leaves!

40. What are the risk factors for the development of pulmonary aspergillosis?

Aspergillus fumigatus is a mold that produces four different types of disease in humans:

Invasive infection in immunocompromised hosts

    Chronic granulomatous disease

    T-cell deficiencies

    Chemotherapy subjects

Allergic disease

    Sensitized individuals with asthma can simply react to *A. fumigatus* as an allergen in the same way that they might react to ragweed.

Mycetoma

    The mold fills an old cavity in the lung (e.g., tuberculosis)

Allergic bronchopulmonary aspergillosis (ABPA)

    ABPA is a hypersensitivity response to saprophytic colonization of diseased airways by the mold. A significant component of the disease is produced by the immune response to *Aspergillus fumigatus* and not the organism itself. This disease tends to affect children with abnormal airways, especially children with cystic fibrosis. In adults, allergic bronchopulmonary aspergillosis is usually associated with asthma but this association is uncommon in childhood.

41. What are the features of allergic bronchopulmonary aspergillosis (ABPA)?

Hyphae in the sputum	Positive serum precipitins
Sputum eosinophilia	Positive immediate and delayed skin tests
Peripheral blood eosinophilia	Transient infiltrates on chest x-ray
Increased serum IgE	Proximal, cylindrical bronchiectasis
Positive IgE antibody test (RAST)	

42. What x-ray findings, signs, and symptoms are suggestive of a foreign body aspiration?

Symptoms and History
    Child less than 4 years old
    Boys twice as common as girls
    Coughing
    Hemoptysis
    A respiratory infection that does not resolve with treatment
    History of choking
    Difficulty in breathing
Signs
    Fixed, localized wheeze
    Generalized wheezing in a child with no prior history of asthma
    Reduced breath sounds over one lung, one lobe or a segment
    Mediastinal shift
    One nipple higher than the other
    Stridor
X-ray Findings
    The chest radiograph may be normal
    Persistent infiltrate
    Obstructive emphysema
    Obstructive atelectasis
    Radiopaque foreign body
    Bronchiectasis (late complication)
    Asymmetry of lung volumes in left and right lateral decubitus views (obstructed side with trapped air does not collapse)

43. What is the scimitar syndrome?

This syndrome is a rare congenital malformation in which a hypoplastic lung is associated with a systemic arterial supply and anomalous pulmonary venous drainage into the inferior vena cava. The "scimitar" refers to the characteristic radiographic appearance of a crescent-shaped shadow adjacent to the right cardiac border due to the presence of the anomalous pulmonary vein.

44. What is Kartagener's syndrome?

Kartagener's syndrome is a clinical syndrome of recurrent pulmonary infections, chronic sinusitis, situs inversus, and infertility in males. This is now recognized to be a clinical manifestation of the immotile cilia syndrome. These syndromes are usually inherited in an autosomal recessive pattern and have recurrent pulmonary infections caused by defective mucociliary clearance. Some of the features are similar to cystic fibrosis but the incidence is approximately 10 times less. Infertility in affected individuals occurs because the tails of the spermatozoa have the same abnormality of ultrastructure as the respiratory cilia. The cause of the situs inversus is not fully understood. It has been suggested that cilia are important for movement of the midgut into the coelomic cavity in the proper orientation, and that derangements of this process may lead to situs inversus.

45. With what conditions are nasal polyps associated?

Pediatric: Nasal polyps are very rare in children except as a manifestation of cystic fibrosis. A sweat test is therefore essential in such patients. Nasal allergies should also be considered as a cause of polyps.

Adolescents: There is a wider range of possible diagnoses such as:

Cystic fibrosis	Triad asthma
Nasal allergies	Asthma
Chronic sinusitis	Nasal polyps
Malignancy	Aspirin sensitivity

46. How may parental smoking affect children?

Effects of Smoking

	FETUS AND NEONATE	HEALTHY CHILD
Well-documented evidence	Decreased birth weight Increased incidences of spontaneous abortions, abruptio placentae, placenta previa, and premature deliveries Increased perinatal mortality	Increased risk of upper and lower respiratory tract infections Slight decrease in lung function
Suggestive evidence	Risk of minimal brain dysfunction and hyperkinesis Reduced lung growth and body size	Independent risk of sudden infant death syndrome Risk of asthma

From Wall MA: Update on the effects of passive smoking in children. J Respir Dis 8:31–36, 1987, with permission.

47. What are the indications for surgical repair of pectus excavatum?

This is a controversial subject. Physiological limitations in pulmonary or cardiac function are the principal indications for surgical repair and these are uncommon except in patients with very large defects. Repair should be considered if the child is embarassed or psychologically affected by the appearance of the lesion. Surgical correction should not be delayed too long, as the operation becomes more difficult as the skeleton matures. A decision concerning surgery should be made by the time that a child is 8–9 years old.

48. Who was Ondine and what is her curse?

Ondine was a legendary water nymph who fell in love with a mortal and put a curse on him that should he ever betray her, he would suffocate by not breathing when he fell asleep. The legend is derived from medieval times and, more recently, was portrayed in the play "Ondine" by the French playwright Jean Giraudoux (1882-1944). Ondine's lover, Hans, did deceive her by falling for the greater charms of Bertha and gets his dues in the third act of the play. The term "Ondine's curse" has been used to describe the syndrome of sleep apnea secondary to reduced respiratory drive. This is a rare condition and it is often associated with other abnormalities of brain stem function. Ondine's curse may be idiopathic or it may be a complication of an earlier insult to the developing brain. These children are treated by mechanical ventilation during sleep; some centers have successfully used phrenic nerve pacing.

Note: "Intern's curse" is the precise opposite. Such mortals are affected by not sleeping while they breathe.

49. Which laboratory tests are useful discriminators of exudates and transudates in pleural effusions?

Laboratory Tests for Pleural Effusions

	EXUDATE	TRANSUDATE
Protein	> 2.6 g%	< 2.6 g%
Pleural:plasma protein ratio*	> 50%	< 50%
LDH	> 200 IU	< 200 IU

Modified from Pagtakhan RD, Chernick V. Liquid and air in the pleural space. In Kendig EL, Chernick V (eds): Disorders of the Respiratory Tract in Children. Philadelphia, W.B. Saunders Co., 1983, pp 483–496.

*The use of the ratio of the pleural fluid protein to the plasma protein is essential in evaluating a hypoproteinemic patient (such as a child with nephrotic syndrome), who may have developed an effusion either from decreased oncotic pressure or from pneumonia.

50. When are chest tubes indicated for the management of pleural fluid?

1. Respiratory distress caused by a large pleural effusion.

2. Empyema (to hasten resolution and to reduce the risk of a thick, pleural "orange peel" developing).

3. A chest tube is occasionally inserted for drainage of chylous effusions. The drainage of a chylothorax can lead to malnutrition and to depletion of T-cells if large volumes of lymph are removed. The conventional management has been the use of a chest tube in combination with a low-fat diet to reduce the formation of chyle.

51. What is the treatment of choice for pneumomediastinum?

The answer to this question depends on the magnitude of the air leak. Small, asymptomatic pneumomediastina are commonly observed in asthmatics and they usually resolve without any intervention. Moderate-sized collections are usually associated with a pneumothorax, and drainage of the pneumothorax by chest tube should relieve the pneumomediastinum. Large collections do not usually cause major symptoms but they may compromise cardiac function, leading to hypotension, muffled heart sounds, and cyanosis. In such circumstances, the best strategy is to insert a drain into the mediastinum using a subxiphoid approach. All air collections in the thorax reabsorb more quickly if the patient is given 100% oxygen to breathe.

52. What are the radiographic signs of pulmonary edema?

Loss of definition of the pulmonary veins, "hilar haze," septal lines (Kerley A and B lines), and fluffy alveolar shadows (alveolar flooding).

53. What are the causes of unilateral pulmonary edema?

1. Rapid removal of air or fluid from the pleural space on one side.

2. Abnormal lymphatic drainage of one lung (e.g., pulmonary lymphangiectasia).

3. Any cause of diffuse pulmonary edema may present as unilateral pulmonary edema if the child is lying in a decubitus position.

54. A child with epiglottitis is intubated and within one-half hour develops severe pulmonary edema. Why?

This is a fairly common clinical scenario. Two explanations have been suggested for the development of pulmonary edema.

1. With severe upper airway obstruction, the intrathoracic pressure swings may become very great with negative pressures as high as 70–80 cm of water. This hydrostatic gradient far exceeds the oncotic pressure of plasma, and water tends to move into the lung interstitium.

2. A better explanation is that the negative intrathoracic pressure causes an increased venous return to the heart with an increase in pulmonary vascular volume and impaired left ventricular ejection fraction. This could cause an increase in the ultrafiltration of fluid into the interstitium, which is masked during the period of obstruction by the very positive pressures

that develop during exhalation. After relief of the obstruction, the patient's own PEEP is removed and the pulmonary edema may become apparent. Pulmonary edema is manifested by pink, frothy secretions when the child is intubated. These secretions may be dispersed by nebulized ethyl alcohol to break up the foam if it is causing airway obstruction.

Reference: Sofer S: Bar-Ziv J, Scharf SM: Pulmonary edema following relief of upper airway obstruction. Chest 86:401–403, 1984.

55. What are the most common pulmonary malignancies in childhood?

Primary malignant tumors of the lung are extremely rare in childhood to the extent that you might be able to publish a case report if you diagnose one! The following tumors are the most common:

Benign

    Hamartoma

    Bronchial adenoma (usually of the carcinoid type)

    Papilloma of the trachea or bronchi: these are usually multiple and associated with laryngeal papillomata. They probably occur secondary to infection of the child's airways at birth with papilloma virus. This virus also causes condylomata (venereal warts) and cervical neoplasia. The prognosis is not good, as the condition is very difficult to eradicate.

Malignant

    Bronchogenic carcinoma

    Leiomyosarcoma (this often arises from the airway smooth muscle)

    Fibrosarcoma

Metastatic Tumors

    Wilms' tumors

    Lymphoma

    Osteogenic sarcoma

    Sarcomas

56. How does the pH of a substance affect the severity of disease in aspiration pneumonia?

A low pH is more harmful than a slightly alkaline or a neutral pH and is more likely to be associated with bronchospasm and pneumonia. The most severe form of pneumonia is seen when gastric contents are aspirated; symptoms may develop in a matter of seconds. If the volume of aspirate is sufficiently large and the pH is less than 2.5, the mortality may exceed 70%. The radiographic picture may be that of an infiltrate or of pulmonary edema. Unilateral pulmonary edema may occur if the child is lying on one side.

57. How should children with aspiration pneumonia be managed?

Aspiration pneumonia is best treated supportively and conservatively. Administration of antibiotics does not appear to improve the prognosis significantly, probably because the pathophysiology is that of a chemical pneumonitis. Cultures of blood and sputum (or tracheal aspirate) should be obtained. Penicillin is the antibiotic of choice for an aspiration pneumonia where secondary infection is suspected. Postural drainage is helpful to remove the inhaled fluid. If gastric acid has been inhaled, a short course of corticosteroids may be helpful if therapy is started within a few hours of the aspiration.

58. What are the most common causes of stridor in the first few days of life?

Laryngomalacia	Congenital subglottic stenosis
Vocal cord paralysis	Vascular ring
Laryngeal web	Hypocalcemia

59. What are the types of vascular malformation that cause obstruction of the airway?

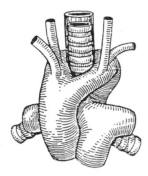

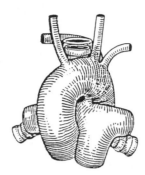

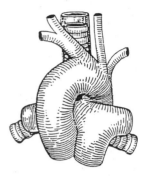

The *double aortic arch malformation* is the most common of the complete vascular rings encircling the trachea and esophagus. It results from persistence of the right ventral fourth arch artery.

An *aberrant right subclavian artery* is the least constricting of the open vascular rings. The artery compresses only the esophagus but may cause respiratory disease secondary to recurrent aspiration.

An *anomalous innominate artery,* another of the open rings, arises farther to the left than is usual and must cross the anterior aspect of the trachea. This in turn may lead to upper airway compromise.

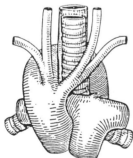

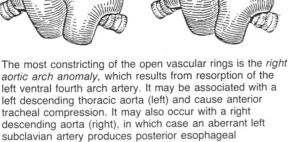

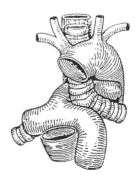

The most constricting of the open vascular rings is the *right aortic arch anomaly,* which results from resorption of the left ventral fourth arch artery. It may be associated with a left descending thoracic aorta (left) and cause anterior tracheal compression. It may also occur with a right descending aorta (right), in which case an aberrant left subclavian artery produces posterior esophageal compression. The anomaly causes problems with respiration and deglutition.

Pulmonary sling is the notable anomaly of the sixth brachial arch artery. An anomalous left pulmonary artery follows a circuitous route between the trachea and esophagus, compressing both.

From Smith RJH, Coombe WT: When congenital vascular anomalies cause airway problems. Contemp Pediatr 2:94–106, 1985, with permission.

60. What are the tumors that may develop in the anterior, middle, or posterior mediastinum in childhood?

Mediastinal Masses in Children

COMMON	RARE
Anterior Mediastinum	
Thymic lesion	Substernal thyroid
Hyperplastic cyst	Thymic tumor
Angiomatous tumor	
Hemangioma	
Lymphangioma	
Teratoma	
Lymphoma	
Hodgkin's disease	
Non-Hodgkin's lymphoma	
Middle Mediastinum	
Lymphoma	Pericardial cyst
Lymphadenopathy	
Bronchogenic cyst	
Granuloma	
Posterior Mediastinum	
Neurogenic tumor	Pheochromocytoma
Duplication cyst	Anterior meningocele
	Hemangioma

From Brecher ML: Pediatric mediastinal masses: Your role in management. J Respir Dis 7:73–87, 1986, with permission.

61. Are steroids or antibiotics useful in the management of smoke inhalation?

There is little place for the use of steroids in the management of smoke inhalation. In fact one study showed that steroids appeared to increase the mortality of smoke inhalation because of an increased risk of infection (Moylan JA, Alexander LG: Diagnosis and treatment of inhalation injury. World J Surg 2:185–191, 1978). Routine, prophylactic antibiotics should not be administered to victims of smoke inhalation, as this practice is ineffective and may predispose to infection with resistant organisms. However, pneumonia is a common complication because the chemicals in smoke, and the smoke particles, interfere with the lung's defense mechanisms. Therefore, a high index of suspicion for infection and a low threshold for performing cultures and commencing antibiotic therapy is appropriate.

62. How are alveolar-arterial oxygen gradients calculated?

The alveolar-arterial oxygen gradient (A-aDO$_2$) is a useful index of the degree of lung disease and is used in the pediatric intensive care unit to monitor changes in gas exchange. The gradient is the difference between the theoretical PO$_2$ in the alveoli (PAO$_2$)—calculated from the barometric pressure (BP), the inspired oxygen concentration (FiO$_2$), the saturated water vapor pressure at 37°C (47 mm Hg), the respiratory quotient (RQ) and the arterial CO$_2$—and the measured arterial oxygen tension (PaO$_2$) according to the following formula:

$$A-aDO_2 = (BP - 47)FiO_2 - \frac{PaCO_2}{RQ} - PaO_2$$

The normal A-aDO$_2$ is 1–9 mm Hg in young adults, with a mean value of 5 mm Hg, and it increases with age to 22–30 at age 70, with a mean value of 26 mm Hg. It should be noted that the normal A-aDO$_2$ increases two- or three-fold when a person is breathing 100% oxygen for reasons that are not fully understood.

Examples:

1. Calculate the A-aDO$_2$ in the following 15-year-old patient: pH 7.42; PaCO$_2$ = 35; PaO$_2$ = 60

Patient is breathing room air and the atmospheric pressure is 760 mm Hg. Assuming a normal RQ of 0.8: A-aDO$_2$ = (713 × 0.21) − 35/0.8 − 60 = 46 mm HG (which is increased).

2. Try to calculate the FiO$_2$ that would have to be administered to a child with a PaO$_2$ of 100 in Denver where the barometric pressure is 630 mm Hg. You will have to rearrange the equation and solve for FiO$_2$. The correct answer is 0.325 (32% oxygen).

63. What are the causes of a decreased arterial blood PaO$_2$ associated with an increased alveolar-arterial oxygen gradient?

Right to left shunting
  Intracardiac
  Abnormal arteriovenous connections
  Perfused airless alveoli (e.g., pneumonia, atelectasis)
Maldistribution of ventilation
  For example: asthma, bronchiolitis, cystic fibrosis
Impaired diffusion
  This mechanism is uncommon, as many of the conditions that have been described
    to have a "diffusion block" such as the respiratory distress syndrome have a
    major component of shunting.
  Impaired diffusion does occur when interstitial edema affects the septal walls.
Decreased central venous oxygen content
  Sluggish circulation, as in shock
  Increased tissue oxygen demands, as in sepsis

64. What are the causes of hypoxemia with a normal A-aDO$_2$?

Hypoxemia can occur in the absence of any lung disease from: hypoventilation (Ondine's curse, narcotic overdose); increased altitude; and breathing hypoxic gas mixtures.

65. What are the best ways to quantitate digital clubbing?

Digital clubbing is caused by the presence of increased amounts of connective tissue under the base of the fingernail. This may be determined by:

1. Visual inspection
2. Rocking the nail on its bed between your finger and thumb (it seems to float). This sign is easy to elicit and takes very little time.
3. Looking for the diamond sign. Normally if the nails of both index fingers or any other two identical fingers are opposed, there is a diamond shaped window present between the nail bases (see figure). This sign is quite sensitive if there is any doubt about the presence of mild finger clubbing.
4. Measurements made on plaster casts or on radiographs of the fingers.

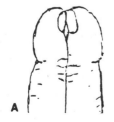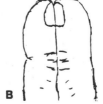

Left, A normal child with a diamond-shaped window present between the nail bases when the fingers are opposed. *Right,* The appearance of digital clubbing where the diamond-shaped window has been obliterated by the increased amount of soft tissue under the base of the nail.

66. What are the causes of clubbing?

Pulmonary
Bronchiectasis
Pulmonary abscesses
Empyema
Chronic infection
Malignant neoplasms
Interstitial fibrosis
Cardiac
Cyanotic congenital heart disease
Subacute bacterial endocarditis
Hepatic
Biliary cirrhosis
Biliary atresia
Gastrointestinal
Ulcerative colitis
Crohn's disease
Chronic infective diarrhea (amebic and bacillary)
Polyposis, multiple
Other
Thyrotoxicosis

Reference: Modified from Waring WW: The history and physical examination. In Kendig EL, Chernick V (eds): Disorders of the Respiratory Tract in Children. Philadelphia, W.B. Saunders Co., 1983, pp 57–78.

67. Why does pulmonary disease cause clubbing?

The answer to this question is unclear. The increased soft tissue under the nail beds that causes digital clubbing is thought to be vascular (possibly multiple arteriovenous connections). These may be caused by the presence of vasoactive substances that are increased either by hypoxia or by decreased lung clearance. A new theory holds that digital clubbing is caused by local release of platelet-derived growth factor because of platelet emboli that are normally trapped by the pulmonary circulation and that are deposited in the digital vessels when there is pulmonary shunting.

Bibliography

1. Abraham WM, Wanner A: Inflammatory mediators of asthma. Pediatr Pulmonol 4:237–247, 1987.
2. Canny GJ, Levison H: The modern management of childhood asthma. Pediatr Rev Commun 1:123–162, 1987.
3. Eggleston DE, Slovis TL, Watts FB: Update on pediatric chest imaging. Pediatr Pulmonol 5:158–175, 1988.
4. Fernald GW, Boat TF: Cystic fibrosis: Overview. Semin Roentgenol 22:87–96, 1987.
5. Kendig EL, Chernick V (eds): Disorders of the Respiratory Tract in Children, 4th ed. Philadelphia, W.B. Saunders, 1983.
6. Koff PB, Eitzman D, Neu J: Neonatal and Pediatric Respiratory Care. St. Louis, C.V. Mosby, 1988.
7. Rossman CM, Newhouse MT: Primary ciliary dyskinesia: Evaluation and management. Pediatr Pulmonol 5:36–50, 1988.
8. Thiebault DW, Gregory G: Neonatal Pulmonary Care. Norwalk, CT, Appleton-Lange, 1986.
9. Wood RE, Boat TF, Doershuck CF: Cystic fibrosis. Am Rev Respir Dis 113:833–878, 1976.

RHEUMATOLOGY

Andrew H. Eichenfield, M.D.

1. What are the most common causes of isolated arthritis (monarticular)?
The most common cause of monarticular arthritis in childhood is post-traumatic synovitis; infectious etiologies are next most common. About one-third of all septic arthritis occurs in the pediatric age group. A bacterial etiology is established in approximately 70% of cases. Most recent series indicate that *Staphylococcus aureus* is the most commonly implicated pathogen overall and is isolated from children of all ages. However, in children aged 6 months to 6 years, *Hemophilus influenzae* type b is the most frequent cause of septic arthritis. *Neisseria gonorrhoeae* must be considered as an etiology in any potentially sexually active child or adolescent.

2. In the initial workup of a child with suspected juvenile rheumatoid arthritis (JRA), what serologic studies and other laboratory tests should be ordered?
Laboratory tests are helpful primarily in excluding other ("reactive," infectious, rheumatic, paraneoplastic) causes of arthritis in childhood, but cannot establish a diagnosis of JRA. In a prospective analysis of 278 Finnish children with arthritis, Kunnamo et al. examined the utility of 22 laboratory tests and came to the conclusion that the following tests are indicated in all children with joint symptoms:

Complete blood count with platelets and differential
Erythrocyte sedimentation rate
C-reactive protein
Urinalysis
Throat culture

Their recommendations for evaluation of children with symptoms lasting >2 weeks include antinuclear antibody and quantitative immunoglobulins. In selected cases, determinations of rheumatoid factor, antistreptolysin O, and antibodies to the Lyme spirochete may be indicated.

Reference: Kunnamo I, et al: Clinical signs and laboratory tests in the differential diagnosis of arthritis in children. Am J Dis Child 141: 34–40, 1987.

3. Is the measurement of rheumatoid factor a good screening test for JRA?
Rheumatoid factor, as measured by the classic latex-fixation test, is an anti-IgG antibody of the IgM class. It is present in the sera of 80% of adults with rheumatoid arthritis, but in only 5–10% of children with JRA (primarily older girls with polyarticular disease). A screening test should have a high sensitivity ("PID, positive in disease" = true positives/all diseased). JRA is a disease with a relatively low prevalence rate, somewhere on the order of 1/1000. Assuming a sensitivity of even 10%, one would have to screen 10,000 children to identify 1 child with JRA and positive RF (assuming 100% specificity). False-positives can be seen in SLE, Sjögren's syndrome, mixed connective tissue disease, viral infections, parasitic infections, malignancies, SBE, and sarcoidosis. The value of measuring RF has recently been subjected to a more formal analysis and found to be of no benefit in ruling JRA in or out.

Reference: Eichenfield AH, et al: Utility of rheumatoid factor in the diagnosis of JRA. Pediatrics 78: 480–484, 1986.

4. What is the current recommendation for first-line therapy in suspected JRA?
The "gold standard" for first-line anti-inflammatory therapy in JRA is not gold, but a derivative of willow bark, acetylsalicylic acid. Aspirin is given four times/day with meals in a dosage of 80 mg/kg/day (it need *not* be given at evenly spaced intervals or equally divided doses). Steady-state levels are usually reached 5–9 days after institution of or change in therapy; levels between 20 and 30 mg/dl are usually effective at decreasing joint pain,

stiffness, and swelling. Levels in excess of 30 mg/dl effect no greater improvement and may engender greater toxicity. At total daily doses $\geq$ 100 mg/kg, increments of 10 mg/kg may result in disproportionately high elevations in salicylate level and toxicity. Signs of acute salicylism include nausea, vomiting, irritability, and hyperpnea. Adverse reactions associated with chronic administration (not related to salicylate level) include hepatotoxicity (AST and ALT should be checked frequently, especially early in therapy), gastritis and ulcers, and renal papillary necrosis. There is a strong association between Reye's syndrome and salicylate therapy during episodes of varicella and influenza. Therefore, it would seem prudent to discontinue aspirin during such intercurrent illnesses.

If aspirin is ineffective (after at least a 6–12 week trial at therapeutic levels) or not tolerated properly, a nonsteroidal anti-inflammatory drug (NSAID) should be tried. Two NSAIDs are available for pediatric use in the U.S.— tolmetin sodium (Tolectin) (20–30 mg/kg/day in three divided doses) and naproxen (Naprosyn) (10–20 mg/kg/day in two divided doses). These are generally less irritating to the gastric mucosa, cause hepatotoxicity less frequently, and are not associated with Reye's syndrome. Ibuprofen is available as an over-the-counter preparation, but is not officially indicated for the treatment of JRA by the Food and Drug Administration.

Reference: Doughty RA, et al: Salicylate therapy in JRA. Am J Dis Child 134: 461–463, 1980.

5. What are the most common signs and symptoms in children with systemic JRA?

Systemic-onset JRA (known as Still's disease to old hands) accounts for approximately 20% of most series of JRA. Children with this form of disease classically present with fevers of unknown origin with single to double quotidian spikes as high as 41°C. The temperature characteristically returns to 37° or lower at other times; continuous fever should suggest other diagnoses. A blotchy, light pink, evanescent macular eruption accompanies the fever in over 90% of cases. The rash of systemic JRA is diagnostic only *after* the diagnosis is made (by exclusion). Other early signs and symptoms include arthralgia, myalgia, neck pain, irritability, generalized lymphadenopathy, hepatosplenomegaly, anemia, and thrombocytosis. Pericarditis and pleuritis may be associated. Arthritis may not be present for the first weeks of illness, but chronic joint involvement follows in most cases.

6. How often is there chronic joint involvement in JRA, and which joints are most often affected?

By definition, all children with JRA have chronic joint involvement (i.e., arthritis for more than 6 weeks without other known etiology). Children are assigned to appropriate subgroups depending on: (1) the presence or absence of fever at presentation; and (2) the number of joints involved in the first 6 months of illness.

JRA Subgroups, Joints Involved, HLA Associations, Eye Findings, and Prognosis

JRA SUBGROUP (% affected)	SEX	NUMBER AND DISTRIBUTION OF JOINTS INVOLVED	HLA	EYE FINDINGS	JOINT DISABILITY
Pauciarticular Type I (35%)	F>M	≤4: Asymmetrical, knee, wrist, ankle	DR5	Chronic uveitis (associated with ANA)	10%
Pauciarticular Type II (15?%	M>F	≤4: Asymmetrical, knee, wrist, ankle, hip, sacroiliac	B27	Acute uveitis	10%
Polyarticular RF-positive (5–10%)	F>M	≥5: Symmetrical, small and large joints	DR4	Rare	50%
Polyarticular RF-negative (20–30%)	F>M	≥5: Symmetrical, small and large joints	?	Rare	15%
Systemic-onset (15–20%)	F=M	40% Pauciarticular course 60% Polyarticular course	?	Rare	25%

7. What percent of patients with JRA go on to chronic debilitating disease and what percentage "outgrow" their arthritis?

Overall, between 75 and 85% of children with JRA are free of arthritis 5 years after diagnosis. However, prognosis varies greatly from one subgroup to the next. Children with pauciarticular disease rarely have persistent problems, although boys with older age onset can develop ankylosing spondylitis. The percentage of children with grade III or IV disability (partially or totally dependent on assistive devices for activities of daily living) are noted in the table above. Poorer prognoses are associated with the presence of rheumatoid factor and unremitting systemic disease.

8. Is there any evidence to suggest JRA has a hereditary, infectious, or traumatic basis?

Unlike SLE, JRA rarely affects other first-degree relatives. Sibling pairs with JRA are decidedly uncommon, with the exception of identical twins. However, there is clearly a genetic component to chronic arthritis in childhood. The preceding table lists the HLA types which have been correlated with the various subgroups. JRA probably represents an abnormal immune response to any number of inciting antigens. Rubella virus has been cultured from the joints of children with chronic arthritis, indicating incomplete clearance of virus in such cases. Other infections may mimic JRA, notably Lyme disease and parvovirus. "Reactive" arthritides follow infections, but causative organisms cannot be isolated from affected joints. Organisms implicated as causes of reactive arthritis include group A streptococci, Salmonella, Yersinia, and meningococcus. Occasionally, a history of antecedent trauma is elicited in a patient subsequently found to have JRA. It is possible that a sprain may "uncover" antigens to which the patient then makes an abnormal immune response; this is more likely if the arthritis is polyarticular and does not involve only the traumatized joint. In most cases, however, it is probable that the trauma calls attention to an otherwise unrecognized arthritis.

9. What are considered poor prognostic factors in JRA?

It is difficult to make sweeping statements regarding poor prognostic features. It is self-evident that a child with pauciarticular disease is likely to fare better than one with more involved joints. However, the presence of latex-agglutinating rheumatoid factor in patients with polyarticular disease confers a poor outcome in up to 50% of cases. Children with systemic-onset disease fare poorly approximately 25% of the time. Those with pauciarticular disease and positive tests for ANA are at high risk (70–90%) for development of chronic iritis and should be screened for asymptomatic changes by slit lamp examination at least every 6 months. (Those with negative tests for ANA are also at risk and should be examined at least yearly.) Prior to the institution of such screening examinations, up to 17% of affected children became totally blind.

10. What are the indications for systemic corticosteroid therapy in children with JRA?

The adrenal glands are better regulators of corticosteroid release than any rheumatologist. Indications for corticosteroid therapy in JRA are few. Children with systemic-onset JRA and pericarditis or myocarditis may require high doses of glucocorticoids. Those with unremitting fever unresponsive to NSAIDs may benefit from addition of a small dose of prednisone (½ mg/kg) on *alternate days*. This is also true of children with unrelenting polyarthritis who become bed- or chair-bound and require intensive physical therapy to achieve ambulatory status. Daily steroid therapy should be avoided at all costs, as it is exceedingly difficult to manage. Rarely, children with aggressive uveitis may not respond to topical therapy and will require systemic corticosteroids. A patient with a single symptomatic joint may benefit from intra-articular corticosteroid.

11. What are the indications for second-line therapy in JRA?

Arthritis that does not respond to conservative management (NSAIDs) for 6 months is the primary indication for a disease-modifying drug. The only slow-acting antirheumatic drug currently approved for use in children is injectable gold. Drugs used in adults with rheumatoid arthritis which are also used in selected children include hydroxychloroquine, auranofin (oral gold), d-penicillamine, azathioprine, sulfasalazine, and methotrexate. Consultation with a pediatric or adult rheumatologist is probably in order before addition of a disease-modifying drug, given the risk-benefit ratio of some of the agents.

12. What is the significance of hyperextensible joints?

Hyperextensible joints predispose some children to recurrent strains and sprains that can mimic JRA. The "benign hypermobile joint syndrome" of childhood is a form of Ehlers-Danlos syndrome, with the following criteria:

1. Passive apposition of the thumbs to the flexor aspect of the forearm.
2. Passive hyperextension of the fingers so they lie parallel to the extensor aspect of the forearms.
3. Hyperextension of the elbows 10°.
4. Hyperextension of the knees 10°.
5. Flexion of the trunk with knees extended so the palms rest on the floor.

Gedalia et al. found that children with episodic joint complaints fulfilled 3 of the criteria more frequently than other children (J Pediatr 107:873–876, 1985).

13. How is ankylosing spondylitis (AS) diagnosed in children?

AS is diagnosed in children as in adults, with difficulty. The *sine qua non* for the diagnosis is radiologic evidence of sacroiliitis.

New York Criteria for Diagnosis of Ankylosing Spondylitis (1966)

Diagnosis

1. Limitation of motion of the lumbar spine in all three planes: anterior flexion, lateral flexion, and extension.
2. History of the presence of pain at the dorsolumbar junction or in the lumbar spine.
3. Limitation of chest expansion to 1 inch or less, measured at the level of the fourth intercostal space.

Grading

Definite AS

1. Grade 3–4 radiographic bilateral sacroiliitis with at least one clinical criterion.
2. Grade 3–4 unilateral sacroiliitis with clinical criterion 1 or with both clinical criteria 2 and 3.

Probable AS

1. Grade 3–4 bilateral sacroiliitis without clinical criteria.

The criteria are rarely fulfilled in childhood. In adults, it takes an average of 5 years from first symptoms to make a diagnosis of AS. Children are more likely to present with a prodrome of oligoarticular asymmetrical arthritis (indistinguishable from pauciarticular JRA Type II) and/or inflammation at the sites of tendon insertions (enthesitis). Sacroiliitis or spondylitic symptoms are uncommon. Furthermore, not all children with pauciarticular Type II JRA go on to develop AS, although both groups have strong HLA-B27 associations.

14. What other conditions mimic the findings of AS?

Other HLA-B27 associated syndromes that share symptoms in common with AS include Reiter's syndrome, "enteric arthropathies" (following infections with Salmonella, Shigella, Yersinia), the arthritis of inflammatory bowel disease, psoriatic arthritis, and pauciarticular JRA (Type II). Frequently, only time distinguishes these entities and all can lead to true AS.

15. What is enthesitis?

The enthesis is the area of attachment of ligaments and tendons to bone. Enthesopathy is unique to the spondyloarthropathies; inflammation results in cellular resorption, bony erosion, and ultimately calcification. This results in pain on motion or palpation of the tendons, including the infrapatellar and Achilles tendons. The heel spurs and "bamboo spine" of AS are a consequence of this process.

16. What are the most common manifestations of systemic lupus erythematosus (SLE) in children?

SLE is the prototypical multisystem autoimmune disease. Its manifestations are protean and virtually any organ system can be involved.

Signs and Symptoms of SLE in Children

SIGNS/SYMPTOMS	APPROX. PREVALENCE
Rash/fever	70%
Arthritis	70%
Renal (proteinuria/casts)*	60%
Anemia, leukopenia, thrombocytopenia	50–75%
Cardiac	25%
CNS (psychosis/seizures)	15%
Other: GI and pulmonary less common	

*Some abnormality probably demonstrable on kidney biopsy in any patient.

17. Which diseases should be considered in the differential diagnosis of children with butterfly rash?

A malar rash is present in 50% of children with SLE and cutaneous involvement. In the typical butterfly rash, the malar areas are prominently involved, with the nasolabial folds being relatively spared. The rash crosses the nasal bridge in a "butterfly" distribution. Occasionally, it is difficult to distinguish from the rash of dermatomyositis (eruption on the extensor surfaces of the fingers is common in dermatomyositis and rare in SLE). Vesiculation should suggest a diagnosis of pemphigus erythematosus or contact dermatitis. A malar flush is clinically distinct and can be seen in individuals with mitral stenosis or hypothyroidism.

18. Which laboratory tests should be ordered in a child suspected of having SLE?

The best screening study for SLE is the fluorescent antinuclear antibody (FANA) test. Antinuclear antibodies are immunoglobulins directed against a variety of nuclear antigens including nucleic acids, histones, non-histone proteins, and the nuclear matrix. Up to 97% of patients with SLE will have positive ANAs at some point in their illness (not necessarily at diagnosis). In a patient with characteristic signs and symptoms, a FANA test may serve to confirm suspicions of SLE. Other antibodies considered to be more specific for the diagnosis of SLE include those to native DNA and the extractable nuclear antigen Sm. The finding of a low C3 and positive anti-native DNA antibody is *100% specific* for SLE.

19. What criteria must be met for diagnosis of SLE?

The 1982 revised American Rheumatism Association criteria for SLE are presented below. Four of the eleven criteria are ultimately present in 96% of patients with SLE, though not necessarily at the time of diagnosis. It should be stressed that these are *not* diagnostic criteria, but were devised for the purposes of defining the illness to facilitate study of its epidemiology, clinical course and prognosis. One can have SLE and not meet 4 criteria; conversely, occasional patients without SLE can meet 4 criteria (primary biliary cirrhosis, chronic active hepatitis).

Revised Criteria for the Classification of Systemic Lupus Erythematosus (ARA 1982)

1. Butterfly rash. Fixed erythema, flat or raised, over malar eminences.
2. Discoid lupus. Erythematous, raised patches with adherent, keratotic scaling and follicular plugging.
3. Photosensitivity.
4. Oral ulceration. Oral or nasal ulcers, usually painless.
5. Arthritis. Non-erosive arthritis.
6. Serositis. Pleuritis or pericarditis.
7. Renal disorder
     Proteinuria (≥0.5 gm/24 hr), or
     Cellular casts.

Continued on next page.

8. Neurologic disorder
   Seizures in the absence of offending drugs or metabolic derangements, or
   Psychosis in the absence of offending drugs.
9. Hematologic disorder
   Hemolytic anemia with reticulocytosis, or
   Leukopenia <4,000/mm³ on 2 or more occasions, or
   Lymphopenia <1,500/mm³ on 2 or more occasions, or
   Thrombocytopenia <100,000/mm³ in the absence of offending drugs.
10. Immunologic
    Positive LE cell preparation, or
    Anti-native DNA antibodies in abnormal titer, or
    Anti-Sm antibody, or
    False-positive serologic test for syphilis for at least 6 months and confirmed by
      TPI or FTA tests.
11. Antinuclear antibody. Abnormal titer at any time in the absence of drugs known to
be associated with the "drug-induced lupus" syndrome.

20. What is the prognosis for children with confirmed SLE?

The prognosis for survival in children with SLE has improved remarkably in the last 20 years. Survival rates at 10 years in excess of 85% can be expected, compared with mortality rates of 75–80% in the early 1960s. It is not at all clear that this outcome is a function of aggressive treatment with corticosteroids and cytotoxic agents; it may well reflect improved general supportive care (intensive care, earlier diagnosis, etc.).

21. What laboratory values are most useful in the monitoring of the effectiveness of anti-lupus therapy?

Sequential serologic studies can provide information regarding the activity of SLE and the effect of therapy on the disease process. The titer of ANA is not well correlated with disease activity: however, antibodies to doublestranded DNA are helpful in this regard. Complement levels (C3, CH_{50}) are inversely related to the levels of anti-DNA antibody and are useful as well in gauging response to therapy.

22. What is the recommended treatment for children with SLE and central nervous system involvement?

As opposed to SLE nephritis, in which there is at least general agreement that corticosteroids and/or immunosuppressive agents are of value, CNS lupus does not appear to respond well to treatment. Seizures are treated with anticonvulsants and psychoses with psychotropic medications. The underlying lupus is managed initially with high doses of corticosteroids (prednisone, 1–2 mg/kg up to 80–100 mg/day) in divided doses. If there is no response, consideration might be given to treatment with "pulse" methylprednisolone. There is as yet no evidence to support the use of cytotoxic agents in SLE patients with CNS disease; the same is true of plasmapheresis.

23. What are the neurologic manifestations of SLE and how frequently do they occur?

Lupus cerebritis is a term that implies an inflammatory etiology of CNS disease. Microscopically, however, widely scattered areas of microinfarction and noninflammatory vasculopathy are seen in brain tissue; actual CNS vasculitis is rare in SLE. Imaging techniques usually reveal brain atrophy. Lumbar punctures may reveal CSF pleocytosis or increased protein, but can be normal. EEGs may similarly be entirely normal. Neuropsychiatric manifestations of SLE are listed in the following table.

Major Manifestations of Primary Neuropsychiatric Dysfunction in SLE

MANIFESTATION	APPROXIMATE FREQUENCY
Organic mental syndrome	20%
Seizure disorder	15%
Cranial neuropathy	12%
Peripheral neuropathy	10%
Movement disorder	4%

From Bluestein HG: Neuropsychiatric disorders in SLE. In Lahita RG: Systemic Lupus Erythematosus. New York, John Wiley and Sons, 1987, with permission.

24. What is the significance of a positive ANA?

A rose is a rose is a rose, but whither the ANA? Chudwin and colleagues reviewed the clinical and laboratory findings of 138 children with positive tests for ANA over a 10 year period. The ANA is a sensitive, but not a specific test. The authors conclude that pediatric patients with a positive ANA should undergo clinical and laboratory investigation for autoimmune or rheumatic diseases.

Significance of a Positive ANA Test

DIAGNOSIS	NO. OF PATIENTS (%)
SLE	37(27)
Discoid LE	2(1.5)
JRA	33(24)
Sjögren's syndrome	9(6.5)
MCTD	7(5)
Dermatomyositis	3(2.2)
?Autoimmune disease	27(20)
IgA deficiency	9(6.5)
Post-infectious (presumed)	10(7.2)
Leukemia	1(0.7)

From Chudwin DS et al: Significance of a positive ANA test in a pediatric population. Am J Dis Child 137:1103–1106, 1983, with permission.

25. Which drugs are known to cause lupus-like signs or symptoms and/or false-positive ANAs?

Drugs for which there is definite proof

Hydralazine ⎫
Procainamide ⎬ Drug-induced LE
Isoniazid ⎭
Methyldopa ⎫
Chlorpromazine ⎭ Drug-induced ANA

Drugs for which there is a possible association

Beta blockers (practolol, atenolol, metoprolol, oxprenolol, acebutolol)
Anticonvulsants (phenytoin, phenobarbital, trimethadione, mephenytoin, ethosuximide)
Anti-thyroid agents (propylthiouracil, methimazole)
Quinidine
d-Penicillamine
Captopril

Adapted from Hess EV: Drug-related lupus: the same or different? In Lahita RG: Systemic Lupus Erythematosus. New York, John Wiley and Sons, 1987.

26. What are the common features of drug-related lupus?
Abrupt onset of symptoms, fever, myalgia/arthralgia ± serositis, resolution of symptoms within weeks of discontinuation, and anti-histone antibodies. The following are *not* associated: multisystem involvement, CNS or renal involvement, low complement levels, antibodies to native DNA, malar rash, alopecia, or oral ulcers.

Note: Approximately 20% of children receiving anticonvulsants develop a positive ANA, so get your ANA before starting anti-seizure therapy, or you'll be wondering whether your patient has CNS lupus all along when she starts to complain of joint pain.

27. What are the ocular manifestations common to the various connective tissue diseases?
When it comes to pediatric rheumatic diseases, the eyes have it. Eye problems (chronic uveitis) are particularly common in children with type I pauciarticular JRA, especially those with a positive ANA. Other manifestations are presented below.

Ocular Manifestations of Pediatric Rheumatic Diseases

OCULAR MANIFESTATION	DISEASE
Uveitis — acute	Pauciarticular JRA (Type II)
	Ankylosing spondylitis
	Arthritis of inflammatory bowel disease
Uveitis — chronic (± band keratopathy)	Pauciarticular JRA (Type I)
Keratoconjunctivitis sicca	Sjögren's syndrome
Retinopathy (cotton wool spots)	SLE
	Polyarteritis nodosa
	Dermatomyositis

28. What are the most common side effects of prolonged corticosteroid therapy in children with rheumatic diseases?
A trip to Stockholm is yours, expenses paid, if you can synthesize an anti-inflammatory steroid without untoward side effects. Commonly encountered problems associated with high-dose corticosteroid therapy in childhood are listed below; they are sometimes worse than the disease itself. Most are minimized if an alternate-day regimen is employed.

Growth retardation	Cataracts
Hypertension	Myopathy
Cushingoid features	Osteoporosis
Dissemination of fungal/viral infections	Avascular necrosis of bone
	Pancreatitis
Masking signs of bacterial infection	Diabetes mellitus
Peptic ulcer	Pseudotumor cerebri

29. In infants born to mothers with SLE, what are the most common manifestations during the neonatal period?
Although relatively rare, this is the most common reason to call a rheumatologist to the nursery, but (s)he will no doubt have been beaten to the consult by a dermatologist or cardiologist. The syndrome of neonatal lupus (NLE) was first described in babies born to mothers with overt SLE or Sjögren's syndrome, but it has since been found that 70–80% of mothers are asymptomatic. The cutaneous manifestations of NLE include erythematous macules, papules, and annular plaques, usually on areas exposed to light. These can be present at birth or develop within the first 2 months of life, usually resolving by 6 months of age. The other major clinical feature, occurring in 50% of infants with NLE, is complete heart block. Although usually an isolated finding, affected infants may also have congenital anomalies (PDA, VSD, TGA). Conduction defects other than complete heart block have also been described.

Watson R: Neonatal lupus syndrome. Pediatr Ann 15:605–621, 1986.

30. What is the pathophysiology of the congenital heart block noted in children born to mothers with SLE?
You can look like a star the next time you encounter a newborn infant with complete heart block (1 in 20,000 deliveries you will attend) by casually inquiring about symptoms of SLE in the baby's mother and sending off her serum for antinuclear and anti-Ro antibodies. Ro is a non-DNA nuclear antigen. Although she is likely to be asymptomatic, the anti-Ro antibody will be positive 80% of the time. It is not yet clear how intimately involved the Ro antibody is in the pathophysiology of the heart block, but Ro antigen has been demonstrated in fetal myocardium. Mothers of babies with heart block can go on to have normal pregnancies subsequently, despite the persistence of the antibody. Therefore, anti-Ro is unlikely to be the only cause of heart block in these infants.

31. Who made the first description of what would later become known as Henoch-Schönlein purpura (HSP)?
People who have nothing better to do than worry about such things will argue that this syndrome should be called Schönlein-Henoch purpura, as Schönlein described the association of purpura and arthralgia in 1837, to which Henoch added associated GI symptoms in 1874 and documented renal involvement in 1899. Actually these Viennese Meisters (whose names few can spell) were preempted by William Heberden in 1806 in his *Commentaries on the History and Cure of Disease* in which he described a 5-year-old boy with joint and abdominal pains, petechiae, hematochezia, and gross hematuria. You can avoid this eponymic boggle if you call it anaphylactoid purpura, and you will remember that the rash starts out looking urticarial.

32. What kind of skin lesions are noted in HSP?
HSP is one of the hypersensitivity vasculitides and, as such, is characterized by leukocytoclastic inflammation of arterioles, capillaries, and venules. Initially, urticarial lesions predominate, which may itch or burn. These develop into pink maculopapules. With damage to vessel walls, there is bleeding into the skin, resulting in nonthrombocytopenic petechiae and palpable purpura.

33. Which etiologic agents are thought to cause HSP?
HSP is probably mediated by immune complexes that require the participation of an inciting antigen. Any number of infectious agents or drugs can fit the bill. The vast majority of children with HSP have a history of prodromal illness, usually an upper respiratory infection. Serologic evidence of antecedent streptococcal infection is present in up to 50% of cases. Drugs associated with HSP include penicillin, tetracycline, sulfonamides, thiazides, and aspirin.

34. Which joints are most often affected in HSP and how is the arthritis managed?
Involvement of the knees, ankles, wrists, and elbows is common, and may present as an additive or migratory arthritis. (If a patient with HSP has migratory arthritis and an elevated ASO titer and ESR, does he have rheumatic fever? Would you recommend penicillin prophylaxis?) When arthritis is present without abdominal pain, salicylates or NSAIDs suffice to control joint pain and swelling. Corticosteroids are indicated for abdominal pain and GI blood loss, and treat the arthritis quite nicely.

35. What visceral organs/systems are most often involved in HSP?
Classically, HSP can involve the joints, GI tract, and/or kidneys. The most common abdominal finding is GI colic (70%), frequently associated with nausea, vomiting, and GI bleeding. These findings may precede the skin rash in up to 30% of cases. Intussusception is a complication that must be borne in mind, especially if steroid therapy is to be introduced, as it may mask signs. Renal involvement occurs in about half of reported cases and is usually apparent early in the course of HSP, ranging in severity from microscopic hematuria to the

nephrotic syndrome. A review of 88 children with renal involvement indicated that those more severely affected tended to be older and have more prolonged systemic manifestations and abdominal pain. (Meadow SR et al: Schönlein-Henoch nephritis. Q J Med 41:241–258, 1972.) While we're in the neighborhood, please note that epididymitis, orchitis, testicular torsion, and scrotal bleeding can occur in HSP.

36. What percentage of children with HSP develop chronic renal disease? Can this outcome be predicted during the acute phase of illness?

A follow-up study of 88 children with Henoch-Schönlein nephritis indicated that 67 had no demonstrable or minor urinary abnormality; 5 had hypertension without urinary abnormality or renal dysfunction; 4 had heavy proteinuria; 8 chronic renal failure; and 4 had died within 25 months of onset. Neither corticosteroid nor cytotoxics, alone or in combination, affected the outcome. Poor outcome was associated, to some degree, with a combination of acute nephritis and nephrosis at presentation and crescents on renal biopsy.

Reference: Counahan R et al: Prognosis of Henoch-Schönlein nephritis in children. Br Med J 2:11–14, 1977.

37. What are the characteristic laboratory findings in HSP?

Acute phase reactants, including the ESR, are commonly elevated and there is frequently a mild leukocytosis. Thrombocytopenia is *never* seen. Microscopic hematuria and proteinuria are indicators of renal involvement. HSP appears to be an IgA-mediated illness. Elevated serum IgA has been noted and it has been demonstrated by immunofluorescence in skin and renal biopsies. (The latter are indistinguishable from Berger's disease, which some people feel is HSP without the P.) Circulating immune complexes and cryoglobulins containing IgA are also found with some regularity.

38. How is the diagnosis of Wegener's granulomatosis made?

Wegener's granulomatosis is a nasty disease that thankfully affects few children. This necrotizing granulomatous vasculitis classically presents a triad of upper respiratory (sinusitis), lower respiratory (pneumonitis), and urinary tract (glomerulonephritis) involvement. Common symptoms of early disease include nasal stuffiness, cough, sinusitis, ulcerating rashes, and arthralgia. The lungs are almost invariably involved, although symptoms may be minimal. Extrarenal manifestations generally precede functional renal impairment, and renal histology varies from focal segmental glomerulosclerosis to rapidly progressive glomerulonephritis. The diagnosis is confirmed by biopsy demonstration of necrotizing granulomatous vasculitis in the respiratory tract. If there are few respiratory symptoms, the illness may be mistaken for HSP.

Reference: Hall SL, et al: Wegener's granulomatosis in pediatric patients. J Pediatr 106:739–744, 1985.

39. Which diseases should be considered in the differential diagnosis of Wegener's granulomatosis?

Wegener's granulomatosis is a pulmonary-renal syndrome. Other diseases that involve these two organ systems include sarcoidosis, Goodpasture's syndrome, and Churg-Strauss disease. Vasculitic syndromes which can be confused with Wegener's granulomatosis include Henoch-Schönlein purpura, SLE, and lymphomatoid granulomatosis.

40. What are the characteristic laboratory and physical findings in mixed connective tissue disease in children?

Mixed connective tissue disease is what it sounds like, a mish-mash of scleroderma, dermatomyositis, rheumatoid arthritis, and SLE first described by Sharp in 1972. Common signs and symptoms include Raynaud's syndrome, esophageal dysmotility, diffuse puffiness of the hands, as well as myositis. Studies in adults emphasize the relative rarity of renal and CNS involvement, but children do not appear to be so spared. Severe vasculitis and thrombocytopenia have been reported in children. The serologic markers which confirm the diagnosis are high-titer speckled ANA (1:1,000–1:1,000,000) and antibodies to the extractable nuclear antigen RNP.

Reference: Singsen BH, et al: Mixed connective tissue disease in childhood: a clinical and serologic survey. J Pediatr 90:893–900, 1977.

41. Are skin infections caused by *Streptococcus pyogenes* capable of causing rheumatic fever?

Acute rheumatic fever follows only a few streptococcal pharyngitides. Streptococcal infections at other sites such as skin have *not* been associated with rheumatic fever.

42. What are the clinical manifestations of rheumatic fever? What are the criteria?

Although some of us weren't around for the original appearances, acute rheumatic fever is back to haunt us. The diagnosis is a clinical one and is based on characteristic signs and symptoms in association with clinical, bacteriologic, or serologic evidence of group A hemolytic streptococcal pharyngitis. T. Duckett Jones proposed "rather strict diagnostic criteria" which have been modified with time in order to: (1) accurately assess the incidence of ARF; (2) aid in interpretation of studies of prevention and treatment; and (3) avoid overdiagnosis. The 1984 revised criteria are presented below; major manifestations offer greater specificity than minor ones. Rheumatic fever can be diagnosed if a patient: (1) fulfills 2 major criteria (Column A) or (2) fulfills 1 major and 2 minor criteria (Column B) with supporting evidence of antecedent streptococcal infection (with 6 you get egg roll).

A. Major Criteria	B. Minor Criteria
Carditis	Fever
Polyarthritis	Arthralgias
Chorea	Previous rheumatic fever
Erythema marginatum	or rheumatic heart disease
Subcutaneous nodules	Elevated ESR, CRP, leukocytosis
	Prolonged PR interval

Plus supporting evidence of preceding streptococcal infection: history of recent scarlet fever; positive throat culture; increased ASO titer or other streptococcal antibodies.

Major Manifestations

1. *Carditis* is diagnosed by the appearance of a significant murmur (mitral insufficiency, Carey-Coombs murmur, aortic insufficiency), changing murmurs, cardiomegaly, congestive heart failure, or pericarditis.

2. *Polyarthritis* is the most frequent major manifestation and is usually migratory. It usually affects larger joints (knees, elbows, ankles, wrists).

3. *Chorea* is characterized by purposeless, involuntary, rapid movements associated with muscle weakness and/or behavioral abnormalities. It can also be seen in SLE and Wilson's disease and can be confused with tics and athetosis. It is frequently a later finding and may not be associated with other rheumatic manifestations or serologic evidence of streptococcal infection.

4. *Erythema marginatum* is an evanescent pink eruption with pale centers and serpiginous margins, occurring mainly on the trunk and proximal extremities, but never on the face. It may be induced by the application of heat.

5. *Subcutaneous nodules* occur over bony prominences including the olecranon, patellae, ulnar and radial styloids, the occiput, and the spinous processes of thoracolumbar vertebrae. They correlate with the presence of carditis.

Minor Manifestations

1. *History of previous rheumatic fever or evidence of preexisting rheumatic heart disease:* The history must be well documented, or the auscultatory evidence absolute.

2. *Arthralgia:* pain without objective signs of inflammation in the joints. If arthritis is a major criterion, you cannot cheat and use this one as a minor.

3. *Fever:* usually at least 39°C.

4. *Acute phase reactants* may be normal in patients with isolated chorea.

5. *PR prolongation* occurs in other inflammatory processes and does not correlate with chronic rheumatic heart disease.

References: Bhattacharya S., Tandon R.: The diagnosis of rheumatic fever—evolution of the Jones criteria. Int J Cardiol 1986; 12:285–294, 1986.

Ad Hoc Committee on Rheumatic Fever and Bacterial Endocarditis of the American Heart Association: Jones criteria (revised) for guidance in the diagnosis of rheumatic fever. Circulation 69:204A–208A, 1984.

43. How quickly can valvular lesions occur in children with rheumatic fever?

In patients with valvular involvement, signs appear within the first 2 weeks of illness in 80% of patients and rarely appear after the second month of illness. The average duration of a rheumatic attack is less than 3 months.

44. What is the incidence of acute rheumatic fever following streptococcal pharyngitis?

Studies during epidemics of exudative group A streptococcal pharyngitis in military recruits indicate that 3% will develop rheumatic fever, regardless of age, race, or ethnic group. Children aged 6–10 years appear to be most susceptible to develop ARF; it is rare in those under 5 years of age. Attack rates in the general population had declined steadily over the last 30 years to approximately 0.5 per 100,000 in 5 to 17 year olds, but the incidence in the Salt Lake City outbreak in 1985 and 1986 was 18.1 per 100,000 comparable to the incidence 30 years previously.

Reference: Veasy LG, et al. Resurgence of acute rheumatic fever in the intermountain area of the United States. N Engl J Med 316:421–427, 1987.

45. What variables concerning the acute streptococcal illness increase a person's chances of developing rheumatic fever?

The severity of pharyngitis correlates to some degree with the attack rate of rheumatic fever. There are a few M serotypes of streptococcus which appear to be rheumatogenic; a mucoid M type 18 strain was implicated in the Salt Lake City outbreak.

46. What is the usual duration of the arthritis associated with acute rheumatic fever?

In the classic rheumatic attack, several joints become affected in succession. A given joint will remain inflamed for less than a week and the entire sequence rarely lasts longer than 4 weeks. The arthritis never occurs more than 35 days from the time of pharyngitis and is virtually always associated with positive streptococcal serology.

47. What percentage of patients with acute rheumatic fever will have positive throat cultures for group A streptococcus?

Less than 50%.

48. Which serologic studies should be ordered in a patient suspected of having rheumatic fever?

The anti-streptolysin O (ASO) titer is the most widely used anti-streptococcal serologic test. Titers peak about 4–5 weeks after the pharyngitis, usually during the second or third week of the rheumatic attack. However, up to 20% of normal school-age children will have ASO titers in the diagnostic range, probably as a consequence of other mild nonpharyngeal streptococcal infections, or non-group A infections. Furthermore, about 20% of patients with a rheumatic attack, especially those who present with chorea, will have low or borderline titers. The Streptozyme is an agglutination test for antibodies to multiple streptococcal extracellular antigens, is quite sensitive, and is a good screening test but has not been well standardized in relation to acute rheumatic fever. Anti-DNAase B tends to remain elevated for longer periods of time and may serve to confirm clinical suspicions.

49. If initially negative, when should serologic testing be done again in an individual with suspected rheumatic fever?

To document recent infection by rising titers, sera should be obtained at 2–4 week intervals and tested simultaneously. A rise in titer of 2 or more dilutions is diagnostic.

50. What immediate and long-term therapy is recommended for a patient with acute rheumatic fever?

Antirheumatic therapy is/was a subject of controversy. Controlled studies have failed to show any contribution of corticosteroids or salicylates in altering the course of a rheumatic attack or preventing cardiac stigmata. They may be useful in providing symptomatic and supportive therapy, but are not curative. In patients with pancarditis and severe symptoms secondary to myocarditis (severe CHF), corticosteroids may prove beneficial. It is agreed that patients with acute rheumatic fever should receive penicillin (either as 1 intramuscular dose of 600,000–900,000 units of benzathine penicillin G in children, 900,000–1,200,000 units in adults, or 200,000–250,000 units of phenoxymethyl penicillin tid–qid for 10 days). Erythromycin is prescribed in the case of penicillin allergy. Continuous prophylaxis should then be undertaken with (1) benzathine penicillin G, 1,200,000 units per month intramuscularly or (2) penicillin, 200,000–250,000 units orally once or twice a day. A streptococcal infection occurring in a rheumatic patient on or off prophylaxis should be treated with 600,000 units of procaine penicillin once or twice daily for 10 days. There is no agreement at present as to how long prophylaxis should be maintained.

51. What is Jaccoud's syndrome?

Jaccoud's syndrome is a "post-rheumatic" periarticular fibrosis and not a synovitis. It results in subluxations of the metacarpophalangeal joints with ulnar deviation. It also occurs in SLE.

52. What distinguishes dermatomyositis and polymyositis in children?

The clinical criteria of Bohan and Peter were developed to aid in diagnosis. A definitive diagnosis of dermatomyositis or polymyositis is made in the presence of 4 criteria.

    1. Symmetrical proximal muscle weakness (Gowers' sign, etc.)
    2. Elevated serum muscle enzymes (CPK, LDH, AST, and/or aldolase)
    3. Abnormal electromyography (increased insertional activity; bizarre, high-frequency discharges)
    4. Inflammation and/or necrosis on muscle biopsy.
    5. Characteristic skin eruption

    Thus, a child has definite juvenile dermatomyositis (JDMS) if (s)he has the rash and 3 of the other 4 criteria (so a biopsy is not necessary if you know what the rash looks like) and possible JDMS if the rash is there and 2 criteria are fulfilled. If there is no rash, there is no dermatomyositis, so definite polymyositis requires a muscle biopsy for diagnosis.

    Reference: Bohan A, Peter JB: Polymyositis and dermatomyositis. N Engl J Med 292:344–347, 1975.

53. What is the rash of dermatomyositis?

The most common cutaneous finding in JDMS is periorbital edema and erythema, which takes on a violaceous (heliotrope) color. It can also mimic the butterfly eruption of SLE and may extend down to the upper chest in a "shawl" distribution. A maculopapular psoriasiform eruption is present over the knuckles, elbows, knees, and other extensor surfaces (Göttron's papules). The children may be photosensitive. Cutaneous vasculitis, while uncommon, does occur.

54. What are the other causes of myositis in children?

Viruses (notably influenza A and B, echoviruses, and Coxsackie viruses) can cause acute myositis. Viral myositis is characterized by severe pain (unusual in dermatomyositis), predilection for the calf muscles, and resolution within 1–4 weeks. Toxoplasmosis and trichinosis should also be considered in the differential diagnosis of myositis. Elevated CPK values are associated with hypocalcemia (rickets, hypoparathyroidism), hypothyroidism, and chronic renal failure.

55. What is the prognosis for children with dermatomyositis and polymyositis?

The advent of corticosteroid therapy has greatly changed the prognosis of JDMS. Before steroids, 1 in 3 children died. The mortality rate is now on the order of 7.2%, a better survival than in adults. The disease can take a monocyclic, polycyclic, or chronic continuous course.

Reference: Pachman LM: Juvenile dermatomyositis. Pediatr Clin North Am 33:1096–1117, 1986.

56. How is scleroderma manifested in childhood?

Scleroderma is rare in childhood and can be divided into localized and systemic forms. Localized scleroderma embraces the following confusing terms:

Morphea: patches of plaque-like, hidebound skin. It may start as a violaceous or erythematous discoloration before hardening and becoming waxy.

Linear scleroderma: like morphea, but in bands.

Scleroderma "en coup de sabre": involvement of the upper face, forehead and scalp; may lead to hemifacial atrophy (Parry-Romberg syndrome).

Localized scleroderma involves all layers of skin and can cause abnormalities of underlying tissue, down to bone. Thus, unilateral linear scleroderma of the leg will lead to shortening of the limb. Although systemic involvement is rare, it is best to evaluate internal organs at intervals.

Systemic sclerosis is diagnosed by the presence of proximal scleroderma, defined as skin changes proximal to the MCP or MTP joints, the single major criterion. Minor criteria include sclerodactyly (what it sounds like), digital pitting at the finger tips or loss of the finger pad, and bibasilar pulmonary fibrosis. (Two minor criteria can fulfill the diagnosis.) Visceral involvement includes:

GI: Esophageal dysmotility, dilatation of small bowel with decreased motility, bowel diverticula, malabsorption (secondary to bacterial overgrowth)

Pulmonary: interstitial pneumonitis

Renal: vasculopathy leading to renovascular hypertension and renal failure

Cardiac: conduction abnormalities, cardiomyopathy secondary to fibrosis

Raynaud's syndrome

Reference: Singsen BH: Scleroderma in childhood. Pediatr Clin North Am 33:1119–1139, 1986.

57. What is Raynaud's phenomenon and what is its significance?

Maurice Raynaud described a triad of episodic pallor, cyanosis on cold exposure with vasoconstriction, and subsequent erythema and hyperemia with subsequent vasodilatation. The following schema has been developed to confuse the matter: Raynaud's *phenomenon* described the above clinical situation. Raynaud's *syndrome* occurs when the phenomenon is associated with a disease (scleroderma, SLE). Raynaud's *disease* is the phenomenon occurring in isolation (present for several years without apparent association). Thus, Raynaud's *syndrome* is seen in 90% of patients with systemic sclerosis.

58. How are children with Raynaud's phenomenon managed?

Children with Raynaud's phenomenon are cautioned to avoid cold exposure (protection of hands and feet). Many can learn to control the temperature of their extremities through biofeedback. Those who cannot and progress to trophic changes may benefit from treatment with nifedipine.

59. What is the differential diagnosis of acute uveitis?

Acute uveitis is seen in a variety of rheumatic and chronic inflammatory conditions including:

Ankylosing spondylitis
Pauciarticular JRA (Type II) } B-27 related
Enteropathic arthritis

Inflammatory bowel disease
Sarcoidosis
Kawasaki disease
Vogt-Koyanagi-Harada syndrome

60. Who was Sydenham?

Thomas Sydenham (1624–89) was educated at Oxford and was the first to revive Hippocratic methods of clinical observation. His reputation today rests upon his descriptions of chorea, hysteria, gout, scarletina, measles, bronchopneumonia, and dysentery.

61. How quickly do the signs and symptoms of serum sickness appear following drug exposure?

Serum sickness occurs after injection of heterologous serum and, as such, is relatively rare. A serum sickness-like reaction occurs after exposure to certain drugs or viruses. In classic serum sickness, fever, urticaria, arthralgia, and lymphadenopathy follow 1–3 weeks after primary antigen exposure.

62. How is serum sickness diagnosed?

Serum sickness is a clinical diagnosis, based on the manifestations noted above. Visceral involvement is unusual. Associated laboratory findings include mild leukocytosis, normal or elevated ESR, eosinophilia, hypergammaglobulinemia, and IgG antibodies against heterologous proteins (''reverse heterophile'').

63. What are the criteria by which Kawasaki disease is diagnosed?

The mnemonic "Feel my conjunctivitis" may prove helpful:

Fever: abrupt onset, >1 week
Exanthem: polymorphous without vesicles or crusts
Extremity changes: reddened palms/soles, indurative edema of hands and feet, desquamation from fingertips or toes
Lymph node: cervical, usually unilateral (50% of cases)
Mucosal changes: dry, chapped lips; strawberry tongue; diffuse reddening of oropharyngeal mucosa
Conjunctivitis: bilateral injection without discharge

Bibliography

1. Brewer EJ, Giannini EH, Kuzmina N, et al: Penicillamine and hydroxychloroquine in the treatment of severe juvenile rheumatoid arthritis. N Engl J Med 314:1269–1276, 1986.
2. Brewer EJ, Giannini EH, Person DA: Juvenile Rheumatoid Arthritis, 2nd ed. Philadelphia, W.B. Saunders, 1982.
3. Cassidy JT: Textbook of Pediatric Rheumatology. New York, John Wiley & Sons, 1982.
4. Golitz LE: The vasculitides and their significance in the pediatric age group. Dermatol Clin 4:117–125, 1986.
5. Kelley WN, Harris ED Jr, Ruddy S, Sledge CB: Textbook of Rheumatology. Philadelphia, W.B. Saunders, 1985.
6. Kunnamo I, Kallio P, Pelkonen, et al: Serum-sickness-like disease is a common cause of acute arthritis in children. Acta Paediatr Scand 75:964–969, 1986.
7. Schumacher HR: Primer on the Rheumatic Diseases, 9th ed. Atlanta, The Arthritis Foundation, 1988.

TOXICOLOGY

Fred M. Henretig, M.D.

1. What percentage of pediatric poisonings are accidental and what percentage are intentional?
Almost all poisonings in those under age 5 are accidental, and most in children over age 12 are intentional. The 6–12 year age range has fewer total exposures, and often the etiology is difficult to ascertain.

2. What are the five most common ingestions for children under 5 years of age?
(1) Pharmaceuticals 40%—especially over-the-counter medications such as aspirin, acetaminophen, vitamin A, iron, cough, and cold preparations; (2) household cleaners and polishes 14%; (3) plants 14%; (4) cosmetics 10%; and (5) pesticides 5%.

3. What is the mechanism of ipecac-induced vomiting?
Ipecac has two sites of action: gastric mucosa as a direct irritant and the chemoreceptor-trigger zone in the medulla.

4. When is ipecac-induced vomiting contraindicated?
Contraindications to the use of ipecac include: coma, convulsions, caustics, and ingestion of household hydrocarbons.

5. What are the alternatives to ipecac for induction of vomiting?
Apomorphine is an alternative, but it must be given parenterally and may cause depressed sensorium and respiration.

6. Following an ingestion what is the volume of lavage fluid necessary to achieve acceptable decontamination?
Toddlers: 1 liter administered in 50–100 ml aliquots of 0.45 or 0.9 N saline. Adolescents: 2 liters administered as 150–200 ml aliquots.

7. What is the value of administering activated charcoal?
Activated charcoal absorbs many chemicals and drugs. It has a long history of safe and effective use. Dose: 15–30 gm in toddlers, 50–100 gm in adolescents. Representative drugs and toxins bound by activated charcoal are:

Acetaminophen	Digitalis	Nicotine
Amphetamine	Ethanol	Organophosphates
Arsenic	Ethchlorvynol	Phenothiazines
Atropine	Glutethimide	Phenylpropanolamine
Barbiturates	Ipecac	Phenytoin
Carbamazepine	Mercuric chloride	Propoxyphene
Cocaine	Methaqualone	Salicylates
Diazepam	Morphine	Sulfonamides

8. In what situations is activated charcoal contraindicated?
In poisonings involving household petroleum distillates (no efficacy and possible increased risk of aspiration) or caustics (obscures burns at endoscopy), immediate need for an oral antidote is anticipated (e.g., late presentation of pure acetaminophen ingestion).

9. Should all children with ingestion be given a cathartic?

Cathartics may help to decrease absorption and lessen constipation caused by charcoal. Magnesium sulfate (250 mg/kg), magnesium citrate (3–5 cc/kg up to 300 cc) or sorbitol (70%, premixed with charcoal) are usual choices. The contraindications are similar to those for activated charcoal. Care must be taken when cathartics are given to smaller children, as large volume loss may result.

10. Following which kinds of ingestions is induced diuresis of value?

Forced diuresis is no longer routinely advocated for treatment of significant overdoses because of the potential risks of pulmonary or cerebral edema from fluid overload. Diuresis can be combined with alkalinization of the urine to enhance phenobarbital and salicylate excretion. Urine pH is more important than urine flow rate. Alkalinization can be attempted by providing sodium bicarbonate (1–2 mEq/kg) every 3–4 hours to achieve a urine pH in the 7.0–8.0 range. Urine acidification has been advocated in the past to enhance excretion of alkaline compounds such as phencyclidine and amphetamines, but is now felt to increase the risk of myoglobinuric renal damage associated with those ingestions. Therefore, acidification is no longer recommended.

11. Which drugs can be removed by hemodialysis or peritoneal dialysis?

Since peritoneal dialysis is only 10–25% as effective as hemodialysis, it is rarely used today.

Common Toxins for which Hemodialysis or Hemoperfusion May Be Useful Adjuncts to Treatment

TOXIN	BLOOD LEVEL (MG/DL)*	PREFERRED METHOD
Phenobarbital	10	HP > H
Other barbiturates	5	HP
Glutethimide	4	HP
Methaqualone	4	HP
Salicylates	80	H
Theophylline	6.0 (60 μg/ml)	HP
Meprobamate	10	HP
Methanol	50	H
Ethylene glycol	50	H
Lithium	3.5 to 4.0 (mEq/L)	H

H=Hemodialysis, HP=hemoperfusion

*Levels at which, in conjunction with clinical picture, H or HP might be considered.

Adapted from Haddad and Winchester: Clinical Management of Poisoning and Drug Overdose. Philadelphia, W.B. Saunders, 1983.

12. What is "intestinal dialysis"?

This new technique of enhancing toxin excretion is far more readily available and much less hazardous to patients than the extracorporeal techniques. This method utilizes repeated doses of activated charcoal to trap toxin in the intestinal lumen by charcoal, creating a diffusion gradient from high toxin concentration in capillary blood to low (free) toxin concentration in the gut lumen. This treatment can be effected by administering charcoal (0.5 g/kg) every 4–6 hours, accompanied by a cathartic with every second or third dose. The method is contraindicated for patients with an ileus or acute abdomen. The comatose patient may have an impaired gag reflex and should be treated with charcoal only if the airway is protected with an endotracheal tube. Reflux and vomiting are common side effects. This technique has proven effective for overdoses with barbiturates, salicylate, theophylline, carbamazepine, and digitoxin. Multiple doses of charcoal are also helpful in tricyclic antidepressant overdoses by interrupting both gastric resecretion and the enterohepatic circulation.

13. What is a toxidrome?

A clinical constellation of signs and symptoms that is very suggestive of a particular poisoning or category of intoxication.

Toxidromes

Atropinics and anticholinergics (atropine, tricyclic antidepressants, phenothiazines, antihistamines)	VS	Fever, tachycardia, hypertension (cardiac arrhythmias–TCA)
	CNS	Delirium/psychosis/convulsions/coma
	Eye	Mydriasis
	Skin	Flushed, hot dry skin
Amphetamines and sympathomimetics (especially in OTC cold preparations and diet pills)	VS	Fever, tachycardia, hypertension
	CNS	Hyperactive to delirious and tremulous, myoclonus, psychosis, convulsions
	Eye	Mydriasis
	Skin	Flushing (mild); sweating (severe)
Opiates and narcotics	VS	Bradycardia, bradypnea, hypotension, hypothermia
	CNS	Euphoria to coma, hyporeflexia
	Eye	Pinpoint pupils
Organophosphate insecticides	VS	Bradycardia or tachycardia; tachypnea (secondary to pulmonary manifestations)
	CNS	Confusion to drowsiness to coma, convulsions, muscle fasciculations, weakness to paralysis
	Eye	Miosis, blurry vision, lacrimation
	Skin	Sweating
	Odor	Garlic
	Misc.	Salivation; bronchorrhea, bronchospasm, and pulmonary edema; urinary frequency and diarrhea
Barbiturates and sedatives/hypnotics	VS	Hypothermia, hypotension, bradypnea
	CNS	Confusion to coma, ataxia
	Eye	Nystagmus, miosis or mydriasis
	Skin	Vesicles, bullae
Salicylates	VS	Fever, tachypnea
	CNS	Lethargy to coma
	Odor	Oil of wintergreen with methylsalicylate
	Misc.	Vomiting
Phenothiazines	VS	Postural hypotension, hypothermia, tachycardia, tachypnea
	CNS	A. Lethargy to coma, tremor, convulsions B. Extrapyramidal syndromes: ataxia, torticollis, back arching, oculogyric crisis, trismus, tongue protrusion or heaviness
	Eye	Miosis (majority of cases)
Theophylline	VS	Tachycardia, arrhythmias, hypotension
	CNS	Headaches, restlessness, muscle twitching to seizure
	Misc.	Vomiting, hematemesis

Adapted from Mofenson and Greensher: Pediatrics 54:336, 1974.

14. A large acetaminophen ingestion is suspected. When should symptoms develop?

Most severe acetaminophen poisonings have minimal symptoms for the first 2–3 days after exposure. Some patients have mild nausea, vomiting, anorexia and abdominal pain during the first 24 hours. In severe cases, 3–5 days after ingestion there are signs of liver failure with right upper quadrant pain, jaundice, coagulopathy, and occasionally encephalopathy. About 10% of cases also have renal impairment.

15. How soon should acetaminophen levels be checked following an ingestion?
Four hours after exposure.

16. What is the value of N-acetylcysteine for acetaminophen removal, and when should it be administered?
N-acetylcysteine (NAC) is a specific antidote for acetaminophen hepatotoxicity which serves as a glutathione-substitute in detoxifying the hepatotoxic metabolites. It should be used for any acetaminophen overdose with a toxic serum acetaminophen level within the first 24 hours after ingestion. If levels are not available on a "stat" basis, or if the time since ingestion is not clear, it is preferable to initiate NAC therapy while awaiting consultation with a toxicologist or Poison Control Center.

17. What are the signs and symptoms of ethanol, methanol, and isopropyl alcohol ingestion?
The common alcohol poisonings all produce coma and varying metabolic complications. Ethanol produces CNS depression in a rostrocaudal progression as the blood alcohol level increases. Moderate metabolic acidosis and severe hypoglycemia may complicate the picture. Methanol causes CNS depression and severe, refractory acidosis. It may also cause severe and permanent retinal damage leading to blindness. Isopropyl alcohol causes CNS depression and gastric irritation. Although ketosis may be present, significant acidosis and/or hypoglycemia do not usually occur.

18. Why is methanol the most dangerous of alcohol ingestions?
Small amounts of methanol (1 ml/kg) may be lethal. Further, the early signs of a methanol poisoning may be fairly subtle despite an ingestion of a lethal or eye-damaging amount.

19. Why is ethanol used as an antidote in methanol ingestions?
Ethanol competitively inhibits the formation of methanol's toxic metabolites, formaldehyde and formic acid, by preferentially serving as substrate for alcohol dehydrogenase.

20. What causes the crystalluria and hypocalcemia associated with ethylene glycol ingestion?
Ethylene glycol, another toxic alcohol, may also cause CNS depression and metabolic acidosis. In addition, it is metabolized to oxalic acid, which causes renal damage via precipitation of calcium oxalate crystals in the renal parenchyma. The calcium oxalate formation also results in hypocalcemia. All alcohol poisonings may be suspected by observing an "osmolal gap." This is the difference between measured (freezing-point depression) osmolality and the expected osmolality utilizing the formula:

$$mOSM = 2\ Na\ (mEq/L) + \frac{BUN}{2.8}(mg\ \%) + \frac{glucose}{18}(mg\ \%)$$

21. Why are thiamine and pyridoxine administration helpful in ethylene glycol poisoning?
Thiamine and pyridoxine are cofactors for the metabolism of ethylene glycol by alternative pathways. These vitamins may help shift the metabolism away from oxalic acid toward other ethylene glycol intermediates.

22. What are the most feared complications of antihistamine overdose?
Antihistamine overdoses may cause a full-blown anticholinergic syndrome with agitation, hallucinations, and seizures; hot, dry, flushed skin; dilated pupils; tachycardia; hypertension and arrhythmias ("Mad as a hatter, hot as Hades, dry as a bone, red as a beet").

23. What quantity of ingested aspirin is cause for concern?

Generally, an acute salicylate overdose of 140 mg/kg will produce symptoms. In chronic salicylism, a dose that averages more than 100 mg/kg/day for several days may also lead to toxic effects.

24. How should children with an acute salicylate ingestion be managed?

The mainstay of salicylate intoxication is careful supportive care with scrupulous attention to fluid and electrolyte balance. Repeated dosing with activated charcoal has recently been shown to be helpful. Urinary alkalinization with bicarbonate may be attempted. (Acetazolamide is currently felt to be contraindicated, since it acidifies blood and tissue compartments, which tends to increase salicylate concentration in target organs, such as the brain.) Very severe cases associated with coma, refractory metabolic acidosis, and/or pulmonary edema may require assisted ventilation or hemodialysis.

25. What is the management plan for suspected ingestion of a soap, detergent, or household cleaner?

Most household soaps and detergent cleansers are mild gastrointestinal irritants, as are most household bleach and ammonia-containing products. A few products (such as electric dishwasher detergents) may have caustic potential.

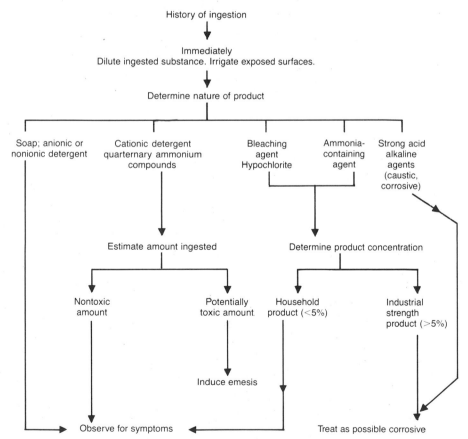

Approach to the management of household cleaning product ingestion. Adapted from Temple and Lovejoy: Cleaning Products and Their Accidental Ingestion. NY, NY, Soap and Detergent Assoc., 1980.

26. When is esophagoscopy indicated in a suspected caustic ingestion?
Esophagoscopy is generally indicated in every patient with a significant caustic ingestion by history and/or physical signs such as oral burns, dysphagia, or drooling, unless the patient is critically ill and too unstable to undergo the procedure.

27. Are acid or alkali ingestions more harmful?
Both acid and alkali ingestions may cause severe esophageal or gastric burns, but alkalis tend to be worse because they produce a relatively more penetrating liquefactive necrosis of the esophagus.

28. Are steroids helpful for caustic ingestions?
Steroids are controversial in the treatment of caustic ingestions. They are purported to reduce scar formation and strictures, but may interfere with wound healing and predispose to perforation. Most authors currently recommend steroids for all significant second degree burns, and advocate their omission for significant full-thickness burns (where their use might be hazardous as well as ineffectual), or first degree burns (which are expected to heal without scarring regardless of treatment).

29. Which hydrocarbons pose the greatest risk for chemical pneumonitis?
The household hydrocarbons with low viscosities pose the greatest aspiration hazard. These include furniture polishes, gasoline and kerosene, turpentine and other paint-thinners, and lighter fuels.

30. Why does ingested gasoline rarely cause systemic symptoms?
Ingested gasoline, and most of the common household hydrocarbons, cause little systemic effect. This may be due to hepatic detoxification from the portal circulation "first pass" effect, or it may simply indicate that significant volumes of gasoline are rarely absorbed because of intense gastric irritation and spontaneous vomiting.

31. Are there any indications for induced emesis in a hydrocarbon ingestion?
Indications for emesis in a child with a hydrocarbon ingestion include: (1) those rare exposures due to inherently toxic compounds (e.g., carbon tetrachloride, toluene, benzene); or (2) the occasional hydrocarbon–toxic compound combination, such as pesticides.

32. Which patients with hydrocarbon ingestions should be admitted?
All patients with significant clinical findings or an abnormal chest x-ray 2 to 4 hours after ingestion should be admitted. Children with a history of exposure are safe to discharge if they have: (1) no symptoms; (2) very transient coughing or gagging; (3) a normal physical exam after 4 hours, and (4) a normal chest x-ray after 4 hours.

33. Are steroids indicated for treatment of hydrocarbon ingestion?
Steroids have no benefit in hydrocarbon aspiration.

34. Where did the "Mad Hatter" get his name?
The encephalopathy of chronic elemental mercury poisoning was an occupational hazard of hat makers, who used mercury to produce felt.

35. What is the pathophysiologic basis for the toxicity in iron ingestions?
Iron is toxic in various ways. It has a direct caustic effect on the gastrointestinal tract, and when absorbed in excess of the total iron-binding capacity, free iron causes shock due to vascular dilation. Hepatotoxicity results from accumulation of free iron in hepatocytes.

36. How do signs and symptoms of acute iron ingestion differ from those of other heavy metal poisonings?

Iron salt ingestion causes early gastrointestinal symptoms, and, in severe cases, hemorrhagic gastritis, shock, and coma. After 24–48 hours, evidence of hepatic damage ensues.

Lead poisoning may cause mild gastrointestinal symptoms; however, encephalopathy with cerebral vasculitis, increased intracranial pressure and coma, seizures, and severe neurologic damage are the most feared complications.

Acute mercury salt poisoning causes both a hemorrhagic gastroenteritis and renal damage. The liver is generally not injured.

Arsenic poisoning affects multiple organs with marked skin and hair changes, neurologic effects (encephalopathy, peripheral neuropathy, tremor, coma, and convulsions), fatty infiltration of the liver, renal tubular and glomerular damage, and cardiac involvement with conduction delays and arrhythmias.

37. What clinical and laboratory features correlate with an acutely elevated serum iron?

Iron levels in the toxic range ($>$ 350 μg/dl) are associated with early (first 6 hours) symptoms such as nausea, vomiting, diarrhea, lethargy or coma, convulsions and/or shock. Laboratory correlates of an elevated iron level include leukocytosis ($>$15,000/mm^3), hyperglycemia ($>$150 mg/dl), and radiopaque tablets on abdominal x-ray.

38. What is the value of a deferoxamine challenge?

Deferoxamine challenge may be occasionally useful as an additional screening test for mild to moderate iron poisoning if "stat" iron levels are not available. In the asymptomatic or mildly symptomatic patient, a dose of 50 mg/kg (up to 1 g maximum) of deferoxamine may be given intramuscularly. A positive test (orange or "vin rose" tint to the urine) signifies the excretion of feroxamine (deferoxamine-iron chelate). All patients with a positive challenge test should be admitted for continuing chelation therapy. A negative challenge test in a patient with *significant* symptoms does not rule out iron toxicity, and should not be relied upon.

39. What are the signs and symptoms of acute and chronic lead intoxication?

Acute lead poisoning is rare in children, and differs from chronic poisoning mainly in the occurrence of a reversible renal Fanconi-like syndrome. In chronic exposure, a glomerulonephritis with hypertension and renal failure may occur. The central nervous system effects are similar, however, and are the most feared consequence of pediatric plumbism. Lead encephalopathy may range from mild behavioral and cognitive dysfunction to severe, life-threatening coma, seizures, cerebral edema, and permanent neurologic sequelae in survivors.

40. What are the environmental sources of lead other than lead-based paint?

Lead-contaminated water, lead dust carried into homes by clothing and shoes of lead-factory workers, improperly glazed "home-made" ceramics, "moonshine" liquor made with lead vats or tubes, and the burning of lead batteries as fuel are uncommon causes of lead poisoning. An organic-lead encephalopathy has also been reported in adolescents who willfully abuse leaded gasoline by chronically inhaling the fumes.

41. What historical features suggest the possibility of lead toxicity in a child?

Testing for lead poisoning is warranted in children with a history of pica and: (1) vague abdominal complaints such as anorexia, recurrent abdominal pain, constipation, and vomiting; (2) vague behavioral effects such as hyperactivity, malaise, or lethargy; (3) a history of unexplained anemia; (4) a history of a sibling with plumbism; or (5) a history of living in a contaminated environment.

42. How should children with an acute iron poisoning be managed?

These patients need careful supportive care. Patients with significant early symptoms, a positive laboratory screen, a positive challenge test and/or a measured serum iron in the toxic range need chelation therapy with deferoxamine.

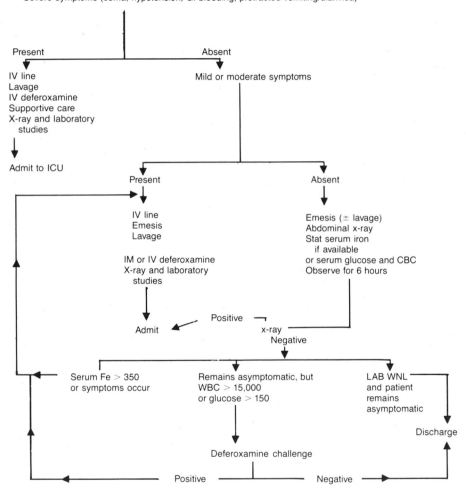

The initial management of the patient ingesting iron. ICU 5 intensive care unit; WNL 5 within normal limits. (Adapted from Henretig FM, Cupit GC, Temple AR: Toxicologic emergencies. In Fleisher, G, Ludwig S (eds): Textbook of Pediatric Emergency Medicine, 2nd ed. Baltimore, Williams and Wilkins, 1988.)

43. What laboratory studies should be ordered in a child with suspected lead toxicity? What are the expected derangements?

A blood lead level and free erythrocyte protoporphyrin (FEP) determination. With acute exposure, the blood lead level rapidly rises to abnormal levels (> 25 µg/dl). Symptoms are associated with levels in 50–70 + µg/dl range. Within a few months of exposure, the FEP will also increase to abnormal levels (35 µg/dl). Most children with encephalopathy have blood lead levels in excess of 100 µg/dl and FEP levels in excess of 190 µg/dl, although occasional cases of "acute" encephalopathy have been reported with elevated but not alarmingly high (e.g., 50–100 μg/dl) FEP levels. Additional tests that may aid in the emergent diagnosis of plumbism include abdominal and long bone films, which may reveal characteristic radiopaque chips of paint, or dense metaphyseal bands ("lead lines"), respectively, a complete blood count demonstrating basophilic stippling, and a urine spot test for coproporphyrins.

44. Which kinds of plants account for the greatest percentage of deaths related to plant poisoning?

Mushrooms account for more than 50% of all deaths due to plant poisoning. The most dreaded variety are the Amanita species, which cause renal and hepatic failure.

45. What are the indications for physostigmine in children who have ingested tricyclic antidepressants?

Physostigmine is currently considered a last resort in the management of tricyclic antidepressant overdoses. While the tricyclics do have some anticholinergic properties, the majority of their toxicity is due to quinidine-like effects on cardiac conduction and to the blockage of catecholamine re-uptake. Current guidelines recommend sodium bicarbonate to alkalinize the blood to a pH of 7.45–7.50, and then specific therapy for persistent seizures. Hypotension may also complicate tricyclic overdoses and usually responds better to norepinephrine (Levophed) than to dopamine, since catechol stores are depleted.

46. Narcan is considered an antidote for which kinds of ingestions?

Narcan (naloxone) is an antidote for the opioid category of drugs. In "low" doses (0.005–0.01 mg/kg), it effectively reverses the CNS and respiratory depression of morphine and heroin. It is also useful in reversing or improving sensorium in overdoses due to many of the synthetic opioids, including propoxyphene, dextromethorphan, codeine, pentazocine, and meperidine. In these cases, a "high" dose is utilized, usually 0.01–0.1 mg/kg. In fact, there is no significant risk to using a high dose of Narcan in any pediatric overdose situation. Many authors now recommend the following regimen for all suspected opioid poisonings: coma without respiratory depression—0.4 mg; coma with respiratory depression—2.0 mg. These doses may be repeated every 5–10 minutes up to a total dose of 8–10 mg before concluding that there is no effect.

47. What are the signs and symptoms of acute digitalis toxicity?

Vomiting, lethargy, bradycardia, and occasionally hypotension. Case reports describe rare instances of life-threatening effects such as arrhythmias and hyperkalemia after massive overdoses.

48. How should children who have ingested a toxic dose of digoxin be managed?

The majority should be managed conservatively with observation, EKG monitoring, and routine supportive care. Most patients with mild symptoms will become asymptomatic within 24 hours. Digoxin levels are a useful screen. Levels greater than 2 ng/ml may correlate with acute or delayed-onset symptoms. Patients who remain asymptomatic for at least 6 hours after ingestion, and who have a normal EKG and digoxin level < 2 ng/ml can probably be discharged. Although the use of Fab fragments of digoxin-specific antibody has been recommended in the rare case of severe digoxin overdose in children, there is no rationale for their routine use in the typical case without life-threatening complications.

49. What are the signs and symptoms of organophosphate poisoning?

Organophosphates inhibit cholinesterase and cause all the signs and symptoms of acetylcholine excess. *Muscarinic effects* include increased oral and tracheal secretions, miosis, salivation, lacrimation, urination, vomiting, cramping, defecation, and bradycardia, and may progress to frank pulmonary edema. *CNS effects* include agitation, delirium, seizures, and/or coma. *Nicotinic effects* including sweating, muscle fasciculations and, ultimately, paralysis. (Mnemonic: salivation, lacrimation, urination, defecation, GI cramps, emesis = SLUDGE)

Differential Diagnosis of Drug-Induced Delirium/Psychosis

	MENTAL STATUS	PUPILS	VITAL/AUTONOMIC SIGNS	OTHER/COMM
PCP	Catatonic, agitated, violent, coma seizures	Variable, nystagmus	Increased BP, PR	Rigidity, increased strength, myoclonus, self-mutilation
LSD, Mescaline, Psilocybin	Oriented × 3, percept/cognitive distortion, hyperalert, panic, hallucinations (auditory, visual)	Usually mydriasis	Increased BP, PR, diaphoresis	Usually PCP on the street
Cannabis	Stimulation or sedation	Variable	Dry mouth, eyes	Conjunctival injection
Amphetamine/PPA/Caffeine	Hyperalert, paranoid hallucinations (auditory, visual)	Mydriasis	Increased BP, PR (sometimes decreased PR), fever, increased bowel sounds, diaphoresis	Tremors, seizures, chronic weight loss, dysrhythmias
Cocaine	Normal or paranoid, hallucinations, tactile "bugs"	Similar to amphetamines/PPA	—	Also: Atrophic nasal mucosa
Alcohol	Lethargy, coma, combativeness	Variable	Decreased temperature, BP, increased or decreased RR	Alcohol on breath, increased serum osmol
Solvents	Similar to alcohol	Variable	Tachydysrhythmias	Solvent odor, increased Pb level
Anticholinergics	Sedation, confusion, agitation, seizures, hallucinations (Lilliputian)	Mydriasis	Increased PR, BP, temperature. Flushed skin, dry skin and mucous membranes. Decreased bowel sounds, urine retention	Dysrhythmias common: (conduction abnormalities)
Withdrawal	Anxiety, restlessness, tremor. Seizures, hallucinations (EtOH, sed-hypnotics)	Usually mydriasis	Increased PR, RR, BP. Fever (EtOH, sed-hypnotics)	Piloerection, cramps, yawning (opioids)
Psychosis	Oriented × 3. Bizarre thought patterns. Systematized paranoid ideation. Hallucinations (auditory)	Normal	Normal	Progressive school failure, loss of friends

From Goldfrank LR, Kirstein R: Amphetamines. In Goldfrank LR (ed): Toxicologic Emergencies: A Comprehensive Handbook in Problem Solving. Norwalk, CT, Appleton-Century-Crofts, 1981, pp 119–120; with permission.

50. What is considered standard therapy for organophosphate poisoning?

Good supportive care, atropine to counteract muscarinic effects, and pralidoxime to effect the regeneration of active cholinesterase. The usual dose of atropine needed in this context is much higher than the standard vagolytic dosage range. The starting dose should be 0.05–0.1 mg/kg IV, with repeated doses of 0.02–0.05 mg/kg every 15 minutes until the desired effect of drying of secretions is achieved. Atropine may have to be given frequently (q 15–60 minutes) over the first several days. In severely poisoned patients, grams of atropine have been required. Pralidoxime is also recommended for all significantly poisoned patients. It is infused at 25–50 mg/kg over 1 hour. In severe cases, the dose may be repeated in 1 hour, and then every 12 hours PRN.

51. What are the signs and symptoms noted with the commonly abused "street" drugs?

"Street" drugs fall into several different categories, and their effects vary widely. In significant exposures, a frequent common denominator is altered mental status. See table on opposite page.

Bibliography

1. Blumer JL, Reed MD (eds): Pediatric toxicology. Pediatr Clin North Am Volume 33:nos. 2 and 3, 1986.
2. Goldfrank LR (ed): Toxicologic Emergencies, 3rd ed. Norwalk, CT, Appleton-Century-Crofts, 1986.
3. Henretig FM, Cupit GC, Temple AR: Toxicologic emergencies. In Fleisher G, Ludwig S (eds): Textbook of Pediatric Emergency Medicine, 2nd ed. Williams and Wilkins, Baltimore, 1988.

INDEX

Page numbers in **boldface type** indicate complete chapters.

Abdominal mass, in neonate, 259
Abdominal trauma, 59
Abuse, child, 56–57
Acetaminophen poisoning, 423–424
Achondroplasia, 135
Acid burns, of the eye, 61
Acid indigestions, 426
Acidosis, 320
  in chronic renal failure, 205–206, 329
  renal tubular, 324–326
Acidurias, organic, 208, 335
Acne, 40–42
Acrodermatitis enteropathica, 34
Acromegaly, 85
Acute lymphoblastic leukemia (ALL), 363–364, 371–372
Acute renal failure, 327–329
Acyclovir, for treatment of genital herpes, 239
Adenoidectomy, indications for, 217
Adenopathy/adenitis, 219
Adolescent growth spurt, 47
Adolescents, alcohol and drug use by, 150
  response to parental divorce, 149
  suicide and, 149
Adrenal response, to stress, 77
Adrenal steroidogenesis, 75
Adrenocortical insufficiency, causes of, 75
Afterload reduction, in treatment of congestive heart failure, 27
Agammaglobulinemia, X-linked, 193
Aganglionic megacolon, 99
Age, gestational, assessment of, 241–242
AIDS, 130, 197–199, 396
  factor VIII and, 161
Airway obstruction, 47
  during asthma attack, 389
Airway pressure, mean, 276
Alactasia, 101
Alagille syndrome, 116
Albinism, 202
Albumin therapy, with exchange transfusion, 261–262
  in nephrotic syndrome, 323
Alcohol, poisonings, 424
  use, adolescent, 150
Alkali, administration, in neonate, 313
  burns, of the eye, 61
  ingestions, 426
Alkalosis, metabolic, 320–321
Alkaptonuria, 202
Allergic bronchopulmonary aspergillosis (ABPA), 397
Allergic contact dermatitis, 38

Allergy, milk protein, 100–101
Alopecia, causes of, 31
Alpha-fetoprotein, increased, cancers associated with, 368
Alpha-1-antitrypsin deficiency, 110
Alveolar-arterial oxygen gradients, 402–403
Ambiguous genitalia, 77–78
Amenorrhea, in anorexia, 86
Amino acids, for neonate, 249
Amniocentesis, 122
Amniotic fluid, 133–134
Ampicillin rash, 231
ANA test, 411
Anemias, 157–159, 166–171, 283–285
Anion gap, 319–320
Ankle sprain, casting of, 384
Ankylosing spondylitis, 109, 408
Anorexia, 23–24, 86, 199
Antibiotic prophylaxis, for endocarditis, 19–22
  for H. influenzae type b, 227
  for lacerations, 52
  for N. meningitidis infections, 226
  for necrotizing enterocolitis, 257
  for otitis media, 216
  for sickle cell disease, 154–155
  for urinary tract infection, 317
  in neonates, 292
  with splenectomy, 372–373
Antibiotic treatment, for acne, 41
  for gastroenteritis, 221
  for impetigo, 37–38
  for infant botulism, 236
  for septic arthritis, 379–380
  for smoke inhalation, 402
Antibiotics, associated with pseudomembranous colitis, 220
Anticonvulsants, 336–340
Antidepressants, tricyclic, overdose of, 429
Antihistamine overdose, 424
Antimicrobial therapy, for gastroenteritis, 221
  for neutropenia, 173
Antipyretic therapy for infection, 215
Antithymocyte globulin, 170–171
Antitoxins, for treatment of infant botulism, 236
Apgar scores, and cerebral palsy, 140–141
Apgar, Virginia, 270
Aplasia, red cell, 169
Aplasia cutis congenita, 32
Aplastic anemias, 169–171
Apnea, 272–273, 398
Appetite, infant, 97
Apt test, 289
Arnold-Chiari, type II, 351

Arsenic poisoning, 427
Arterial blood gas sampling, 390
Arthritis, 40, 109–110, 119, 378–380, 405–408
Arthrogryposis multiplex congenita, 310–311
Ascites, diagnosis of, 111, 258–259
Aspergillus infections, 233, 396–397
Asphyxia, 270–271, 309–310
Aspiration, of foreign body, 397
Aspiration pneumonia, 400
Aspirin, for Kawasaki disease, 230–231
  overdose of, 425
Asthma, 50–51, 389–392, 395
Ataxia, 344
Ataxia-telangiectasia, 194
Atherosclerosis, premature, 22
Atopic dermatitis, 34–36
Atresia, intestinal, 118
Atrial beats, premature, 15
Atrial flutter, causes of, 16
Atrial gallop, 10
Atrial tachycardia, paroxysmal, 282
Atropine, 47–48
Attention deficit disorder, 147
Auspitz sign, 40
Autism, 143–144
Autoimmune disorders, with selective IgA
  deficiency, 194
Autoimmune polyendocrinopathy syndromes, 73
Autosomal trisomies, features of, 121
Azidothymidine (AZT), 199
Azotemia, prerenal, 318

B-cell deficiencies, 192
Babinski response, 345–346
Bacille Calmette-Guerin (BCG) vaccine, 185
Bacteremia, 52, 153–154, 218–219
Bacterial endocarditis, 19–21, 236
Bacterial inhibition test, Guthrie, 202
Bacterial meningitis, 225
Bactrim, contraindications for, 234
Balloon atrial septostomy, 1
Banding, chromosome, 124
Bart's hemoglobin, 285
Bartter's syndrome, 321
Beckwith's syndrome, 269
Bedside cold agglutinin test, 233
Behavior, **145–150**
  common problems of, 145
  IQ and, 125
Behcet's syndrome, 239
Berloque dermatitis, 39
Bile duct paucity, syndromic, 116
Biliary atresia, 116
Biliary system, neonatal, 260–265
Bilirubin, 117, 260–264
Binocular fixation, development of, 141
Birth defects, 123
Birth weight, low-risk factors for, 247
Bites, dog and cat, 239–240
  human, 53
Blackheads, 40

Bladder aspiration, 332–333
Bladder control, daytime, 315–316
Blalock-Taussig shunt, 1, 5
Bleeding, upper vs. lower GI, 113–114
Bleeding disorders, 162. See also specific
  disorders
Blindness, post-measles, 237
Blood, for transfusion, HIV testing in, 198
  cultures, diagnosis of endocarditis by, 20
  for pneumonia, 232, 396
  glucose, monitoring of, 80
  oxygen, content of, 275
    saturation of, 275
  PO_2 of, 275
  transfusions, exchange, 159, 261–262, 303
Blount's disease, 386
Blue diaper syndrome, 204
Blue sclera, 135–136
Body, proportions of, 138
Bone. See also Fractures
  marrow transplantation, 365
  remodeling, 384
  scan, 382
  tumors, 369
Bornholm disease, 234
Botulism, 236, 357–358
Bowel resection in neonate, 256
Boxer's fracture, 384
Brachial plexus injury, 311–312
Brachial plexus palsy, neonatal, 312
Brain death, criteria for, 336
Brain tumors, 361, 373
Breast development, in pubertal males, 83–84
Breast milk, 96–97, 197, 250–252
  jaundice, 251–252
  protective elements in, 251
  viruses transmissible by, 251
Breastfeeding, 96–97
  contraindications to, 252
  and oral poliovirus vaccine, 181
Breathholding spells, 145, 341
Breathing, periodic, 272
  rates of, in infants, 270
Bronchiolitis, 50, 394–395
Bronchopulmonary dysplasia, 277
Bronze baby syndrome, 264
Brown fat, 244
Bruit, intracranial, 12
Bruton's agammaglobulinemia, 193
BT shunt, 1, 5
Buckley's syndrome, 195
Bulimia, 119
Burkitt's lymphoma, 199, 366
Burn injuries, 55
Burns, alkali and acid, of the eye, 61
Burst suppression, in EEG, 350
Butterfly rash, 409

C-reactive protein, derivation of, 238
C1 esterase inhibitor deficiency, 197

Cafe-au-lait spots, syndromes associated with, 45
Caffeine, for apnea of prematurity, 273
Calcifications, cerebral, 347–349
  renal, 328–329
Calcium, for resuscitation, 48
  given during exchange transfusion, 261
  given to neonate, 243
  imbalance, 14–15
Calorie-nitrogen ratio, 93, 265
Calories, required for preterm infant, 248
Cancer. See also Oncology and Tumors
  congenital, 368
  incidence in black and white children, 371
Candidiasis, systemic, 301
Caput succedaneum, 311
Carbohydrate malabsorption, 102
Carbohydrate requirements, 93–94
Carbon monoxide poisoning, 51
Carcinogens, transplacental, 371
Cardiac. See also Heart
  anatomy, 9–10
  catheterization, 17–18
  disease, in neonate, 280–282
  examination, 10–17
  heave, 10
  output, 4, 19
  pharmacologic agents, 25–27
  resuscitation, emergency drips for, 24
  surgical procedures, 25
  toxicity, with chemotherapy, 363
Cardiology, **1–28**
Cardiomegaly, without heart murmur, diagnosis of, 7–8
Cardiomyopathy, 270
Cardiopulmonary resuscitation (CPR), 47–49, 271
Cardiothoracic postoperative syndromes, 25
Cardiovascular system, neonatal, 4, 280–283
Carditis, rheumatic, 24
Casting, ankle sprain, 384
Cat bites, 239–240
Cat-scratch disease, 240
Catecholamine infusions, preparation of, 24
Cathartics, 422
Catheter-related sepsis, 292
Catheterization, cardiac, 17–18
Catheters, umbilical, 291
Cavernous sinus, 354
Celiac disease, 102–103
Cellulitis, 217, 219
Central nervous system, disorders of, vs. CP, 141
  tumors of, 373
Cephalhematoma, 311
Cephalosporins, indications for, 235
Cereals, dietary, 103
Cerebral calcifications, 301, 347–349
Cerebral palsy, 140–141
  Apgar scores and, 141
  immunization and, 178

Cerebrospinal fluid, 227, 294–295, 346–347
Cerumen, in diagnosis of otitis media, 216
CH_{50}, 196
Chagas' disease, 236
Chalazion, 61–62
Chamber enlargement, EKG criteria for, 13–14
Chancre, 239
Chancroid, 239
Charcoal, activated, use in poisonings, 421
CHARGE, 127, 133
Chemical pneumonitis, 426
Chemotherapy, 363, 371–372
Cherry-red spots, 343
Chest pain, occurrence and causes of, 22
Chest tubes, for management of pleural fluid, 399
Chest x-ray, in wheezing child, 50
Chickenpox, 237
  vaccine, 182
Child abuse, indicators of, 56–57
Chlamydial pneumonia, congenital, 232–233
Chloramphenicol, 225–226
Chocolate, effect on acne, 41
Cholestasis, hyperalimentation-induced, 265
Cholesterol, 210–211
Chromosome, abnormalities, 121–126
  analysis, maternal age and, 122
  banding, 124
  sex, 125
  translocation, 123
Chronic illness, 148
Chronic lymphocytic thyroiditis (CLT), 68
Chronic pulmonary insufficiency of prematurity (CPIC), 278
Chronic renal failure, 329
Circulation, fetal and neonatal, 3
Circumcision, 331–332
Cis-retinoic acid, oral, side effects and toxicity of, 41
Clavicular fracture, 384
Cleft lip and palate, 135
Clinitest, urine, 328
Clostridium difficile carriage, 220–221
Clubbing, digital, 403–404
Clubfoot, 386
Clue cells, 238–239
Coagulation disorders, 164–165
Cognitive handicap, 139–140
Cold agglutinins, 233, 395
Cold injury, neonatal, 265
Colic, 146
Colitis, 108–109, 220–221
Colles' fracture, 384
Colloid, treatment of hypotension, 58
Colobomas, of the iris, syndromes associated with, 133
Coma, doll's eye and, 342
  Glasgow scale, 49–50
  hyperglycemic, 52
Complement deficiencies, 195–196
Compressive head wrapping, 310

Concanavalin-A (con-A), 195
Condyloma acuminatum, 33–34, 239
Congenital adrenal hyperplasia, 75
Congenital anomalies, common, 129
Congenital heart disease. *See* Heart and specific
    type
Congenital hip dislocation (CHD), 377
Congenital limb hemihypertrophy, 130
Congestive heart failure, 6–8, 27
Conjunctivitis, causes of, 62
    gonococcal, 302
Consent, parental, for immunizations, 177
Constipation, Hirschsprung's disease and, 99
Contact dermatitis, 38
Continuous positive airway pressure (CPAP),
    276
Convulsion, 341
Coombs' test, 289
Copper, deficiency, 44, 250
    metabolism, defect of, 212
Coprolalia, in Tourette's syndrome, 147
Corticosteroids, for juvenile rheumatoid arthritis,
    407
    for treatment of asthma, 51
    for treatment of hemangiomas, 32
    side effects of, 412
    topical, potency of, 29
Cough, chronic, 390
CPR, 47–49, 271
Cradle cap, 34
Cranial irradiation, 363
Cranial ultrasound, for preterm infants, 309
Craniopharyngioma, 355–356
Craniosynostosis, 381
Craniotabes, 387
Cranium, at birth, 137
Creatinine clearance, 318–319
Cri du chat syndrome, 124–125
"Critical thermal maximum", 56
Crohn's disease, 106–109
Cromolyn sodium, for treatment of asthma, 391
CROTCHS, 297
Croup, 50, 231–232, 395–396
Crying time, average, 146
Crystalloid, treatment of hypotension, 58
Crystalluria, with ethylene glycol ingestion, 424
Cushing's disease, 75
Cushing's law, 351
Cushing's syndrome, 75–76
Cushing's triad, 351
Cutis aplasia, of the scalp, 32
Cutis marmorata, 30
Cyanosis, 274, 280–281
Cyanotic heart disease, 4–6
Cystic fibrosis, 110, 132, 392–94
Cystinosis, 207
Cystinuria, 207
Cystitis, 318
Cystourethrograms, 317
Cytomegalovirus (CMV) infection, 228–229,
    262, 347

Daily energy requirements, 93–94
Damocles syndrome, 148
Damrosch criteria, 227
"Dazzle reflex", 345
Death, comprehension of, by child, 148
Decongestants, for treatment of otitis media,
    216
Deferoxamine challenge, 427
Defibrillation, 48
Dehydration, 57
Delirium, drug-induced, 430
Delivery, "traumatic", commonly injured
    systems after, 245
Denis-Browne splint, 386
Dental emergencies, 58–59
Denver Developmental Screening Test, 139
Depth perception, development of, 141
Dermatitis, 32–36, 38–39. *See also specific
    types*
Dermatoglyphics, 131
Dermatology, **29–45**
Dermatomyositis, 45, 417–418
Dermatoses, of the feet, 38
Dermographism, 36
Detergent, ingestion of, 425
Development, prematurity and, 139–140
Developmental delay, 139
Developmental milestones, 138–139
    in children with Down syndrome, 124
Dextrocardia, conditions associated with, 13
Diabetes, 80–81
    complications of, 81
    insipidus, 88–89
    maternal, 270
    mellitus, 371–372
    role of diet and exercise in, 80
    transient neonatal, 270
Diabetic ketoacidosis (DKA), 78–79
Dialysis, 59, 328, 422
Diamond-Blackfan syndrome, 168–169
Diaper dermatitis, 32–33
Diapers, cloth vs. disposables, 33
Diaphragmatic paralysis, 313
Diarrhea, 100, 102–104, 220–222, 263
    milk protein allergy and, 100–101
Diet, Feingold, 147–148
    role in diabetes, 80
Dietary deficiencies, in eczematous
    dermatitis, 35
DiFabrizio theorem of medical education, 62
DiGeorge syndrome, 192–193
Digestive system, neonatal, 254–260
Digital clubbing, 403–404
Digitalis toxicity, 26–27, 429
Digoxin, 25–26
    overdose, 429
Diphenylhydantoin, exposure, in utero, 129
Diphtheria vaccine, 180
Dipstick, urine, 322
Disaccharidases, 257
Dislocation, 384

Disseminated intravascular coagulation (DIC), 163–165, 288–290
Diuresis, induced, following ingestion, 422
Diuretics, 319
Diurnal enuresis, 315–316
Diving seal reflex, 255
Divorce, effects on children, 149
Dobutamine, indications for, 27
Dog bites, 239–240
"Doll's eyes" reflex, 342
Dopamine, indications for, 27
Doppler echocardiography, 19
Down syndrome, 121–124, 362
    hematologic abnormalities in, 155
DPT vaccine, 178–180
Drowning, near, 57
Drugs, abuse, 149–150, 431
    delirium/psychosis from, 430
    overdose, antidote for, 429
    "street", 431
    teratogenic, 127
    withdrawal from, in neonate, 266–267
D^u antigen, 289
Dubowitz scoring system, for gestational age assessment, 241–242
Ductus arteriosus, 1, 3–4, 282
Dwarfism, 135, 387
Dysraphic state, 351
Dysrhythmias, atrial and ventricular, treatment of, 26

E. coli, 393
Ears, low-set, 132
Ecchymosis, color changes in, 61
Echocardiography, 18–20, 282
Eczema, 34–36
Ehlers-Danlos syndrome, 387
Ejection click, 10
Electrocardiography (EKG), criteria for chamber enlargement, 13–14
    developmental changes in, 14
    diagnosis of calcium imbalance by, 14–15
    diagnosis of magnesium imbalance by, 14–15
    diagnosis of potassium imbalance by, 14–15
    diagnosis of right ventricular hypertrophy by, 14
    findings in congenital heart malformations, 13
    findings in Pompe's disease, 210
    neonatal, 280
    signs of digitalis toxicity, 26–27
Electroencephalography (EEG), burst suppression pattern in, 350–351
    for febrile seizure, 337
    for herpes simplex disease, 237
    for neonatal seizures, 306
Electrolyte solution, WHO oral, 223
Elliptocytosis, hereditary, 159
Embden-Meyerhof pathway, 166
Emergency medicine, **47–63**
Emesis, in hydrocarbon ingestion, 426
Encephalitis, 237

Encephalopathy, hypoxic-ischemic, 271
Endocarditis, 19–21, 236
Endocrinology, **65–90**, 265–270
Endomyocardial biopsy, indications for, 25
Endotracheal tube, 47–48, 271–272
Energy requirements, 93–94
Enterocolitis, necrotizing, 251, 254–257
Enthesitis, 408
Enuresis, diurnal, 315–316
Eosinophilia, 174–175
Epidermolysis bullosa, 43
Epiglottitis, 50, 231, 395–396, 399–400
Epilepsy, 337–341
Epinephrine, 47, 53, 271
Epistaxis, cause of, 60, 164
E/PUFA ratio, 249
Epstein-Barr virus infections, 223–225
Erb's paralysis, 312
Erikson's life-cycle crises of psychosocial development, 149
Erythema infectiosum, 237
Erythema nodosum, 44
Erythema toxicum, 30–31, 42
Erythrocyte sedimentation rate (ESR), 173–174
Erythrocytosis, 373
Erythromycin, for pertussis infections, 234
    gonococcal conjunctivitis following, 301
Esophageal atresia, 259
Esophagoscopy, 426
Essential fatty acids, 96, 249
Ethylene glycol ingestion, 424
Ewing's tumor, 371
Exanthematous illnesses, 237
Exchange transfusion, 159, 261–262, 303
Exercise, role in diabetes, 80
Exercise testing, 19
Exophthalmos, in Graves' disease, 72
Extracranial hemorrhage, 311
Eye, alkali and acid burns of, 61. See also Pupils
    screening examination of, for retinopathy of prematurity, 245

Fabry's disease, 213
Facial nerve injury, traumatic, prognosis in, 313
Factor VIII, concentrates, 160–162
    deficiency, 162, 165
Factor IX deficiency, 162
Familial hypercholesterolemia, 211
Fanconi syndrome, 171, 202, 362
Fasciculation, muscle, 356–357
Fat absorption, neonatal, 257
"Fat baby" syndromes, 128
Fat requirements, 93–94
Febrile seizures, 336–338
Feeding, of neonate, 248–255
Feet, dermatoses of, 38
    "sweaty", odor of, in isovaleric acidemia, 204
Feingold diet, 147–148
Felon, 62

Femoral anteversion, 385
Femoral epiphysis, slipped, 377
Femur, fracture of, 384
Ferric chloride test, 202–203
Fetal AIDS syndrome, 130
Fetal alcohol syndrome, 127–128
Fetal circulation, 3
Fetal hydantoin syndrome, 129
Fetus, growth, assessment of, 137, 246–249
Fever, with bacterial meningitis, 227
    management of, 52, 218–219
    of unknown origin (FUO), 229
Fibrillation, cardiac, 16
    muscular, 356–357
Fibula, 386
Fifth disease, 237
Finger, laceration, nerve injury with, 54
Fitz-Hugh–Curtis syndrome, 60
Fluid requirements, for asthma patients, 390
    for neonates, 243
Fluoride supplementation, for neonates, 250
Fontan procedure, 5–6
Fontanelles, 137–138, 248
Food poisoning, 219–220
Foot disorders, 38, 385–386
Foramen ovale, 283
Foreign body, aspiration of, 397
Formula feeding, 252–255
Fractures, 245, 382–384
    skull, 54
Fragile X syndrome, 126
Fructose intolerance, hereditary, 208
Functional asplenia, occurring with sickle cell
    disease, 153
Fundoplication, 118
Furosemide, 277, 304, 319, 323
Furosemide-resistant hypercalcemia, 74

G6PD deficiency, 166
Galactosemia, 207–208
Gammaglobulin, in idiopathic thrombocytopenic
    purpura, 155–156
Gancyclovir, 228
Gasoline, ingestion of, 426
Gastric aspirates, 294
Gastric fluid, in neonate, 257
Gastroenteritis, 119, 181, 221–222
Gastroenterology, 93–120
Gastroesophageal reflux (GER), 117
Gastrointestinal hemorrhage, 112–113, 258
    in hepatic failure, 106
Gastroschisis, 134, 259
Gaucher's disease, 213
"Genetic-lethal" disease, 132
Genetics, 121–136
    acronyms used in, 126–127
Genitalia, ambiguous, evaluation and
    management of, 77–78
Genitourinary trauma, 331
Germ cell tumors, 370
Gestational age, determination of, 241–242

Gianotti-Crosti syndrome, 38
Giardiasis, 222
Gigantism, 85
Gilles de la Tourette's syndrome, 146–147
Gingivitis, 235
Glasgow coma scale, 49–50
Glomerulonephritis, 324, 329
Glucose, blood, home monitoring of, 80
Glucose-6-phosphate dehydrogenase
    deficiency, 166
Glucosuria, 328
Gluten-sensitive enteropathy, 102
Glycogen storage diseases, 209–210
Goat's milk, anemia and, 165
Goiter, congenital, 67
Gonococcal conjunctivitis, 301
Gonococcus, in pelvic inflammatory disease, 60
Gottron's papules, 45
Gower hemoglobin, 285–286
Graft versus host reaction, 197
Gram stains, urine, 332
Grand mal seizures, 338–340
Granulocyte transfusion, 302, 363
Granulomatous disease, chronic, 195, 414
Graves' disease, 68–72
Group B streptococcal (GBS) disease, 295–296
Growth, of fetus and neonate, 137, 246–249
    of head, 349–350
    rate, of boys and girls, 138
    retardation, in Crohn's disease, 109
        intrauterine, 137, 246–247
    spurts, 144
Growth and development, 137–144
Growth arrest lines, 363
Growth hormone excess, 84–85
Grunting, in infants, 277
Guthrie bacterial inhibition test, 201
Gynecomastia, in pubertal males, 83–84

H. influenzae type b, 225–228
Hair loss, classification of, 31
Haldane hypothesis, 131
Hand preference, 346
Haptic perception, 142
"Harlequin color change", 30
Hashimoto's disease, 68
Head banging, 146
Head growth, of premature infant, 349–350
Head trauma, 54–55
Headache, 55, 352
Hearing loss, with meningitis, 227
Hearing test, indications for, 143
Heart. See also Cardiac and Cardiology
    block, 413
    chamber enlargement, 13–14
    contraction of, 3
    defects, 21–23
    disease, 1–2, 4–7, 9, 23–24, 280–282
        afterload reduction in treatment of, 27
        with Wilm's tumor, 368
    malformations, congenital, 13

Heart *(Continued)*
  monitors, 16–17
  murmurs, 10–13
  neonatal, 3–4, 280–282
  pressure and oxygen saturation values of, 17
  sounds, 10–11
  rate, of newborn, 4
  transplantation, survival rate in, 25
Heart-lung machine, 1
Heat loss, 61
Heatstroke, 56
Height, 138
Heiner's syndrome, 101
Heinz bodies, 167
Hemangiomas, 32
Hematology, **151–175**
Hematuria, 368
Hemihypertrophy, limb, 130, 362
Hemiplegia, 346
Hemodialysis, 328, 422
Hemoglobin, in neonates, 285–286
  unstable, identification of, 167
Hemoglobin H disease, 167
Hemoglobin level, normal, 171
Hemoglobinopathies, testing for, 152–153
Hemoglobinuria, 327
Hemolytic anemia syndrome, 25
Hemolytic-uremic syndrome (HUS), 327
Hemoperfusion, drugs removed by, 422
Hemophilia, 160–162
Hemophilus influenzae type b, 182, 225–227
Hemophilus vaccines, 182–183
Hemoptysis, in cystic fibrosis, 394
Hemorrhage, extracranial, 311
  gastrointestinal, 106, 112–113, 258
  intracranial, 308
  intraventricular, 308–310
  subarachnoid, 307
  subdural, 306–307
  subependymal, 308
Hemorrhagic disease, of newborn, 289–290
Henoch-Schonlein purpura (HSP), 413–414
Heparin therapy, for disseminated intravascular
    coagulopathy, 164
Hepatic disease, 104–106, 115, 164–165, 290
Hepatic encephalopathy, 106
Hepatic failure, 104–105
Hepatitis, acute, 105
Hepatitis B immunoglobulin, 185
Hepatitis B infection, 38, 300
  vaccine, 185–186
Hepatitis e antigen, 301
Hepatomegaly, 115–116
Hepatorenal syndrome, 106
Hereditary angioneurotic edema (HANE), 197
Hereditary diseases, occurring with congenital
    heart disease, 1–2
  pedigree chart for, 130
Hernia, inguinal, 260
Herpangina, 235
Herpes, 237, 239, 299, 347–348

Heterophile test, 224
Hip, dislocation, congenital, 377
  painful, cause of, 377
Hirschsprung's disease, 99
Histiocytosis "X" syndromes, 33, 374
HIV-infected child, 197–199
  factor VIII and, 161
  vaccination recommendations for, 187
Hodgkin's lymphoma, 365–367, 371
Holter monitors, 16–17
Home monitoring, of apnea, 273–274
  of blood glucose, 80
Homocystinuria, 206–207
Hordeolum, 61–62
Hormones, fetal, 246
Household cleaner, ingestion of, 425
Howell-Jolly bodies, 167
HTLV-III infection, 300
Human diploid cell vaccine, 186
Hutchinson's triad, 239
Hydantoin, exposure in utero, 129
Hydrocarbon ingestion, 426
Hydrocephalus, 309–310, 351
Hydrocortisone, for treatment of asthma, 51
Hydrops fetalis, 291
Hyper IgE syndrome, 195
Hyperactivity, 147–148
Hyperalimentation, 97–98, 265
Hyperammonemia, neonatal, 213
Hyperbilirubinemia, 116–117, 260–261
  intralipid use in, 253
Hypercalcemia, 74, 374
Hypercholesterolemia, 211
Hypercoagulability, nephrotic syndrome
    and, 324
Hyperextensible joints, 408
Hyperglycemic coma, 52
Hyperkalemia, 321–322
Hyperlipidemias, 22, 210–211, 322
Hyperoxia test, 277
Hyperphenylalanemia, 201
Hyperpigmentation, 44
Hyperpnea, in neonate, 272
Hypersensitivity reactions, types of, 196
Hypertelorism, 136
Hypertension, 23, 111–112, 243
Hyperthyroidism, 165, 268
Hypertrophy, ventricular, EKG criteria for,
    13–14, 280
Hyperuricemia, 374
Hyperventilation, adverse consequences of, 279
  to induce seizure, 339
Hyperviscosity, 286
Hypocalcemia, 265–266, 424
Hypocomplementemia, 329
Hypogammaglobulinemia, transient, 191
Hypoglycemia, 82–83, 268–269
Hypokalemia, 321–322
Hypomagnesemia, 266
Hypoparathyroidism, 72
Hypophosphatemia, 208

Hypoplastic left heart syndrome, 136
Hypospadias, 330–331
Hypotension, treatment of, 58
Hypothalamic-pituitary dysfunction, 85–86
Hypothermia, 61, 244
Hypothyroidism, 66–71, 165, 268
Hypothyroxinemia, transient, 268
Hypotonia, 358
Hypoxemia, 403
Hypoxia, 271

Icteric leptospirosis, 236
Idiopathic nephrosis, 323–324
Idiopathic thrombocytopenic purpura (ITP),
    155–156
IgA deficiency, 194–195
IgM levels, in serum, 297
Ileocolic intussusception, 114
Illness, response of children to, 148
Immunization, **177–189.** *See also* Vaccines
    injection location, 178
    of children receiving chemotherapy, 372
    of children with cerebral palsy, 178
    of children with febrile and nonfebrile
        illnesses, 177
    of premature babies, 178
    parental permission for, 177
    recommended schedule for, 177
    schedule, for previously unimmunized
        patients, 187–188
    simultaneous, 187
Immunodeficiency, 191–194, 196
Immunoglobulin, in breast milk, 197
    deficiencies, 192
    levels, by age, 191
Immunology, **191–199**
Impetigo, 37–38
Inborn errors of metabolism, **201–214**
In-toeing gait, 385
Indomethacin, indications for, in neonate, 283
Infantile cortical hyperostosis, 387
Infection. *See also* Sepsis
    antipyretic therapy for, 215
    chronic perinatal, 298
    congenital, 297–299
    early-onset, 292
    enteric, 220
    fever in infants and, 218–219
Infectious diseases, **215–241**
Inflammatory bowel disease (IBD), 106–110
Influenza vaccine, 186
Inherited disorders. *See* Genetics and specific
    types
Ingestion, toxic. *See* Toxicology
Injection, of air bolus, 58
    intramuscular, 178
Inotropic agents, 25–27
Insensible water loss (IWL), 263, 279
Insulin, 78–80
Intelligence quotient, measurement of, 140
Intensive care, cardiac, 24

Intestinal atresia, 118
Intestine, malrotation of, 118
Intracranial bruit, 12
Intracranial pressure, increased, after head
    trauma, 54–55
Intralipid usage, 253
Intraosseous line, 48
Intrauterine growth retardation, 246–247
Intrauterine infection, late sequelae of, 299
Intravenous access, time needed for, 48
Intravenous hyperalimentation, 97–98, 265
Intravenous pyelogram, for abdominal
    trauma, 59
Intraventricular hemorrhage, 308–310
Intussusception, 113–114
Iodide, radioactive, treatment of Graves' disease
    with, 71
Ipecac-induced vomiting, 421
IQ, measurement of, 140
Iris colobomas, syndromes associated with, 133
Iron, deficiency, 157–158
    ingestions, 426–428
    supplementation, 250, 285
    therapy, 157
Ischemia, 271
Isolette, humidity in, 245
Isoproterenol, indications for, 27
Isovaleric acidemia, 204

Jaccoud's syndrome, 417
Janeway lesions, 235
Jatene operation, 5
Jaundice, 116, 251–252, 260–263
Jaw-thrust maneuver, 47
Jaw-winking phenomenon, 343
Jitteriness, vs. seizures, 305
Job's syndrome, 195
Joint disease, with inflammatory bowel disease,
    109–110. *See also* Rheumatology
Joints, hyperextensible, 408
Juvenile rheumatoid arthritis (JRA), 405–408

Kartagener's syndrome, 397
Kasabach-Merritt syndrome, 32
Kasai procedure, 116
Kawasaki disease, 229–230, 419
Kehr's sign, 62
Kernicterus, in neonate, 264
Kidney, of neonate, 303. *See also* Renal
Kidney disease, polycystic, 328
Kinky hair syndrome, Menkes', 44
Kleihauer-Betke test, 289
Klinefelter's syndrome, cancers associated
    with, 362
Klumpke's palsy, 312
Koebner reaction, 38
Kupffer cells, 197
Kwashiorkor, 96

Labor, length of, and sex of baby, 137
Lacerations, 52–54

Lactose intolerance, 101
Landry-Guillain-Barre syndrome, 358–359
Language, development of, 142–143
Lasix therapy, in nephrotic syndrome, 323
"Last gasp", 272
Lavage fluid, required following ingestion, 421
Lead toxicity, 162–163, 427–428
Learning disability, vs. attention deficit
    disorder, 147
Leg length discrepancy, 386
Legg-Calve-Perthes (LCP) disease, 381
LEOPARD, 127
Leptospiral infection, 236
Lesch-Nyhan syndrome, 207
Leukemia, 170, 361, 363–366, 371–372
Leukemic lines, 363
Leukemoid reaction, 164
Leukocoria, 370
Leukocyte counts, normal, 172
Life cycles, Erikson's, 149
Ligaments, sprained, 384
Liley's zones, 264
Limb hemihypertrophy, 130
Linoleic acid, 94, 96
Lip pits, 135
Lipid infusions, 253
Lipid screening, for premature
    atherosclerosis, 22
Lipid storage disorders, 213
Lipids, drugs producing elevated, 213
Lipoproteins, drugs producing elevated, 213
Listeriosis, neonatal, 302
Liver, neonatal, 260–265
Liver disease, 104–106, 115, 164–165, 290
Liver span, normal, by age, 114–115
Livor mortis, 49
Loop diuretics, 319
Low birth weight, risk factors for, 246–247
Lowe syndrome, 202
L-thyroxine, 67
Ludwig's angina, 235
Lumbar puncture, 218–219, 228, 294, 308,
    310, 346
Lumirubin, 263
Lung, maturity, prenatal testing of, 277–278
    metastases, 374, 400
    neonatal, pressures required to inflate, 270
Lupus erythematosus, systemic, 409–413
Lymph node biopsy, 219
Lymphadenitis, 219
Lymphadenopathy, 371
Lymphocytes, distribution of, 197
Lymphocytic interstitial pneumonitis (LIP), 199
Lymphocytosis, atypical, cause of, 159
Lyon hypothesis, 131

Macrocephaly, syndromes associated with, 129
"Mad hatter", 426
Magnesium imbalance, 14–15
Malar rash, 409
Malformation, major and minor, 133

Malnutrition, 95–96, 237
Malrotation, intestinal, 118
Mantoux test, 181, 184–185
Marasmus, 96
Marcus-Gunn pupil, 343
Marcus-Gunn reflex, 343
Marfan syndrome, 22, 206
Marrow, tumors capable of replacing, 363
MAST trousers, 58
Mastoiditis, 215–216
McCune-Albright syndrome, 74, 381
Mean cell volume, normal, 171
Measles, 237, 348
Measles, mumps and rubella (MMR) vaccine,
    181–182, 237
Mechanical ventilation, 274–276
    for asthma, 391
Meckel's diverticulum, 118–119
Meckel's scan, 119
Meconium, 254, 264
Mediastinal tumors, 402
Megacolon, toxic, 109
Melanosis, transient neonatal pustular, 31
Membrane disorders, 165
Membranous glomerulonephritis, 324
Meningeal irritation, 347
Meningism, 347
Meningismus, 347
Meningitis, 225–228, 294–295, 301, 347
Meningococcal vaccines, 183–184
Menkes' kinky hair syndrome, 44
Mental retardation, 140
Mentzer index, 159
Mercury poisoning, 426–427
Metabolic acidosis, in neonate, 205–206,
    267, 320
Metabolic alkalosis, 320–321
Metabolic disease, vitamin-responsive, 204–205
Metabolism, in neonate, 265–270
    inborn errors of, **201–214**
Metatarsus adductus, 385
Methanol ingestion, 424
Methemoglobinemia, 163–164, 286
Methylcrotonylglycinuria, 206
Microcephaly, syndromes associated with, 129
Microcytosis, 158, 162–163
Migraine headaches, 352
Milia, 42
Miliaria, 42
Milk, breast. See Breast milk
    heating by microwave oven, 97
Milk protein allergy, 100–101
Miscarriage, 123
Mitogens, 195
Mitral valve prolapse (MVP), 21–22
Mixed connective tissue disease, 414–415
Mobius syndrome, 313
"Mongolian spots", 45
Mononucleosis, Epstein-Barr virus induced, 223
Monoplegia, 346
Mosaicism, 124

Motor deficit, causes of, 141
Motor skills, development of, 138–139
Mucha-Habermann disease, 40
Mucoid pseudomonas, 393
Multiple endocrine neoplasia (MEN) syndrome, 73
Mumps, 238
Murmur, heart, 7–8, 10–13
MURCS, 127
Muscle, fibrillation and fasciculation, 356–357
Myasthenia gravis, neonatal, 357
Mycoplasmal infections, 395
Mycoplasmal pneumonia, 233
Myelogenous leukemia, 364–365
Myelomeningocele, 312, 351–352
Myocarditis, 23–24
Myoglobinuria, 327
Myositis, 417–418

N-acetylcysteine, for acetaminophen hepatotoxicity, 424
N. meningitidis infections, 226
Naloxone, as antidote for opioid overdose, 429
Nasal polyps, 398
Nasal trauma, 60
Nasopharyngeal cultures, 396
Near-drowning, 57
Necrotizing enterocolitis (NEC), 251, 254–257
Nelson's syndrome, 85
Neonatology, 241–313
Nephritis, 324
Nephrology, 315–333
Nephrosis, idiopathic, 323–324
Nephrotic syndrome, 322–324
Nervous system, in neonate, 304–313
Neural tube defects, 312–313
Neuroblastoma, 362–363, 367
Neurofibromatosis, 128, 355
Neurology, 335–360
Neuropathies, 359–360
Neutropenia, 172–173, 196, 294
Neutrophil index, 293–294
Neutrophils, 172, 196
Nevi, congenital pigmented, malignant risk of, 42
Nevus flammeus, 32
Nezelof's syndrome, 192
Night terrors, 145–146
Night waking, 146
Nightmares, 146
Nikolsky's sign, 37
Non-Hodgkin's lymphomas, 365
Nontuberculous mycobacterium, 217
Noonan's syndrome, 126
    vs. Turner's, 126
Nose, trauma to, 60
Nosebleeds, 60, 164
Nursemaid's elbow, 381
Nutrition, 93–120, 248–253
Nutritional requirements, 93–84
Nutritional status, assessment of, 94–95
Nystagmus, 344–345

Obesity, 119, 128
Occult bacteremia, 52
Ocular manifestations, of rheumatic diseases, 412
Oculovestibular reflex, 342
Odor, cat urine, 206
    sweaty feet, 204
    See also specific diseases
Oligohydramnios, 133–134, 247–248
Oliguria, 303–304
Omphalocele, 134, 259
Oncology, 361–375. See also Tumors and Cancer
"Ondine's curse", 398
Opioid overdose, 429
Opsoclonus-myoclonus, 343–344
Oral bronchodilators, 391
Oral poliovirus vaccine (OPV), 181–182
Organic acidemias, 213
Organophosphate poisoning, 429, 431
Orthopedics, 377–388
Osgood-Schlatter disease, 380
Osler's nodes, 235
Osmotic fragility test, 165–166
Osteochondritis dissecans, 382
Osteochondroses, 380
Osteogenesis imperfecta, 135–136, 380
Osteogenic sarcoma, 369
Osteoid osteoma, 382
Osteomyelitis, 296, 379–380
Osteopenia, of prematurity, 249
Osteoporosis, 380
Osteosarcoma, 369
Otitis media, 216–217
Ovarian dysgenesis, chromosome abnormalities in females with, 126
Ovarian tumor, 371
Oxygen saturation values, in heart and great vessels, 17

P_{50}, 284
Pacemakers, 17
Paganini, Nicolo, 387
Painful crisis, in sickle cell disease, 151
Palsy, peripheral seventh nerve, 360
Panhypogammaglobulinemia, 193
PaO_2, 403
Paralysis, in mechanically ventilated neonate, 275
Paraplegia, 346
Paronychia, 62
Paroxysmal atrial tachycardia, 282
Parrot's paralysis, 301
Partial thromboplastin time (PTT), 288
Patent ductus arteriosus, 1, 3–4, 282
Paternal age, advanced, syndromes associated with, 122–123
Pavor nocturnus, 145
PCO_2, 4, 275
Pectus excavatum, surgical repair of, 398
Pedigree chart, 130
PEEP, optimal, 276

Pellagra, 119
Pelvic fracture, 59
Pelvic inflammatory disease (PID), 60
Penred's syndrome, 68, 267
Pentamidine, for *Pneumocystis carinii*
    infections, 234
Peptic ulcers, neonatal, 257
Perianal disease, with inflammatory bowel
    disease, 108
Pericarditis, 23
Periodic lateralized epileptiform discharges, 237
Periodontitis, 235
Periorbital cellulitis, 219
Peripheral pulmonic stenosis (PPS), 13
Peripheral seventh nerve palsy, 360
Peritoneal dialysis, 59, 328, 422
Peritonitis, with nephrotic syndrome, 324
Peritonsillar abscess, 217, 395
Peroxisomal disorders, 213–214
Persistent fetal circulation (PFC), 283
Persistent pulmonary hypertension, 279
Pertussis, infection, 234
    vaccine, 178–180
Pes cavus, 386
Petit mal epilepsy, 338–340
pH, changes in, in newborn, 4
Phagocytic disorders, 195
Pharyngitis, 217–218
Phenobarbital, 225, 260–261
Phenylalanine restriction, 135
Phenylketonuria (PKU), 135, 201
Phenytoin, 225, 340
Photoallergic reactions, drugs causing, 39
Photosensitivity disorders, 39
Phototherapy, 260–264
Phototoxic reactions, drugs causing, 39
Phrenic nerve paralysis, 313
Phytohemagglutinin (PHA), 195
Pi typing, 110–111
Pig-Bel, 255
Pigeon toeing, 385
Pits, syndromes associated with, 129
Plant poisoning, 429
Platelet function, congenital disorders of, 156
Platelet transfusions, 155–156, 288
Pleural effusions, 232, 399
PLEVA (pityriasis lichenoides et varioliformis
    acuta), 40
Pneumatic anti-shock garments (PASGs), 58
Pneumatosis, 257
Pneumaturia, 330
Pneumococcal vaccine, 154–155, 183
Pneumocystis carinii pneumonia, 233–234
Pneumomediastinum, 399
Pneumonia, 232–234, 396, 400
Pneumonitis, lymphocytic interstitial, 199
Pneumothorax, 279
PO$_2$, 4, 275, 284
Poison ivy, 38
Poisoning. *See* Toxicology *and* specific poisons
Pokeweed mitogen (PWM), 195
Poliovirus vaccine, 180–181

Polycystic kidney disease, 328
Polycythemia, in neonate, 286–287
Polyendocrine disorders, 73
Polyhydramnios, syndromes associated with,
    133–134
Polymorphonuclear cell, 197
Polymorphous light eruption, 39
Polymyositis, 417–418
Polyneuropathy, 359
Polyunsaturated fatty acids, 249
Pompe's disease, 210
Ponderal index, 247
Porphyrias, classification of, 211–212
Port-wine stains, 32
Portal hypertension, 111–112
Portocaval shunts, complications of, 111
Positive end-expiratory pressure (PEEP),
    optimal, 276
Postcoarctectomy syndrome, 25
Posterior fossa tumor, 373
Postperfusion syndrome, 25
Postpericardiotomy syndrome, 25
Potassium requirements, 14–15, 243, 330
Potter's syndrome, 134
Preauricular tags, syndromes associated
    with, 129
Precocious puberty, 89–90
Precordial thump, 47
Pregnancy, vaccines and, 178
Premature atrial contractions (PACs), 15
Premature ventricular contractions (PVCs), 16
Prematurity, apnea of, 272–273
    development and, 139
    immunization and, 178
    osteopenia of, 249
    retinopathy of, 245
Prerenal azotemia, 318
"Prickly heat", 42
Promyelocytic leukemia, 364
Prostaglandins, 4, 283
Protein requirements, 93–94, 249
Proteinuria, 213, 322, 328
Proteus, UTI and, 328
Prothrombin time (PT), 288
Prune belly syndrome, 304
Pseudomembranous colitis, 220–221
Pseudoparalysis, Parrot's, 301
Pseudoseizure, 340
Pseudotumor cerebri, 354–355
Psoriasis, 40
Psoriatic arthritis, 40
Psychosis, drug-induced, 430
Ptosis, 343
Puberty, precocious, 89–90
Pulmonary aspergillus infections, 233
Pulmonary edema, 399–400
Pulmonary function test, for asthma, 390
Pulmonary hypertension, causes of, 6
Pulmonary interstitial emphysema (PIE),
    278–279
Pulmonary malignancies, 400
Pulmonary vascular resistance, at birth, 270

Pulmonology, **389–404**
Pulse patterns, 13
Pulsus alternans, 13
Pulsus paradoxus, 13
Pupils, changes in, in asystolic child, 48
   constriction and dilation of, 345
   Marcus-Gunn, 343
   pinpoint, 342
   size of, 345
Purified protein derivative (PPD), 184, 300
Purified protein derivative tuberculin
   (PPDT), 184
Purpura, idiopathic thrombocytopenic, 155–156
Pyelonephritis, 318
Pyknodysostosis, 387
Pyloric stenosis, 254
Pyridoxine, for ethylene glycol ingestion, 424
Pyridoxine-dependent seizures, in neonate, 309
Pyruvate kinase deficiency, 166

Qo-Tc, measurement and clinical significance
   of, 15
Qp/Qs, calculation of, 17
QT interval, 15
QTc, measurement and clinical significance
   of, 15
Quetelet's index, 144
Quinsy, 217

Rabies, 240
   human diploid cell vaccine (HDCV) for, 186
Radii, absent, 378
Raji cell, 199
Rash, ampicillin, 231
   butterfly, 409
   in hepatitis B infection, 38
   in poison ivy, 38
Raynaud's phenomenon, 418
Rebuck skin window, 196
Recommended dietary allowances, for
   vitamins, 249
Rectal prolapse, in cystic fibrosis, 393
Red blood cell, aplasia, 169
   casts, in urine, 329
   enzymopathy, 166
   membrane, 165
   morphology, disorders of, 159
   targets, 165
   washed, 165
Reflexes, 356
   dazzle, 345
   doll's eye, 342
   primitive neonatal, 138
Reflux, 257, 317–318
Refractive capacity, 142
Rehydration solution, WHO oral, 223
Reimplantation, 54
Renal abnormality, physical findings indicating,
   333
Renal agenesis, 304
Renal biopsy, for nephrosis, 323–324

Renal calculi, 328–329
Renal failure, 303–304, 318, 327–329
Renal papillary necrosis, 329
Renal trauma, 331
Renal tubular acidosis (RTA), 324–326
Renal vein thrombosis, 303–304, 327
Respiration, periodic, 272
   rate of, in infants, 270
Respiratory distress syndrome, 253, 274, 292
Respiratory syncytial virus, 395
Respiratory system, neonatal, 270–279
Respiratory tract infections, 231, 394–404
Restriction analysis, 237
Resuscitation, 47–49, 271
Retardation, IQ and, 140
Retinoblastoma, 134–135, 369–370
Retinopathy of prematurity, 245
Retropharyngeal abscess, 395
Rett syndrome, 350
Rh complex, 289
Rhabdomyosarcomas, 369
Rheumatic carditis, minimal, 24
Rheumatic fever, 218, 415–417
Rheumatoid factor, 405
Rheumatology, **405–419**
Rhinorrhea, watery, 60
Rhus dermatitis, 38
Ribavirin therapy, in bronchiolitis, 395
Rickets, 249, 380
Rifampin, 226–227
Right ventricular hypertrophy (RVH), 14
Rigor mortis, 49
Rings, vascular, 9
Risus sardonicus, 236
Robertsonian translocation, 123
Rocky Mountain spotted fever, 238
Rolandic epilepsy, 341
Romaña sign, 236
Rotator cuff, 387
RSV pneumonitis, 6
Rubella, 348
Rubella vaccine, 181–182

Sabin vaccine, 181
Salicylate overdose, 425
Salicylate therapy for Kawasaki disease,
   230–231
Salmon patches, 32, 45
Salmonella gastroenteritis, 221–222
Salter-Harris fracture, 382–383
Scabies, treatment of, 42–43
School refusal, 149
Schwartz formula for creatinine clearance,
   318–319
Scimitar syndrome, 397
Sclera, blue, 136–137
Scleredema, 30
Sclerema neonatorum, 30
Scleroderma, 418
Sclerosis, tuberous, 45, 355

Scoliosis, 378–379
Seborrheic dermatitis, 34, 36
Sedimentation rate, 173–174
Seizure-like behaviors, 304
Seizures, epileptic, 338–341
  febrile, 336–338
  neonatal, 305–306, 309–310, 338
  vs. breathholding spell, 145
Sella turcica, 84
Senile-like appearance, syndromes characterized by, 132
Sepsis, neonatal, 218–219, 291–303. *See also* Infection
  TPN and, 97–98
Septra, contraindications for, 234
Sequestration crisis, management of, 154
Serum iron levels, decrease of, during infections, 215
Serum magnesium concentration, in neonate, 266
Serum sickness, 199, 419
Severe combined immunodeficiency disease (SCID), 193
Sex chromosome abnormality syndromes, 125
Sex maturity stages, 89
Sexual abuse, 56–57
Shagreen patch, 355
"Shaken baby" syndrome, 56
Shwachman-Diamond syndrome, 170
Shin splints, 385
Shivering, in infants, 244
Shock, 58, 244
Shoe dermatitis, 38
Short stature, 86–88, 126
Siamese twins, 245
Sibling deprivation, 148
Sick sinus syndrome (SSS), 16
Sickle cell disease, 151–155
Sickle cell trait, 153
Sideroblastic anemias, 158–159
Silver nitrate, gonococcal conjunctivitis following, 301
Simian crease, 121
Sinus, cavernous, 354
Sinus tachycardias, 282
Sinus thrombosis, lateral, 354
Sinusitis, 215–216
Skeletal dysplasia syndromes, 135
Skin, effect of ultraviolet radiation on, 38
Skin tests, 196
Skull fractures, management of, 54
Sleep apnea, 398
Sleeptalking, 146
Sleepwalking, 146
Slings, vascular, 9–10
Small pox, 238
  vaccine, 186–187
Smoke inhalation, 55–56, 402
Smoking, parental, 398
Soap, ingestion of, 425
Sodium, for neonate, 243

Sodium bicarbonate, for metabolic acidosis in neonate, 267
  for resuscitation of newborn, 271
Spasmus nutans, 342
Spastic quadriplegia, 346
Speech, development of, 142–143
Spherocytosis, congenital, 159, 167–168
Spinal cord compression, 55, 352
Spinal cord tumors, 373
Spinal tap. *See* Lumbar puncture
Spitzer's laws of neonatology, 245–246
Spleen, in sickle cell disease, 153–155
Splenectomy, 155–156, 372–373
Splenic tear, 59
Splenomegaly, 168, 371
Spondylitis, ankylosing, 109, 408
Spondylolisthesis, 379
Sprengel's deformity, 378
Staphylococcal impetigo, 37
STARCH, 127
Statue of Liberty splint, 312
Sternal edema, 238
Steroids, for asthma, 51
  for bronchopulmonary dysplasia, 277
  for caustic infections, 426
  for croup, 231
  for cystic fibrosis, 394
  for Epstein-Barr virus infections, 224
  for hydrocarbon ingestion, 426
  for idiopathic thrombocytopenic purpura, 155–156
  for management of smoke inhalation, 402
  for myocarditis, 23
  for shock, 58
  for sunburn, 39
  potency of, 29, 77
  tapering of, 76–77
  topical, 29
Strawberry hemangiomas, 32
Streptococcal impetigo, 37
Streptococcal infection, 217–218, 415–416
Stress, adrenal response to, 77
Stridor, 400
Stroke volume, of newborn, 4
Stuttering, 143
Sty, 61–62
Subacute bacterial endocarditis (SBE), 19–21
Subarachnoid hemorrhage (SAH), 307
Subcutaneous fat necrosis, 30
Subdural effusions, in bacterial meningitis, 227
Subdural hemorrhage, neonatal, 306–307
Subdural tap, 307
Subependymal-intraventricular hemorrhage, 308
Subgaleal hematoma, 311
Subluxation, 384
Submersion, 57, 61
Suicide, adolescent, 149
Sunburn and sunscreens, 3, 39
Superior vena cava syndrome, 372
Suprapubic bladder aspiration, 332–333
Surfactants, 277

Sutures, 53, 381
Sweat, inability of preterm infants to, 244
Sweat tests, 392
"Sweaty feet" odor, in isovaleric acidemia, 204
"Swimmer's itch", 43
Sydenham, Thomas, 419
Syncope, 341
Syndrome of inappropriate antidiuretic hormone (SIADH), 375
Synovitis, toxic, 378
Syphilis, 239, 301
Syphilitic meningoencephalitis, 301
Systemic diseases, associated with photosensitivity disorders,. 39
Systemic lupus erythematosus (SLE), 409–413

T-cell deficiencies, 193
T-lymphocyte/B-lymphocyte ratio, 197
Tachycardias, 16, 282
Tachypnea, in neonate, 272
Talking. See Speech
Tamm-Horsfall protein, 328
Tanner staging system, 89, 144
TAR syndrome, 287
Taste, in infant, 141
Tay-Sachs disease, 343
Technetium brain scan, 309
Teeth, primary and secondary, 142
Telangiectasia, ataxia and, 194
Television watching, effects of, 148
Temperature, lowering of, and cardiovascular changes, 61
Teratogenic drugs, 127, 336
Testicles, undescended, 333
Testicular torsion, 62
"Tet" spell, 5
Tetanus, 236
Tetanus toxoid vaccine, 53, 180
Tetany, classic neonatal, 266
Tetralogy of Fallot, 5
Tetraplegia, 346
TGA repair, 1
Thalassemia, 167
THAM, 267
Thanatophoric dwarfism, 135
Theophylline, for apnea of prematurity, 273
    for asthma, 391–392
Thermogenesis, in infants, 244
Thiamine, for ethylene glycol ingestion, 424
Thiazide diuretics, 319
13q-syndrome, 362
Three glass test, 327–328
Throat culture, for pneumonia, 232
Throgmorton's sign, 245
Thrombin time (TT), 288
Thrombocytopenia, neonatal, 287–288
Thrombocytosis, 159–160
Thrust, cardiac, 10
Thumb-sucking, race and culture variations, 145
Thurston-Holland sign, 383
Thyroid disease, 65, 72
    hematologic manifestations of, 165

Thyroiditis, chronic lymphocytic, 68
Ticks, diseases transmitted by, 240
Tics, 146
Tidal volume, normal, 61
Tine test, 181, 184
Tinea capitis, cause and treatment of, 42
Tinea versicolor, 29
Toilet training, 144
Tolazoline, adverse consequences of, 279
Tonsillectomy, 217, 395
Topical steroids, 29
TORCH, 127, 296–297
Torticollis, 350, 379
Total parenteral nutrition (TPN), complications of, 97–98
Toulouse-Lautrec, Henri, 387
Tourette's syndrome, 146–147
Toxic megacolon, 109
Toxic shock syndrome, 238
Toxicara canis, 240
Toxicology, 51, **421–431**
Toxidrome, 423
Toxocara infection, 240
Toxoplasmosis, 349
Tracheoesophageal fistula, 259
Transfusion, complications of, 159
    exchange, 159, 261–262, 303
    granulocyte, 302, 363
    idiopathic thrombocytopenic purpura, 155–156
    of washed red cells, 165
    platelet, 155–156, 288
Transient erythroblastopenia of childhood (TEC), 168–169
Transient hypogammaglobulinemia of infancy, 191
Transient neonatal pustular melanosis, 31
Transient neutropenia, 196
Transient tachypnea of the newborn (TTN), 278
Transient tyrosinemia, 202
Translocation, 123
Transposition of great arteries (TGA), repair of, 1
Trauma. See specific types.
Tremors, in neonate, 305
Trendelenburg test, 387
Tricyclic antidepressant overdoses, 429
Triglycerides, 93–94, 96, 210–211
Trimethoprim-sulfamethoxazole, contraindications for, 234
Tris (hydroxymethyl) aminomethane (THAM), 267
Trisomies, autosomal, 121
Trisomy, 21, 122. See also Down Syndrome
Tuberculosis, 181, 184–185, 300
Tuberous sclerosis, 45, 355
Tularemia, types of, 240
Tumor lysis syndrome, 367
Tumors. See also Oncology; Cancer and under names of tumors
    capable of replacing marrow, 363
    secondary, 369–370

Turner syndrome, 126
  vs. Noonan, 126
Twins, verbal and motor delay in, 139
Tympanocentesis, 217
Tyrosinemia, transient, 202
Tzanck prep, 239

Ulcerative colitis, 106–109
Ulcers, peptic, in neonate, 257
Ultrasound, 309
Ultraviolet radiation, adverse effects of, 38–39
Umbilical catheter, 291
Upper respiratory infections, 231
Urea cycle disorders, 213, 335
Urinary system, in neonate, 303–304
Urinary tract infection, 304, 316–317, 328, 332
Urine, alkaline, 328
  black, 328
  blue, 330
  brown, 328
  cat, odor of, 206
  dipstick in testing of, 322
  green, 330
  milky, 330
  output, neonatal, 304
  production, fetal, 133–134
  red, 330
  red cell casts in, 329
  specific gravity of, 328
  testing of, 202–204, 328, 332
  white cell casts in, 329
Urine metabolic screening tests, 203–204
Urine-reducing substances, false positive tests for, 213
Urticaria, in hepatitis B infection, 38
Urticaria pigmentosa, 44
Usher regimen, 274
Uveitis, 418–419

Vaccines, **177–189**
See also Immunization *and* specific vaccines
  for HIV-infected child, 187
  given during pregnancy, 178
  indications for, 188
  live virus, 178
  simultaneous administration of, 187
Vaginal bleeding, diagnosis of, 60–61
Valgus deformities, 387
Valproate, for seizures, 340
Varicella zoster, congenital, 299–300
Varus deformities, 387
Vascular lesions, 416
Vascular malformation, 401
Vascular rings and slings, cardiac, 9
VATER syndrome, 126
Vectorcardiogram, 16
Ventilation, mechanical, 274–276
  for asthma, 391
Ventricular contractions, premature, 16
Ventricular gallop, 10

Ventricular hypertrophy, in neonate, 14, 280
Ventricular tachycardia, 16
Ventriculomegaly, 309–310
Vestibular nystagmus, 344
Vigintiphobia, 261
Virilization, associated with cancer, 370
Visceral larval migrans, 240
Vision, 141–142
Vital signs, for neonates, 242–243
Vitamin A deficiency, measles and, 237
Vitamin C, 201
Vitamin E deficiency, neonatal, 249
Vitamin K deficiency, coagulation abnormalities in, 164–165
Vitamin-responsive metabolic diseases, 204–205
Vitamins, recommended dietary allowances for, 249
Vomiting, induction of, 421
von Gierke's disease, 210
von Recklinghausen's neurofibromatosis, 355
von Willebrand's disease, 160
Vowel sounds, infant, 142

Water loss, 263, 279
Weaning, 97
Wegener's granulomatosis, 414
Weil's disease, 236
Weil-Felix test, 238
Werdnig-Hoffmann disease, 360
Westergren sedimentation rate, 174
Western Blot test, for AIDS, 198–199
Wetting, daytime, 315–316
Wheezing, 50–51, 390, 395
Whey/casein ratio, in infant formulas, 252
White blood cell counts, in diagnosing bacterial sepsis, 293–294
White cell casts, in urine, 329
Whiteheads, 40
WHO oral electrolyte solution, 223
Wilm's tumor, 368, 371
Wilson's disease, 212
Wilson-Mikity syndrome, 278
Wintrobe sedimentation rate, 174
Wiskott-Aldrich syndrome, 194
Withdrawal, drug, in neonate, 266–267
World Health Organization, 223, 238
Wound botulism, incubation period for, 236

X-linked agammaglobulinemia, 193
X-ray, for congenital heart malformations, 13
  for head trauma, 54
  for malrotation of intestine, 118
  for wheezing children, 50–51
Xylocaine, 53

Z-E bilirubin, 263
Zellweger syndrome, 214
Zinc deficiency, neonatal, 250
Zinc sulfate, for Wilson's disease, 212
Zollinger-Ellison (ZE) syndrome, 100
ZZ bilirubin, 263